RECOLLECTIONS OF MY LIFE

Santiago Ramón y Cajal

PLATE 1

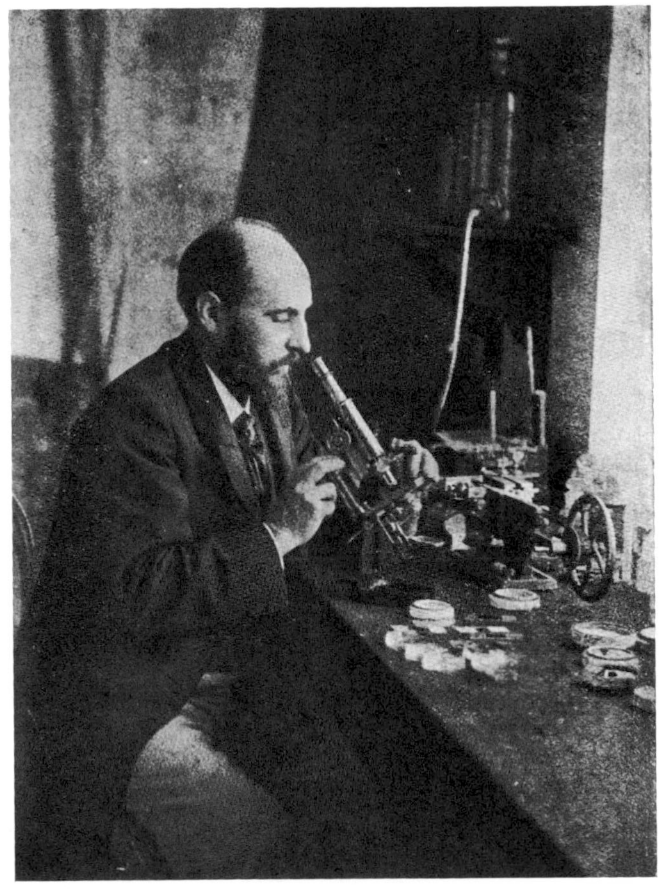

PORTRAIT OF THE AUTHOR AT THE AGE OF FORTY, shortly after becoming Professor of Histology in Madrid.

RECOLLECTIONS OF MY LIFE

Santiago Ramón y Cajal

TRANSLATED BY

E. HORNE CRAIGIE

Associate Professor of Anatomy and Neurology
University of Toronto

WITH THE ASSISTANCE OF

JUAN CANO

Associate Professor of Spanish
University of Toronto

The MIT Press
Cambridge, Massachusetts
London, England

First MIT Press paperback edition, 1989

Published by arrangement with the American Philosophical Society, Philadelphia. Originally published as *Recuerdos de Mi Vida* in Madrid, 1901–1917. First published in English as Volume 8 of *Memoirs of the American Philosophical Society,* 1937. Reprinted, 1966 by The MIT Press.

Library of Congress Cataloging-in-Publication Data

Ramón y Cajal, Santiago, 1852–1934.
[Recuerdos de mi vida. English]
Recollections of my life / Santiago Ramón y Cajal ; translated by E. Horne Craigie, with the assistance of Juan Cano.—1st MIT Press paperback ed.
p. cm.
Translation of: Recuerdos de mi vida.
Reprint. Originally published: Philadelphia : American Philosophical Society, 1937.
ISBN 0-262-68060-2
1. Ramón y Cajal, Santiago, 1852–1934. 2. Anatomists—Spain—Biography. I. Title.
QM16.R3A3 1989
611′.0092—dc20
[B]

Foreword to Paperback Edition

W. M. Cowan

Until the recent spate of biographical memoirs sponsored by the Sloan Foundation, there had been surprisingly few autobiographies by biologists. It is hard to believe that biologists are more modest or self-effacing than, say, physicists or psychologists, but the fact remains that the number of memorable biographies by biologists of note can probably be counted on the fingers of one hand. Without speculating about the reasons for this (except to guess that biologists are more likely to know Thomas Henry Huxley's famous dictum that "autobiography is a special branch of fiction"), I can think offhand of only two autobiographies by biologists from the period before World War II that are still worth reading. The first, of course, is Charles Darwin's delightful memoir, written originally for the entertainment of his children but still poignant in its modesty and disarming simplicity. The other is Santiago Ramón y Cajal's *Recollections of My Life*. I still recall with pleasure the sense of surprise and amazement with which I first read it in E. Horne Craigie's excellent English translation. On innumerable occasions since that time, I have had occasion to browse through it again, always with enjoyment and wonder. And until it went out of print, I made a point of giving copies of it to my graduate students in the hope that they would be inspired and challenged by this astonishingly frank and engaging account of one man's single-minded endeavor to understand the most complex of all biological issues, the organization and function of the nervous system.

By any measure, Ramón y Cajal was a remarkable man. Starting from the most humble of beginnings that gave little promise of intellectual achievement, he was to become not only Spain's most distinguished scientist but also, arguably, the founder of the discipline we now know as neuroscience. How this came about is engagingly recounted in his autobiography.

The son of a county surgeon better known for his strongmindedness than the soundness of his judgment, Cajal (as he is usually referred to in the English-speaking world) grew up in one of the poorest districts of upper Arragon, in a family and among townsfolk for whom "intellectual pleasures which make life agreeable and make up for its brevity" simply did not exist. He was taught to read and write at an early age by his father, but almost from the beginning of his formal education he chaffed at the mindless discipline and insensitivity of his teachers. Even if one allows for a degree of exaggeration in the account of his many childhood scrapes with authority, it is evident that even as a boy he displayed the rebelliousness and determination that later would be channeled so effectively in his scientific work.

His first love was art, not science. And had it not been for the callous insensitivity of his father, he might well have become a painter in the tradition of Goya and Velásquez. As it was, his father forbade him to paint or draw in his home, and it was not until he had begun his scientific career that he was to find an outlet for his extraordinary artistic gifts. Just how gifted he was can be judged by even the most cursory examination of any of his published works: no one, before or since, has produced illustrations of the organization of the nervous system that remotely rival Cajal's pen-and-ink drawings that grace almost every page.

After being apprenticed for about a year to a shoemaker, his father considered him sufficiently disciplined to enter college and later medical school at Zaragoza, where he came under the influence of an otherwise forgotten chemistry teacher, one Don Bruno Solano, whose flights of imagination and verbal excesses were occasionally to find their echo in Cajal's own speech and writings: ". . . the adventures of oxygen, a kind of Don Juan, a passionate and irresistible conqueror of the virginity of elements; the revenges of hydrogen, a jealous lover responsible for so much molecular widowhood. . . ." But it was anatomy that most appealed to his growing interest in science, and it was to anatomy that he would return when, after graduation and a period of compulsory military service in Cuba, he took up his first academic appointment. Setting up a microscopy laboratory, he became captivated by the "life of the infinitely small." "There was presented to me," he wrote, "a marvelous field for exploration, full of the most delightful surprises."

If during his "honeymoon with the microscope" he considered himself little more than a "fascinated spectator," his discovery of the Golgi method for impregnating nervous tissue was to transform him into the most remarkable of all explorers of the nervous system. As he describes it, it was a psychiatric colleague at Valencia, Luis Simarro, who first drew his attention to Golgi's work. He was so impressed by the potential of Golgi's method that he redirected the entire work of his laboratory to its perfection and to its use on the nervous system of every class of vertebrate (and, toward the end of his career, most classes of invertebrates). The appeal of the method was obvious: "The exclusive coloration of some few cells or fibers which stand out in the midst of extensive masses of cells that are uncolored . . . [makes it possible] to follow a nervous conductor from its origin to its termination." This was especially true when the method was applied to embryonic or fetal tissue, and almost as a revelation his life's work seemed laid out for him. "If the brain and other adult central organs of man and other vertebrates are too complex to permit of scrutinizing their structural plan by [the methods available] why not apply the [Golgi] method systematically to lower vertebrates or to the early stages of ontogenetic development, in which the nervous system should present a simple and, so to speak, diagrammatic organization." Realizing that he had struck a rich vein, ready to be mined, in his own words he "proceeded to take advantage of it, dedicating myself to work, no longer merely with earnestness, but with fury."

Frustrated at the slowness of publication (a problem, one might point out, that is a good deal more troublesome today then in the late 1880s), he chose to publish his own journal. Looking at his bibliography, one can only be astounded at the rapidity with which work flowed from his fertile mind in those formative years. In 1881 he had published only a single paper; in 1887 there were five research reports; in 1888 there were nine, including two monograph-length works; in 1889 he published eleven more original works together with a full-scale translation of his monograph on the avian retina; and in 1890 there were no fewer than nineteen reports and larger works. Never had the field witnessed such an intellectual assault.

To Cajal's chagrin all too often his work (originally published in his native Spanish) seemed to attract little or no attention from recognized leaders in the field. In an attempt to overcome this, he translated his works into French and had them published in the leading French and German journals. But it was not until he attended the German Anatomical Society's annual meeting in Berlin in the fall of 1889 that he finally gained the attention of his peers. At the congress he virtually held hostage the leaders in the field—His, Retzius, and especially Kölliker, the acknowledged doyen of German anatomy. Not until they had examined his Golgi preparations and had personally confirmed the correctness of his interpretations would he let them go. His efforts did not go unrewarded. "The results you have obtained are so beautiful," Kölliker was to tell him toward the end of the meeting, "that I intend to undertake a series of confirmatory studies immediately . . . I have discovered you, and I wish to make my discovery known in Germany." More than this, Kölliker learned Spanish so as to be able to read Cajal's other works as soon as they appeared, and he later undertook the translation of one of Cajal's major works (on the hippocampus) into German for publication in his own journal.

From 1890 Cajal's scientific career was to witness one triumph after another. He had progressed rapidly up the recognized ladder of Spanish institutions—from Zaragoza to Valencia, to Barcelona, and finally to Madrid, where a proud nation was to create an institute in his name. Almost every academic distinction that Spain could offer was bestowed on him between 1895 and 1907, and international honors followed rapidly. In 1894 he gave the Croonian lecture before the Royal Society, in 1900 he received the prestigious Moscow prize (which included sufficient funds—6,000 francs—to enable him to purchase his first microtome), in 1905 he was awarded the Helmholtz Gold Medal of the Imperial Academy of Sciences, and in 1906 he was to share the Nobel Prize for Physiology/Medicine with the Italian histologist Camillo Golgi. Honorary degrees, honorary memberships in academic societies throughout Europe and the United States, followed with a profusion that almost rivaled his own rate of publication. By the time of his death in 1934 he was universally recognized as the greatest Spaniard of his generation and as a scientist of the first rank. Today, more than fifty years later, we still pay homage to his genius.

I recall some years ago hearing Sir John Eccles say that he had often wondered who was the greater scientist: Sir Charles Sherrington, the great British neurophysiologist under whom he had trained, or Ramón y Cajal. "Reluctantly," he said, "I've come to the conclusion that Cajal was probably the greater." "After all," he added with a grin, "Cajal did not have the benefit of a Cambridge education." While this may say more about British chauvinism than about the relative merits of these twin founders of modern neuroscience, it is a not unfitting tribute to Cajal's monumental contribution to the field.

This is hardly the place to attempt to summarize Cajal's

fundamental and enduring contributions. Just mentioning a few of his more outstanding discoveries may suggest a measure of his originality, but it is the totality of his work that is the real measure of the man. The sheer volume of his published scientific work is overwhelming. To say that he published almost 300 major works gives no real indication of his prolificacy, since many of these works are book-length monographs. And his great treatise *Histologie du Système Nerveux de l'Homme et des Vertébrés*—best known in its French translation—is not only monumental in length (consisting of two large and profusely illustrated volumes, each about 1,000 pages in length) but also remains as *the* definitive work on the morphology of the vertebrate nervous system. I can think of no other biological publication of comparable scope (save perhaps *The Origin of Species*) that has endured so well and is still consulted so regularly. As recently as 1982 my friend Professor Reinoso-Suarez estimated that Cajal's work (most commonly the *Histologie*) is quoted, on average, in eleven neuroscience papers every week! No one who has had occasion to refer to Cajal's magnum opus can fail to be impressed not only by its exhaustiveness—it covers almost every neural system in each of the major classes of vertebrates—but also by its accuracy. In fact if a neuroanatomist ever has occasion to disagree with Cajal, his immediate (and persisting) concern is that there may be something wrong with his own observations! To paraphrase another great man, "Never was so much written, about so many subjects, with so few errors."

One might say the same about several of his other monographs. His last great work, *Neuron Theory or Reticular Theory,* finally laid to rest the issue whether the nervous system was formed by structurally independent units or was a more or less continuous syncytial network, as a vocal generation of his contemporaries had believed. His two-volume work, *Degeneration and Regeneration in the Nervous System,* is all too often overlooked by those working in the currently fashionable field of "neuromorphological plasticity." In fact almost every important conceptual issue is foreshadowed in Cajal's work—and it usually contains (if one is willing to search for it) some of the best experimental evidence for such plasticity. His collected writings on neural development, which have been repeatedly translated, contain, again, the kernel of most of the important ideas that currently inform the field. The following is only a partial listing: the notion that the axon is an outgrowth of the nerve cell body, the functions of the growth cone, the probable role of chemical factors in axon guidance and target selection, and the exuberant early production of neuronal processes and their later refinement.

Among the discoveries in which he took greatest pride were, first, the initial description of the climbing fibers of the cerebellum, which originally convinced him of the correctness of the "neuron doctrine." Second, the discovery of the growth cone, which with characteristic flamboyance he described as a "living battering ram, soft and flexible, which advances, pushing aside mechanically the obstacles which it finds in its way, until it reaches the area of its peripheral distribution." And third, the concept of the "dynamic polarity" of the neuron, by which he meant the essentially unidirectional flow of information within neurons from their receptive surface (commonly the dendrites), through or past the cell body to the axon, and hence to its terminal branches and synaptic endings.

To this we could add several more, including an anticipation of the later discovery of axonal transport, the prescient prediction that, since neurons are not static but dynamic structures, new synapses may be formed throughout life and that this could be the physical basis of learning and memory, and the long-forgotten fact that even adult central axons are capable of regeneration after injury.

Since it is as a scientist that Cajal is principally remembered, I have chosen to focus my remarks on his scientific career and on the abiding value of his published works. One of the great charms of his autobiography, however, is how much attention he gives to his nonscientific life. His great concern for the glory of his native land, his love for the Spanish countryside and his frustration with the backwardness of its political and educational leaders, his affection for his family, his awareness of his own weaknesses (the section dealing with his preoccupation with chess, which for a period threatened to exclude almost everything else from his life, is one of the most amusing chapters in his autobiography). What is less apparent—and barely known outside of Spain—was his lifelong fascination with photography (he was to write one of the first books dealing with color photography) and his felicitous gift for popular writing on an astonishing range of topics from politics to psychology, from literary criticism to what he disarmingly called "coffee-shop chats." His oft-repeated remarks about women and their role in society are today perhaps best forgotten but really only reflect the tenor of his times. In a more sober moment he was to remark, "Let society concede to all . . . young women the same kind of education and instruction as men, relieving . . . them also of the preoccupation and care of bringing up children, and then we can discuss [whether women are intellectually inferior to men]."

When in 1937 the American Philosophical Society published Craigie's translation of Cajal's *Recuerdos de Mi Vida* (done with the assistance of a Spanish-speaking colleague, Dr. Juan Cano), it brought this fascinating autobiography (which had first appeared in Madrid in several installments between 1901 and 1917) to the attention of English readers. The entire translation was later published in one volume by The MIT Press. Regrettably the work has been out of print for several years, and the relatively few copies still extant are so jealously guarded by their owners that to all intents and purposes it has been lost to a whole generation of young neuroscientists. The decision of The MIT Press to reissue the volume at this time is much to be applauded. I can only hope that those who read this new edition will derive as much pleasure and enjoyment from it as I and so many of my colleagues derived from reading the first edition. And if it encourages the readers to go back to reexamining the *Histologie* or any of Cajal's other works, it will only enrich future work in the field. I say this fully cognizant of Cajal's own comment, "There are people for whom nothing is accomplished in this world without the original sin of recommendation."

Bethesda, December 1988

RECOLLECTIONS OF MY LIFE

Santiago Ramón y Cajal

TABLE OF CONTENTS

TRANSLATOR'S PREFACE

The preparation of the English version of the present work has been inspired by the belief that it is at the same time a document of considerable value for the history of science and a book containing much which will interest not only biologists and physicians but also a rather wide circle of readers in many different walks of life. The author was one of the greatest figures in the scientific world of his day and probably the most remarkable and impressive figure whom the translator has ever been privileged to know.

The author tells us in his preface that his purpose was to present not only the usual human document but "a case of individual psychology and a reasoned critique of our educational system." "This book will contain, rather than a narrative of activities, an exposition of feelings and ideas. In it will be reflected synthetically the series of mental reactions provoked in the author by the clash with the reality of the world and of men."

The value of the work lies less in the events which it narrates, interesting and instructive as these may be, than in the revelation of the character and personality of a great man enshrined in its pages. In this belief, the aim of the translator has been to reproduce the text as precisely as it is possible to do in another language. The result will undoubtedly be criticized, probably severely, for having adhered too closely to a literal translation. Nevertheless, so much of the personality of the author is contained in his very diction and phraseology, that it was felt best to risk sacrificing to some extent the values of literary English in order to try to give as precise rendition as possible of each word or phrase of the original.

The translation has been made from the third Spanish edition (except one sentence added from the first edition), published in 1923. No cuts have been made in the first part, but in the second the summaries of the author's scientific publications have been considerably curtailed. It has been necessary also to reduce the number of scientific illustrations. Otherwise the text of the third edition has been followed exactly. Unfortunately, the original illustrations were reported to have been extensively damaged and it was necessary to reproduce the figures directly from those printed in the Spanish volume.

The English version, including the alterations just mentioned, was prepared with the permission of the author during his life-time, and the translator wishes to express his gratitude to the late author, as well as to his son Dr. Jorge Ramón and to the new Director of the Instituto Cajal, Dr. Francisco Tello, the two latter having confirmed the permission to publish the translation and illustrations.

The translator is deeply indebted to Dr. Juan Cano, who went over the whole manuscript and gave much assistance in the effort to attain an accurate translation. He is also much indebted to Dr. William A. Hilton, of Pomona College, who had an English version partly prepared and generously turned over his whole manuscript and drawings to the present writer.

Deep gratitude is due also to the American Philosophical Society for publishing the work and to Dr. Arthur W. Goodspeed for his editorial labours.

TORONTO, June, 1936

ILLUSTRATIONS

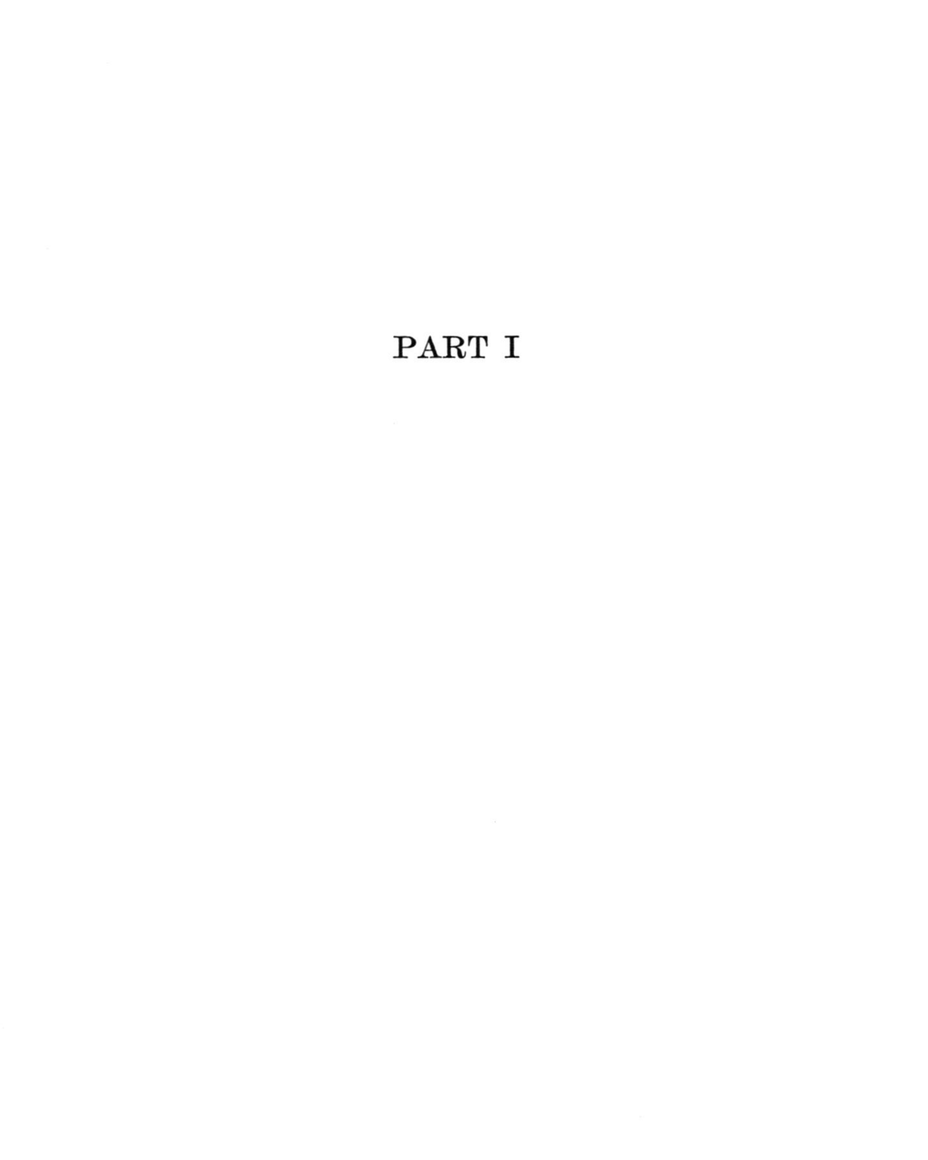

PART I

CHAPTER I

My parents, my birthplace and my early childhood

I was born on the first of May, 1852, in Petilla de Aragon, a small town of Navarre, situated, by a strange geographical freak, in the centre of the province of Zaragoza not far from Sos. The uncertainties of the medical profession took my father, Justo Ramón Casasús, a pure-blooded Aragonese, and a modest surgeon[1] at the time, to the insignificant village which was my birthplace, and where I passed the first two years of my life.

My father was a man of great energy, an extraordinarily hard worker, and full of noble ambition. Depressed during the early years of his professional life because he had been unable, through lack of funds, to complete his medical studies, he resolved, when already established and supporting a family, to save enough to complete his academic career, even at the cost of great privations. This enabled him to substitute for the humble title of second-class surgeon the brilliant diploma of physician and surgeon.

Only when I was nearly six years old, did he attain this laudable ambition. About 1849 and 1850 his whole desire was to become a real and great surgeon. He attained his aim, for the fame of his cures soon spread through a great part of Navarre and of upper Aragon, and brought him good and ever-increasing returns, besides the satisfaction of personal honour.

The medical district of Petilla was one of those which doctors call a spur-district; it had dependencies, and the necessity of passing daily through the wild and wooded countryside of his circuit, full of abundant and varied game, awakened in my father the love of the chase, so that he devoted himself to hunting hares, rabbits, and partridges

[1] Not a physician but one performing minor operations. (Translator.)

with the same earnestness and persistence which he put into all his undertakings. It was not long, then, before he monopolized both the scalpel and the gun through the whole neighbourhood.

With the returns from these two, the partridges and the patients, he was able, after two years in Petilla, to furnish a modest house and marry a girl from his own town with whom he had been in love for many years.

My mother, according to those who knew her in her youth, was a beautiful and robust highland woman, born and brought up in the village of Larrés, near Jaca, close to the road to Panticosa. They had known each other as children (my father also came from Larrés), became increasingly attached in their youth, and decided to marry as soon as it should be permitted by their modest capital, which was to grow by work and thrift.

Unfortunately, I have no pictures of my parents in their youth, nor even in their maturer years. The accompanying photographs were taken when they were already of advanced age—more than seventy years old.

Of the beauty of my mother and of her excellent qualities, not a single trace was transmitted to any of the four brothers and sisters who were, both physically and morally, almost exact reproductions of our father; a circumstance that has condemned us in our family life to a sentimental and ideological atmosphere both monotonous and annoying.

But I cannot complain of my biological inheritance from my father. He was a man of vigorous mentality, in whom the finest qualities found their highest expression. With his blood he transmitted to me traits of character to which I owe everything that I am: a profound belief in the sovereign will; faith in work; the conviction that a persevering and deliberate effort is capable of moulding and organizing everything, from the muscle to the brain, making up the deficiencies of nature and even overcoming the mischances of character—the most difficult thing in life. From him I acquired also the beautiful ambition to be something worth while, and the determination to spare no sacrifice for the

PLATE 2

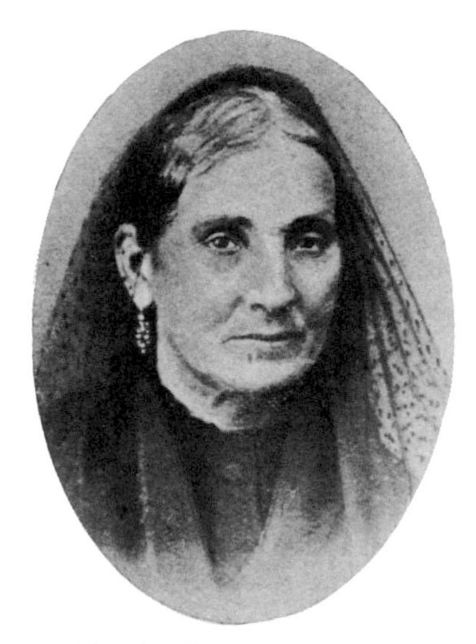

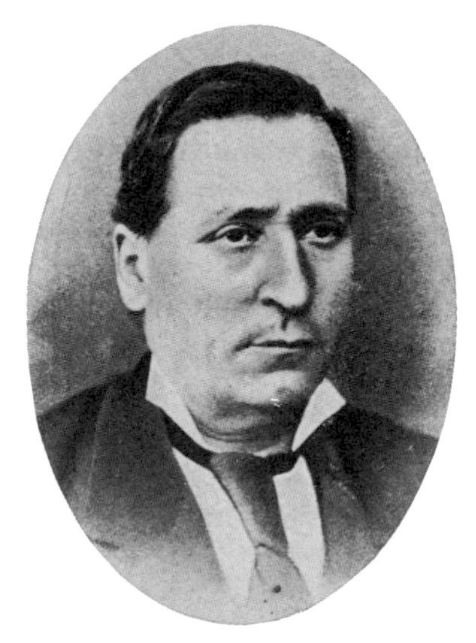

FIG. 1. PORTRAITS OF MY PARENTS. These photographs were taken when my progenitors were over seventy. Unskilful retouching has largely deprived the likenesses of character.

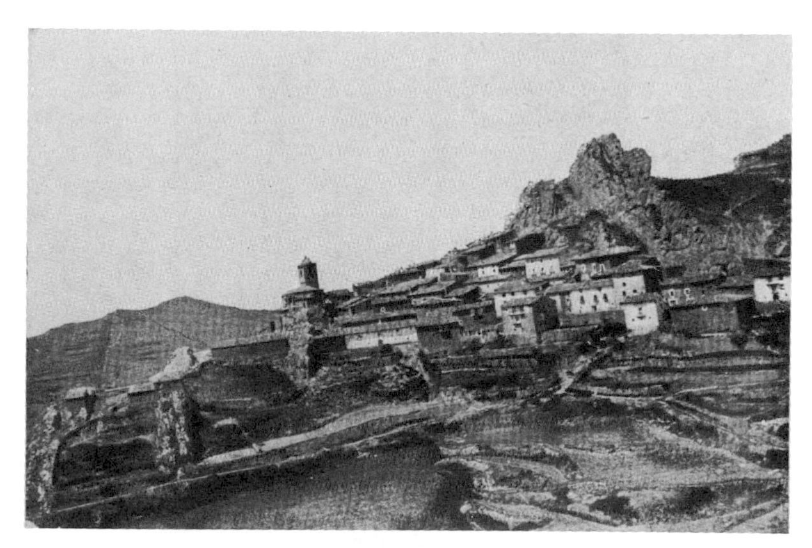

FIG. 2. PETILLA DE ARAGÓN FROM THE SOUTH. Photograph taken about the end of the nineteenth century by the Navaraise Commission.

PLATE 3

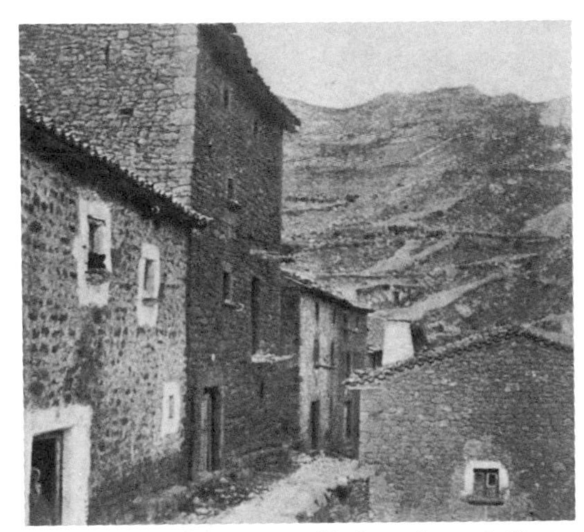

FIG. 3. PETILLA. The high, poor, tumble-down house half way along the street is where I was born.

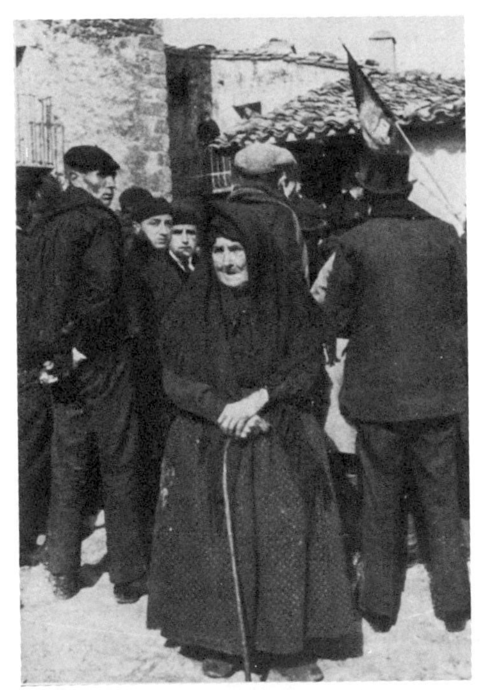

FIG. 4. MY NURSE, IN 1892, AT THE AGE OF EIGHTY-SEVEN. I reproduce this picture as a tribute to the venerable old woman, who knew my parents in their youth and endured the impertinences and caprices of a little devil of a few months old.

fulfilment of my aspirations, nor ever to deviate from the direct path on account of secondary motives or minor reasons. Nevertheless, I lacked what was perhaps his finest mental quality, his extraordinary memory. This was so great that, as a student, he could recite by heart works on pathology in several volumes and was able to retain after hearing them once lists with hundreds of words taken at random. Great as was his natural or organic retentiveness, he increased it still farther by means of ingenious associations which remind one of the famous and highly artificial ones of the Abbé Moigno.

To illustrate the will-power of my father, I shall tell his life story in a few words. A son of modest farmers of Larrés (Huesca), with older brothers who by law had the right to inherit and cultivate the fields of the scanty patrimony, he had to abandon the paternal home when very young, and apprenticed himself to a certain surgeon of Javierre de Latre, a village on the banks of the Gállego, not very far from Anzánigo. There he learned the trade of barber and blood-letter, spending eight or ten years with his master, a worthy "romancista" surgeon.

Anyone else than my father would have considered his career definitely ended or would have tried, as the ideal and crown of his ambitions, to obtain the humble title of a male nurse. The brilliant cures performed by his master, the assiduous study of all the books on surgery upon which he could lay his hands (of these there was a rich collection on his master's shelves), the care and assistance of the numerous patients whom his master, who recognized the exceptional earnestness of his assistant, entrusted to him, awakened in him a decided vocation for the practice of medicine.

Resolved, then, to emancipate himself from his poor and humble position, one day when he was already nearly twenty-two, he shocked his master by asking him for payment of his modest salary. Taking leave of him, and provided with some money lent by relatives, he undertook on foot the journey to Barcelona, where finally, after many days of privation (in Sarriá), he found a barber shop, the owner of which allowed him while working there to attend the university and study for the career of surgeon.

Refraining from all pleasures, submitting to a regimen of unbelievable austerity, and without any income other than his salary and tips at the barber shop, my father obtained the coveted diploma of a surgeon with first class standing in all subjects, having been an outstanding example of application and good behaviour. There, in his quiet and obscure struggle for spiritual and physical nourishment, breathing that atmosphere of indifference and coldness which surrounds the talent of the unprotected poor, my father learned the terror of poverty and the rather exclusive worship of utilitarian science, which later, as a result of the mental reaction of his sons, was to cause him and us so much trouble.

Some years afterwards, when he was already married and father of four children, while practicing temporarily in the district of Valpalmas, province of Zaragoza, he realized his ideal by graduating as a doctor of medicine.

I relate these events of my father's life because, besides being so highly honourable to him, they are also the necessary antecedents of my own history. There is no doubt that, aside from hereditary influence, the ideas and example of a father are factors of decisive importance in the education of his children, and therefore are essential determinants of their tastes and inclinations.

Of my native town, and of the years passed in Larrés and Luna, medical districts where my father practised between 1850 and 1856, I remember almost nothing. My first recollections, quite vague and indefinite, are of the town of Larrés, to which my father moved two years after my birth, greatly pleased with the thought of carrying on his profession in his native town, near his friends and relatives. These hazy recollections have as their scene the weaver's shop of my maternal grandfather, to whom I gave much trouble by tangling his threads and shuttles. For, according to my relatives, I was a restless little devil, wilful and

PLATE 4

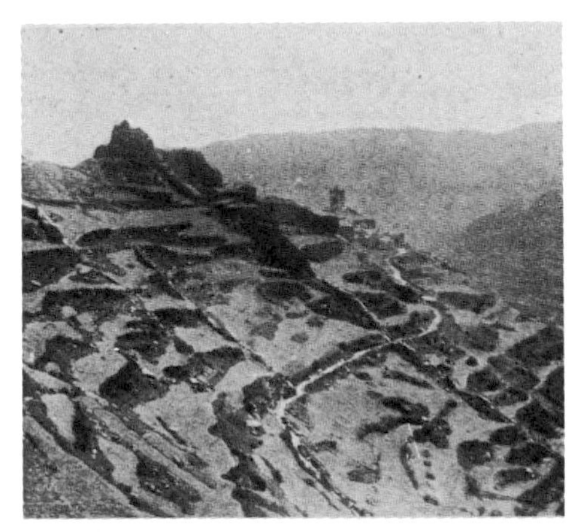

FIG. 5. PETILLA FROM THE NORTH. Observe the poverty of the slopes, cut up by ruined retaining walls which support narrow and irregular terraces for cultivation.

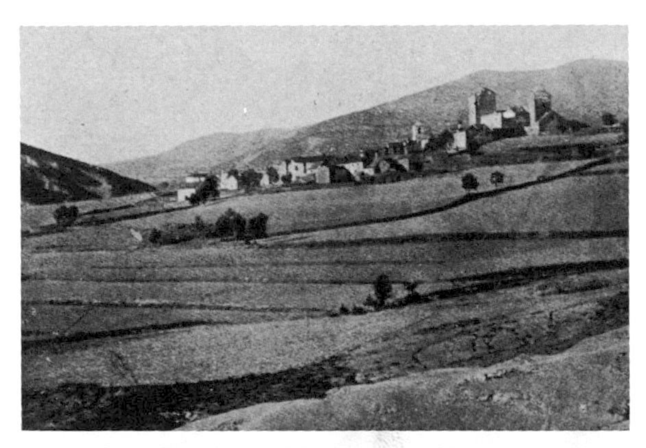

FIG. 6. LARRÉS, A BIRD'S-EYE VIEW OF THE VILLAGE WHERE MY PARENTS WERE BORN. This photograph does not show the snow-covered Pyrenees which cut off the horizon on the north.

unbearable. In Larrés was born my brother Pedro, the present professor in the Faculty of Medicine of Zaragoza.

A certain piece of mischief perpetrated when I was about three or four years old might have put a tragic end to my life. It was in the town of Luna. I was playing on a threshing floor on the town common when I had the devilish idea of beating a horse. The animal, somewhat wild and vicious, gave me a terrible kick on the forehead, so that I fell senseless, bleeding profusely and in such a plight that they thought me dead. The wound was very serious; but I recovered, after making my parents pass days of great anxiety. This was my first mischief; we shall see later that it was not my last.

CHAPTER II

A belated trip to my birthplace. The poverty of my fellow townsmen. A poor and isolated town which appears like a symbol of Spain.

Although it may change and mutilate the good order of my story, I will tell something now of my native town, which as I have already related, I left at about two years of age. Of my birthplace, for that reason, I retain no recollection. Besides, my later relations with the place have not been such as to relieve this ignorance, since they have been reduced simply to the requesting, receiving, and paying for an endless series of certificates of baptism. I lack, then an exactly defined native province by reason of the peculiar fact already mentioned that Petilla belongs to Navarre although it is situated in Aragon. This was the disagreeable outcome of the contrariety with which I had been dealt the cards by politics; but was an advantage for my patriotic feelings which have had freer scope on behalf of the broad and noble cause of Spain as a whole.

Nevertheless, while I confess that my love for my native country surpassed greatly that for my birthplace, I have felt more than once strong desires to make the acquaintance of the little town where I was born. I regret that I did not first see the light in a great city, adorned with splendid monuments and illuminated by geniuses, but I could not choose and I had to content myself with my sad and humble little village, which will always have for me a supreme dignity in having been the scene of my first cries, and the austere decoration with which nature stimulated my newborn eyes and enlivened my brain.

Impelled then by such natural feelings I undertook eighteen years ago a journey to Petilla. After determining carefully its geographical position, which was an arduous task, and studying the difficult itinerary, so remote and inaccessible is my town, I set out. My first stage was Jaca, the second Verdún y Tiermas, a country town on the banks of the Aragon celebrated for its thermal baths, and the third and last Petilla.

To Verdún y Tiermas there is a beautiful road which is traversed in the coach which runs from Jaca to Pamplona, but the way from Tiermas to Petilla, more than three leagues, is a bridle path, through precipitous mountains cut up and almost entirely obliterated in many places by dry ravines and gorges.

Mounted upon a mule and conducted by a man on foot who was familiar with the district, I set forth one August morning. As we left behind the relatively green banks of the Aragon, there appeared to me the characteristic desolate and dismal Spanish country side. The systematic clearing of the woods had left the mountains denuded of vegetable mold. It is well known that in these unhappy districts every watercourse, instead of being the hope of the tiller of the soil constitutes a tragic menace. Just two days before, there had occurred a devastating storm, fields previously fertile were seen covered with clayey mud and the denudation of the slopes and valleys had converted streams and rivulets into ravines filled with stones.

As I approached my native village there took possession of me an inexplicable melancholy which reached its height when my guide made me listen to the sound of the bell, as strange to my ear as if I had never heard it before. My state of mind continued in fact to be somewhat peculiar. Upon returning to his birthplace every man tastes in anticipation the pleasure of embracing the comrades of his childhood and youth; his mind enjoys the pleasant recollection of common amusements and pranks; everyone, in short, is eager to revisit again the streets, the church, the fountain, and the surroundings of the place where every tree and every stone calls forth an emotion and a pleasant recollection. I, I said to myself, will have only the sad privilege of finding as my sole reception upon my arrival curiosity, perhaps somewhat hostile, and the coldness of hearts. No one awaits me for nobody knows me.

Nevertheless, I was mistaken, the priest and the mayor had been forewarned of my visit and awaited me in the square of the town. There was besides a moving episode. At the foot of the elevation which is crowned by the village, a certain old woman, who had not had any notice of my visit and who was busy washing clothes at the edge of a stream, turned her face, then suddenly left her work and facing me and staring exclaimed: "Señor, if you are not Don Justo himself, you must be the son of Don Justo! It is a miracle! The same face as his father! Do not deny it! Is Señora Antonia still alive? How good and how beautiful she was!" I congratulated the poor old woman[1] upon her remarkable memory and kindly sentiments and, pressing a piece of money into her hands, I continued my ascent to Petilla.

Petilla is one of the poorest and most desolate towns in upper Aragon, without roads connecting it with the neighboring Aragonese villages of Sos and Un Castillo, or with the more distant Aoiz, the county town of the district to which it belongs. Only rough and narrow tracks lead to the humble village, the natives of which are ignorant even of the use of the cart. It rises almost on the crest of a very precipitous hill, a spur of the neighboring lofty range which is derived in turn, according to observations made on the spot, from the cordillera of La Peña and Gratal.

The panorama which strikes the eyes from the railing of the church could not be more romantic and at the same time more gloomy and desolate. Rather than the home of hardy and happy peasants, it seems like a place of punishment and expiation. As may be seen in the accompanying

[1] A photograph of this good woman was taken in Petilla by the Navarraise commission formed by prominent representatives of all the activities of the region, which, on the occasion of my retirement from the university had the courtesy to proceed to my town to place a memorial tablet on the house where I was born and to celebrate my modest scientific accomplishments in charming and extremely complimentary terms. A portrait of my nurse is reproduced here as she appeared at the age of eighty-seven.

picture, a great mountain, rocky and jagged, with steep and eroded slopes, fills almost the whole horizon with its huge bulk; at the foot of the giant, a brook, which arises in the adjacent hills, runs musically along the narrow valley-floor beside the dangerous path which leads to the place. The sides and spurs of the mountain, the only arable land available to the people of Petilla, appear streaked with innumerable narrow fields laid out in terraces laboriously defended against washouts and torrential rains by stout buttresses and thick walls. Upon the peak, as if defending the town from the cold north winds, colossal rocks shut off the horizon and rise imposingly like sharp sickles, a kind of cyclopean wall raised there by the force of some geological cataclysm. In the protection of this natural defence, reinforced further by a feudal castle now in ruins, the poor and humble houses of the place, between forty and sixty in number, are built upon rocks and separated by irregular streets, the transit of which is hindered by crevices, stairs, and furrows opened in the rock by the violent erosion of the torrential waters. Looking at such miserable cottages, one feels profound sadness. Not a flower pot in the windows, not the smallest decoration on the fronts of the houses, nothing in a word, to indicate the slightest feeling for beauty or the slightest aspiration to convenience or to comfort.

It is easy to see as one passes along in the shade of such miserable dwellings, that the country people who inhabit them are condemned to a hard existence with no other interest than to procure by rude labour the most frugal daily nourishment.

Unfortunately my town is no exception to the rule; the great majority of our villagers also live thus with trifling differences. Their ignorance is the result of their poverty. For them the intellectual pleasures which make life agreeable and make up for its brevity do not exist.

Oh, the heroic rustics of our barren plateaux! Let us love them sincerely. They have performed the miracle of populating sterile regions from which the well-fed Frenchman or the rubicund and lymphatic German would have fled as from the plague. And in passing let us repulse indignantly the brutal injustice with which certain French, Italian, English, and German writers, and in general the happy people of naturally fertile countries, disparage or disdain the lean, dried up, sun-burned, but energetic inhabitants of the harsh Castilian, Estremenian, and Aragonese tablelands, as if those humble tillers of the soil were to blame for having seen the light beneath a sun of fire and a sky implacably blue for half the year.

But, distracted by my thoughts, I am forgetting to talk of my visit to my birthplace. I must say, then, that upon my arrival I was received most affectionately by the acting priest to whom the regular priest, who resided elsewhere and knew of my visit, had recommended me. Various other people treated me with fine and generous hospitality, especially some of the older residents who remembered my father, whom they found me to resemble surprisingly. All were eager to show me their good will and to shower me with friendly attentions, for which I was sincerely grateful. To make my brief visit agreeable, they arranged some picnics in the open country. I remember among them the exploration of the ruins of the ancient castle, the outing to the age-old woods of the neighbouring sierra, and the visit to a modest hermitage, situated a short distance from the town, which is held in great reverence and about which extends a delicious and flowery oasis, where it was arranged that we should refresh ourselves with a tasty and well-served afternoon repast. They showed me also the humble house in which I was born, a ruinous and almost abandoned structure inhabited by nomadic beggars.[2]

Some old women of the place, who boasted kindly of having held me in their arms, told me of the vigour of my first months, the tireless industry of my mother, and the accomplishments in surgery and in hunting of my father, whose fame as a nimrod still endured.

[2] I am told that the house has recently been repaired and made respectable.

Upon taking leave of the rough but honourable mountaineers, my fellow townsmen, my heart was oppressed. A vehement desire of my soul had been satisfied but I bore away with me a great sadness. A voice within told me that I should never return to these places,[3] that the romantic scenery which caressed my eyes and my brain when they were opened for the first time upon the spectacle of the world would not again impress my retina, that those hands of old men ennobled by the honourable calluses of hard work would not again be pressed effusively in mine.

[3] And in fact, I have not returned, in spite of the sympathy with which my fellow townsmen inspired me, and, what is worse, I cannot return; overwork must be paid for with the heavy price of premature senility and its accompanying indispositions.

CHAPTER III

My early childhood. My father's vocation for teaching. My character and tendencies. Love of nature and passion for birds.

The early years of my childhood, with the exception of the two passed in Petilla and one in Larrés, were spent partly in Luna, a populous town of the province of Zaragoza near Monlora, a pine-clad hill crowned with the ruins of an ancient monastery, and partly in Valpalmas, a less important town of the same province, not more than three leagues distant from Luna. In the latter my family lived four years from 1856–60 and there were born my two sisters Paula and Jorja.

My education and instruction began in Valpalmas when I was four years old. It was in the modest school of the place that I learned the first rudiments of letters, but in reality my true master was my father who took upon himself the task of teaching me to read and write and of inculcating elementary ideas of geography, physics, arithmetic, and grammar.

Such a vexatious undertaking was for him more than an unavoidable duty, it was an irresistible necessity for his spirit, so strong was his natural vocation to give instruction.

He experienced an incomprehensible pleasure in awakening childish curiosity and hastening intellectual development, which is so slow at times in some children. Of my father may be said justly what Socrates boasted of himself: that he was an excellent accoucheur of intellects.

There is actually in the function of the teacher something of the arrogant satisfaction of the breaker of colts; but there enters also the kindly curiosity of the gardener who eagerly awaits the spring to find out the colour of the flower he has sown and to test the success of his methods of cultivation. I hold for my part that to develop an embryonic understanding, recreating oneself in its advance and individualizing it progressively, is to attain the most lofty and noble paternity; it is as if to correct and perfect the work of nature. To construct original brains, that is the great triumph of the pedagogue.

This didactic function my father performed not only for his own children but for any child with whom he came in contact, because for him ignorance was the greatest of all misfortunes, and teaching the most noble of duties.

I remember well the enthusiasm which, in spite of my tender age, he put into teaching me French. The study of this language took place in a certain abandoned shepherd's cave, not far from the town (Valpalmas), to which we were in the habit of retreating to concentrate on the work and avoid visits and interruptions. As a result of this curious circumstance, whenever I see a copy of Telemachus, there rises in my memory the image of the cave referred to, the recesses and windings of which I still see after sixty-five years as if they were before me now.

Thanks to the efforts of my father, I progressed so far and so quickly that at six years of age I wrote readily and in a fair hand and possessed some ideas of geography, French, and arithmetic. As a result of this relative precocity I came to be the amanuensis and secretary of the household, and so when a year later my father went to Madrid to complete his course and to graduate as a doctor of medicine and surgery, I was intrusted with the correspondence of the family and with reporting to him the events of his medical district which was in charge for the time being of a locum tenens. My progress caused my parents, full of that optimism so natural in all such, to foresee a brilliant future for their son, a little hastily, as we shall soon see.

In the realm of the inclinations and tendencies of my mind, I was, like the majority of the youngsters brought up in the small towns, an enthusiast for the open-air life and a tireless cultivator of games of strength and agility, in which I already excelled amongst the boys of my age.

Among my natural inclinations there were two which predominated, which lent to my character a somewhat strange aspect. They were the investigation and contemplation of natural phenomena and a certain incomprehensible antipathy for social intercourse.

My bashfulness and diffidence when among older people were a great annoyance to my parents. To acknowledge it at once, I was in my childhood a wayward creature, excessively mysterious, secretive and unlikeable. Even to-day, conscious of my defects and after having worked heroically to correct them, I retain some of that shy unsociability so much regretted by my parents and friends.

It must be recognized that there is a refined egotism in meditation upon one's own ideas and in the cowardly avoidance of intellectual intercourse with other people. It brings a certain morbid pleasure. Far from human society, we create for ourselves the illusion of complete freedom. Solitude produces thus something like the feeling of being the owner of oneself. When a conversation is commenced our words respond to the thoughts of others. Mental initiative and the command of our actions are lost. The associations of ideas succeed each other in the order indicated by the interlocutor, who is, in a way, the master of our mind and of our emotions. We cannot long prevent him from evoking with his indiscreet or impertinent chat, distressing recollections, which bring into action trains of thought which we would prefer to bury in the shadows of the unconscious. How often we go to the café or to the club in search of distraction and come away with a dejection of the spirit, with a repression of the will, which sterilizes or makes impossible its daily labor sometimes for a considerable time.

But let us leave irrelevant reflections and resume the narrative.

The admiration of nature constituted, as I have said, one of the unbridled tendencies of my spirit. I never tired of contemplating the splendours of the sun, the magic of the twilight, the alternations of the vegetation, with its

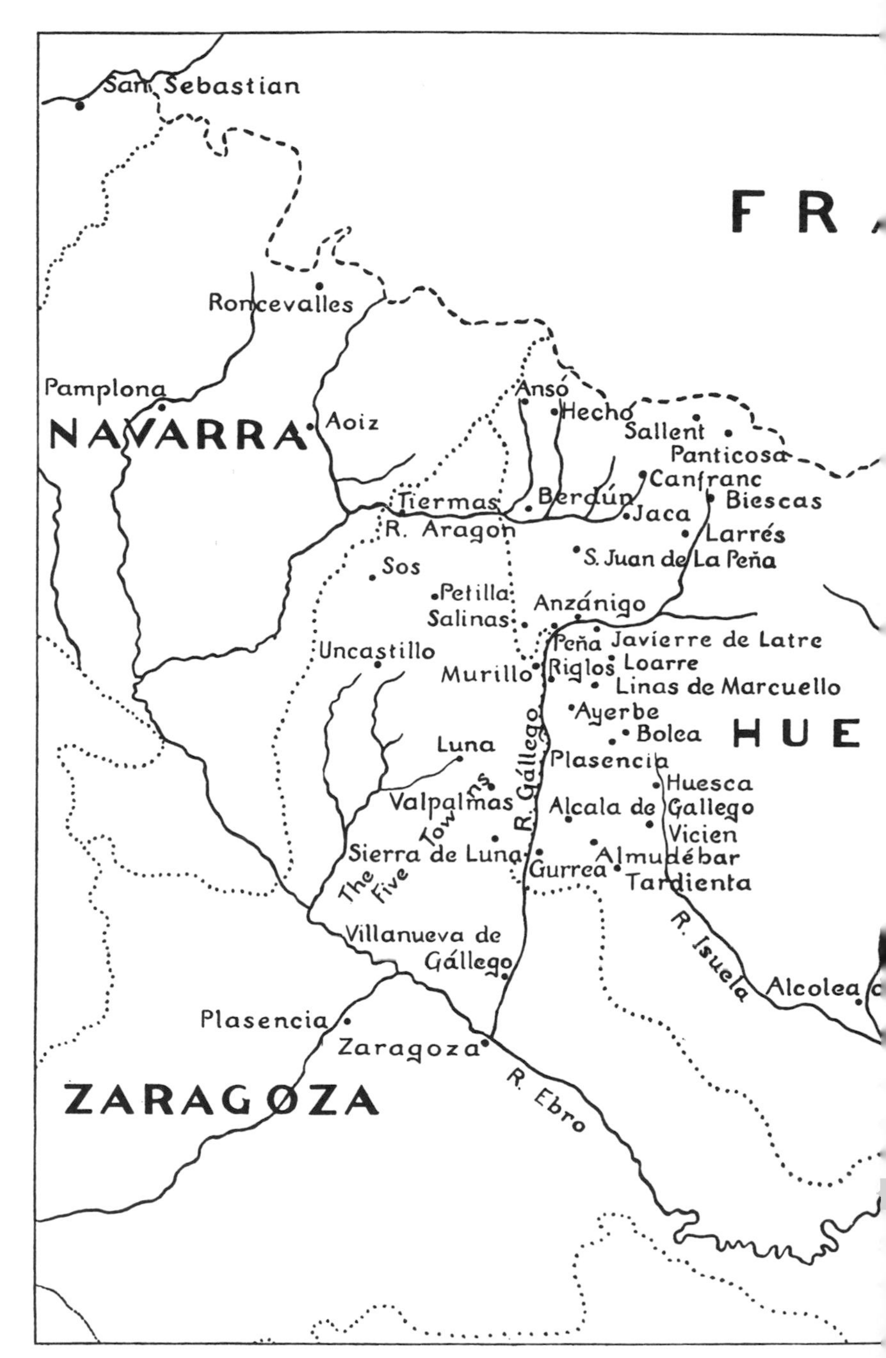

FIG. 7. MAP OF THE NORTHEASTERN PART OF SPAIN.

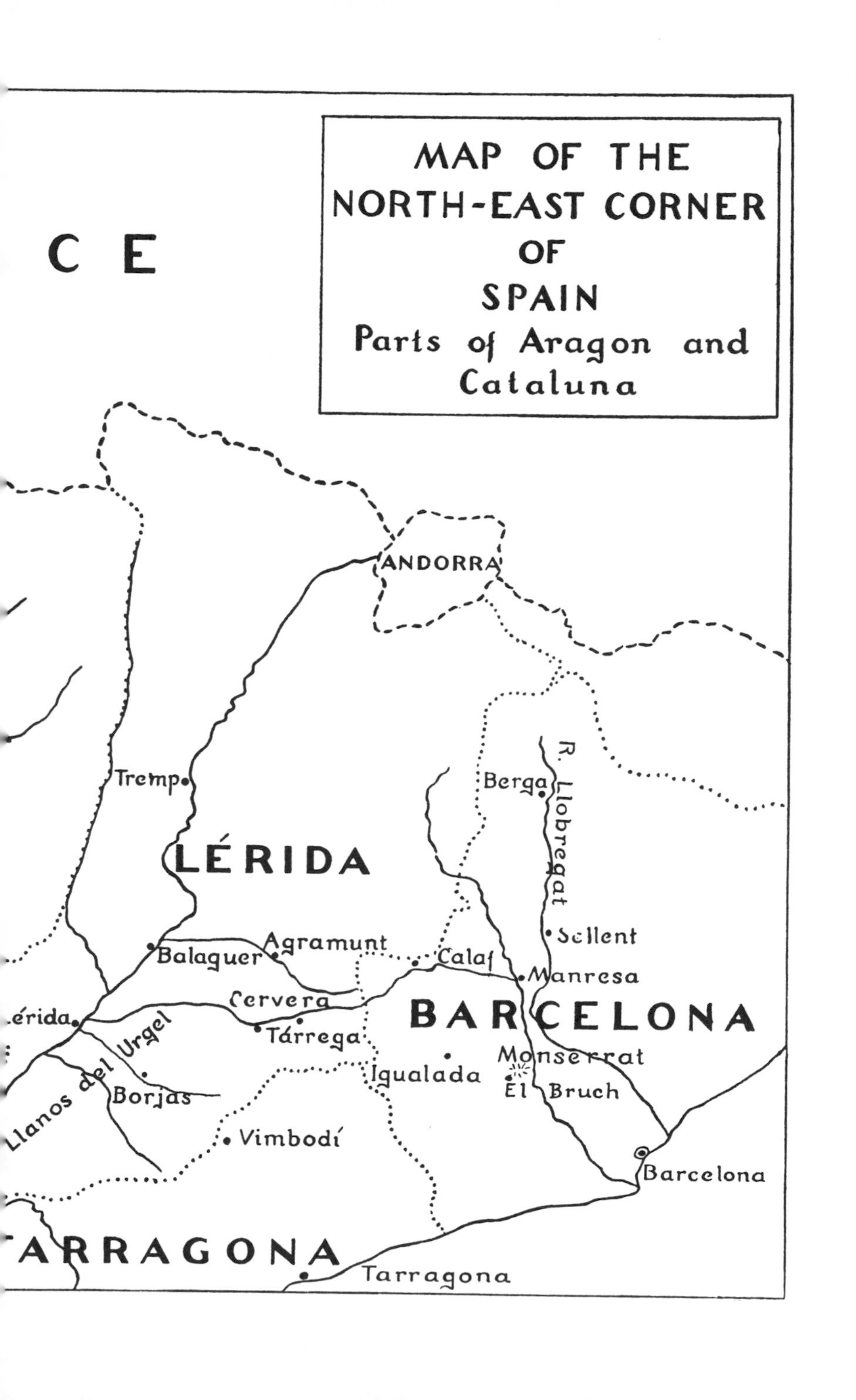
MAP OF THE
NORTH-EAST CORNER
OF
SPAIN
Parts of Aragon and
Cataluna
C E
ANDORRA
Tremp
LÉRIDA
R. Llobregat
Berga
Sellent
Agramunt
Balaguer
Calaf
Manresa
Cervera
BARCELONA
Tárrega
Llanos del Urgel
Monserrat
Igualada
El Bruch
Borjas
Vimbodí
Barcelona
TARRAGONA
Tarragona

gaudy spring festivals, the mystery of the resurrection of the insects, and the varied and picturesque scenery of the mountains. All the hours of freedom which my studies left me were spent in wandering about the outskirts of the town exploring glorious ravines, flood-plains, springs, rocks, and hills, with great anxiety on the part of my mother, who always feared some accident during my long absences.

As an outgrowth of these tastes, there soon developed in me the love of animals, especially of birds, of which I kept many. I delighted in caring for them as nestlings, in building for them cages of osiers or of reeds, and in lavishing upon them all kinds of caresses and attentions.

My passion for birds and for nests was so extreme that some springs I came to know more than twenty of the latter belonging to different species of birds. This instinctive inclination toward ornithology increased still more later on.[1] I remember that when I was nearly thirteen I took a notion to make a collection of eggs of all kinds of birds carefully classified. In order to help my collection (upon which my father looked favourably) I offered the boys and the farm labourers a cuaderna[2] for each nest which they showed me. In this way the collection was rapidly enriched, attaining a total of thirty different specimens. I showed it proudly to my playmates as if it were an inestimable treasure. Unfortunately my collection, which I kept carefully in a special pasteboard box divided into labeled compartments, had an untimely end. The heat of the month of August ruined my treasure, causing the decay of the yolks and the cracking of the shells. Great was my distress when I realized the full extent of the irreparable damage! I was inconsolable when I saw that the eggs of the wagtail, the thrush, the sparrow, the linnet, the chaffinch, lark, *cudiblanca,* black bird, heron, goldfinch, cuckoo, nightingale, quail, etc., exuded through their cracked shells,

[1] I refer to my stay some years later in Sierra de Luna, a town of the province of Zaragoza.

[2] Roughly an American cent or an English halfpenny. (Translator's note.)

a corrupt and malodorous liquid. Such interests accentuated my feelings of forbearance towards animals. I liked to raise them so as to enjoy their graceful movements and to discover their curious instincts, but I never tortured them by using them as playthings as so many other boys do.

In hunting them I preferred the methods which permitted their capture alive: bird lime, *lienas*[3] with deep holes, nets, etc.

When I had collected so many that I could not look after them and care for them properly, I released them or returned them, still featherless nestlings, to their nests and the care of their mothers. Into these amusements there entered nothing of gastronomic interest or of the vanity of the hunter, but only the instinct of the naturalist. It was sufficient for my satisfaction to watch the marvelous process of incubation and the hatching of the little birds; to follow step by step the metamorphosis of the newly born, discovering first the appearance of the feathers in the bare skin of the tiny little creatures, later the timid flapping of the bird which tries its strength and stretches its wings, and finally the rapid flight with which it takes possession of the expanse of space.

[3] Traps made with a flat stone and some little sticks easily dislodged by the bird in pecking the bait.

CHAPTER IV

My sojourn in Valpalmas. The three decisive events of my childhood—the festivities in celebration of our victories in Africa, the striking of the school by lightning, and the eclipse of the sun in the year 1860.

During the last years, which I spent in Valpalmas there occurred three events which had a decisive influence upon my later ideas and feelings. These were the commemoration of the glorious victories in Africa, the falling of a thunderbolt upon the school and the church of the town, and the famous eclipse of the sun in 1860. I was seven or eight years old at the time.

The festivities arranged by the officials of Valpalmas to celebrate the triumphs of our brave soldiers in Africa were magnificent and proportional to the patriotic enthusiasm which reigned at that time throughout Spain. "At last," I heard it said, "the lances and swords which often have been directed against ourselves have been turned against the hated enemies of our race." It was such a long time since the glorious banner of Spain had floated over the walls of a foreign city. There was no doubt about it, the Spanish race had returned to itself, regaining consciousness of its own value. Those were the same valiant infantrymen as at Pavia, Saint Quentin, and Flanders.

With what hearty and ingenuous enthusiasm we acclaimed the brave soldiers of Africa and especially the generals Prim and O'Donnell! How proud we were of the defeat of Muley-el-Abbas and of the sanguinary capture of Tetuan, and how indignant we were with English diplomacy for having stopped, by an attitude of pride and disapproval, the triumphal advance of our troops—perfidious Albion as they used to say then, forgetting the priceless service which she had done us in our war with the French. I did not then have any very clear idea of the nature of the offences received, of the legitimacy of and necessity for vengeance, nor of the moral and material advantages which the war might bring us; but at the sight of joy and enthusiasm everywhere, I was fired and exhilarated also, taking my part in the celebrations with which our rough but patriotic magistrates of Valpalmas wished to demonstrate the great satisfaction and noble pride overflowing in the hearts of all.

Among the festivities prepared to celebrate the entry of our troops into Tetuan I remember the marches, onesteps, and jotas performed with more fervor than skill by a street band brought from I know not where, and a tremendous bonfire kindled in the public square, in the coals of which many sheep and fowls were roasted and baked, as in the account by Cervantes of the nuptials of Camacho. In time with the noisy and unpleasant orchestra, there circulated ceaselessly from hand to hand leather bottles overflowing with old wine and savory chunks of meat, which, as will be well understood, were not distasteful to us children; thus, excited by the festivities and boisterousness and inspired by this kind of patriotic communion, we gorged ourselves with meat and became half fuddled with wine.

This was the first time that there arose in my mind with any clearness a feeling for my country and its historic peoples. Generally speaking, patriotism is a passion which develops late, taking possession of the spirit during adolescence when the sensibilities are penetrated by the first definite ideas of national history and geography. These ideas surpass and expand the narrow concept of the family and, without lessening our love of our own neighborhood, teach us that beyond its boundaries there dwell millions of our brothers who love, hope, struggle, and hate in common with ourselves, who speak the same language and have similar lineage and destiny. Such a sense of solidarity arises in the child when he reads the story of the deeds of his elders; these tales inspire in him admiration and fervent adoration for the national heroes, the defenders of the land against foreign agressors, and arouse the noble desire to emulate the great figures of history and to sacrifice himself, if necessary, upon the sacred altar of his country.

It is well known that patriotic feeling is two-sided; it is compounded of loves and hates. On the one side is the love of the territory and of the culture of one's own country; on the other, the hatred of foreigners with whom the nation has to contend in defence of its independence. Both these forms of patriotism, and especially the negative one, reigned at that time in Aragon, as in most of Spain. I did not then realize how instinctive and natural to us was our abhorrence of the ferocious Moroccan, the legendary enemy of Christianity, and how excusable was our dislike for the French, whose invincible power and riches had prevented our expansion in Europe. Nevertheless, this involved an injustice which I corrected later on. As time passed and I gained in understanding, I came to realize that, in respect of unjust and impetuous aggressions, all peoples are alike. We have all made wars both just and unjust, and in the end have prevailed not the bravest, but the richest, the most industrious, and the most intelligent. It is not to be wondered at, then, that later on I repudiated my dislike and antipathy for foreigners so as to cultivate only the positive aspect of patriotism, that is to say, the disinterested love of the race and fervent desire that my country should act a brilliant part in the history of the world and the enterprises of European civilization.

Certainly, without ignoring the fact that many factors have contributed to my patriotic fire, it appears certain that the event just described had a definite influence, being the very thing to inflame the souls of the young and to sow seeds of enthusiasm which would blossom richly in maturity.

The second event to which I referred, namely the striking of the school by lightning, with extraordinarily dramatic results, also left a broad stamp upon my memory. For the first time there appeared to me in all its irresistible majesty, that blind and ungovernable force of the universe, which is indifferent to suffering and seems not to distinguish between the innocent and the guilty.

This was the tragic occurrence. We children were assembled one afternoon in the school, engaged in prayers under the leadership of the mistress (the master being confined to bed that day). When the afternoon was already advanced, the sky became rapidly overcast and there were several violent thunder-claps, which did not alarm us; then suddenly, in the midst of the deep abstraction of the prayer, our lips in the act of uttering the words of supplication: "Lord deliver us from all evil," there sounded a terrific crash which shook the building to its foundations, froze the blood in our veins, and cut short abruptly the petition which we had commenced. Dense dust mingled with debris and fragments of plaster dislodged from the ceiling, obscured our eyes, and an acrid smell of burned sulphur spread through the place. Terrified and running like mad creatures, half blind with the cloud of dust, tumbling over each other under the shower of falling fragments, we anxiously sought the way out without finding it for a while. More fortunate or less paralyzed by fear than the others, one of the children reached the door and the rest rushed after him in terror. The vivid fear which we felt did not allow us to realize what had occurred. We thought that a mine had exploded, that the house had caved in, that the church had fallen down on to the school, everything occurred to us except a lightning stroke.

Some good women who saw us running distractedly came at once to our assistance, gave us water, cleaned off the dusty perspiration which gave us the appearance of ghosts and bandaged temporarily those who had been hurt. A voice coming from among the crowd called our attention to a strange, blackish figure hanging on the railing of the bell tower. In fact, there, beneath the bell, enveloped in dense smoke, his head hanging over the wall lifelessly, lay the poor priest, who had thought that he would be able to ward off the threatening danger by the imprudent tolling of the bell. Several men climbed up to help him and found him with his clothes on fire and with a terrible wound in his neck from which he died a few days later. The bolt had passed through him, mutilating him horribly. In the school, the mistress lay senseless upon her dais, also struck by the lightning but without serious injuries.

Little by little we took in what had happened. A bolt or flash of lightning had struck the tower, partly melting the bell and electrocuting the priest; afterwards, continuing its capricious path, it had entered the school through a window, had pierced the ceiling of the lower floor where we children were, shattering a great part of the ceiling, had passed behind the mistress, whom it deprived of sensibility, and, after destroying a picture of the Saviour hanging upon the wall, had disappeared through the floor, by a gap, a sort of mouse hole close to the wall.

It is unnecessary to emphasize how stupefied I was by this tragic event. For the first time there crossed my mind, already deeply moved, the idea of disorder and lack of harmony. Everyone knows that for the child nature is a perpetual marvel. The scientific conception of law penetrates the infantile brain very slowly with the revolutionary doctrines of physics and astronomy. This capricious course of phenomena does not disquiet the child. That is prevented by the profound optimism of all beginning life and especially by the certainty acquired from the teaching of the catechism that there exists on high a Good God who watches piously over the march of the great cosmic mechanism and imposes and maintains order among the elements. Parents and teachers have shown him also that the Psychological Principle of the Universe is besides a most tender father and a sublime artist. In His infinite power He adapts ingeniously the vicissitudes of the seasons to the necessities of life, and, descending from the highest heaven, deigns to compose and preserve superb pictures for the edification and pleasure of human sensibilities: the sky and its red painted cloud effects; the fields and meadows of springtime sown with poppies and scattered with butterflies; the dark night adorned with stars; the trees and the grapevines laden with fruit.

But here, of a sudden, this beautiful conception which I, like all children, had adopted was rudely shaken. The smiling palette of the artist became darkened; unexpectedly the idyl was transformed to tragedy. My mind floated in a sea of confusion and anxious questions came in quick succession without finding any satisfactory answer.

Fortunately, the age of eight years is not one at which philosophy flourishes nor which grasps broad abstractions. In the dawn of life deep feeling is fairly transient, for no event, however moving it may be, can disturb in an enduring manner the serenity of the child who is taken up by an irresistible instinct with moulding and developing the body by play and spontaneous gymnastics and with enriching and strengthening the mind by continuous observation of the spectacle of nature.

The third occurrence which also produced upon me an important moral effect was the eclipse of the sun in the year 1860. Having been announced in the newspapers, it was awaited eagerly by the townspeople, many of whom, their eyes protected by smoked glasses, ascended a neighboring hill to observe the surprising phenomenon comfortably. My father had explained the theory of eclipse to me and I had understood fairly well, but a little distrust lingered in my mind. Will the moon not forget the course indicated by the calculation? Will science be mistaken? Was human intelligence, which could not foresee the striking of my school by lightning, capable nevertheless of predicting phenomena occurring millions of miles from the earth? In a word, could human intellect, though incapable of explaining many nearby things, things so intimate as our life and thought, nevertheless enjoy the remarkable privilege of understanding and foretelling that distant event which could interest us much less from the practical point of view? Obviously these questions were not formulated thus in my mind, but I believe that they represent well my feelings at that time.

It is but just to recall that the chaste Diana came to the rendezvous, carrying out her programme conscientiously and with admirable precision. It seemed as if the astronomers, besides being prophets, must have been to some extent accomplices, pushing the moon with the levers of their enormous telescopes to the place in the sky where they had agreed to examine the phenomenon. During the eclipse my father drew my attention to the kind of fear and of indefinable anxiety which takes possession of the whole of nature, which is accustomed to be regulated in all its activities by the regular rhythm of light and darkness, heat and cold, resulting from the eternal spinning of the earth. For animals and plants the eclipse seems to be opposed to reason, something like an inexplicable mistake in the cosmic mechanism, heedless of the permanent interests of life.

It will be readily understood that the eclipse of 1860 was a brilliant revelation for my youthful intelligence. I now realized that man, helpless and unarmed before the irresistible power of cosmic forces, possesses in science a heroic redeemer and a powerful and universal instrument of foresight and dominion.

CHAPTER V

Ayerbe. Games and pranks of childhood. Warlike and artistic instincts. My first experimental notions concerning optics, ballistics, and the art of warfare.

When I was eight years old my father applied for and obtained the medical practice of Ayerbe, a town of which the richness and populousness promised him higher professional prestige and wider scope for his surgical prowess than Valpalmas, besides better facilities for the education of his children.

Ayerbe is an important town of the province of Huesca, famous for its wines throughout the Somontano.[1] It is situated on the road from Huesca to Jaca and Panticosa not far from the Sierra de Gratal, the first spur of the Aragonese Pyrenees. Its picturesque houses are spread out at the foot of a high mountain with two peaks, one of them crowned with the ruins, still imposing, of a very ancient feudal castle. In the center of the town, two large and regular squares provide ample space for its merchants and its fairs, which are famous through the whole district. Separating and adorning the two squares stands an opulent mansion which formerly belonged to the Marquises of Ayerbe.

My appearance in the public square of Ayerbe was hailed with general mockery by the boys. From mockery they passed to serious abuse. Whenever several of them were together and believed themselves certain of impunity, they insulted me, struck me with their fists, or tormented me by throwing stones at me. How brutal we boys of Ayerbe were!

Why is this idiotic aversion for the strange child? I

[1] The Somontano is one of the richest districts in the province of Huesca, situated at the foot of the Sierras of Guara, Sevil, and Alquézar and traversed by the river Alcanadre. (Translator's note.)

PLATE 5

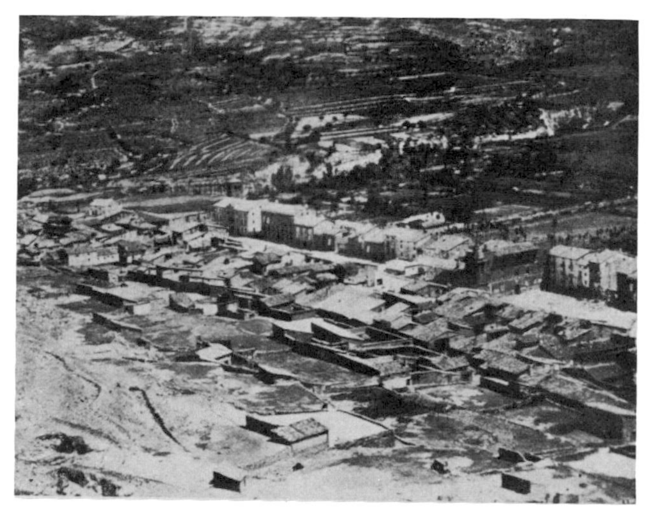

FIG. 8. VIEW OF AYERBE FROM THE SLOPES OF THE CASTLE HILL. Observe the two squares, separated by the palace of the Marquises.

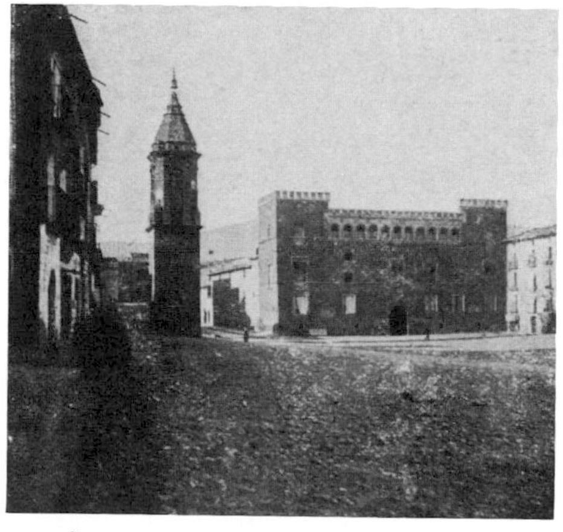

FIG. 9. THE LOWER SQUARE OF AYERBE with the clock tower and the palace of the Marquises, now turned into a tenement.

did not understand it, and even to-day it is not clear to me. I believe, nevertheless, that I see in it an effect of that repressed hatred, not often translated into action, which the poor labourer feels towards the burger and the professional man; restrained in men by prudence, it bursts out violently in lads, in whom the arts of dissimulation have not curbed even the more savage impulses. To such ill will rusticity, envy, and ignorance doubtless contributed.

My appearance, nevertheless, could not inspire misgivings in the children of the town. Dressed simply—for the strict economy which ruled in my home permitted no luxuries—with a swarthy face and a lean appearance which, even at a distance, proclaimed long hours in the sun and air, no one would have taken me for the son of a well-to-do citizen; but I did not wear breeches nor sandals, nor bind my head with a handkerchief and that was enough to make me pass among those clowns for a little gentleman.

The feeling of strangeness caused by my language also contributed to this antipathy. At that time there was spoken in Ayerbe a peculiar dialect, a disorderly jumble of French, Castilian, Catalan, and archaic Aragonese words and phrases. There they said, *forato* for *agujero* (a hole), *no pas* for *no* (not), *tiengo* and *en tiengo* for *tengo* and *tengo de eso* (I have some), *aivan* for *adelante* (forward), *muller* for *mujer* (woman), *fierro* and *ferrero* for *hierro* (iron) and *herrero* (blacksmith), *chiqué* and *mocete* for *chico* (young boy) and *mocito* (young man), *abrios* for *caballerias* (riding horses), *dámene* for *dame de eso* (give me some), *en ta allá* for *hacia allá* (in that direction), *m'en voy* for *me voy de aqui* (I am going from here), and many other expressions of that kind, which I have now forgotten.[2] In the mouths of the people of Ayerbe even the articles had suffered unbelievable omission in that *el, la, lo,* had been converted into *o, a,* and *o* respectively. One would have said that we were in Portugal.

To the rascals of Ayerbe on the other hand the relatively

[2] I cite these because this old Aragonese jargon has now disappeared almost entirely and possesses therefore the philological interest of dead dialects.

pure Castilian which I used,—that is to say that spoken in Valpalmas and Cinco Villas,—appeared to be insufferable gabbling, and they made fun of me calling me the *forano* (*forastero*—foreigner).

Little by little, however, we came to understand each other, and as there could be no question of many learning the language of one, the reverse had to take place and I finally accommodated myself to their slovenly jargon, cramming my memory with barbarous terms and atrocious solecisms.

I have said more than once that I was particularly fond of solitary places and of excursions into the outlying regions; but in Ayerbe, once I had satisfied my curiosity about its mountains, its little river, held back by a high dam and bordered by leafy orchards, and especially about its romantic, ruined castle, which seemed from the mountain top to be telling us of heroic legends and long past greatness, I felt the necessity of plunging into the social life and taking part in the common games, in the races and fights of the gangs, and in all sorts of destructive pastimes with which the small boys of the town used to occupy the hours of play.

The games of children, and especially the social games, in which physical exercise and mental activity are combined in due proportion, have a high educative value. In those competitions of agility and strength, in those contests which exalt bravery, daring, and astuteness, abilities are evaluated and compared, the body is tempered and strengthened, and the mind is prepared for the hard struggle for existence in manhood. It is not strange then that many educationists have said that the whole future of a man is determined in his childhood, and that Rod, Froëbel, Gros, France, etc., and in our country Giner, Letamendi, Castillejo, and many others have attributed to the play of children great importance for physiological development, and for the regular training of the senses and the formation of character.

"To play," says Thomas, "is to apply one's organs, to

feel oneself live, and to procure for oneself the opportunity to become familiar with the objects which surround the child, objects which are for him a perpetual marvel.'' For my part, I have always believed that the games of children are an absolutely essential preparation for life; thanks to them the infantile brain hastens its development, receiving, according to the hobbies preferred and the amusements carried on, a definite moral and intellectual stamp upon which the future will largely depend.

As the ill will of the boys towards me relaxed, then, I joined in their sports and skirmishes, and took part in the games of spinning tops, of quoits, of *espandiella*, of *marro*,[3] not to forget the races, fights, and jumping contests; finding in all these diversions the healthy pleasure which comes from the stimulation of all our organs and the feeling of increasing muscular energy and sensory acuity. Aristotle said—and many teachers, especially Bouillier, have repeated it—''there is pleasure whenever the activity of the being is exercised in accordance with its nature and in the line of its conservation and development.'' Who does not know that to keep still is the worst torture for a child? Pain itself is preferred to rest. Besides, there is positive delight in the consciousness of our physical and mental development and in observing how, in that daily conflict of stratagems, the regular resort in every struggle among boys, the attention is sharpened and the ability to repulse unforeseen and unjust aggressions is increased.

But the boys of Ayerbe did not amuse themselves only with innocent games; quoits and *marro* alternated with diversions somewhat more risky and wicked. Stone throwing, pillaging, and robbery, without consideration for anybody or anything, were the natural occupations of my mischievous comrades. To crack each other's crowns by stone throwing, to break lamps and lanterns, to attack orchards, and at the time of the grape harvest to steal grapes, figs, and peaches; such were the favorite occupations of the

[3] A kind of game of tag played between two organized groups of children, and governed by special rules. (Translator's note.)

youths among whom I soon had the unenviable honor of counting myself.

I have attempted many times to understand this tendency to marauding by which boys amuse themselves with such satisfaction without being able to explain it to myself adequately. To such dangerous conduct there must contribute, doubtless, the desire for delicacies natural to children, which demands the daily consumption of a large quantity of sweets indispensable for the repair of the continuous expenditure of muscular energy (oxidized sugar produces heat and motor energy); but that does not appear sufficient. Almost all of us youngsters who took part in the robbery of the orchards and vineyards had in our homes fruit in plenty. Besides, as for my case, my family possessed a fertile orchard and during summer and autumn there was rarely a day when patients grateful for my father's medical services did not bring some gift of fruit or vegetables. Nevertheless, reading the books which treat of the great problem of education and of the psychology of games, I think that I have found the main key to the engima: the desire for excitement, the irresistible attraction of danger.

Educators rightly point out that the child in his games and other undertakings likes constantly to border upon danger: thus when he goes for a walk, he prefers climbing over walls and rocks to walking on the level road; and likewise when he plays, he enjoys those diversions in which only his agility, coolness, or strength enable him to avoid an accident.

From another point of view the child may be considered as a representative of that beautiful golden age when, as Cervantes says, the meaning of the words thine and mine was unknown. In the bottom of every juvenile head there is a perfect anarchist and communist. Even to the form of his features and the disproportion of his members, the child resembles the savage, as was remarked by Herbert Spencer. Like the wild Indian, the child is all determination. He acts before he thinks, without caring a straw for the consequences. Before his tyrannical will, his absorbing individualism, affirmed constantly in acts of pillage and vandalism, laws are meaningless, and property rights a mere fiction maintained by judges and governors.

To the anarchistic instincts of the child must be added two others: cruelty and the inclination to dominate. Very often, in spite of the rules of morality and good breeding, childhood is pleased to abuse its powers, maltreating the weak and subjecting them to its sovereign autocracy, which it exercises without other limits than those set by its powers and its daring. I will not say with Rousseau "that the heart of the child feels nothing, is untouched by piety, and understands only justice"; but I am bound to confess that the sentiments of humanity, charity, and compassion are in an embryonic state, and even the conception of justice is rather vague and questionable.

I made some resistance at first to the brutal games and to the undesirable escapades of climbing into orchards and stealing fruits. But the spirit of imitation was more powerful in me than the wise counsel of my parents and the commandments of the Decalogue. There was one respect, however, in spite of this, in which my natural chivalry never transgressed, namely in the abuse of strength against the weak, or unjust and cruel aggression.

Pablos was told by his uncle, the executioner of Segovia, "Look here, son, with your knowledge of Latin and rhetoric you will be outstanding in the executioner's art." This amusing remark of Quevedo, while it appears as a joke, contains a fountain of truth. The rapid steps which I made in the violent occupations of stoning, assaulting, and attacking public and private property proved, no doubt, that the geography, grammar, cosmography, and rudiments of physics with which my father had enlightened my turbid understanding counted for something in my youthful activities. I believe that this knowledge, acquired early, produced a certain habit of reflection which enabled me rapidly to come to the front among the ignorant urchins about me, surpassing many of them in the contrivance of tricks, roguery, and mischief, as well as in the realm of games and more or less brutal struggles.

Soon I had enthusiastic supporters, companions in glory and in fatigue, who emulated my accomplishments; I remember among them Tolosana, Pena, Fenollo, Sanclemente, Caputillo, and others, who were joined later by my brother Pedro, two years my junior. Thanks to constant gymnastics, my muscles acquired strength, my joints suppleness, and my vision clearness. I jumped like a grasshopper, climbed like a monkey, ran like a buck, scaled a wall with the celerity of a lizard, without ever feeling dizziness at great heights, even on the eaves of the roofs or in the branches of the walnut trees, and I handled the cudgel, the arrow, and especially the sling with exceptional dexterity.

So many and such profitable accomplishments of this kind could not lie idle. My facility in scaling walls and climbing trees soon brought me unpleasant fame. Like Quevedo's *buscon,*[4] I exacted taxes, tithes, and first-fruits from the beanfields, orchards, vineyards, and olive groves. The most delicious apricots, the finest figs, and the most luscious peaches were produced for the benefit of the gang of which I was captain. From our communistic confiscations, applied according to principles of strict equity, was exempt neither the orchard of the priest nor that of the mayor. For neither authority, the ecclesiastical nor the civil, did we care a straw.

In a word, I contrived to join in and surpass the escapades, knaveries, and rascalities of the boys of Ayerbe so much that I quickly had the honour of figuring in the *Index of Bad Companions* drawn up by the God-fearing fathers of families.

While I showed myself so active and interested in all kinds of mischief and depredation, there were some, especially those into which there entered a mechanical element, in which my superiority was acknowledged by all. My assistance, then, was sought by many and for no good ends.

[4] *El Buscon,* literally *the great seeker,* is translated *the great rascal.*

Was there occasion to organize a charivari for an old man or a widow married for the second or third time? Then there was I getting ready the drums and cow-bells and preparing the flutes and whistles, which I made of cane, with their proper stops, reeds, and even keys. Careful observation, enriched by much practice, had shown me the distances at which the holes should be made to produce tones and semitones, as well as the shape and sizes of the reeds. I remember that some of my flutes, which had a range of about two octaves, sounded with the quality and intensity of the clarinet. Sometimes when I was playing some popular tunes by ear I was taken for a wandering minstrel.

Was a fight with stones in the neighboring threshing floors [5] or the road to the fountain being arranged? Then I was entrusted with the delicate commission of making the slings, which I constructed of hemp and pieces of goat-skin provided by my playmates. More than once it occurred that, lacking old leather, we had to make use of the material of our boots, the height of which, naturally, diminished progressively. Who could recount the indignation of our parents upon observing that retrograde evolution of our footwear, as a result of which what had been brand-new boots became dilapidated and effeminate slippers!

Did we play at ancient wars? Then it was my industry that provided the helmets and cuirasses, which I manufactured from cardboard or old tins, and especially the arrows, in the fashioning of which I attained great proficiency. In fact my arrows not only had a great range, but flew without swerving or turning from their course. The observant mind developed in connection with these amusements soon caused me to notice that the shaft of the arrow must weigh less than the head and must be perfectly smooth and straight in order that the projectile should not waver and deviate from its initial path. Following this practical rule, I made the shafts of bamboo and substituted for the nails and pins which others used as heads broken shoemaker's

[5] The threshing floors are usually in the outskirts of the town. (Translator's note.)

awls. This iron or spike has the shape of a lance, weighs sufficient, and, when suitably sharpened and firmly bound to the shaft of cane with tarred pack-thread, makes an excellent dart. As for the bow, I employed large and strong pieces of green boxwood, laboriously bent, of the excellent qualities of which in respect of strength and elasticity I assured myself by making a comparative study of bows made of almost every kind of wood to be found in the district. Needless to say, in order to procure the raw materials (the broken awls), I established commercial relations with all the shoemakers' apprentices in the community. These provided me also, at times, with leather for the slings in exchange for a gift of one of them.

The reader will understand that such arrows, upon the tips of which I used to put balls when fighting with my playmates, so as not to injure them seriously, were not used exclusively in frivolous imitations of old-time wars; they served also more utilitarian purposes. We hunted birds and hens with them and did not disdain dogs, cats, and rabbits if they appeared within range.

These risky exploits in the chase cost me tremendous whippings and countless troubles and persecutions. Although my whole gang took part in the deeds, no partridge was killed, no decoy-bird in its cage, no rabbit or hen in the corral, but the responsibility was laid upon my shoulders either as the material author or as the contriver of the crime, or else as the instigator of its commission.

Whether deserved or not, my fame as a mischievous rascal grew from day to day, with a good deal of sorrow to my parents, who were seized with righteous indignation whenever they received complaints from injured neighbors. Chastisement at home came frequently to reinforce that received at the even less merciful hands of those whom I had offended. I was thus fated to pay for not only my own crimes but also those of many others, much to the satisfaction of my accomplices, who used to run away, constantly leaving me in the lurch.

Nevertheless, in spite of everything, I was not so bad

after all. My misdeeds were inspired more by vain-gloriousness and complacency than by ill will, and when I caused an injury I regretted it with sincere repentance. But the mad desire to excel and to assuage my spirit with strong emotions obsessed me, and after a few weeks of quietness and contrition, the diabolical instigations of my friends made me return to my activities, confident that my future misdeeds would remain secret and would not cause my parents any displeasure.

CHAPTER VI

The unfolding of my artistic tendencies. The dictum of a house painter regarding my ability. Good-bye to my dreams of being an artist. Utilitarianism and Idealism. My father decides to make me study medicine and to send me to Jaca.

About that time, if my memory does not deceive me, my artistic instincts began or at any rate showed a great increase. When I was about eight or nine years old, I suppose, I already had an irresistible mania for scribbling on paper, drawing ornaments in books, daubing on walls, gates, doors, and recently painted facades, all sorts of designs, warlike scenes, and incidents of the bull ring. A smooth white wall exercised upon me an irresistible fascination. Whenever I got hold of a few cents I bought paper or pencils; but, as I could not draw at home because my parents considered painting a sinful amusement, I went out into the country, and sitting upon a bank at the side of the road, drew carts, horses, villagers, and whatever objects of the countryside interested me. Of all these I made a great collection, which I guarded like a treasure of gold. I took pleasure also in adorning my drawings with colours, which I obtained by scraping the paint from the walls or by soaking the bright red or dark blue bindings of the little books of cigarette paper, which at that time were painted with soluble colours. I remember that I attained great skill in extracting the dye from coloured papers, which I employed also in place of brushes damped and rolled up in the shape of a stump; an occupation which was forced upon me by the lack of a box of paints and of money to buy them.

My artistic tastes, ever more definite and absorbing, led me to habits of solitude and contributed not a little to the shy character which so much distressed my parents. In reality, my habitual reclusiveness did not spring from aversion to social intercourse, since, as we have already seen, that of the boys contented and satisfied me; it sprang from the need of removing myself during my artistic efforts and my clandestine manufacture of instruments of music and of war from the severe vigilance of older people.

My father, who was more laborious and studious than most people, had grown up with a mental hiatus; he was almost completely lacking in artistic sense and he repudiated or despised all culture of a literary or of a purely ornamental or recreative nature. He had formed an extremely severe and rigid ideal of life. He was what educationists call a pure intellectualist. Man he regarded as a mere machine for knowledge and production, which had to be trained very early in order to be ready for the possible contingencies and reverses of life. This somewhat positivistic tendency I believe to have been not innate but acquired; it was an extreme adaptation brought about by the gloomy spiritual atmosphere which surrounded his youth. That incurable fear of poverty often represents the bitter lees left in the heart by the harsh struggle with misery, injustice, and neglect.

In the family circle this utilitarian and decidedly pessimistic outlook had two consequences—overwork and the most rigid economy. My poor mother, who was already very economical and a good manager by nature, made incredible sacrifices to obviate any superfluous expenditure and to conform with this system of exaggerated foresight. It was necessary to economize at all costs.

Far be it from me to censure a course of conduct which made it possible for my parents to amass the funds necessary for moving to Zaragoza, for providing a career for their sons, and for creating for themselves a position, if not brilliant and showy, at least comfortable and free from anxiety; but it must be recognized that the spirit of economy has commonsense limits which it is rather dangerous to exceed. Excessive saving declines rapidly into miserliness, falling into the absurdity of considering even necessaries superfluous; it banishes from the hearth the happiness which ordinarily springs from the satisfaction of a thousand innocent caprices and the possession of inexpensive trifles which would not be burdensome; it prevents the desirable relaxations of the novel, the theater, painting, and music, which are not vices but instinctive necessities for young people, for which every wise and well-regulated education must provide; and it loosens in the family the bonds of affection, for the children get the habit of regarding their parents as the perpetual preventers of present happiness. Nor may it be forgotten that every age has its pleasures as well as its troubles, and that it is a very harsh rule of conduct which sacrifices entirely those of youth for the sake of the distant and problematical enjoyments of maturity.

I trust that the reader will find it natural that I reacted obstinately against so gloomy an ideal of life, which killed in flower all my boyish illusions and cut off sharply the impulses of my budding fantasy. Certainly, without the mysterious attractiveness of forbidden fruit the wings of my imagination would have extended, but they would perhaps not have reached the hypertrophic development which they attained. Dissatisfied with the world around me, I took refuge within myself. In the theater of my feverish imagination, I substituted for the common beings who work and economize, ideal people with no other occupation than the serene contemplation of youth and beauty. Translating my dreams on to paper, with my pencil as a magic wand, I constructed a world according to my own fancy, containing all those things which nourished my dreams. Dantesque countrysides, pleasant and smiling valleys, devastating wars, Greek and Roman heroes, the great events of history all flowed from my restless pencil, which paid little attention to common scenes, to ordinary nature, or to the activities of every day life. My specialty was the terrible incidents of war; and so in a moment I covered a wall with sinking ships, with sailors rescued on planks, with ancient heroes covered with shining harness and protected by plumed helmets, with catapults, battlements, moats, horses, and riders. It is unnecessary to say that, being drawn from memory, these scenes did not pass beyond the category of pretentious and grotesque scrawls or lifeless mannikins.

I very seldom drew modern soldiers: I found them insignificant, prosaic, laden with a knapsack and a blanket which gives them the air of porters, with their ugly shakos, a poor parody of the knightly and majestic casque, and with their short and almost inoffensive bayonets, a sort of spit without a handle, a ridiculous caricature of the elegant and efficient sword. Besides, modern war, with firearms, I considered inartistic and cowardly. I believed that in it the most gallant, intrepid, and bold warrior could no longer win, but rather the most faint-hearted and mean, who fired his gun from a protected spot, and without risk. I regarded such a manner of fighting as more liable to degrade the human race than to improve it: truly a selection of the least fit. Doubtless old-time wars were death dealing, but they had the prestige of elegance of gesture and of apparel. In accordance with the principle of evolution, the laurel almost always crowned in them the supreme artists of energy, form, and rhythm. To-day the enemies' bullet decimates in preference the big, the brave, and the bold, and respects the small, the weak, and the faint-hearted. Henceforth, I said to myself, not the Greeks but the Persians will triumph; unarmed heroism will be overcome by wealth and cold calculation; the fox will disarm the lion; and those imposing athletes with strong arms hardened in a thousand glorious combats, who, like Milo of Crotona, were the shield and bulwark of their country and the light and glory of the human race, will remain relegated to the sad and base condition of the strong man in a side show. Obviously, in my ignorance, I was not capable of formulating these thoughts, but they represent my state of mind during that period.

From warlike interests I turned to the lives of the saints. But when I painted saints I preferred the active to the contemplative ones; I adored those who were fighters, among whom, as the reader will easily guess, my own saint, that is to say Santiago (St. James) the apostle, the patron of Spain and the terror of the Moor, enjoyed all my sympathies. I delighted in representing him as I had seen him in prints, or else galloping intrepidly over a large surface thickly covered with Moorish corpses, his blood-stained sword in his right hand and his shield in his left. With what pious care I coloured the helmet with a little gamboge and passed a band of blue along the sword, and lingered over the black beards, which I made long and wavy as I supposed that those of the Apostles must be!

One of the copies of the Apostle St. James drawn on paper and illuminated with certain colors which I was able to "snitch" from the church, was the cause of a serious grief and of my father, who was already averse to all kinds of aesthetic tendencies, becoming the declared enemy of my artistic inclinations. Wearied, no doubt, of depriving me of pencils and drawings and seeing the ardent vocation towards painting which I exhibited, he decided to determine whether those scrawls had any merit and promised for their author the glories of a Velazquez or the failures of an Orbaneja. As there was no one in the town sufficiently qualified as a critic of drawing, the author of my days turned to a certain plasterer and decorator from somewhere else, who arrived about that time in Ayerbe, where the chapter had engaged him to whitewash and paint the walls of the church, damaged and scorched by a recent fire.

When I arrived in the presence of the Aristarch, I timidly displayed my picture, which was incorrect enough; the house painter looked at it and looked at it again; and after moving his head significantly and adopting a solemn and judicial attitude he exclaimed, "What a daub! Neither is this an Apostle, nor has the figure proportions, nor are the draperies right—nor will the child ever be an artist." I remained stricken dumb by the categorical verdict.[1] My father dared to reply, "But does the boy really show no aptitude for art?" "None, my friend," replied the wall scraper inexorably, and turning to me, he added, "Come

[1] And to think that those crude sketches could pass to-day for one of the quite tolerable manifestations of modern painting! But then, classicism reigned and was indeed a truly fanatical cult.

PLATE 6

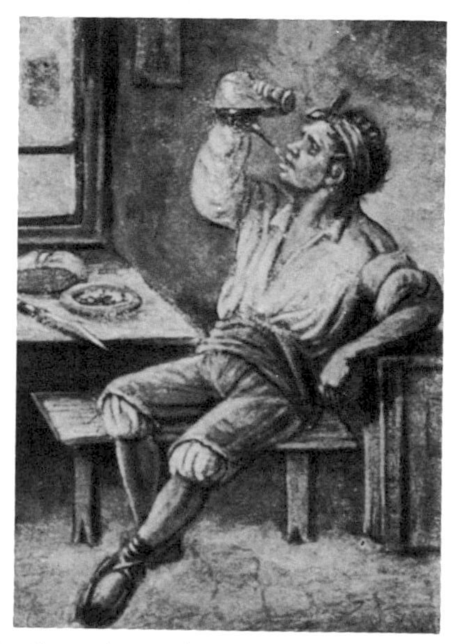

FIG. 10. For those who are interested in such trifles, I reproduce here two water-colors found among my old papers. They were drawn from memory when I was nine or ten years old, shortly after the time of my dismissal by the house-painter. Both, especially the first, show obvious defects of draughtsmanship and of proportion. The former represents a certain labourer of Ayerbe drinking in the tavern. There will be observed a decided tendency towards caricature and an ignorance of anatomy, a tendency which many modernist and futurist painters to-day cultivate systematically with rapturous applause from superficial critics. The second sketch (Fig. 11) represents the Hermitage of the Virgin of Casabas, in los Anguiles, near Ayerbe.

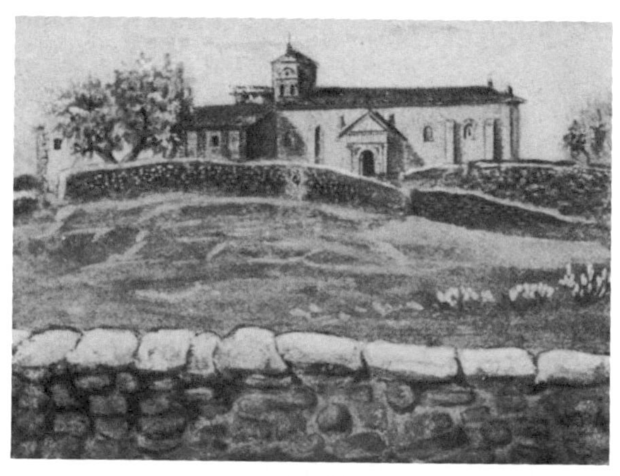

FIG. 11.

here, Mr. Painter of mannikins, and look at the large hands of your apostle. They are like a glove maker's samples! Look at the shortness of the body, where the eight heads' length prescribed by the canons have diminished to a bare seven, and, finally, look at the horse, which appears to have been taken from a merry-go-round!"

Choked with disappointment, I proffered some timid excuses; but the cultivator of red ochre and white lead spoke *ex cathedra* and gave me up with finality. The significant silence of my father told me clearly that all was lost. In fact, the opinion of the dauber of walls was received in my family like the pronouncement of an Academy of Fine Arts. It was decided, therefore, that I should renounce my madness over drawing and prepare myself to follow a medical career. The persecution of my poor pencils, charcoals, and papers was consequently redoubled, and I had to employ all the arts of dissimulation to hide them and to conceal myself when, swept away by my favorite passion, I amused myself with sketching bulls, horses, soldiers, and landscapes. I still preserve some of those childish efforts so much disliked by the famous plasterer. As a sample of my drawings of that period, I reproduce an aquarelle in which serious defects in proportion are immediately evident. It is a somewhat grotesque representation of an Aragonese working-man in a tavern, grasping the classic porron.[2] But who draws well at eight years of age without guidance or methodical studies? I add another drawing saved from the injuries of time and reproduced by the indulgent and admirable writer, Don Luis Zulueta.[3]

Thus there began between my parents and me a silent war of duty against desire. Thus there arose in my father the most obstinate opposition to a vocation which was so clearly indicated; an opposition which was to continue for ten or twelve years and as a result of which, if all my ar-

[2] A wine bottle with a long side spout from which the wine is poured into the mouth. (Translator's note.)

[3] "Cuando yo era nino."

tistic tendencies were not entirely wrecked, at least all my aspirations died out for good.

Farewell to ambitious dreams of glory, illusions of future greatness! I must exchange the magic palette of the painter for the nasty and prosaic bag of surgical instruments! The enchanted brush, the creator of life, must be given up for the cruel scalpel, which wards off death; the maulstick of the painter, like the scepter of a king, for the knotted walking-stick of a village doctor!

My studies meanwhile progressed poorly. I went to school, but paid little attention and did not learn much. My elementary knowledge was really good enough, thanks to the lessons of my father, who now sent me to the municipal school with the idea more of subduing than of enlightening me. This prudent bridle upon my liberty was made advisable by my waywardness and my tendency to play truant. My father would have liked to keep watch over me and to chastise me upon the first transgression, but was prevented by his extensive practice in the town and especially by his frequent visits to the adjacent villages of Linás, Riglos, Los Anguiles, and Fontellas. The oversight of my actions and the punishment of my trespasses was therefore placed in the hands of the schoolmaster and of my mother, who, being already sufficiently occupied with the care of the younger children and the management of the household, could not devote to her first born all the attention desired.

In spite of the precaution taken, the devil often tempted me. Whenever an opportunity presented itself, we mischief-makers of the school took full advantage of it, celebrating it sometimes with battles staged in the suburbs; at others with exploring and climbing the ruins of the historic castle, where we delighted in reproducing the struggles of olden days; and sometimes plunging into the neighboring "*sarda*," an ancient wood of live-oaks, where we spent long hours shooting arrows at the birds and hunting for magpies' nests.

It was in this last occupation that I once suffered a painful accident. I had climbed up into a live-oak and undertaken the examination of a magpie's nest when I touched something soft and furry, and quickly withdrew my hand covered with blood and bitten painfully. A family of rats, which had taken possession of the nest and devoured the eggs, had turned furiously against the intruder who came to disturb them in the peaceful possession of their stolen home.

On another occasion my craze for nests placed me in a very dangerous situation. I was anxious to examine an eagle's nest, so climbed with difficulty down a series of ledges on a tremendous cliff in the Sierra de Linás and looked from close at hand at the still naked eaglets, which stared at me with terror. I could not actually reach them, however. Fearing attack by the eagles, of which I thought that I could hear the screeches, I tried to escape from the projecting ledge where I was perched, but upon attempting the ascent I met with insurmountable difficulties. The shelf to which I had got down by a foolhardy jump projected from a lofty and almost smooth wall. There I remained for hours, caught as in a trap, consumed by terrible anxiety, with a burning sun overhead, and in danger of death from hunger and thirst, as there was no one to help me in these solitudes. Industrious use of the clasp-knife which I always carried saved me at last. Thanks to this implement and to the relative softness of the rock, I was able to enlarge some narrow cracks until they provided sufficient hold for my hands and feet and thus set me at liberty. How many such rash actions I could relate did I not fear to abuse the reader's patience!

Upon his return from the outlying villages, my father would inquire into the misdeeds and excesses of his sons and, rising in anger, would favor us with a formidable thrashing, besides reproaching my poor mother (a thing which distressed us greatly) for what he called her carelessness and excessive softness towards us.

The announcement of these paternal floggings, which, by a logical progression and in suitable adaptation to the hardening of our skins, began with a whip and ended with cudgels and tongs, inspired us with absolute terror; and so it happened upon one occasion that, to avoid this rather vigorous paternal caress, we ran away from home, thereby causing deep grief to our mother, who sought us anxiously throughout the town.

I remember that my brother and I, having played truant one afternoon and knowing that someone had told our severe progenitor, resolved to escape to the hills, where we remained for several days, pillaging the fields and living on fruits and roots, until one night, when we were already beginning to enjoy the wild life, our father, who was looking for us in every hiding-place in the neighbouring woods, discovered us sleeping peacefully in a lime kiln. He shook us violently, bound us arm to arm, and led us in that shameful attitude back to the town, where we had to endure the jeers of the women and children in the streets.

As the reader will have gathered, beatings and thrashings were the usual conclusion of our escapades, but, as a result of the process of adaptation already mentioned, the rods made us smart but did not correct us. While the bruises were fresh, we refrained successfully from backsliding, but once they had vanished we forgot our intentions of reformation. In fact, natural impulses, when they are very strong, may be modified somewhat, and often conceal themselves, but are never obliterated. Thwarted in our natural tastes, deprived of the pleasure of camping among the crags and ravines, there to exercise the artist's pencil, the warrior's arrow, or the naturalist's net, we sullenly attended school, without being corrected or made reliable. All that was accomplished was to change the scene of our misdeeds: the sketches of the countryside were replaced by caricatures of the master; the battles in the open air were changed to skirmishes among the benches, in which paper pellets, cabbage-stalks, haws, chick peas, and kidney beans served as projectiles; and, in default of paper for drawings, I made use of the wide margins of the catechism, which were filled with tasteless ornamentations, conceits, and puppets, some having reference to the pious text, others rather irreverent and profane.

In school, my caricatures, which passed from hand to hand, and my unsuppressible chatter with my fellows exasperated the master so much that more than once he had recourse, in the effort to daunt me, to locking me up in the classical dark chamber—a room almost underground, overrun with mice, of which the youngsters felt a superstitious terror, but which I regarded as an opportunity for recreation, since it provided me with the calm and concentration necessary for planning my escapades of the next day.

There, in the darkness of the school prison, with no other light than that which filtered faintly through the cracks of the rickety window shutter, it fell to my lot to make a tremendous discovery in physics, which, in my utter ignorance, I supposed entirely new. I refer to the camera obscura, wrongly ascribed to Porta, though its real discoverer was Leonardo da Vinci.

The curious fact which I observed was as follows: The little shuttered window of my prison faced the square, which was bathed in sunlight and full of people. Having nothing to do, I happened to look at the ceiling and noticed with surprise that a slender beam of light projected upon it, head downwards and in natural colors, the people and the beasts of burden which passed outside. I widened the hole and found that the figures became vague and nebulous, I reduced the size of the opening with paper moistened in saliva, and observed with satisfaction that, corresponding with the reduction, the clearness and detail of the figures increased. Thence I concluded that the rays of light, as a result of their absolute straightness, paint an image of their source, whenever they are made to pass through a small hole. Naturally my theory lacked precision, ignorant as I was of the rudiments of optics. In any case, that simple and well-known experiment gave me a most exalted idea of physics, which I at once came to regard as the science of marvels. Of course I did not forget the wonders of the railway, of photography (recently invented at that time), of balloon ascents, etc. And my enthusiasm did not deceive me, for to physics we owe the glories of European civilization. If the laws and applications of that science could be extracted from the heritage of human knowledge, the race would step back at one stride to the condition of the cave men.

For the time being, very far from appreciating the magnificent perspectives which the study of natural forces opens to the spirit, I proposed to profit by my unexpected discovery; and, mounted upon a chair, I amused myself by tracing on paper the bright and living images which appeared to console me, like a caress, in the solitude of my prison. "What does the loss of liberty matter to me?" I thought. "I am prevented from rambling about the square, but in compensation the square comes to visit me. All these luminous shades are a faithful reproduction of reality and better than it is, since they are harmless." From my cell I watched the games of the children, followed their quarrels, observed their gestures, and, in fact, enjoyed their play as if I were taking part in it.

Proud of my discovery, I became daily more attached to the realm of shadows. But I was so simple as to tell my comrades in confinement of my discovery, and they, laughing at my foolishness, assured me that the phenomenon was of no importance, since it was a natural thing and, as it were, a trick which the light plays when it enters dark rooms. How many interesting facts fail to be converted into fertile discoveries because their first observers regard them as natural and ordinary things, unworthy of thought and analysis! Oh that unlucky mental inertia, the lack of wonder of the ignorant! How it has delayed our acquaintance with the universe!

It is strange to see how the populace, which nourishes its imagination with tales of witches or saints, mysterious events and extraordinary occurrences, disdains the world around it as commonplace, monotonous and prosaic, without suspecting that at bottom it is all secret, mystery, and marvel.

For the rest, I have already said that my brilliant physical discovery could not gain me the honor of priority. Centuries earlier it had been made by the great Leonardo, who was not only a distinguished painter but also an illustrious physicist; and it may be presumed that in more distant times many others had observed the surprising phenomenon, though they published no account of it.

CHAPTER VII

My removal to Jaca. The picturesque banks of the Gállego. My uncle Juan and the vegetarian diet. Latin and the dominies. Vain effort of the friars to subdue me. Return to my madness over painting.

The year 1861 passed by. As I was nearly ten years old, my father decided to take me to study for my *baccalaureate* [1] at Jaca, where there was a College of Esculapian fathers which enjoyed the reputation of teaching Latin well and of educating and subduing wonderfully boys who were froward and rebellious.

When the matter was brought up in the family circle, I protested timidly: I said to my father that, as I felt a decided vocation for painting, I should prefer to pursue my secondary education in Huesca or in Zaragoza, cities where there were schools of art; and added that I did not like medicine and that, considering my tastes and inclinations, I did not expect to display any aptitude for Latin; so that I should be wasting time and money. My father, however, would not listen to arguments and was sceptical about my vocation, which he perhaps took for the caprice of a headstrong and fickle child.

I have already made it clear that my father was an extreme utilitarian and intellectualist and far from being a sentimental person. His judgment was warped by a certain mistaken conception of art as a profession. In his view, painting, sculpture, music, and even literature did not constitute serious ways of making a living, but were uncertain, irregular, occupations, suitable only for people of unsteady character, loafers, and vagrants and which could end, with rare exceptions, only in misery and social failure. To him,

[1] Degree given at the end of a course of seven years at an *Instituto,* corresponding approximately with the end of the second year in an American university. (Translator's note.)

the artistic obsession of some young people was something like a developmental defect, which it is necessary to combat resolutely with the discipline of methodical work.

In order to persuade me and lead me into what he considered the better way, he told me stories about people he had known, unsuccessful artists, painters of historical pictures with too much history and little money; of writers who thought themselves geniuses and ended as miserable reporters or as hungry clerks of town councils; of musicians who were resolved to emulate Beethoven and Mozart but who ended as defeated and greasy village organists. As a final argument and by way of consolation, he promised me that when I should be a doctor, that is to say at twenty-one years of age, when my economic position would be assured, I should be able to wander as much as I would through the chimerical regions of art; but meanwhile his duty was to provide me with an honest and peaceful manner of life capable of keeping me from want.

My forebear was not one of those who, having once taken a firm resolution, may go back upon it, and least of all in response to the comments of his children. Thus I had to submit and prepared myself for the study of hateful Latin and for making the acquaintance of the friars. During the days which followed, which were the last of September, my father wrote to Jaca announcing to some honorable and hard-working relatives the decision he had taken and asking them to receive his son as a boarder during the period of his studies. Consent was received, as was to be expected, considering the relationship of my uncle Juan and the feelings of affection and gratitude which linked him to my family.

My excellent uncle Juan, my mother's brother, was a skilful weaver in Jaca, where he enjoyed a well-established reputation as a just and hard-working man. His financial position, however, which in former years had been comfortable, had recently suffered reverses, which had been further aggravated by the death of his wife and the abandonment of his eldest son, who had been his right arm in the workshop and without whom he could not get on very well. These family misfortunes obliged him to incur some debts, my father being the principal creditor, although a disinterested one.

I relate these details in order that my peculiar position in my uncle's house may be better understood. My father being anxious to have the loan refunded, he agreed with my relative to pay him a small monthly sum for my board, the remaining part of the value of this being directed to pay off the debt. In this peculiar method of collecting his dues, he committed a grave mistake, for, however well the relationship and the goodness of my hosts might allay any suspicion of bad faith, it was impossible that my uncle, being in very reduced circumstances and in poor health for working, should sacrifice himself without sufficient and immediate financial compensation, in order to procure for his nephew the food and comforts which he would desire for himself.

When everything was arranged for my departure, I took a regretful leave of my friends, the companions of so many pranks and escapades. I said good-bye to the schoolmaster whom I had made to suffer so much and, one beautiful September morning, I set out for the frontier city accompanied by my father, who wished to present me personally to the Esculapians. We travelled in the carrier's cart, in which a soft mattress had been spread over the baggage. I placed myself at the very front of the wagon in order to watch the landscape comfortably. The first two hours of the trip passed slowly and sadly. It was the first time that I had gone away from home and a vague feeling of melancholy weighed down my spirits. I thought of the sobs of my mother at parting from her son and of the advice with which she had tried to urge upon me the affection and obedience due to my relations and the respect and veneration to my future masters.

By degrees, however, my sadness faded away, as it soon does in children. My instinctive delight in the picturesque overcame my languor and depression. The road is somewhat monotonous from Ayerbe to Murillo but becomes more interesting from that town towards Jaca. During a great part of the journey, the highway winds along the banks of the Gállego, which is a broad and shallow stream at some points while at others its waters are gathered together and rush tumultuously between huge rocks or half hidden in narrow gorges.

I did not grow tired of admiring the thousand picturesque details revealed by each turn of the road and each elevation laboriously climbed. Among other details of the panorama, there remained deeply engraved upon my memory the huge "mallets" of the mountain of Riglos, like the columns of a palace of Titans, the great rock of Lapeña, which threatens to plunge down upon the town and at the foot of which the noisy Gállego runs hidden at the bottom of a very deep ravine; the lofty and sombre Mount Pano, of which the formidable crest appears in the west not far from Anzánigo; and lastly the gloomy and fantastic Uruel, with its red peak which dominates the valley of Jaca and looks like a collosal sphinx guarding the entrance to the valley of the Aragon.

My curiosity delighted excessively in such beautiful and varied scenery and so I continually questioned my father, who knew the district thoroughly, about the details of the villages, mountains, and rivers by which we passed. Not only did he satisfy my curiosity, but he told me many anecdotes and episodes of his youth, spent in these regions, and some historical events of which the banks of the Gállego were the scene during the first civil war.

When we arrived at Jaca and were installed in my uncle's house, my father's first care was to present me to the reverend Esculapians, to whom he recommended me highly. He charged them that they should watch my conduct carefully, and punish me without consideration whenever I should offend in the least.

The director of the college satisfied my father fully upon this point and to set his mind at rest introduced us to Father Jacinto, the professor of elementary Latin, who was at that time the terrible horse breaker of the community, and whom, according to report, no rebel had yet been able to resist. In truth I was somewhat alarmed, though only a little, at the sight of the gigantic stature, the broad shoulders, and the massive fists of the dominie, who seemed to have been built expressly to overcome untamed colts. I restricted myself to saying under my breath, "Well, we shall see."

Some days later, I underwent the entrance examination. So satisfactory was the result that the friars considered me one of those pupils who were better prepared for secondary education. My father being tranquilized by the satisfactory course of events and hoping that I would pay with exemplary application for the anxiety and sacrifices which he imposed upon himself, returned to Ayerbe and I remained delivered over to my own free will, which was the same as if I had been delivered over to the devil himself.

I have already said that my uncle was very old and in poor health. He lived almost alone, since of his two sons, only the younger, my cousin Timoteo, at that time an apprentice in a chocolate factory, bore him compnay. Busy with his loom, he paid little attention to the house, which he turned over to the care of an old servant. The culinary skill of this good woman could not have been simpler nor better calculated to avoid waste and indigestion. Cabbages, turnips, and potatoes were the essential dishes and the pieces de resistance; occasionally we had meat; but in just compensation there was a disgusting superabundance of corn meal porridge, there called *farinetas*. Our regular dessert was apples, a fruit of which excellent varieties are grown at Jaca. On festival days the housekeeper prepared for us a pleasant surprise. She added to the ordinary porridge juicy pieces of fat pork. What gestures of disgust my cousin and I made when the blind lottery of the serving spoon favored us with only one prize, reserving the majority of the savory fragments for the others at the table!

Hunger, however, we did not suffer. When our unsatisfied stomachs demanded something more, we found it in the heaps of sweet apples in the barn and in the improvization of a dish of potatoes in their skins, which we prepared by roasting the tubers in hot ashes and flavouring the golden substance with a few grains of salt and drops of vinegar.

Thanks to the diet of farinetas and the fasts of punishment of which I shall speak later, I became as thin as a rail. I believe that even my understanding, which was not very wide awake, declined somewhat. One would have said that the paste of maize seeped into my head and occupied the place of my brains, since, as we shall soon see, the best efforts of the Friars were unavailing to impress upon them some elements of Latin.

I must add that at the end of that year the treatment of my guardian improved very much. One of my cousins, Victoriano Cajal, returned from his travels and took up his residence in the home of his father, soon afterwards entering into marriage with an exceedingly kindly and intelligent girl. With this unhoped for reinforcement, the government of the house was restored to order and the menu became more varied and appetizing. I cannot say whether or not the lack of affection and the austerity of my masters aggravated my inborn rebelliousness and ruined my promises of good behaviour. Probably they had some influence. I imagine, nevertheless, that they were not the primary determinants of my escapades. The imagination, with which my father had not reckoned, and which from day to day increased in power, contributed considerably more to my increasing foolish and rash activities.

My madness over art reappeared vigorously. I conceived a loathing for Latin grammar, where I saw nothing but an irritating downpour of rules which were made valueless by innumerable exceptions and which I had to drive into my head whether I wished or not, by sheer force, like a nail into a wall. I was disgusted also with the comfortless aridity of the didactic style, dry and harsh like a dusty road in summer.

Along with this antipathy to grammar, there was established within me that silent and persistent physical and moral struggle between brain and book in which the latter always comes out worst; for of the wise precepts of the text, few or none penetrate the mind, but, on the other hand, the wanderings and the dreams of the imagination invade the pages of the text, of which the margins become covered with parasitic growths of verses, landscapes, warlike episodes, and merry caricatures. My Latin books—Cornelius Nepos, the Ars Poetica of Horace, etc.—vanquished in this battle, were rapidly transformed into albums where my overflowing imagination deposited daily its fantastic progeny and as the margins of the book became rather too narrow to contain comfortably all my happy "escapes into the ideal," I exclaimed more than once, "What a pity that grammar is not all margins."

But if my Nebrija [2] taught me almost nothing it was of value on the other hand for the amusement of my comrades. Whenever I arrived at the class they surrounded me eagerly to see my illustrations of the text, which were passed from hand to hand and were more handled and passed to and fro than the rolling pin of a wafermaker.

[2] Nebrija. Spanish author who wrote a Latin grammar at the end of the fifteenth century. (Translator's note.)

CHAPTER VIII

Father Jacinto, my Latin master. Carthaginians and Romans. The reign of terror. My hatred of studying. The increase of my artistic and romantic fever. The River Aragon, symbol of a people.

I shall not try to excuse my mistakes. I confess publicly that for the ill success of my studies, I alone am responsible. My body occupied a place in the school rooms, but my mind wandered continually through the spaces of imagination. In vain the energetic exhortations of the teacher, accompanied by furious blows with the strap, recalled me to reality and fought to wrest me from my distractions; the blows sounded in my head like those of the door knocker in an empty house. All the efforts of Father Jacinto, who made my case a matter of personal pride, failed lamentably. Having made this confession, it may be permissible for me to declare also that to my dislike for study there contributed in considerable degree the system of teaching and of rewards and punishments employed by these Esculapian fathers. As the sole pedagogical method, pure memorization reigned supreme.[1] Their aim was to create stored heads rather than thinking heads. To mold a mental individuality, to consent that the pupil, sacrificing the letter for the spirit, should be permitted to change the form of the recitations—that was not to be thought of. There, as still happens to-day in many school rooms, the only person who knew the lesson was he who recited it like a phonograph, that is to say, discharging it in a continuous stream with great vivacity and fidelity. The scholar who stopped the stream for a moment, or wavered in the expression, or changed the order of the state-

[1] Unfortunately the same thing took place in the institutes. (See note on p. 48.) The system was general—what do I say? It still is.

ments, did not know it and was in consequence severely punished.

As infallible stimulants for sluggish memories or backward intelligences, were employed the pointer, a strap, a cat-of-nine-tails, a prison, the *reyes de gallos*,[2] and other coercive and outrageous methods.

As may be seen, the old adage that knowledge enters with pain, ruled unquestioned among those good fathers; but in my case, knowledge slipped through my head without engraving itself upon my brain. On the other hand, many pupils conceived a decided aversion for Latin literature and dislike for the masters. Thus there was lost entirely that cordial intimacy, a mingling of friendship and respect, between master and pupils without which the labor of the educator is the greatest of martyrdoms.

I should be committing a great injustice if I were to say that all the friars applied these pedagogical principles with equal rigor; we had some teachers who were excellent and even kind and sympathetic. But I did not have the happiness to come into contact with them because they took charge of the higher classes and I was obliged, for reasons which I shall explain shortly, to leave the Esculapian school when I was in the second grade. Among these amiable masters, I remember Father Juan, the teacher of geography and an excellent pedagogue. He did not whip the boys, but instead he knew how to arouse their curiosity and captivate their attention.

Following, doubtless, the principle of the skilful knife-sharpener, which is to grind the knife first with the coarsest whetstone and to finish it by further treatment with finer and softer ones, the cloister of Jaca very wisely entrusted the rough-hewing of the first-year students to the harshest breaker-in of intelligences. In fact, we poor wretches of the beginners' class in Latin were handled by the most severe of all the friars, Father Jacinto, of whom I have already spoken in the preceding chapter. He was a native of

2 Literally the kings of cocks. This punishment is explained later on (p. 66).

Egea and had the strength and aggressiveness of the imposing youths of the Five Towns. His huge and stentorian voice stunned the class, thundering in our ears like the roaring of a lion. Into the power of this Herod fell about forty of us unhappy lads, gathered from various mountain towns, and still homesick for the attention of our mothers. An elevated bench formed his throne; his scepter was the cat-of-nine-tails; his ministers were two favorite pupils who were entrusted with keeping watch on the others.

We were divided into two bands or groups, called Carthaginians and Romans, as was announced by placards posted on each side of the schoolroom. It fell to my lot to be a Carthaginian, and I soon came to merit the name, in that I was beaten by Scipio, that is to say by the formidable dominie, who was capable of destroying all the Carthaginians and Romans single handed. For me, then, Carthage fell every day without the triumphs of Hannibal ever being experienced, and still less the pleasures of Capua.

Cowed by this reign of terror, we entered the classroom trembling, and when the lessons commenced we felt such dread that we did not remember a single thing. Woe to him who got mixed in the conjugation of a verb or who stumbled in the declension of *quisnam, quaenam, quodnam* or of the no less peculiar *quicumque!* The blows of the strap rained upon him like a cloudburst, confusing him more and more and inhibiting his weak memory completely. When we left the schoolroom our faces shone with the boisterous joy of liberation; we did not stop to consider, poor children, that on the next day, the flogging would be renewed, and that our wrists, from which the swellings of the day before had not yet completely disappeared, would be delivered again to the terrible strapping of the master.

The teacher who begins to punish early runs the risk of never finishing it. The exclusive use of force, without the wise alternatives of kindness, indulgence, and even cajolery, quickly blunts the sensibilities, both physical and moral, and kills in the child every vestige of the sense of honour and personal dignity. From hearing himself so frequently called stupid, he finally believes that he is so, and that his stupidity is beyond remedy. This was what happened to me and to many of my comrades. Insulted and lashed from the very first, and convinced that such treatment would continue, we had to accept philosophically our rôles as slothful fellows and as helpless victims seeking a remedy in accustoming ourselves to chastisement. In our ingenuousness, we thought that the best way to avenge ourselves was to do the opposite of what the master told us.

Apart from my lack of interest, I grew up with a defect which, under the prevailing pedagogical rule, was fatal: my verbal memory was untrustworthy; I always lacked—and of this I shall speak again—that quickness, certainty, and clearness in the use of words which are the outstanding characteristics of oratorical temperaments. And to add to my misfortune, this difficulty in speaking was exaggerated enormously by emotion. On the other hand, my memory for ideas, without being remarkable, was fairly good and my understanding was quite up to the average. My father had already observed these characteristics of mine, and used to warn my preceptors, telling them, "Be careful with the youngster. He will learn all the principles, but do not expect him to be word-perfect in his lessons, for he is timid and backward in expressing himself. Excuse him if he changes the words in the definitions and uses unsuitable terms. Allow him to explain himself and he will explain himself." Unfortunately few teachers took this prudent advice into consideration; they never waited for me to explain before they judged me.

The evil springs, as Herbert Spencer well remarks, from the fact that the schoolmaster ought to be an expert psychologist, whereas, unfortunately, he is generally nothing but a routine reciter of texts and traditional formulae. According to the law of inheritance he usually carries on in his pupils the bad work which his masters did in him. And in speaking thus, I refer not only to my teachers at Jaca, but to those of the majority of our scholastic institutions. Of this serious defect, however, I shall speak again later.

One consequence of this didactic attitude is a certain mistaken valuation of abilities. Suggestibility and nervous automatism are regarded as desirable and praiseworthy qualities, while spontaneity of thought and a critical mind are considered to be odious defects, deserving correction and condemnation. The usual attitude of this tribe of schoolmasters is to take quickness for cleverness, memory for ability, and submissiveness for righteousness.

I cannot deny, certainly, that verbal readiness and a quick and tenacious memory are often associated and suggest exceptional understanding; more than that, I consider that there is no outstanding talent which is not rooted in the ground of an excellent memory; but, as experience has shown, one also finds frequently a considerable separation of understanding and retentiveness. This circumstance did not escape our own Huarte, who in his "Treatise on the Talents," calls attention to the fact that young people who are endowed with great mnemonic powers, and who learn languages easily, usually display only mediocre ability for science and philosophy. It would be easy to recall other testimony to this effect, that of Locke, for example.

I have mentioned several times the terror which Father Jacinto inspired in us. Although it is emphasizing the same subject again, I shall recall an incident which illustrates the great strength of this cassocked giant. He launched such a blow at a miserable boy, named Barba, who, in his terror and confusion, made some foolish answer, that he hurled the poor wretch against a blackboard at least seven feet away. The collision was so violent that it knocked down the blackboard, broke the trestle which supported it, and by the rebound of the former and the flying splinters of the latter, hurt two other unfortunates.

Such a system of intimidation and harsh punishments produced results the opposite of those intended. Our conduct grew daily worse. We were too much accustomed to disgrace and our sense of honour was blunted. We fell so low that we lost hope of and even the wish for improvement. For those pupils, the teacher was no longer the fatherly guide, but was the enemy who abused his powers and against whose physical superiority they could revenge themselves only by impassiveness and disobedience. The partisans of moral orthopedics may say what they like, but the discreet and preferential use of humoring and persuasion, with explanation of the reasons for each command, and above all a real or pretended confidence in the potential ability of the child, a talent which is only awaiting a favorable opportunity to manifest itself, these are pedagogical methods far superior to corporal punishment.

Fortunately, I found great consolation in the cultivation of art and in the contemplation of nature. Before the grandeur of the tremendous mountains which surround the historic city on the Aragon I forgot my humiliations, discouragements, and sorrows.

The panorama of the valley of Jaca is one of the most beautiful and varied in the whole of the Pyrenees. To the north, the horizon is cut off by the majestic height of el Pirineo, crowned with perpetual snows; to the west, separated from the city by a pleasant and fertile plain, Mount Pano lifts its rugged head, while in its western slope, drenched more than once with the blood of the followers of Mahommed, opens the sacred cavern which was in olden days the cradle and the altar of the independence of Aragon; to the east, are discerned the mountains of Biescas, above which emerge the white-shrouded peaks of Panticosa and Sallent; and to the south, closing the path of the mild breezes from the plain, there rises proudly to the clouds the fantastic Uruel, mute witness of the legendary exploits of the race, its red head seeming to look obstinately southward as if pointing out for the hardy warrior the way to glory.

The city itself held for me unspeakable enchantment. I delighted in admiring at leisure the beauties of its old cathedral, in climbing its walls and exploring the towers and battlements. How often, seated in a bastion and sweeping the plain from the narrow loopholes, pretending to be a watchman in the Middle Ages, I gave rein joyfully to my romantic dreams and consoled myself for my sentimental solitude! From time to time the appearance of a sun-loving lizard or the flight of a kite would draw me out of my abstraction, awakening my enthusiasm as a naturalist. For these wanderings above the roofs, my host's house gave me excellent facilities, the orchard abutting upon a tower of the city wall.

Naturally, I found in Jaca also friends and playmates with whom to share in games and mischief. As the climate there is very cold, our favourite winter sport was throwing snowballs at each other, even the young women taking part in this amusement, hurling their projectiles from windows and balconies. When the icy north winds of January formed great snowbanks against the walls, the game we liked best consisted in digging within their thickness rooms and corridors. At other times, we built with packed snow houses, castles upon rocks, and caverns of troglodytes. The habit of struggling daily with snow and ice soon rendered me insensible to the cold, hardening my skin and adapting me perfectly to the rigorous mountain climate.

Nevertheless, social games did not interest me so much as solitary walks and excursions. One of my favourite outings was to go down to the river Aragon and ramble along by the edge of its deep and rocky bed, going up stream until I was tired. Sitting at the water's edge, I delighted in the contemplation of the crystal ripples and in watching through the restless waters the silvery little fish and the painted pebbles of the river bed. More than once, looking at some great rock loosened from the mountain side, I tried, though in vain, to copy faithfully in my sketch book the fugitive play of light from the waves and the brightly colored stones which emerged at intervals covered with green moss.

Often, through long hours of contemplation I fell into a sweet lethargy; the gentle murmur of the ripples and the splashing of the water as it glided over the pebbles paralyzed my pencil, insensibly clouded my eyes, and produced in my brain a state of subconsciousness favorable for fantastic recallings of the past. The sound of the stream acquired little by little a quality of martial trumpets and the swish of the wind seemed to bear from the blue shores of the past the voice of tradition overflowing with heroic ballads and golden legends.

This, I thought in my day dream, is the sacred river of ancient Aragon; that which fertilized the lands conquered by our forebears; that which gave a name to a great people, and which symbolizes to-day the whole of its history. Born in the valleys of el Pirineo with the melting of the snow and the abundance of ice cold springs, it increases richly through the valley of Jaca and pours a great stream into the Ebro. Thus the race of the mountain people which grew humbly, but brave and free, in the narrow valleys of the Pyrenees spread through the broad river bed of the Aragonese fatherland, in its turn flowing also, inspired by high political motives, into the broad sea of the Spanish nation. Its cold currents tempered the steel of the heroes of the reconquest; they are perhaps those which, circulating through our veins, temper the resilience of the obstinate will of the race.

My supreme desire was to follow the sacred river upwards to discover its sources and lakes and to scale the peaks of el Pirineo, a perennial temptation to my greediness for new panoramas and unlimited horizons. What will there be, I often asked myself, beyond these giant peaks, white, silent, and immutable? Will one see France perhaps, with its green hills, its fertile valleys, and its lovely cities? Who knows if from the giant summit of the "Col de Ladrones" or from the divided crest of the "Sumport" there will not appear crystal and placid lakes bordered by lofty cliffs of painted rock over the steps of which there fling themselves rainbow cascades. What more enchanting subjects could there be for a romantic pencil? Unfortunately, I had neither the money nor the freedom to undertake such extensive and dangerous excursions. Nevertheless, so determined was I to satisfy my frantic love of the mountains that upon one occasion I set out along the road to Canfranc and arrived, passing over Villanua, at the foot of the celebrated Col de Ladrones. But as night was near, and I was told by a shepherd that it would require at least another four hours to gain the summit, I had the disappointment of being obliged to give up the attempt and to return sad and mournful.

Another time I proposed to climb to the crest of Uruel, but, lacking the time, I was only able to reach the first counterforts, covered with age-old forests. In my eagerness for mad adventure, I would have given anything to meet some monstrous bear or wild boar, or even some inoffensive fallow deer; but unfortunately, disappointed in all my hopes, I had to return home footsore, covered with perspiration, hungry and with torn clothes and shoes, and, what most distressed me, without being able to tell my friends of any extraordinary experience.

Of some other expeditions somewhat more extensive and comfortable, as, for example, that to San Juan de la Peña, we shall treat on a more opportune occasion.

CHAPTER IX

My heedlessness continues. Confinement and fasting. The expedients which I used to escape. My examinations. My return to Ayerbe and resumption of my former ways.

I have already explained that I did not feel the least interest in those studies which are called classical and particularly in Latin, philology, and grammar. I was still at the happy age when the child feels more admiration for the works of nature than for those of man; the pleasant time when his sole preoccupation is to explore and to become familiar with the external world. Much time had still to pass before this contemplative phase of my mental development would be replaced by the reflective and my intellect, mature enough to comprehend the abstract, would be able to enjoy the excellencies and beauties of classical literature, mathematics, and philosophy. That period arrived too, but very slowly, as we shall see later. For the time being, as I have already indicated, the picturesque surroundings of the city, the general topography of which (highways, roads, paths, ravines, rivers, springs, rills, and ponds), with its flora and fauna, I came to know perfectly, to the smallest detail, attracted me more than the insufferable hammering of the conjugations and the difficult rules of Latin construction.

A man of inflexible character, Father Jacinto, had given his solemn word to break the colt and he proposed to accomplish it at any cost. It was found necessary, however, to change the tactics. Seeing the uselessness of whipping, against which I was found perfectly immunized, the masters decided to try with me the punishment of starvation. All my misdeeds were set down in a special book carried by one of the favorite pupils, the leader of the band of Carthaginians. Unfortunately, my debits increased continuously and, as they could be paid only by one fast per day, it was seriously feared that the whole course would not be long enough to wipe out the deficit. With the object then of lightening the debt, some of the fasts were commuted in consideration of periodical strappings and even of exhibitions of ignominy; but all the expedients were in vain.

It was already April and my debt had hardly diminished in spite of the sharpness of my shoulders and the sufferings of my stomach. Each day, as I have already said, I had to carry out my penance. When lessons were over, I was shut up in the schoolroom and remained without eating until night. Little by little I was transformed into a person eating only once in twenty-four hours.

At the beginning, my stomach protested somewhat but, following the example of my skin, it finally adapted itself. Of amendment there was not a particle.

What do I say! Things happened quite the other way. Reflecting with the logic of the lazy, I considered that, having reached the limit of punishment, I might as well sin a hundred times as once, and since I felt the irremediable sentence—the terrible failure in examinations—to be already certain, I ended by turning my back upon all sense of shame and gave myself over violently to disturbing and talking in class, to distracting my comrades with grotesque caricatures, and to plotting all sorts of tricks and outrages.

When several months of this dietetic restriction had passed thus, I wondered if it would not be possible to return sometime to the natural alimentary rhythm, eating in the middle of the day like everybody else, and thus avoiding the gastric distention brought about by the necessity of concentrating in one filling and at one meal, more or less warmed over, the materials of two meals and two digestive efforts. The project was worth trying and I tried it. Thus, profiting one day by the lack of vigilance of the school, brought about by the savory banquet with which the fathers were celebrating some festival, I tried to move the spring of the lock of my prison with various implements. A pencil served me as a lever. The spring yielded, the bolt slipped back quickly and I was free. Eureka! I had discovered the secret of dining daily. When I arrived at the house my landlady was much surprised, having already become accustomed to passing over my share in the common repast. But joy does not last long in the house of the poor. In spite of my caution, my escapes were discovered and I was severely castigated and, besides, obliged to suffer the disgrace of being dressed in the *rey de gallos.*

I was decked out with a grotesque robe and crowned with an enormous mitre decorated with many-coloured feathers. I looked like a wild Indian. My cynical tranquility at being paraded among my comrades exasperated Father Jacinto, who added for good measure some blows with the fist and slaps on the neck. I looked at him with calm indignation without blinking an eyelid. My animosity or, if you prefer it, my outraged dignity would not let me cry. What better vengeance could I take against my oppressors?

In the days which followed, the lock was changed and watch was kept in such a manner that all my expedients were frustrated.

I remember that one Thursday the worthy friars forgot to free me at night, and so I had to pass the night in the school room stretched out on a bench, shivering with cold, without eating or drinking for thirty-two hours. On the following day, when the class was over, they let me go to dinner, apologizing for the omission. It is useless to say how much I was angered by the negligence of my guardians.

I vowed that I would not risk such suffering again, and so during the hours of the next incarceration, I concentrated my attention upon devising a way of liberating myself from my daily starvation. The room in which I was shut up was on the first floor and had a narrow window opening, overlooking the garden of the college. Climbing up on the teacher's dais, I put my head out at the window and surveyed the topography of the garden, the height of the adobe-walls, and the position of the trees. This rapid examination suggested to me a plan, daring and dangerous but feasible, which I determined to put into practice the next day. It consisted of making in the wall below the window a sort of stair of spikes and crevices which would permit me to descend to the top of an arbor constructed against the wall. To carry out my enterprise, I scaled the garden wall by moonlight, and, creeping along the paths, reached the foot of my prison wall, climbed quickly to the top of the arbor, and mounted on its solid framework, scraped away the mortar between the bricks in two or three places, driving in two short stakes at different heights for greater safety. My plan worked out as desired.

The next day, while the Esculapians were dining in the refectory, I slipped out by inserting my toes in the crevices and resting on the stakes in the wall, reached the garden, crossed to a courtyard communicating with it, and was finally able to renew triumphantly the healthful custom of eating at home, to the great surprise of my uncle, who, having very bad reports about me, wondered greatly at such sudden reformation. To obviate suspicion, as soon as I had had my dinner, and before my teachers had finished their table chat, I returned to my prison, where they found me in the afternoon placid and resigned.

A good many days passed thus without mishap. I was very proud of the scheme, by virtue of which I had regularized my gastronomic arrangements. But the devil, who confounds everything, brought it to pass that some of my comrades, who were just about as bad as I, and who were also condemned to imprisonment from time to time, learned of my method of evasion and proposed to take advantage of it, without studying thoroughly the lay-out of the garden and the details of the wall. Against my advice, they would not wait for the proper time to escape, got into difficulties in the negotiation of the stakes in the wall and, caught in the act just as they reached the courtyard, were severely flogged and confessed their transgression and the way in which it was carried out. Moreover, the ingrates denounced the originator of the scheme.

The indignation of the friars against me was extreme; they talked of expelling me and of forming a disciplinary court to deal with me. I was in consternation at the thought of their dreadful retaliation. Finally, I stopped going to school and wrote to my father an account of what had happened.

It is impossible to describe the displeasure of my father upon hearing of my neglect of my work and the bad opinion which my preceptors had of me. He was tempted to abandon me to the mercies of the masters if they would consent to take me back into the college. However, his paternal sensibilities prevailed and he wrote to the Esculapians requesting them to mitigate their harshness with me, as my health was seriously weakened by the system of daily fasts and excessive chastisements.

To the moral effect of the letter was added the personal appeal of my uncle who enjoyed the friendship of the dominies. These requests made some impression; at least my incarcerations ceased. In my abdomen the bells rang out in thanksgiving. Thus, during the last part of the term, I had the pleasure of eating like other people, although such an unaccustomed habit surprised my stomach, as it was now resigned to dealing with large amounts at long intervals, like the gizzard of a vulture.

After the foregoing, the fatal dénouement was certain. Failure in examination appeared unavoidable. But to ward off that blow, if possible, my father sought introductions to the professors of the Institute at Huesca, upon whom rested the responsibility of conducting the examinations at Jaca. Just at the time, one of these gentlemen was Don Vicente Ventura, who was a great friend of his. This savior of mine was indebted to the surgical skill of Don Justo for having cured his wife of a very serious illness which required a dangerous operation.

When the examination arrived, the friars, as was to be expected, proposed my rejection; but the teachers from Huesca, relying upon a just judgment and remembering that pupils as lazy as, or worse than I—though somewhat more docile—had been passed, procured my pardon.

CHAPTER X

My return to Ayerbe. New warlike exploits. The wooden cannon. Three days in prison. The symbolic musket.

When I returned to Ayerbe for the ensuing vacation, my poor mother hardly knew me, so much had I been reduced by the reign of terror and the dietetic restriction. Of me it could have been truly said, as Quevedo states in his *Gran Tacano*[1] of the pupils of the dominie Cabre: dried up, wiry, with angular face and sunken eyes, shanks long and knotted, nose and chin sharp pointed, I seemed to be in the last stage of consumption. Thanks to the solicitous care of my mother, the open-air life, and the nutritious food, I soon recovered my strength. And feeling myself once more cheerful and robust, I returned to take part in the skirmishes and battles of the lads of Ayerbe.

That summer my favourite amusements were martial, particularly contests with slings and arrows, and boxing. Soon, however, I found these dull and childish. I craved greater exploits; I aspired to the shotgun and the cannon. And I proposed to manufacture these by hook or by crook. To carry out the difficult undertaking, I took possession of a piece of a beam left over from some construction work at my home, and with the help of a large carpenter's auger, and by dint of labor and patience, I bored a tube in the center of the log, smoothing it afterwards as thoroughly as I could with a sort of ramrod wrapped in sandpaper. To increase the strength of the cannon, I reinforced it outside with wire and tarred cord; and, in order to prevent the priming-hole from being enlarged when the powder was ignited and the charge coming out through it, I reinforced it with a close fitting tube of tin from an old oil can.

[1] Usually called "El Buscon" (the Great Rascal), sometimes "Don Pablo." One chapter contains a bitter caricature of boarding school life. (Translator's note.)

I was very proud and satisfied with my cannon, which my friends praised extravagantly. We were all consumed with eagerness to try it out. It was my intention to add wheels to it before the official test, but my play-mates would not consent, so lively was their impatience to load it and see its formidable effects.

After mature deliberation we decided to hoist the cannon on to the wall of my orchard and try it upon the brand-new gate of a neighboring garden, which opened upon a narrow lane with high walls at each side that was little frequented.

The home-made piece of artillery was carefully loaded, a large handful of powder being put in first, followed by a stout wad, and the bore finally being filled with tacks and cobble stones. In the priming hole, which was also filled with powder, was inserted a large fuse of touchwood. The moments passed in excited and anxious expectation. The fuse was lighted by means of a match on the end of a wire, after which we all withdrew with beating hearts to await the terrible explosion at a safe distance.

The report was terrific and deafening, but, contrary to the prognostications of the pessimists, the cannon did not blow up; instead, it performed its impressive function honorably and dutifully. A broad gap opened in the new gate, through which there appeared shortly afterwards the wrathful and menacing head of the gardener, showed us the material and moral effects of the discharge, which, as the reader will guess, was not repeated that day. It must be confessed that we took to our heels, abandoning in our flight the instrument of the crime. It was a great piece of good luck that the gate was so smashed up and obstructed by the shower of splinters that it would not open at once, despite the furious jerks of the enraged owner of the garden. Thanks to this fortunate circumstance, we had a great advantage over him in our flight, although not sufficient to prevent us from being hit on the legs by some stones hurled by the infuriated man.

My prank had disagreeable consequences for me in any

case. The worthy peasant complained bitterly to the mayor, to whom he showed the evidence of guilt, in other words the ponderous timber with which the exploit had been carried out. The petty official, who had already complaints of other damage which I had done, took advantage of the occasion presented to teach me an unforgettable lesson and, coming to my house with the constable, consigned me to the local jail. This took place with the sanction of my father, who considered that my imprisonment would be a good and efficacious treatment for my correction; he even went so far as to order that I should be deprived of food throughout the duration of my confinement.

I protested on the way against the many slanderous rumors about me which were current. Almost all the offences which were attributed to me had been committed by other scamps. I did not deny the damage done to the gate, but excused myself by declaring that I had never dreamt of producing such great destruction; and finally I urged the injustice which resulted from the procedure of punishing me alone for faults committed by several playmates.

My excuses, however, were of no avail and the sentence of the municipal authority was executed at once. As I heard the creaking of the bolt which locked me away for I knew not how long and the indistinct sound of the receding footsteps of my jailer, I lost my serenity. I understood at last that my imprisonment was a real sentence. I was soon aroused from my stupor by the footsteps of people approaching the prison; and at once a swarm of children and women crowded round the bottom of the grating to look and laugh at the prisoner. This I could not endure and, emerging from my apathy, I laid hold of a rough piece of stone and threatened to crack the crowns of all who came up to the grating.

I knew then, at that early age (eleven years), how exact are those well-known expressions in which Cervantes characterizes the annoyances which embitter the existence of him who lies in prison; there, in fact, "every discomfort has its seat and every outcry of misery its natural habitation."

Once I was free of the ridicule of the curious, it seemed to me desirable to explore the stinking enclosure. After assuring myself of the solidity of the door and of the impossibility of forcing the bolts, I noted with disgust that my couch was no more than a pallet of mouldy straw where grew and flourished an overflowing flora and fauna. This effervescence of hungry life filled my mind with dread; for there the *Aspergillus niger* spread its dusky carpets and the jumping flea, the night walking bed-bug, the vile louse, and even the insignificant cockroach—the plague of kitchens and bakeshops—walked about freely or made themselves at home. All these table companions, which had been waiting for months for the ever-postponed feast, seemed to tremble with delight at scenting the new prey. Considering that it would be too foolish to nourish with my skin such ravenous parasites, when night came I stretched myself on the hard flagstones in a relatively clean place.

Although my tranquility may be surprising, I will confess that I slept somewhat, in spite of the tickling sensation in my empty stomach and the gloomy thoughts which passed through my mind.

Three or four days passed in this way. The matter of starvation, however, was only a threat, not because my father repented of the hard sentence which he had delivered, but because of the commiseration of a certain kind lady of our acquaintance, Doña Bernardina de Normante, who, with the connivance of my mother, doubtless, broke the severe order, sending me from the day following my imprisonment excellent viands and delicious fruits. The shame of my situation was not such as to make me disregard the generous solicitude of Doña Bernardina; the chops, pies, biscuits,[2] and cakes were to me like a taste of heaven. However sincere was the remorse which I felt, the Lord knows it did not deprive me of my appetite.

[2] *Sequillos* and *coscaranas*, kinds of spice cakes made in Ayerbe and other towns of upper Aragon.

The patient reader will be entirely mistaken if he assumes that this misfortune would make me hate firearms; on the contrary it farther excited my interest in ballistics. The sole effect of the chastisement was to make me more cautious in my later misdeeds. Another cannon was constructed, which we discharged against the side of a hill, but this time, the firearm, which was loaded to the mouth, was blown to pieces, filling the air with splinters. We were incorrigible.

Finally, if I did not fear to weary the reader altogether, I should like to tell the details of an accident from which we were saved miraculously. For this new experiment a large bronze pipe was used, loaded to the mouth. But, instead of the charge coming out at the mouth, the cannon exploded into a thousand pieces and, in spite of the precautions we had taken, both my brother and I were hurt slightly. I do not know how it is that I did not lose my sight, since a particle of metal entered one of my eyes, produced a serious inflammation and left a permanent scar in the iris. Not even this mischance cooled my love for gunpowder, only, in place of using wooden cannons, we found a way to get real muskets.

Our greatest delight was to go out into the country armed with a certain musket, which we fired at the birds and, when there were none of them, at stones and tree trunks. Naturally my father kept locked up the splendid gun which he used for hunting, as well as his ammunition; but our industry supplied everything. We procured the coveted arm in this way.

We were passing through a period of political repression, a suspicious and jealous government which saw conspirators everywhere persecuted and imprisoned all who were reported to be liberals or were suspected of being in touch with the exiled generals. The collection of weapons and requisition of horses were frequent proceedings.

My father, having been severely punished by the high-handed seizure of a certain very fine musket which he had innocently surrendered to the police, procured a huge dirty gun which was supposed to have a flint lock but was unprovided with a flint carrier and was consequently useless. Such was the weapon which my father kept for the requisitions. I need not say how faithfully the inoffensive musket was always returned to him when the troubles were past.

This was the firearm which my brother and I proposed to use in our hunting expeditions. We provided it with a kind of key of brass as a holder for tinder, adjusted the pan, cleaned the barrel and the priming hole, manufactured the necessary powder, made bullets and bird-shot with pieces of lead, and, when all our preparations were complete, set out for the haunt of birds, partridges, and rabbits.

We were very proud with our ancient carbine, which we would not have exchanged for the best shotgun in the world; we imagined besides, in our childish innocence, that that formidable weapon gave us a terrifying aspect. I remember that once, in the outskirts, an overgrown fellow threatened me with a small carbine but I, far from being overawed, covered him with my imposing blunderbuss. The effect was instantaneous. At the sight of the wide mouth of the firearm, threatening to pour forth a cloud of grape-shot, our brave man beat a prudent retreat. If my antagonist had fired, I should have been in great difficulty to reply.

Nothing could have been more comical than our appearance when we climbed down from the wall of the orchard harnessed to our terrifically heavy gun and set out upon the road in search of adventure.

Whenever we caught sight of a bird, we made a halt; I lighted the fuse, aimed the unwieldy weapon at the bird, and gravely pulled the trigger,—that is to say the lower part of the fuse holder. Then there began in the pan a spluttering of wet powder and, finally, after the passage of half a minute or more and when the bird had already flown away, the terrific report was produced which filled us with delight and pride. Beautiful simplicity of childhood! How happy we felt with that huge, inoffensive musket!

We never killed anything and yet we placed in it the highest hopes and the most fervid enthusiasm. It is true that in adult life almost the same thing happens.

At the bottom of my interest in firearms, there existed, besides the desire for excitement, a sincere and lively admiration for science and an insatiable curiosity regarding the forces of nature. The mysterious energy concealed in the gunpowder caused me an indefinable surprise. Every discharge of a skyrocket, every report of a firearm was for me a stupendous miracle. Lacking money to buy gunpowder, I sought to find out how to make it and finally by experiments I succeeded in the attempt. I used to procure the sulphur in the shop, the saltpeter in the cellar of the house, the charcoal in charred soft wood. Having prepared the mixture, I sifted it with the greatest care and dried it in the sun; except once when, becoming impatient of the excessive humidity of the atmosphere, I placed the earthen pot with the ingredients in a water-bath and the devil decreed that a spark should catch in the powder, which was not yet quite dry, and produce a great flame. Fortunately all these operations of alchemy were carried out on the roof of the house to avoid indiscretions. If they had been performed inside, heaven knows what might have happened!

CHAPTER XI

My father arranges to send me to Huesca to continue my studies. Exploration of the city. The cathedral, San Pedro, San Jorge, and Mount Aragon. Our instructors.

It was in January or February, 1864, that my father, undeceived regarding the teaching methods of the friars, resolved finally to transfer my further education to the Institute of Huesca, changing his plans since he concluded—probably with good reason—that his son would never master Latin now that he had been removed from the Esculapians.

Goethe remarks very fittingly that every father desires for his children that which he himself has not been privileged to attain. Mine, who had not had the opportunity in his youth to study the language of Latium, desired very keenly that his first born should develop into a great Latin scholar and an accomplished humanist. Such aspirations were in contradiction to his severely utilitarian principles only in appearance. Wide experience of life had taught him that the social prestige of the physician proceeds more from his courtesy, from the distinction of his manners, and above all from his general culture, than from his science. It would have been a strange coincidence if those whose talents had been nurtured upon the classics had not almost always been very eminent writers and orators, and sometimes philosophers and scientists of the first order.

Yielding then, as I have said, to my desires, my progenitor arranged for my transfer to Huesca. Soon afterwards, he accompanied me to the ancient capital of the kingdom of Aragon, where he installed me in a modest boarding house, a quiet and peaceful place which was a regular lodging and stopping place for priests and seminarists. It was situated near the cathedral in the so-called *arco del Obispo* (bishop's arch), and was conducted by a widow of very religious character and excellent disposition.

I soon got to know my schoolfellows, among whom I found warm friends. The most important of these was the son of the mistress of the house, a fine boy, who was pursuing proficiently an ecclesiastical training, and Don Leandro Castro, a native of Ayerbe, who had been refused the priesthood but was intelligent and a competent Latin scholar. To the latter, who was a great friend of ours, my father confided the task of giving me daily lessons, initiating me into the mysteries of translation, and told him not to let me out of his hands until I should have mastered the difficulties of the concise and expressive language of Horace and Virgil.

It is needless to say with how much pleasure and satisfaction I made my entry into the famous and very ancient *Osca* (Huesca), celebrated on account of the deeds of Sertorio. My delight was due largely to the enthusiastic descriptions which some students from Ayerbe gave me of the institute and of the city. From them I learned that the teachers of Latin did not spend their time beating their pupils, even if they made the grossest errors, and that the surroundings of the city were supremely picturesque and suitable for delightful rambles. I took great pleasure in confirming personally the enthusiastic accounts of my companions. Considering my tastes, it was natural that my first visits should be to the famous thrashing-floors of Cascaro, the town common, and the customary scene of games, contests, and fights of the students; to the leafy woodland paths and groves of the Isuela, a paradise of butterflies and songbirds, among which shone the dainty golden oriole; and, finally, to the ancient and decayed walls of the city, the usual theater of warlike escapades of scamps and students.

When my father had returned home and I remained absolute master of my actions and of a few reals,[1] my first

[1] A real is twenty-five centimos or about five cents of American money at par. There is now no such coin, but the word is still much used, especially in reckoning small sums of money. (Translator's note.)

care was to buy paper and a box of paints in order to translate in water colours my latest artistic impressions.

At twelve years of age, to be suddenly plunged into city life is a revolutionary lesson about the world and a ferment which generates many new ideas. Everything is different, both qualitatively and quantitatively, in the village and in the city; the streets become wider and cleaner; the houses are higher and more decorative; the shops are more specialized, tempting the ingenuous villager and the sweet-toothed stripling with fascinating trifles; the sober romanesque churches are transformed into sumptuous cathedrals; and finally, for the first time, book shops appear. With these last, a broad window is opened upon the universe. The new and varied spectacle enriches at the same time the sensibilities and the understanding. To the types of the peasant, the priest, and the schoolmaster—the only forms of humanity to be seen in the village—are now added an infinitude of kinds and varieties of professions, previously unknown. In fact, the boy's intellectual horizon expands through space because of the multitude of new facts which come to his attention, and through time because every city constitutes, as is well known, a repository of historical monuments. For if the village is the shell in which is dormant the protoplasm of the race, only in the city dwells the spirit.

Before the foaming torrent of new impressions, the youth has to bring into action regions of his brain which hitherto lay fallow. A significant indication of the great mental crisis, of this functional struggle between old and new ideas which is stirred up in the mind, is the bewilderment which seizes us during the first days of exploring a city. In the end, order is established. The plastic adaptation once completed, the cerebral organization is enriched and refined; one knows more and one's judgment is improved accordingly. From this it is evident that there is much truth in the claim that a man's intellectual capacity is related to the size of the city in which he passed his childhood and his adolescence. The vigor of the plant depends in large degree upon the size of the flower pot.

At that time I was very far from reflecting in such a manner. My over-excited sensibilities led me on irresistibly to investigate things rather than people. Guided by my natural inclinations to the romantic, I began my explorations with the monuments of the ancient city, in the study of which I was much aided by the beautiful work of Quedrado, "Recuerdos y Bellezas de España," a folio which was in the library of the Institute, and of which the delightful descriptions and artistic lithographs captivated me.

Without attaining the sovereign majesty of the Gothic temples of Burgos, Salamanca, Leon and Toledo, the cathedral of Huesca is an admirable creation of the art of the pointed arch, worthy of attention of the artist. The lofty clock tower which flanks the beautiful façade carved in the fourteenth century by the Biscayan, Juan de Olózaga; the majestic Gothic doorway, decorated with seven arches of decreasing size, ornamented with sculptures of apostles, prophets and martyrs, and separated by florid canopies and pedestals, the triangular pediment adorned with a huge rose-window like filigree in stone; the unusual height of the central nave and of the transept; the bold grace of the columns, of which the capitals break up, towards the vault, into ribs capriciously interlaced; the arabesques and exquisite fretwork of the capitals and rosettes; and above all the unsurpassable creation of the sculptor Forment, the marvellous altar-piece of alabaster, which one might think the delicate embroidery wrought by fairies, filled me with simple and profound admiration.

Very different was the impression produced upon me when I visited the church of San Pedro el viejo (Old St. Peter's), the oldest, probably, of all the churches in Huesca. According to tradition, it served as a chapel for the Mozárabes [2] during the sad times of the Mussulman conquest. This very ancient building is in the byzantine

[2] The Mozárabes were the Christian Moors. (Translator's note.)

style, with little ornamentation and low vaulting, but firm and rugged as the faith of its founders. Not without a certain religious awe did I venture into its gloomy and mysterious cloisters, impaired by dampness and half buried in rubbish. By the dim light of a lamp I gazed upon the tombs where rulers and princes of Aragon sleep their eternal sleep, among them the monk-king, the sombre protagonist of the legend of the famous bell.[3]

There, in the midst of those soul-stirring ruins, as I considered the effacement of the inscriptions, the erosion and crumbling away of the marble tablets, my heart was wounded, perhaps for the first time, by the desolating thought of the transience and vanity of all pomp and greatness. There I discovered at close range that perpetual conflict between the spirit which aspires to eternity and the blind and destructive force of natural agencies.

After the examination of the most important monuments, came the exploration of other structures rich in historical associations: the ancient walls, rotting with the dampness and overgrown with grass, nettles, and wild figs, and from the bastions of which, still partly preserved, tradition has it that the Mohammedan arrow sped to wound Sancho Ramírez[4] mortally as he besieged the city; the castle of the ancient kings of Aragon, converted into a university by Pedro IV and now transformed into the provincial institute, and in the gloomy cellars of which is still preserved the famous bell where, according to the legend, the monk-king ordered the execution of the Levantine nobles of Aragon; the Casas Consistoriales, crowned with lofty towers, in the halls of which the Chief Justice of the city used to pronounce his judgments; the romanesque church

[3] Ramiro II, King of Aragon, 1134–1154. The legend of the bell relates that in 1136 he called together the disaffected nobles to witness the casting of a bell which would be heard throughout the kingdom. They were taken singly into the small vaulted chamber which is still shown, and beheaded, their heads were arranged in a ring on the floor, and the head of the prelate Ordás was hung in the center as the clapper of the "bell." (Translator's note.)

[4] 1045–1094. King of Aragon and Navarre, father of the monk-king. (Translator's note.)

PLATE 7

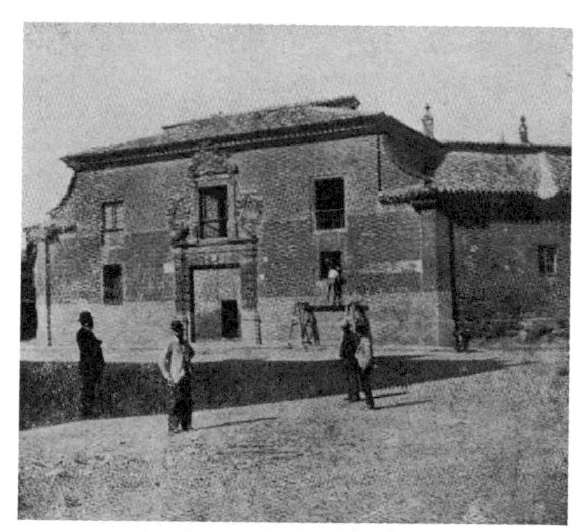

FIG. 12. FACADE OF THE INSTITUTE AT HUESCA.

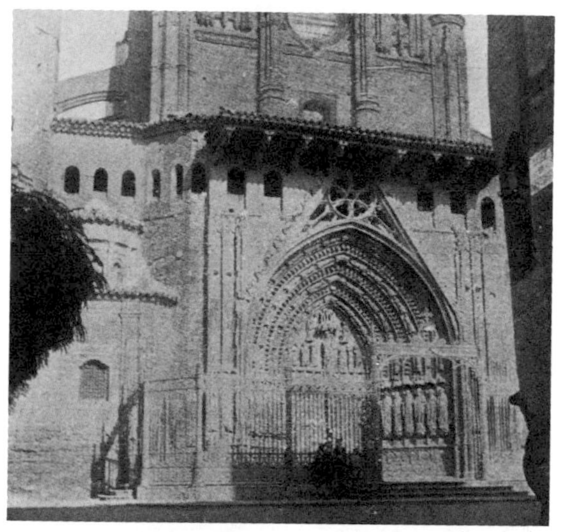

FIG. 13. THE MAIN DOORWAY OF THE CATHEDRAL AT HUESCA.

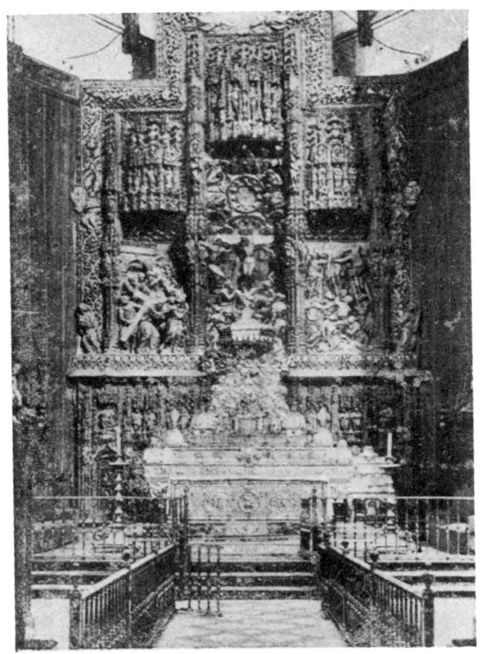

Fig. 14. The High Altar of the Cathedral at Huesca, carved in alabaster by Forment.

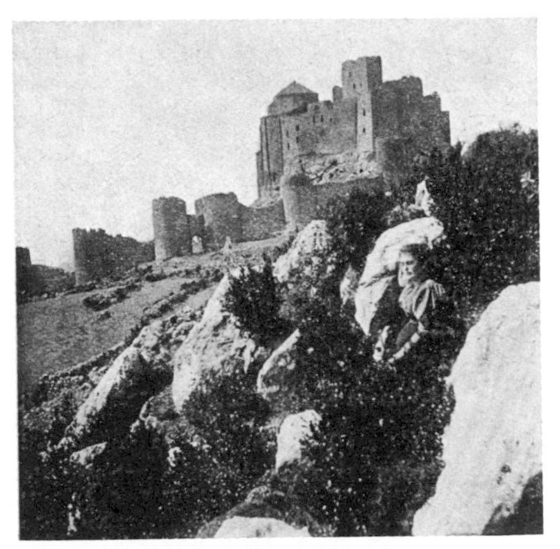

Fig. 15. The Castle of Loarre, the objective of my rambles and archaeological researches in my adolescence. In my romantic fever I delighted in contemplating the ruins of the fortress-palace of Sancho Ramírez, one of the most interesting monuments in Upper Aragón.

of San Miguel, which rises on the right bank of the Isuela, and in the porch of which, in not very distant times, the jurors dispensed justice; the historic hermitage of San Jorge, founded on the battlefields of Alcaraz in memory of the triumph of the Christians over the Mohammedans; the grandiose baroque church of San Lorenzo, erected in honor of the holy martyrs; the little sanctuary of Cillas, situated not far from the Fountain of Health, the favorite gossiping-place of the Huescans; and, finally, the imposing castle of Mount Aragon, an outpost and bulwark against the hosts of the Moors erected in the early years of the reconquest, and of which the ruddy and ruined walls, pierced by great windows, seem to preserve to this day the heat of the terrible conflagration which razed the proud structure to the ground.

But now that I have disposed of these common historical notes and reminiscences, it is time that I spoke of my teachers and companions.

Don Antonio Aquilué, the Latin master, was the complete antithesis of the terrible Father Jacinto. Hard-working, but very old, kindly, and almost blind, he lacked the firmness necessary to control those little twelve-year-old devils. In his class the boys used to run riot, scribbled, read novels and doggerel, smoked, threw paper pellets, played cards—in fact did everything except pay attention to the learned and deliberate lecture of the master, who had to shout to make himself heard in the midst of the uproar.

A detailed account of the pranks carried out there would be an endless story and, besides, a repetition of things already well known. For example, I may mention the disagreeable joke of a certain pupil who opened in class a box full of mice, the terrified flight of which spread disorder through the schoolroom. At a propitious moment, birds and even bats, liberated by unseen hands, sped through the air. At other times, we turned our attention to the spectacles or the hat of the dominie, which, guided by a thread in the hand of some young scamp, gently left the platform, seeming to acquiesce, following the caprice of the shameless pupil, in the arguments of the teacher. Projected by rubber bands, pellets of paper flew towards the platform, often hitting the venerable old man on the cap or on his bald head, so that more than once, angry and indignant at such disrespect and impudence, he turned us out furiously into the street.

I was far from being guiltless, but I was not one of the boldest and most insolent. A certain noble pity for the good old man, who was full of kindness and simplicity, restrained my malevolent impulses. Nevertheless, I was obliged more than once, in company with more impudent companions, to expiate our common misdemeanors in a certain school prison, a kind of stable arranged long since for the incarceration during twenty-four hours of the more perverse rebels. When this happened, far from wearying me, the prison permitted me to give joyful vent to my pictorial craze, drawing on the walls with chalk and charcoal pitched battles between beadles and schoolboys, in which the former, as the reader will suppose, always had the worst of it.

Forming a marked and significant contrast, nobody so much as whispered in the class of the teacher of geography. The latter was a blonde young man of strong physique, with acute senses, grave and serious in his words, and very severe and just in examination. He inspired us with respect and fear. The pupil who disturbed or amused himself by chattering to his neighbours was immediately ejected from the schoolroom. We were restrained by the knowledge that failures of attention or respect were carefully recorded and that they often cost failure in examination. He made his explanations simply, clearly, and methodically and was successful in interesting us in his lessons.

Although I had come well prepared by the paternal instruction, I profited greatly by the explanations of geography, and in this I was greatly assisted by my ability in drawing, since the teacher, an excellent pedagogue, made us copy islands and continents, rivers, lakes, and mountain ranges from the atlas which was prescribed as text-book.

In this way our attention was stimulated and the mental images of the objects were strengthened. This method of teaching appealed to me so much and I made such progress that I would cover a paper with the map of Europe in a moment, tracing the boundaries of many countries with their provinces from memory, without going astray even in the complicated geography of the German confederation or in the difficult outlines of the Spanish-American republics.

The contrasting behaviour of the scholars in the two classes mentioned showed me two facts, which later observations have confirmed fully. The first is that the instructor of pupils of from ten to fourteen years old must necessarily be young, energetic, and with keen senses; old men, however learned they may be, are the pitiful victims of the insolence and lack of consideration of lads for whom quietness and self-restraint are real torture. The second is that children who are too young show little inclination—with notable exceptions—for the study of languages and mathematics. Only the fear of punishment can make rascals who are still in the muscular and sensory period of life endure steadfastly long strings of irregular Latin verbs and endless lists of binomials and polynomials. All this eventually becomes interesting, but only later on, after the fourteenth or fifteenth year.

Experience confirms the view that, except in cases of unusual precocity, the boy recently entered upon his secondary education enjoys studying only those subjects which are capable of enlarging his rudimentary objective experience of the world, which he commenced at home—subjects such as cosmography, geography, and elementary arithmetic, physics, and natural history. Why do not teachers and organizers of educational systems take this fact into account? The dead languages, grammar, psychology, logic, algebra, trigonometry, and physics with difficult formulae should be reserved for the later courses, that is to say, for the period between the fourteenth and the seventeenth years, which is the time when the reflective phase of mental development really begins.

To this pedagogical error, which is sanctioned by the law, are added furthermore the serious defects of the dry and excessively abstract manner in which the subjects are commonly presented. Too much concerned with the logical precision of definitions and corollaries, the master often forgets a most important point, namely, to excite the curiosity of the budding minds, gaining at the same time for his didactic task the intellect and the interest of the pupil; but concerning this matter, which is of the utmost importance in education, I shall say more later on.

CHAPTER XII

My new playmates. Student quarrels. Serious consequences of wearing a long overcoat. Accident in a pond. The fascination of colour and the chromatic dictionary. No rose without a thorn.

In spite of the best intentions, my artistic tendencies, as well as the urge for incessant activity and dramatic excitement, rose with a crescendo, since I found in Huesca many companions who shared my tastes and were ready to join in the most preposterous mischief. Dreamy sentimentality and a proud, punctilious character which did not readily brook insults or humiliations, were the cause of several mischances, and even of real dangers, from which only my robust constitution was able to save me.

I shall pass over most of the unfortunate episodes of that year, otherwise my narrative would be interminable. In order not to try the reader's patience too much, and to adhere to the plan adopted, I shall confine myself to relating some of the events and incidents which remained most deeply engraved upon my memory.

Fortunately, initiations were not customary at the Institute of Huesca, but instead there was something as deplorable as they are; namely, the irritating abuse of strength against the weak, with bullying which regulated the games and the mutual relations of the boys. Every recent arrival who displeased the coxcombs of the upper years, whether by his appearance, by his attire, or by his character, found himself obliged, if he would escape persecution, either to remain prudently indoors during the hours of play or to solicit the protection of some big fellow who could stand up against the insolent bullies.

I had the misfortune to appear unpleasing to the aforesaid braves, so that, for no particular reason, they maltreated me by word and deed from my first appearance in the courtyards of the Institute, forcing me to take part in rows and disputes, from which I nearly always emerged in bad condition. Among those who most abused their strength with me, I recall a fellow called Azcón, a native of Alcalá de Gállego, a chronic loafer, whose studies had been interrupted several times in consequence. He was eighteen or nineteen years old, and his square and robust figure, his coarse red neck, and his vigorous brown arms betrayed at a glance the rustic who had hardened his muscles by guiding the plough and wielding the spade.

This savage recognized at once the weakness in my character and, always ready to cast slurs and in any way amuse himself at my expense, whenever he met me about the Institute he loaded me with insults. Among other epithets which I, in my simplicity, deemed mortifying, he applied to me those of Dago and Goatflesh. (The latter term was at that time applied in ridicule to everyone from Ayerbe.)

The term Dago requires explanation. My good mother, extraordinarily frugal and economical, made for me a roomy winter overcoat from the cloth of an old great-coat of my father's. The unfortunate part was that, considering my rapid growth and foreseeing a continuation thereof, she left the skirts of the coat considerably longer than was fashionable at the time. It must be acknowledged that my appearance was somewhat reminiscent of that of the strolling Savoyards who at that time used to wander about the Peninsula playing the harp or making bears or monkeys dance to the sound of the drum.

Among those young gentlemen, dressed in *le dernier cri*, the sudden apparition of my strange overcoat produced delighted amazement. One harsh and dominating voice—that of the above-mentioned Azcón—put into words the vague idea which welled up in that chorus of wags—"Look at the Dago."

"That is what he is," repeated his laughing cronies.

"He only needs the harp," cried one. "Where has he left his monkey?" exclaimed another.

The crescendo of jokes and jests would have gone on if anger and desperation, which I had with difficulty restrained hitherto, had not impelled me to fight for what I considered my outraged dignity. Without a word of response, I sprang like a tiger upon Azcón and his insolent friends, dealing blows and kicks on all sides.

A wiser and less hot-headed lad would have adopted the procedure, which is best in such cases, of saying nothing or taking it all as a joke. In this case the epithet would soon have been forgotten; but I, who was unacquainted with the well-known counsel, "be the first to laugh at your own defects, if you would not have them flung in your face," took the matter very seriously. The result was that, once they had recovered from their surprise, those whom I had attacked retaliated with interest, and gave me a never-to-be-forgotten beating. Thoroughly did they revenge themselves! For not only did they pound me with kicks, but flinging me to the ground, they rolled on my back, crushing me for a long time, until I was in danger of suffocation. When they were tired of thrashing me, I picked myself up as well as I could, collected the remains of my books, cleaned myself, and went home, aching all over, limping, and vowing vengeance.

The reader will probably expect that after such an impressive lesson my bile would remain pacified, taking up thenceforth an attitude of submission and meekness. Quite the contrary. A few days afterwards, upon leaving the classroom, I came upon the same group of wags who, taking advantage of the presence of Azcón, hurled the hated nickname in my face in cowardly fashion. Seized with blind fury, I boldly attacked the insolent fellows, who closed in upon me with the same deplorable results as in the previous case. And this went on for two or three months. My chums did not know which to be most surprised at, the cruelty of Azcón and his followers or the persistence and impetuosity with which I responded to their abuse. How often, as I returned home sad and depressed, with my hat dented, my chest heaving with excitement, and my eyes red and damp with passion and hatred, I said to myself philosophically "And to think that all this happens to me on account of a few inches of cloth which could have been cut off in the first place!"

In making this sad reflection I was entirely mistaken. What happened to me occurred also, although in a less degree—thanks to their prudence—to other beginners in the lower years, although they were dressed in the latest fashion. A pretext was never lacking, only there were combined in me two features which sooner or later would have attracted to me the animosity of those savages: the well earned fame for boldness and daring which I had brought from Ayerbe, the home of madcaps and a regular hotbed of bullies, and the indignation which injustice and the abuse of strength had always produced in me.

All these boyish conflicts, which to many will appear mere childishness, have a decisive importance not only for the formation of character but even for later conduct in adult life. The most proper and peaceable student, obliged to suffer such iniquitous attacks, ends in adopting according to his temperament one of three attitudes; either fauning and flattery towards his persecutors, the invocation of superior authority, or the most violent use of the muscles accompanied by cunning. The last was the method chosen by me. The two former I considered dishonorable. "In order to keep the strong at bay," I thought, "it is necessary to surpass them, or at least to equal them in vigour."

But how was I to attain this superiority and especially to attain it quickly? My insolent enemies admittedly were older than I, and besides they were many and I was one. Bah! I said to myself, if I can only beat Azcón all the rest will become my allies. And that is exactly what happened.

Fortunately, I knew well the highly strengthening effects of gymnastics and of obligatory work. I had observed how great an advantage in contests, fights, races, and jumping, had the strong and swarthy boys who had recently arrived from the villages and were accustomed to the weight of the spade compared with the tall, pale, young gentlemen with narrow chests and long slender shanks brought up in the sheltered city streets and in the gentle warmth of their mothers' laps.

Consequently, I resolved to engage in systematic physical exercises, to which end I spent hours and hours alone in the groves and thickets of the Isuela, climbing trees, jumping over ditches, lifting heavy stones by hand, and performing, in fact, all the actions which I believed would tend to hasten my muscular development, raising it to the greatest strength possible at my age. I hoped that by the end of a few months, or at any rate by the next scholastic year, things would change radically and that even the proudest bullies would have to treat me with respect. This consoling hope, thought illusory at first sight, was largely realized in the succeeding sessions.

As the reader will see further on, persistent gymnastics and exasperated self-love performed miracles. With all my serious defects, I was always ready to learn by experience, which, in connection with this and other similar cases, is summed up in the common maxim "If you wish to triumph in difficult undertakings, put into them your whole will, preparing yourself with more time and work than are obviously necessary." In the long run, surplus strength is never a loss but rather finds an adequate use in other ways, while an insufficiency, even if very slight, exposes one to distressing failures.

The results of my physical training were splendid. From the third year, my ability with my fists and my skill in the use of the sling and the cudgel inspired respect in the bullies of the upper years, and even the athletic Azcón had to capitulate and finally made friends with me. The fact of the matter is that I had informed him that whenever he was insolent towards me, I should imbed a stone in his skull. And my threat did not sound to him like an idle boast because he observed my prowess with the sling every day and so was convinced that I was capable of making good my promise. Needless to say, my humiliating nickname was forgotten.

An event of a very different nature from those described taught me a bitter lesson about the selfishness of children and the fear of the police which seems to be inborn in Spaniards.

One January day, I was playing with a group of friends, romping and skating on a mill pond. It was freezing quite hard and the ice on the pool was thick enough to support our weight quite safely. A little distance from the shore, some young rascals amused themselves by hurling large stones at the ice until they broke a great hole, through which the water came up, its dark green colour suggesting its considerable depth. Confident in my agility, and tempted by the devil, I suggested to my companions that we jump over the broad opening and, to lead them on, I took the first leap. My evil star decreed that, in one of my jumps, I should land on a loose piece of ice and, falling backwards, tumble right into the water. I was dreadfully frightened for, although I was able to swim, I found myself beneath the thick crust of ice and consequently, as I could not locate the opening, unable to breathe. Struggling frantically, I happened upon the hole, clutched the broken points along the edge, which broke off in my hands, and finally, with a supreme effort, managed to raise up my head and get a breath. Then I was horrified to see that my playmates, believing me certainly drowned, had fled. In that uncomfortable position, stiff and, as it were, paralyzed with cold, I could not scramble out without assistance; to do so would have required what in the jargon of gymnasts is called a *dominación doble;* and the bottom was too far down to be reached by my feet. By good luck, as I kicked and reached about in all directions, my foot came in contact with a stake which provided me with the desired support and at last I was able to draw my body from the water and free myself from the prospect of perishing miserably.

Soaked through, and pierced by the icy cold, I set out for home, but soon I noticed that the water in my trousers was beginning to solidify so much as to hinder walking. In fear of freezing, I undressed completely, wrang as much water as I could from my clothes, and spread them out to dry beside a property where I was sheltered from the bitter north wind. Meanwhile, coughing and shivering, I took refuge behind a barn, bathed in the rays of the setting sun, which had hardly enough warmth to dry my half-frozen skin. To warm myself, I started to run round and round in the adjacent ploughed land, continuing this for about an hour, by which time my shirt had dried somewhat. Soon afterwards (it would be about five o'clock in the afternoon) I finally dressed myself and ran home, changed my damp clothes, and was as well as ever.

The reader who has perused the preceding narrative will doubtless imagine that the polar adventure described would have serious consequences for my health, bringing about some of the many inflammations resulting from chills that are catalogued and described minutely in the books on pathology. Well, I did not even catch cold!

There is no unpleasant experience from which some useful lesson cannot be extracted; and I drew two maxims from my tremendous soaking, one physiological, the other psychological. First, whatever the pathologists may say, cold alone does not cause "colds" or pneumonia; and second, the feelings of philanthropy and compassion in young people are so fragile that they are destroyed by the risk of wetting the cuffs of a shirt or the danger of having to make a statement before a judge if anything serious should happen.

The need of developing my strength to repulse the continual aggressions of the boys had no tendency to make me forget the cultivation of the beautiful; rather my pictorial inclinations found food and encouragement in my new manner of living. Before what we might call the muscular period of my life, my artistic imaginings held man as their preferred subject. But now, as a result of my solitary walks through the groves and gardens of the Isuela, I began to admire the sovereign beauty of the vegetable kingdom and of the insects and to listen to the low and mysterious whispers of animal life in its everlasting rebirths.

It is a common truth that man copies what he loves, and in the world of life, as in that of the spirit, to love is to reproduce. He is lacking in sincere enthusiasm who does not eliminate common and antiesthetic images from his mind by an act of inhibition so as to make his favourite idea stand out clearly; that idea which is something his very own, since he has embellished it with the best of his sensibilities and his creative imagination.

In accordance with this psychological law, I painted whatever charmed my eyes. The pages of my sketch book were filled with drawings of rocks and trees, sprays of wild flowers, butterflies in showy liveries, and brooks gliding among pebbles, rushes, and white water lilies.

My drawings, nevertheless, were very far from satisfying me from the technical point of view. The form and the light and shade I was able to capture fairly easily, but the color eluded me. The chromatic crudity of my reproductions paralleled the lack of atmospheric perspective. I was oppressed above all by the inexhaustible richness of tints in the earth, masses of foliage, flowers, and human beings. Like the majority of inexperienced amateurs, I saw clearly the fundamental quality, but I was ignorant of the difficult use of gray and did not know that nature seldom presents an absolutely pure colour. It is well known that in the chromatic effect of a landscape, as in auditory sensation, there are only varied harmonies; with the color there are always mingled white and black, in varying proportions, somewhat as silence and noise are mingled in auditory perception.

Such deficiencies of perception are inevitable in the child. He simplifies and schematizes the colour unconsciously. After the manner of the musical performer playing by ear, who reproduces only the melody and is oblivious of the harmony, so the embryo painter copies exclusively the dominant colour tone. Who does not remember the atrocious colouring of beginners at sketching? And when visiting an exhibition of pictures, who does not detect at the first glance, by the loudness of its colouring, the unfortunate product of the unskilled painter or the dissident modernist, who from snobbery pays homage to the "loud" school, slipping back unwittingly to the infantile phase of art?

In my experience, I fell into all these deplorable errors. Nevertheless, I improved in the course of my efforts, and finally came to discriminate in part the harmonious tones. For example, in the scale of the greens, which originally I reduced to the clear green of grass, I eventually attained the differentiation of the blue-green of the olive tree, the yellow-green of the boxwood, the gray-green of the evergreen oak and of the pine, and the dark green of the cypress. These modest advances led me to sharpen my observation of nature and to distrust memory, which tends invariably to simplify forms and shades of colour.

Indeed, in connection with these studies of colour, I conceived a childish project at which I worked ardently for some time. As an exercise, I undertook to reproduce in a large sketchbook all the various tints presented by natural objects, making a sort of pictorial dictionary in which, though lacking a name, each complex colour would appear with a number indicating its position in the scale. By way of example I added a picture of the corresponding object. It was something like the well known colour scale of Chevreuil (with which I was not then acquainted), but more complete, since it contained, besides the simple colours in various degrees of saturation, the products of mixing all the colours, including naturally white and black.

The making of this album was carried out just as I desired so long as I chose for reproduction rocks, insects, and wild flowers; but when I came to cultivated flowers, I met unexpected difficulties. Carnations, roses, hyacinths, geraniums, zinnias, pansies, gillyflowers, etc., were not free, they had owners and were private property, and since I had no money, I had to pilfer them from gardens and from flower pots.

As was to be expected, some disagreeable experiences came to me in consequence. Of these I shall mention only two, related, by the irony of fate, to the preparation of the chapter on roses. One of my chums, to whom I had confided my tastes and aspirations, when he saw that I was vexed because of the lack of specimens of a beautiful variety called in Huesca the rose of Alexandria,—a flower notable alike for its colour and for its fragrance—proposed to me a raid upon a certain garden where this and other very fine flowers were abundant. I agreed readily to the suggestion, which held for me the added attraction of a dangerous adventure, and we arranged to carry it out at nine o'clock the next night. When the time came, my friend appeared punctually, accompanied by two playmates who were likewise attracted by the innocent and poetic booty, and we stole silently and cautiously up to the walls of the garden, above which a high grape-trellis extended and sprays of magnificient climbing roses shone at intervals. It was important, before commencing to break in, to ascertain whether the owners, or possibly the gardener, were living in the house; so, in order to make sure, we resorted to the simple expedient of throwing two or three stones at the roof. There was no response to the clatter, not a voice, not a sound. Encouraged by the silence, we approached the wall at a place where it was easily scaled, clambered up quickly, got over the bars of the trellis, and jumped down, not without a thrill, upon the path round the garden.

Hardly had we grasped a few of the coveted roses when there emerged from the house two peasants, each armed with a stick, who rushed at us furiously. Recovering from the disagreeable surprise, we started to run round and round through the avenues of the garden. But how were we to escape? The gates were closed and the walls of the enclosure were so high that it was impossible to climb out of reach before the enraged gardeners should catch us with their formidable cudgels. In this critical situation, instinct suggested to us the strategy of running breathlessly about the garden so as to tire its custodians, or at least to gain such an advantage over them as would allow us the few seconds necessary for scaling the wall. But, alas, we fed ourselves with vain hopes! In truth, for the first quarter of an hour things did not go badly at all; much practice in running and the spur of fear enabled us to preserve an advantage over our enemies of perhaps twenty metres or more. But after fifteen minutes had passed the distance grew progressively less; in twenty minutes or so it was less than ten metres. We were wracked with terror. Nevertheless, we did not despair in the desperate struggle for space and time. In such an extreme danger, it seemed that our spirits had entered into our muscles, and our hearts, which are muscles too, worked at full capacity, preferring to burst rather than surrender.

But alas! The sturdy musculature of our rustic pursuers was not yet wearied, and our forces, on the other hand, began to flag; our hearts palpitated dizzily and our parched throats cried out for unobtainable refreshment. And still the distance diminished alarmingly. Paralyzed with exhaustion, one of my comrades fell, and his cries and howls in our ears served as the final spur. The capture of our playmate gave us a respite, allowing us to get our breath and to regain some of our advantage. Hope was born anew, but only, alas, to vanish again soon; for our enemies, exasperated by such persistence and anxious to trap us surely, divided their forces; one of them kept running straight on, while the other went round in a circle. We were going to be caught between two fires.

There was no time to lose. I had a plan which I had developed during the brief moments when, as I turned the corners, I was out of sight of my pursuers and could examine conveniently the trees and walls of the place. Taking advantage, then, of one of these pauses, I made a supreme effort and jumped up into the branches of an apple tree, from which I gained the wall and so reached freedom. This was real good fortune, for only a few seconds later heartrending groans were heard. It was my poor companions in misfortune who had been caught by the fierce gardeners and bit the dust beneath a rain of blows. Indignant at the abuse of which I considered my friends the victims, I had the impudence to climb back to the top of the wall for long enough to hurl four or five heavy stones at the enraged wielders of the cudgels, some of which must have reached their mark, for the men turned towards me furiously. I had, naturally, the prudence to escape.

Thus was concluded the famous adventure of the roses of Alexandria. The beating which my companions received was so severe that they were absent from school for several days: one of the victims, if I remember correctly, was seriously ill. In truth it was a dreadful whipping and was entirely out of proportion to the insignificance of the offence.

The other episode, which was staged in the garden of the railway station, had more of a comic than a dramatic flavour. Some specially fine tea roses were grown there, of which the graceful shape and delicate perfume daily excited my cupidity. Unable to resist the temptation to complete my collection of drawings with pictures of such exquisite specimens, one afternoon, I took advantage of the absence of the guard to jump over the fence and possess myself of the roses. My evil star willed, however, that when I was already outside the paling, the brakeman should surprise me and start to chase me, musket in hand and determination in his manner. In vain he shouted at me to stop and ordered me to surrender discreetly to avoid a peppering. I paid no attention and kept on as fast as I could across the country.

In a few minutes I considered myself safe when, as ill luck would have it, in jumping over a broad ditch with banks of mud at each side, the drying of the surface of which gave them a deceptive appearance of solidity, I fell on the opposite side and sank into the slime up to my middle. I struggled anxiously to get out of the mire. Unfortunately each contorsion only drove me farther into the slime, where I was held as firmly as a bird in bird lime. Providentially, some poor and charitable women, who were washing not far away, came to my assistance. They pulled me out of the mud in a pitiful state. I was absolutely unfit to be seen. Hence I undressed so as to wash my clothes, but my charitable rescuers would not permit it, taking possession of my belongings and cleaning them carefully for me. During this operation I had to remain in hiding, crouching in my shirt under a willow tree. I forgot to say that before this the enraged guard arrived and seeing me in such a state and not knowing how to take hold of me without spoiling his clean uniform, ended by bursting out laughing and holding his nose. As a matter of fact my armour of foul slime made me invulnerable.

The episodes described, and others which I will not relate, so as to avoid undue prolixity, will appear improbable nowadays. What boy or youth, however romantic, would risk his skin today for the pleasure of possessing a rose and enriching an album?

Not without reason was I considered by my fellow students as unbalanced or utterly silly. More than once I heard myself described as "the crazy Navarran." I was probably so regarded by the more sensible, studious and clever of my companions, among whom stood out Arizón, Salillas, Monreal, Tobeñas, and others whom I have forgotten. I may be permitted to say that, in spite of being good fellows, they avoided my company. Upon my word, I greatly regretted it, for I have always rendered to talent and application the homage of cordial sympathy.

CHAPTER XIII

The holidays. Funereal pictures. Discovery of a library of novels. My romantic ardour flames up anew. Robinson Crusoe and Don Quixote.

It has often been said that happiness and monotony are incompatible; even relative felicity requires a certain rhythm of antagonistic perceptions and emotions, or at least ones which differ to some extent. The law of contrast or of complimentary colors, which contributes so much to the beauty of pictures, holds good likewise in the realm of the intellect. For rest (which is the zero point in the scale of sensibility) does not constitute true pleasure. To enjoy is to exercise without hindrance the sensory capacities of our minds; in the same way that the limited outlook in the valley makes us desire the broad expanse of the plain or of the sea, the excessive tension of study incites the unrestrained expansion of the lower activities of the brain.

These reflections occur to me as I write of the joyful and hilarious enthusiasm with which I celebrated the summer of 1864 after the June examinations, in which, if I did not deserve honour diplomas, neither did I encounter the dreaded failure.

Upon my arrival at Ayerbe, my first thought was to get into touch with my old playmates, to whom I proudly related my adventures and exhibited my drawings and sketches.

When I had satisfied my thirst for friendly expressions of welcome and for running wildly about the town, my father called me to order and informed me of his decision that I must give up foolish pastimes and absurd artistic caprices and devote the summer to study, first reviewing all the work in which I had recently passed the examinations, though I had learned it but mediocrely, and then attacking the texts prescribed for the following session. He believed that this exercise which he had planned would make the next year's tasks much easier. Such a decision was like a jug of cold water poured over my head, which was aflame with eagerness to give joyful rein to my natural inclinations.

I had no alternative but submission to the paternal advice and I even believe that I sincerely intended to comply with it; but the demon of rebellion, which had never been overcome, and my determined and troublesome artistic tendencies broke down these sensible intentions.

It often happens that wilful boys, even though fundamentally good, are transformed into artful hypocrites by the desire to spare their parents pain. On the pretext that my assiduous reading required absolute silence and freedom from disturbance, which could not be had in the study, I asked and obtained my father's permission to equip as a work room the pigeon house, a room adjoining the barn, which had a window opening upon the roof of the next house. From the door of my retreat I could conveniently keep a lookout for those who were watching my conduct. The stratagem succeeded perfectly, as we are about to see.

As the ultimate step in caution, I constructed a sort of confessional or niche out of boards, rough sticks, and brushwood on the roof of the neighbouring house, behind a chimney, where it was screened from prying eyes; and beneath the seat in this I secreted the forbidden papers, pencils, colours, and novels. From time to time, in order to carry out the deception, I returned to the pigeon house (especially when I heard the sound of footsteps) and began very seriously to translate Cornelius Nepos, or to study the psychology of Monlau and the algebra of Vallín y Bustillo. Apart from these brief moments, my retreat was the cage on the roof, where I spent my time drawing, my favourite amusement. I do not remember exactly the subjects which my brush profaned that summer, but I recall that for the time my work had mostly a lugubrious and melancholy atmosphere.

It is manifest to the world that in the fickle interests

of youth an important part is played by suggestion and imitation. Someone (I think it was in Huesca) had lent me a volume of gloomy and funereal poetry, among which I remember the hackneyed and commonplace verses attributed groundlessly to Espronceda and entitled "Despair" and the famous "Mournful nights" of Cadalso.

Influenced by such depressing reading, I imagined it to be my inevitable duty to attune myself with the sombre temper of the poets, affecting the deepest melancholy in both my words and my sketches. And so my brush, which showed the fluctuations of my morbid sensibilities as the pointer of a galvanometer indicates the direction of electric currents, dwelt joyfully upon winter landscapes, desolate wastes, the sufferings of the shipwrecked, and macabre views of cemeteries.

If my memory does not deceive me, it was at the end of that summer that there happened an event which had a decisive influence in directing my future literary and artistic tastes.

I have already mentioned that in my home books of recreation were not permitted. It is true that my father possessed a few works of fiction, but he concealed them from our wild curiosity, as if they were deadly poison. In his opinion, young people should not distract their imagination with frivolous reading during the formative period. In spite of the prohibition, my mother, unknown to the head of the house, allowed us to read some cheap romantic novels which she had kept in the bottom of a trunk since before she was married. There were, I well remember, *El solitario del monte salvaje, La extranjera, La cana* of Balzac, *Catalina Howard, Genoveva de Brabante,* and a few others which have slipped my memory. It is superfluous to say that my brothers and sisters as well as I read them with immediate enthusiasm, evading the jealous vigilance of the head of the family.

Aside from these novels, my reading for pleasure up to that time had been reduced to some poems of Espronceda, of whom I was a fervent admirer, and a certain collection of old time ballads and stories of knight errantry which in those days were sold for a few coppers by the blind and by the dealers in religious prints and writing materials. At that period, as I have already said, I was a romantic though ignorant of romanticism. No book by Rousseau, Chateaubriand, Victor Hugo, etc., had fallen into my hands.

But accident often becomes the accomplice of our desires. One day, when I was exploring at random my secret domain above the tiles, I looked in at the window of a garret belonging to the neighbouring confectioner[1] and beheld—oh, delightful surprise!—beside old pieces of furniture and frames covered with sweetmeats and dried fruits, a rich and varied collection of novels, stories and histories, collections of poetry, and books of travel. There were to be seen, tempting my burning curiosity, the celebrated *Count of Monte Cristo* and *The Three Musketeers* of Dumas père; *María or the daughter of a laborer* by E. Sué; *Men Rodríguez de Sanabría* by Fernándex y González; *The Martyrs, Atala and Chactas,* and *René* by Chateaubriand; *Graziella* by Lamartine; *Notre Dame de Paris* and *Ninety-three* by Victor Hugo; *Gil Blas de Santillana* by Le Sage; *History of Spain* by Mariana; *The comedies of Calderón;* several books and poems by Quevedo, *The voyages of Captain Cook, Robinson Crusoe, Don Quixote,* and innumerable books of less importance of which I have not a detailed recollection. It was obvious that the confectioner was a man of taste and that he did not reckon his happiness solely in terms of making caramels and cakes.

Excitement at such a fortunate occurrence held me spellbound for several minutes. Then, recovering from my surprise, I determined to make the most of my good luck and considered how best to take advantage of that inestimable treasure. It was essential to obviate all suspicions of the owner and to avoid leaving any tell-tale traces of my visits to the garret. The most elementary caution told me to leave alone, for the present the delicious and appetizing

[1] This man, R. Cuideras, was a man of culture, and gave a good education to his sons, with whom I was always on the best of terms.

candies on the frames, for I was sure that, if the manufacturer missed any of his candied pears and plums, he would close the window or put a grating over it and leave me out in the cold. After careful consideration I decided to strike the first blow early in the morning, while the occupants of the house were asleep, and to take the coveted books one at a time, replacing each volume in its own place on the shelves.

Thanks to these precautions, I enjoyed in peace the most interesting works in the library, without the worthy pastry-cook being aware of the abuse, and without my parents discovering my absences from the pigeon house. Who could enhance the enjoyment which I experienced in reading these delightful books! So great were my enthusiasm and pleasure that I forgot entirely the common occupations of every-day life.

What exquisite artistic sensations those admirable novels brought me! What fascinating new types of humanity they revealed to me! The brilliant descriptions in *Atala* of the virgin forests of America, where the abounding plant life seems to smother man in his insignificance; the tender and chaste loves of Cimodocea in *The Martyrs;* the exquisite and angelic form of *Graziella;* the exalted and almost monstrous passion of Quasimodo, in *Notre Dame de Paris;* the nobility, magnanimity, and punctilious bravery of the incomparable d'Artagnan, Porthos, and Aramis, in *The Three Musketeers;* and finally the cold, inexorable, and carefully planned vengeance of the leading character in the *Count of Monte Cristo,* captivated and aroused my sympathies in an extraordinary fashion.

At last, though by illicit means, I made the acquaintance of the splendid creatures of the imagination; superb and magnificent beings, all energy and determination, with overgrown hearts shaken by superhuman passions. It is true that nearly all the novels which I devoured at that time belonged to the romantic school, which was then in fashion, and of which the heroes seem to be designed expressly to carry away the young, who are always thirsty for extraordinary events and marvellous adventures.[2]

It would be difficult for me to tell now, after the passage of so many years, the books which impressed me most. I believe, however, that I am not going far astray when I state that I was most excited and fascinated by the delightful novels of action and intrigue of Dumas (père) and the utra-romantic stories of Victor Hugo, which I then rated higher than *Faust, Gil Blas de Santillana* and even—I blush to confess it—the marvellous *Don Quixote.*

There is a certain psychological aspect of childhood and adolescence which is perhaps insufficiently studied by the specialists.[3] It has rightly been said that young people are extremists in everything, but if we understood them properly we should be less surprised by some of their aberrations of taste. The adolescent loves hyperbole; when he paints, he exaggerates the colour; if he is telling a story, he amplifies and expands; he admires in writers an emphatic, vehement, declamatory style, and in politicians extreme and radical theories. He prefers the particular to the general, the ideal to the real, actions to words. He is carried away by the musical and sonorous qualities of poetry, the pomp of the imagery, and the effect of vigorous and high-sounding epithets. Just as, in the realm of science, he rates the objective sciences more highly than the so-called abstract disciplines, so in the sphere of art, he hates reflection and moralizing and is left cold by the sentimental analyses of the psychological school. As if he saw the world through a magnifying glass, everything appears to him enlarged

[2] It is well known that today the whole product of romanticism is accused, perhaps rightly, of insincerity, of sentimental and linguistic ostentation, while its authors are regarded as hyperbolical play-actors, of limited intelligence, overflowing with words but poor in ideas, in fact systematic falsifiers of nature. We must agree, however, that the lurid imaginations of young people of fourteen to twenty will always prefer this literature to that of all the well-balanced depictors of actual emotions or of coldly natural scenes.

[3] When this was written, my acquaintance with psychological literature was somewhat defective. Important, though not always coherent data on this point are to be found in the studies of Stanley Hall, Ribot, Ferrier, Dewey, James, Hutchinson, etc.

and with a rainbow halo; in contrast to old age, which seems to see things through a concave lens, that reduces and debases everything.

Before finishing this chapter, however, I should like to say a few words about the impression made upon me by *Robinson Crusoe* and *Don Quixote.*

Robinson Crusoe (which I reread later on with true delight) revealed to me the sovereign power of man over nature. But what impressed me most of all was the noble pride of the man who, by his own unaided efforts, found that an uninhabited island, full of dangers and pitfalls, was capable of being transformed, by the miracles of determination and intelligent effort, into a delectable paradise. "What a supreme triumph it must be," I thought, "to explore a virgin territory, to gaze upon scenes untouched by the hand of man, adorned with their original flora and fauna, which seem created expressly for the discoverer, as a reward for his outstanding heroism!"

Although I was not yet in a position to appreciate fully the supreme worth of the inestimable jewel of Cervantes, I yet enjoyed greatly the epic adventure of Don Quixote and the delicious colloquies of the knight and his squire. But to be candid, I must say that I disliked the philosophy which is dispensed by this masterpiece of fiction. How could its profoundly realistic viewpoint please me when it went contrary to my incorrigible idealism! I took the figure of Don Quixote seriously, and so felt keenly the damaged state in which the valiant knight emerged from nearly all his quarrels and adventures.

Besides—why should I not acknowledge it?—that melancholy rout at Barcelona at the hands of the vulgar Sansón Carrasco caused me great disillusion. "Not that"! I exclaimed in my romantic raptures—the hero of La Mancha did not deserve to be vanquished. It is all very well for the vulgar champions of common sense to triumph in the world of reality; but in a work of art designed to exalt courage and glorify virtue, the protagonist should float over the vileness of his moral surroundings and rise to a glorious apotheosis."

Of course, my limited understanding failed to grasp the central idea of the tremendous conception of Cervantes: to banish the follies and extravagances of the novels of chivalry so as to found artistic work upon the solid groundwork of experience. In the long run only the artistic narratives of probable events, ingeniously interwoven with elements of actual life, attain the lofty privilege of teaching, edifying, and pleasing.

From the foregoing sentences, which translate somewhat freely the emotions of my youth and immaturity, the reader will understand that the strong and robust realism of Don Quixote did not appeal to me. Only later, when I was cured of the cloying romanticism from which I suffered, did I learn to enjoy the spirit of the book, to take pleasure in the richness, charm, and elegance of style, and to appreciate at its true worth the marvellous harmony resulting from the contrast between the superb types of Don Quixote and Sancho; personages who—as has often been said—while loftily ideal, are the most real and universal imaginable, because they symbolize and incarnate the two extremes of human thought and feeling.

But let us abandon idle reflection and resume the thread of the story.

CHAPTER XIV

My heedless and foolish actions increasing, my father establishes me as apprentice in a barber shop. My brother Pedro. Señor Acisclo. Boasters and conspirators. The stonings. Skirmish with the police. The pleasure of the gods. Public alarm in connection with the stonings.

There are hazy pictures and even actual gaps in the cinematograph of memory, corresponding to the periods when the attention, like photography on a dull day, had not enough energy to impress the film of the brain. If, by an energetic evocation, some event is brought up out of the black depths of the unconscious, it appears isolated, like a star shining alone in a cloudy sky. The action which has risen may usually be placed definitely in space but with difficulty in time; it can be referred more or less indefinitely to a period, but not to a precise page of the almanack.

To this category of discontinuous and hazy memories belong my recollections of the years 1865 and 1866. I am certain, however, that in 1865 my studies were interrupted because my father considered that his son lacked either the maturity or the ability requisite for an understanding of the fundamentals of the languages and sciences; and I think that probably the main incidents, if not all those with which we are about to concern ourselves in this chapter belong to the year 1866, that is to the third session of my course for the bachelor's degree, which at that time embraced the general and regional history of Spain, algebra, trigonometry, and Greek, which was introduced into secondary education as a result of a transitory decree.

One thing of which I am quite sure is that the aforesaid third session was the most disturbed and unfortunate period of my student life. I remember also that it was then that my brother accompanied me to the Institute at Huesca to commence his studies. Pedro was a boy who was as docile and attentive as he was diligent and punctilious. He possessed, no doubt, artistic inclinations and a passion for warlike games; but these tastes were not strong enough to lead him out of the way in which he should go.

My father, who built high hopes upon his seriousness and obedience, feared, no doubt, the contagion of my rebelliousness and had the foresight to separate the brothers, establishing us in different houses. Pedro was lodged decently in a quiet boarding house; I, in recompense for my sins, had to put up with being apprentice in a barber shop. In taking such an extreme decision with regard to me, my father aimed at two ends: for the present to tie me closely, depriving me of the leisure necessary for rambles and raids and besides to teach me a trade which might some day make a living for me in case my inability should prove irremediable or I should be prematurely orphaned. For it must be acknowledged that, although my father had been so optimistic about my future when I was a child, he was beginning to believe that I had an essential incapacity for a literary career.

I do not now regret my father's decision, which was repeated afterward in Zaragoza, as we shall see in the course of this story. It placed me in contact with the soul of the people, which I learned to know and admire, and, overcoming my inborn pride, it developed in me that feeling of humility and modesty which is associated with hardworking poverty. Then, however, I felt my slavery to be an excessive punishment. And at what a time! Exactly when my soul was still vibrating with the tremendous jolt which it had received from its sudden impact with the romantic! I, who then dreamt of the brilliant heroes of Dumas, Chateaubriand, and Victor Hugo; who, convinced of my artistic ability, believed myself capable of emulating the glories of Titian, Raphael, or Velasquez, to see myself compelled to grasp the dirty and soapy shaving brush of a barber! It was to die of shame!

But what could I do? I had, then, to submit in silence to what, in my stupid vanity, I considered intolerable humiliation and debasement. Fortunately, at fourteen the human mechanism is so plastic that it quickly adapts itself to everything.

Señor Acisclo (this was the name of my master[1]), however, was not an ogre, in spite of his reputation as a grumbler and the severity and ill temper which his hard features and bilious color suggested; rather he was with me very considerate and affable. Sympathetic at seeing my gloomy face, he tried to console me with such words as these: "Take heart, lad! All beginnings are difficult, but you will soon get used to it. Forget your pride and pay attention to lathering beards and if, as I expect, you become used to this business, within a short time you will rise to be a fully qualified barber and will enjoy the wonderful pay of three dollars a month in addition to the tips." What a charming future!

Señor Acisclo was more than right. I finally adapted myself to the new manner of life and even came to find my masters congenial and my subjection tolerable. Besides, after a few weeks, I became friendly with the barber's assistant, a ruddy and good-natured fellow, a great guitar player and a joyous wooer of maids and seamstresses, who in my master's absence excused me from the prosaic duties of my position and allowed me to scribble on papers and draw figures. He took a liking to me because I served him as secretary, writing endearing notes and pretentious verses in his name to a certain servant girl. In return for my kindness, he wished to teach me to play the guitar; but I, who never had any love for music, did not get beyond playing the jota in mediocre fashion and strumming stiffly a few simple polkas.

The psychology of the barber is too well known for me to fall into the temptation to explain it to my readers. Nobody is unaware that the authentic wielders of the razor are chatterers, meddlers, enthusiasts of the bull-ring, play-

[1] My master died many years ago and I have no reason to conceal his name. His establishment, which has now disappeared, was in the Calle de la Correría, not far from the Plaza de la Catedral.

ers of the guitar or of the bandore; but it is not so generally known that most of them profess republican or even socialistic principles. The rule was broken in my master, however, since he neither played the guitar nor was a free talker; on the other hand he was a member of the regular flock in respect of his political radicalism and his ostentatiously revolutionary views. He was also adorned by another quality, not common among tradespeople; he professed the religion of swashbuckling. When his comrades of sprees and nocturnal rambles came to be shaved, nothing was talked of in the shop but scuffles, quarrels, stabbings, slashing in the face, and greeting the dawn. More than one of these habitués had been imprisoned and a number displayed on their chests honorable scars from knife-wounds received in hand to hand combat. Without being vain-glorious or a babbler, my master, when the occasion was opportune and he was in the humour for confidences, spoke seriously and compacently of rows and conflicts in which he had taken part, and in which he had given a good account of himself in self-defence and always in fair combat. As he used to say, "Either do something worth while or keep quiet; I am not quarrelsome, but the man who looks for me finds me."

His associates approved of his ideas and applauded his boasts. Through the tokens of admiration and respect which they paid him, I recognized that Señor Acisclo had a bad temper. Moreover, he was the authorized arbitrator of grievances among these folk, and the final judge in questions of honour and of street chivalry.

The conversation between master-barber and clients often turned upon politics. At times they talked in whispers, passing on some sensational news or other. Our curiosity, however, overcame all their secrecy. We had information about the conspiracies of Prim, Moriones, and Pierrad, exiled generals who, according to the members of our circle, were on the point of crossing the frontier at the head of a large company of carbineers and bold mountaineers from Jaca, Hecho, and Ansó, to proclaim the revolution and overthrow what at that time were called the *ominous* institutions.

Those harmless arm-chair patriots rubbed their hands with glee, tasting in anticipation the unequivocal triumph of the sovereignty of the people and the disgraceful rout of menials and moderates.

While all this was going on, the barber's unhappy wife, who did not share in the hopes of the conspirators, but rather feared denunciation by some base confidant, lived in a perpetual state of alarm. She was afraid that some night, as often happened in those days, the police would search the house and carry off her husband into exile to Fernando Po.

As a matter of fact, I did not understand one iota of politics, but I was carried away by disturbances, scuffles, and rows. I would have given something, at that time, to take part in an insurrection or to be present at the construction and defence of a barricade. Besides, I was instinctively attracted by the so-called democratic creed, which fitted in admirably with my exaggerated individualism and my inborn dislike for the principle of authority. As in the story of the friar, the prior disgusted me merely by being prior.

To flatter my master and at the same time demonstrate to him my liberal sympathies, I made copies of the busts of the rebel military leaders of the period, particularly of Prim and Pierrad. It is certain that, besides my simple devotion to the fighter, what most attracted me in this last leader were the classic lines of his portrait and his beautiful, patriarchal beard. While these sketches were pretty crude and inaccurate, I earned warm praises with them, to which some clumsy verses,[2] dedicated to liberty and written below the portraits, also contributed. In all this, there was a certain amount of calculation on my part; for my master, delighted with the precociously revolutionary sentiments and with the graphic dexterity of his apprentice, gave him bet-

[2] *Décimas.* A décima is a stanza of ten lines with eight syllables in each. (Translator's note.)

ter treatment every day. He let me off not only at the regular hours for classes, but also nearly every afternoon when business was quiet. Hence the plan of my progenitor was entirely frustrated.

The chance finding of a little treasure by my brother and me further excited my bellicose tendencies. One day when walking near the Hermitage of the Martyrs, my brother Pedro noticed something shiny in a rubbish pile. We picked it up and rubbed it to remove the dirt, when, to our surprise and delight, it turned out to be a five dollar gold piece. By good luck, there were still current in those days *onzas,* those famous double doubloons,[3] which have now, unfortunately, been turned into rare museum pieces. To assure ourselves that the doubloon was good, we changed it at some shop, and once we were in possession of a sum so respectable, and for us so unlikely, we agreed to expend it in the purchase of a certain large and imposing pistol which for a long time had been tempting our cupidity daily in the window of an old gunsmith's shop. Providing ourselves with a supply of powder, bullets, and bird-shot, we began to practice using the weapon, with very uncertain results. However, by dint of practice, we succeeded in improving our aim and sometimes hitting the mark.

In providing ourselves with a weapon so unsuitable for boys, it was our intention, besides giving ourselves the appearance of terrible revolutionaries, to revive our old irresistible inclinations for hunting and to sally forth in pursuit of thrushs, partridges, and rabbits. But, just as happened with the formidable musket in our earlier days, we never took anything worth while; only some sparrow that had recently left the nest and was unskilled in flight fell into our hands.

I think it was in that year, 1866, that I made myself feared among my school-fellows by my progress in the manipulation of the sling. I remember that among other proofs of my skill I was able to pierce a hat thrown into the air at a distance of twenty paces. I was not content merely

[3] *Peluconas.*

with improving my aim, but developed also the range and especially the speed of discharge, in which I had a marked advantage over my rivals. While they were shooting one stone I shot four or five. This was the time when the insolent Azcón submitted and when my supremacy in warlike games received general recognition. As is natural, I was spontaneously offered the leadership of the bands in combat. I accepted, as might be assumed, the chieftaincy of the democratic band, since already at that time we boys played at being liberals and reactionaries.

My prestige was not founded upon mere skill and the blind courage of one who is ignorant of the danger and hence is inflamed by the noise of battle. It would be only right for me to confess, although my reputation for bravery should suffer in consequence, that in my boldness there was a large element of the theatrical and considerable observation of child psychology. During my wide experience of student brawls, I had noticed that boldness and pugnacious fury, when they are perfectly feigned, inspire the enemy with panic almost infallibly. Besides, I was always aggressive.

It is not to the point to analyze here the mechanism of suggestion through which a lion-like mien and fearless daring, cleverly feigned, arouse terror in our adversaries. There is something atavistic in this theatrical braggadocio, which, moreover, is practised by savages and was even resorted to by the heroes of the Iliad. Modern psychologists [4] discourse upon it very learnedly, and point out how important, for the understanding and reproduction so far as possible of an affective state, is the exact imitation of the gestures and attitudes characteristic of its natural expression. I do not know whether the feigned and, as it were, instinctive reproduction of the appearance of fearless valor produced the corresponding emotional condition in me by a sort of autosuggestion; but I solemnly declare that if I

[4] The classic example of Campanella, cited by James, will be recalled: "to understand a person's mental condition, imitate his expressions."

put on a ferocious expression and advanced intrepidly against my adversaries, they regularly took to flight.

I am running the risk of making myself tedious by lingering too long over these insignificant boyish struggles. Nevertheless, besides their anthropological significance, concerning which the English psychologists have written so well, there are useful lessons in them for grown men. The ingenuousness of the mind of the child makes admirably clear the means and aims, which are often obscure, of the conflicts of men and of nations. Apart from their instinctive character, which seems to reproduce ancestral conditions, the contests of boys involve a praiseworthy sentiment, namely, the love of glory, the desire for the approval and admiration of ones peers. Never—and this alone would be enough to make one sympathetic towards children—is there any sordid self-interest.

Another lesson is to be derived from the conflicts of youngsters. There is revealed in them, better even than in the competitions of adults, how important and decisive for a favourable outcome is the part played by a strong will and an unquenchable determination to succeed. He who takes things as a joke is always overcome by him who takes them in earnest; the mere amateur has to yield to the professional; he who brings to the palisade only a trivial desire to satisfy his vanity is always routed by the one who puts his whole soul into the undertaking and prepares himself beforehand by strengthening his muscles and tempering his weapons.

Being thoroughly in earnest, I ultimately became very highly skilled in the use of the sling. My observations enabled me to improve the weapon; I used silk for the cords and leather for the strap and selected heavy spherical pebbles as projectiles. I went so far as to compile for the use of my friends an illustrated book with the pretentious title *Lapidary Strategy,* in which were contained practical rules for avoiding systematically various projectiles which might endanger one.

The reader will imagine without difficulty that before

attaining such mastery I had been hurt many times, and this was so true that my head was covered with old scars. Sometimes, when I left school and put on my hat, I found that it did not fit because the lump on my head, which had been almost imperceptible before I entered the classroom, had increased during the lesson, when it was free from the restraint of my cap.

But I must not insist upon a matter which I have already discussed repeatedly. I must conform so far as possible with the well known *non bis in idem* of the Latins. I may be permitted only to recount two relatively interesting episodes before finally abandoning the narration of stonings.

The hero of the first event, which was more comic than dramatic, was my brother. We were contending peacefully in a certain narrow lane near the Institute, the regular scene of our battles, when, after almost the first exchange of projectiles, I saw with surprise that our adversaries had fled from the field precipitately. Suspecting a ruse, perhaps an attack from the rear, I detached two of my band to make an encircling movement, explore the vicinity, and report to me what had happened. But before my emissaries returned the mystery was suddenly explained. At the other end of the lane, where our opponents had been a few moments before, there appeared four policemen, sabre in hand, who advanced threateningly with a shout of, "Wait, you scoundrels!" I guessed then what had happened: the opposing army, surprised by the police, had fled in disorder and, perhaps pursued by the cops, had been subjected to the usual blows with the flat of the sabre.

The situation was critical. We knew well enough that in the end we should have to take to flight, but so as to gain time and to delay or disconcert the officers somewhat, I ordered my followers to halt and, before retreating, to make a general discharge. Daring was of service to us once more. The cops, who were rushing upon us, stopped dead, and one of them fell to the ground, hurling coarse abuse at us.

What had occurred? My stone, taken from the bag of

sure hitters, struck one of our tormentors on the thigh so violently that, transfixed with pain, he fell to his knees on the ground; another pebble found a mark on the shoulder of the second officer; while my brother's projectile, hurled with great force, by a strange chance hit the blade of the third policeman's sword, breaking off the steel at the hilt. The fellow stood in the grotesque attitude which may be imagined, flourishing challengingly a pure and simple brass haft. Only one of our adversaries was not hit. There followed, as has been mentioned, a moment of stupefaction, by which we profited fully in taking to our heels. By the time when the angry cops invaded our territory it was already too late to overtake us; we had reached the threshing floors of Cáscaro, surmounted the old wall, descended by its projecting stones and finally crossed the river and the grove.[5]

The adventure might have cost us dear. It was reported that one of the policemen was confined to bed for several days. We were sought persistently everywhere, but fortunately none of the company gave us away. Although the police wished to make an admonitory example of the presumptive ringleaders of the transgression against authority, they were not successful, at least so far as I was concerned; for my master, cognizant of the occurrence and a bitter enemy of the cops, against whom he had some old grievance, hid me for several days in the house of one of his confrères.

The other dramatic incident has remained imprinted upon my memory under the title the *beating by the mountaineer*. I was fighting alone from a field near the road against eight or ten students who were fortified on the top of the city wall, a position of vantage which was necessitated by my notable marksmanship with the sling, in order to equalize the conditions. In the thickest of the struggle, and just when I had hit the hat of one of the enemy, I saw coming towards me, with an air by no means reassur-

[5] Trees being relatively rare in Aragon and Castile, many towns have a plantation or grove of poplar trees, usually near the stream, and called *la alameda*. (Translator's note.)

ing and flourishing a formidable cudgel, a highland mule driver who a few minutes before had passed on the road peacefully leading his train. I waited him with mingled confidence and distrust, uncertain what attitude to assume, until his first words led me to guess what had happened, namely that he had been hit by a stone cast by those on the top of the wall, and hearing the sound of my sling and discovering my attitude of aggression, he believed me to be guilty of the attack. In vain I protested my innocence and pointed out to him the situation of my adversaries, who, as my ill luck would have it, were not visible during those critical moments. Without paying any attention to my explanations, he seized me by the collar and meted out to me a memorable beating. Having given vent to his indignation, he returned to his mule train and left me bruised and exhausted.

Boiling with wrath, I vowed revenge for the outrage, and for this the lie of the land was in my favour. Limping with the pain, I scaled the nearby wall, as well as I could; returned to the threshing-floors of Cáscaro, slipped along the ruined battlements so as to place myself in front of the choleric highlander, who was proceeding peacefully along the road, blissfully ignorant of the storm which awaited him. In a jiffy I collected ten or a dozen large pebbles and discharged them with dizzy speed at the man from the Valley of Ansó. The train took fright, running in all directions. The fury of the lusty peasant as he saw himself the gainer by three or four projectiles of large size was indescribable! The unhappy fellow, who could neither climb the wall, nor leave his mules, nor withdraw himself behind any shelter, stamped and swore like one possessed.

As soon as he reached the inn he entered a complaint with the mayor, but the authorities could not ascertain the name of the aggressor and the event did not have the disagreeable consequences which were to be feared.

My bad reputation had spread through the district to such an extent that even the girls leaving school hid when they saw me in fear of some clandestine stone throwing.

It is a fact that among the girls who regarded me with most horror, I remember a certain fair and slender little thing with great sea-green eyes, lips and cheeks like geraniums, and huge braids the colour of honey. Her uncle and her father, whom our daily disturbances prevented from enjoying their siesta, had said terrible things about Santiago, the child of the physician of Ayerbe, and the poor little creature ran away in terror whenever she met me, until she reached the safety of her home in the Calle del Hospital.

Caprices of fate! That pretty, timorous child whom I hardly noticed then, was to become, later on, the mother of my children!

CHAPTER XV

Dislike of my professor of Greek. My father decides to punish me severely, changing me to a shoemaker's apprentice. My prowess in shoemaking. The attack on Linás. Reflections upon death.

After what has been related, it is needless to state that my scientific and literary education progressed very little during the session of 1866. Latin and Greek bored me excessively and the history of the world and of Spain, which consisted of an intolerable string of dates and a wearisome list of names of kings and of battles won or lost according to the favour or anger of Providence, had no interest for me.

In spite of everything, the session would have been completed without mishap if the professor of Greek, a worthy gentleman who was as peevish as he was suspicious, had not made me the target of his ill humour. Certainly, my zeal and attentiveness were not extreme, nor did his lessons, pronounced with a crude Catalan accent, laborious and sibilant, inspire me with great enthusiasm; but my inattention was not the chief cause of his grudge, which was due rather to a certain physiological defect of which I have never been able to cure myself.

Like savages and women, I have always suffered from an undue readiness to burst out laughing—a provoking remark, an unexpected gesture, some joke or other were enough to excite my noisy hilarity, without my being restrained by the seriousness of the place or the solemnity of the occasion. Laughter spread upon my thin and mobile countenance like the surge of the sea whipped up by the breeze. Unfortunately, moreover, through a certain diabolical character of my features, my spontaneous smile of simple amusement acquired in some people's eyes a sarcastic, irritating, and provocative quality.

The worthy master, however, was not aware of Dumas' dictum: "Only knaves do not laugh," and became angry every time he noticed my mirth, in which, with his excessive suspiciousness, he saw satirical and mischievous intent. His choler was not disarmed by my assurances that I was not laughing at him, whom I sincerely respected, but at the jests and sallies of some chattering companions. As his irritation increased progressively, he developed a mania for mortifying me daily by comparing me with common animals and making ridiculous comments.

In treating me in this fashion, my masters adopted entirely the wrong method to cure me. At bottom I was unhappy, and had a frank nature, though I was the victim of idealistic tendencies and unruly sensibilities. Both my father and my professors would have been wiser if they had employed with me methods of persuasion and kindness instead of inflicting upon me corrections which were sometimes excessive and always exasperating.

But to return to my austere professor of Greek, his campaign of jibes and thrusts of wit, which I considered unjust, wore out my patience, and, considering myself already lost, I resolved upon reprisals. I determined, then, to torment the poor gentleman with all sorts of offensive jokes, not stopping at the limits of insolence. In order to wound him to the quick, namely in his deep convictions regarding ultramontanism,[1] I passed round grotesque caricatures in which he appeared wearing the uniform of the national militia, with the words "Long live the Constitution," issuing from his mouth, or walking upon all fours, wearing on his head an enormous *boina*,[2] and (this was the bitterest insult) ridden by Espartero,[3] who seemed to be

[1] The clerical and absolutist view in politics. (Translator's note.)

[2] Beret. A flat, round woolen cap generally worn in Navarre and Biscay. This was worn by the Carlists as a distinctive mark. (Translator's note.)

[3] Espartero was a man of low birth who rose to be regent of Spain twice during the minority of Queen Isabel II, when her mother, Queen Christina, was driven out by popular revolt. At the time referred to in the text he was living in retirement. In 1870 he was a candidate for the throne, Queen Isabel having been deposed two years before, but withdrew and later became a supporter of Alfonso XII. He died in January, 1879. (Translator's note.)

singing the *trágala,*[4] in his ear. Such grotesque figures delighted and excited the boys, who listened to the irascible teacher as one listens to the rain.

With these and other offensive, clownish jests, I covered myself with such odium that, when he was about to return to his native Cataluña, he seized the occasion of his farewell address to deplore bitterly being obliged to depart without having had the pleasure of punishing my insolence. "Although my just colleagues will know how to avenge me," he added. I was there to reply to him "Bon voyage!" but I restrained myself so as not to make my already desperate situation any worse.

Serious in every way were the consequences of my folly. Daunted by the threat just mentioned, which was delivered in the month of May, I deemed failure certain and did not dare to present myself at the examination. As a result of this, and of having obtained only mediocre marks in the other subjects, my father was furious and threatened me with exemplary and radical punishment. Resolved to eradicate my artistic inclinations entirely, he considered and put into execution a plan of therapeusis not lacking ingeniousness and efficacy, which consisted of the application of the well known medical principle: *contraria contrariis.* "What," my parent must have asked himself, "is most diametrically opposite, in the professional and aesthetic order, to sweet poetry and the emotions and beauties of pictorial art. Well, the humble functions of the ropemaker, the chimney-sweep, or the cobler." This last profession especially seemed to him suitable to overcome my romantic impulses and finally to cure my rebelliousness.

I thought at first that it would all end in threats, but I deceived myself entirely. Before the end of June—we were then living in Gurrea de Gállego[5]—he put his plan into

[4] A political song against the absolutists and in favour of the constitution. (Translator's note.)

[5] At the end of 1865, as a result of a dispute with the municipal authorities, my father gave up his practice at Ayerbe, removing first to Sierra de Luna and soon afterwards to Gurrea de Gállego. Two years later, having finally made peace with the corporation of Ayerbe, he returned to his former

execution, apprenticing me to a certain shoemaker, a man of few words, coarse, and of evil countenance, who, with the connivance of my father, made me endure torture. He forced me to swallow a vile stew, to sleep in a dark and bare garret full of mice and cobwebs, and made me besides perform the most menial and dirty tasks in the shop. I was deprived of pencils and paper and was even prohibited from decorating the walls of the barn with charcoal. My imagination, being deprived of any instrument of expression, lived within itself and evoked in my mind the most brilliant and delightful fabrications. Never did I live more prosaically or dream more beautiful, noble, and consoling dreams. Whenever I had finished supper, I eagerly hastened to my little room and, until I fell asleep, spent my time giving form and life to the jumble of stains on the wall and the cobwebs of the ceiling, which I transformed, by the power of thought, into the wings of a magic stage, across which filed the cavalcade of my fantasies.

This treatment of spiritual isolation and restricted nutrition would have ended by converting me into an exalted mystic—like a lover of the desert—if my mother, fearful of the debilitating effects of the cabbages and the wretched stew, had not secretly sent me savory pies and juicy pieces of meat. At the end of that summer, I secured pencil and paper also, bought thanks to a generous tip received from the daughter of the Count and Countess of Parcent, a charming young lady of fourteen who deigned one day to visit the shop and entrust to the humble apprentice the repair of an elegant and diminutive boot which had been ripped during a recent hunting party.[6]

practice, to which he was bound by a well-established professional reputation and even some landed property.

[6] The counts of Parcent used at that time to spend the summers in Gurrea, the centre of their vast estates, where they had a magnificent palace. I still remember with delight the gorgeous hunting parties, with the accompaniment of huntsmen's horns, tents, luxurious habits, etc., which took place in the neighbouring woods and to which my father was graciously invited as being the best shot in the district. It is a fact that the Count's brother painted in oils rather well. There is even preserved in my house a portrait of my father with vigorous and well blended colouring, which was presented to him by the aristocratic amateur.

When my family returned to Ayerbe, I had a change of master, entering the service of one Pedrín, of the family of the Coarasas de Loarre, a shoemaker who was cheerful, noisy, and witty, but severe and harsh with his apprentices. I had at that time extreme gastronomic peculiarities (such as an invincible dislike for stew, squash, tomatoes, onions, etc.) which annoyed my parents very much. Hence my progenitor was determined that Pedrín should cure radically such vexatious fancies, besides treating me without consideration and like an ogre, as the saying is. Just as in Gurrea, the most antiesthetic tasks were to fall to my lot.

Senor Pedrín (who, in spite of his reputation for ill-humour, was an excellent person and a good friend of my family) was delighted with my progress, as well as with the patient humility with which I endured the degradation and prosaicness of my work and the deliberate modifications of the menu.

One day he said to my father: "Don Justo, your youngster is a jewel; he is dexterous, and does everything well. Since he has got on so well, I am going soon to put him at making new boots."

"And what about his food?"

"He eats up everything: squash, tomatoes, turnips, stew —he devours everything without making a face."

"I doubt it; watch him closely and don't let the youngster cheat you. He is very deceitful."

Thus prepared, the master watched me during supper without letting it be seen and was not long in discovering my artifices and stratagems. When the dish was not to my liking, I deceitfully hid the food either in my trousers pocket, which was lined for this purpose, or on a handkerchief hidden between my knees. He condemned my disobedience severely and took as a personal matter the democratization of my stomach and the task of making me eat quantities of even the most abominable scraps. He did not succeed, however. His well-intended persistence only served to weaken me and to convert me, by inevitable alimentary compensation, into a ravenous eater of bread.[7]

My rapid advance in the art of shoemaking having become known in the town, one Fenollo, a master shoemaker and the owner of the best shop in the community, proposed to engage me for a certain number of years, on condition that, if I should give up the business before the end of the first season, my father must indemnify him *a posteriori* with two reals a day. When the contract was completed and I was installed in the new workshop (a brighter and more spacious one than that of Pedrín, situated on the beautiful Plaza Baja), I put a cheerful face on my misfortune.

I was not long in getting to know the master's son, a congenial boy of my own age and tastes, and I acquired such skill in the use of the awl that in a few months I was doing all the different kinds of sewing, making new boots of the kind then called *abotinados*,[8] trimming coquettish heels, mastering the open work and ornamentation of the toecaps, and all the fine work of the craft. My progress was much commended by my new master, who promised to pay me a wage of two reals a day if I continued to do as well, with meals and clothing provided. At the same time, in order to encourage and honour my skill, he entrusted to me the boots of the most fastidious and vain young ladies, boots on the high and graceful heels of which I worked delicate ornaments. What! The Ars Poetica of Horace and my artistic leanings had to serve some purpose!

That year (1867) there occurred the famous attempt at revolution by Moriones and Pierrad, which had a gory epilogue in the skirmish at Linás de Marcuello. Discontent with the government was general. Hatred towards the conservatives, on account of the deportation and shooting of liberals, had reached even the most isolated villages.

7 Senor Pedrín was still alive in 1917, and directed a high class shoe factory in Huesca, where he was very highly regarded. Some years ago, soon after a certain fortunate triumph of mine had been made public, he came to receive me at the station at Huesca, and embraced me with tears in his eyes, exclaiming: "And I thought that you had exceptional aptitude for business!"

8 Literally "shaped like gaiters," *i.e.*, high boots. (Translator's note.)

Everything seemed to indicate the imminence of a storm, of which the aforementioned skirmish at Linás was the first threatening lightning flash.

There was almost universal jubilation in Ayerbe upon the news of the insurrection of the generals, whose triumph was believed to be at hand. Many hastened to enlist in the ranks of the rebels. In our own town and Bolea alone there were involved, according to report, over 500 men, who awaited only arms and equipment to join the revolutionary ranks. The news spread at length that the liberal army, composed of carbineers and highlanders from upper Aragon had spent the night at Murillo, Lapeña and Riglos, from which towns they proceeded easily towards Linás de Marcuello, a village situated at the foot of the neighbouring Gratel range. Intense excitement reigned in Ayerbe; some considered the triumphal entry of the insurgents imminent.

Suddenly there appeared in the Plaza Baja the column of General Manso de Zúñiga, made up of a considerable strength of infantry and fifty superb and showy cuirassiers, who aroused the enthusiasm of the boys with their martial air and shining armour. I never tired of admiring the burnished cuirasses and plumed helmets, defences recalling the stout harness of ancient warriors and the epic struggles of the reconquest. I was enraptured above all by the admirable sight presented by the squadrons in correct formation. When the horses moved, all that mass of polished metal reflected the sun like the sea stirred by the breeze: dazzling flashes of lightening shot from the naked swords, and the dust raised by the stamping of the sorrel steeds seemed to sketch about each warrior a glorious halo of light.

Impatient for the combat, the general ordered the mayor to bring along the baggage immediately and, without waiting longer than was absolutely necessary to give the soldiers their rations, departed in the direction of Linás, which he expected to reach early in the afternoon. Only a short time passed before we heard the distant and muffled sound of shooting, re-echoed by the mountains round about.

Little groups of gossipers gathered in the squares and

were joined by us youngsters, bursting with curiosity. Among the men remarks were exchanged in whispers about the battle going on in these anxious moments between liberty and reaction. At the same time, a good many neighbours compromised in the uprising had fled into the mountains to await the outcome and avoid possible reprisals. All of us were consumed with anxiety and impatience to know what had happened. Our eagerness for news was so great that some of us boys ran away across the fields to the scene of battle. Reaching the crest of a little hill overlooking the village of Linás from the south, we witnessed a pitiful and moving sight. The loyal troops were falling back at that moment towards Ayerbe, with evident signs of discouragement, while the rebels, who occupied excellent positions in the houses of the town and its immediate surroundings, were beginning to move along the foot of the range, disdaining to harass the enemy, perhaps so as not to shed Spanish blood uselessly.

Then we climbed a hill near the road along which the troops were going. Great was our surprise to observe that those cuirassiers who had been so gallant and imposing a few hours before now marched silently and in disorder, with their casques dented and their uniforms stained with blood. Some, who had lost their horses in the fray, were going on foot, drooping and miserable. Mounted, or better exposed, upon baggage animals, and escorted by teamsters and soldiers, came numerous wounded men, whose pitiful groans, brought forth by every stumble on the rough road, rent the heart. And in the midst of that melancholy train rose up, like a tragic ghost, the pale figure of General Manso de Zúñiga, dying or dead, held up on his horse by the faithful arms of an aide. Deep was the impression made upon me by the sight of uniforms soiled with dust and blood, the pale and downcast faces of the funereal company, and above all, the intensely white face of the unfortunate commander, who, a few hours before, had been overflowing with energy and proud resolution.

I confess that that brutally realistic picture of warfare cooled my bellicose enthusiasm a good deal. In no book had I read that bullet-wounds were so bitterly painful, nor that the injured moaned so pitifully. Evidently, either historians have not witnessed battles, or they deliberately omit, as taken for granted, the physical and mental torture of the victims!

When they reached the town the soldiers related the details of the encounter. The insurgents (numbering 1600 men), being informed of the paucity of the forces of General Manso, awaited him posted in advantageous positions among the hills surrounding Linás. As soon as they sighted the enemy, the loyal troops took up a position on the heights nearest the town and the first shots were exchanged. Annoyed by the unexpected resistance of forces which he supposed undisciplined, the queen's leader ordered his troops to advance, whereupon they were met with a heavy volley. A movement of uncertainty could not be avoided, on account, perhaps, of the disorder of the cavalry, which was unable to manoeuvre in the narrow space and on the broken ground; and then the brave general, so as to set an example to his men, and carried away by his fearlessness, put spurs to his horse and advanced a long way towards the enemy. The loyal troops regained confidence, galloping as for a charge to overtake the gallant general; but unfortunately, before they arrived to support him, a shot laid him low with a mortal wound. It is said that at that tragic moment, a colossal fellow from the Valley of Ansó, a fellow seven feet high and hardly nineteen years of age, darted rashly towards the fallen man with the aim of disarming him and taking him prisoner; but his intention was frustrated, for a well-aimed bullet entered his heart and dropped him beside the leader. Their general lost and their numbers inadequate for continuing the attack, the queen's troops retired at last, after gathering up the numerous wounded men, who were given attention and medical treatment in the hospital of Ayerbe.[9]

[9] I do not vouch for the absolute exactitude of the preceding narrative. I am interpreting exclusively my own personal recollections and the account, stripped of anecdotes and improbable hypotheses, which was current in Ayerbe at the time.

As was to be expected, those days brought my father not a little to do with the daily treatment of the soldiers wounded in the encounter and the secret care of others, belonging to the rebel forces, who were in hiding in various villages and even the more inaccessible parts of the neighbouring Sierra de Gratal.

The contemplation on the following day, in the fields of Linás, of the unfortunates who fell in the sanguinary combat, and the examination shortly afterwards of the victims of another unexpected action, which took place near Ayerbe[10] between carbineers[11] and smugglers, brought home to my mind for the first time the terrible lesson of death, the most profound and awful of all the realities of life. It is true that, before these events, I had seen the remains of deceased people and been present at the heart-rending spectacle of the death-agony; but my emotion had been rather mild and had passed like the foam on a wave.

In the morning of life, the idea of death seems so absurd that it hardly arouses even a passing reflection. Who thinks of dying when he feels the blood pulsing furiously through his young heart and sees before him in the blue distance of time an endless series of years of luminous

[10] This conflict took place near Plasencia, on the road from Ayerbe to Huesca. A certain company of smugglers, from whom a very valuable load had been captured as they were crossing the Pyrenees, with the loss of a prominent contrabandist, desiring to avenge themselves and recover the booty, followed at a short distance the wagons bearing the captured goods, concealing themselves easily from the escort of carbineers and infantry which guarded them. When they had arrived beyond Ayerbe, they took advantage of a moment when the escort of infantry had gone on too far ahead and only a dozen carbineers remained with the wagons; surprised these, who were marching carelessly; killed six or seven unfortunates and drove off the others, and quickly loaded the contraband on their beasts. When the company of infantry which was leading the convoy learned of the bold and sanguinary stroke, it was already impossible to overtake the smugglers, who took the road to Zaragoza, by paths known only to themselves. The autopsy upon the bodies was carried out under my father's direction, and led away by curiosity, I accompanied him to help in his funereal task. As I learned later on (in 1910) from the *chief of the district* himself (in Ansó), the men from Ansó had also some casualties, whom they hid in farmyards and villages.

[11] Military customs officers. (Translator's note.)

existence! It is the great privilege of children to die without knowing that they are dying.

The melancholy conviction of annihilation, with its train of awful and formidable enigmas, takes possession of us at a mature age when we are confronted with the death of parents and friends, and especially when distressing internal sensations, unequivocal indications of the progressive wear and tear of the vital machine, warn us for a longer or shorter time of the inevitable denouement.

This fear, which is so profoundly human (happier than we, the animals seem to be unaware of it), is further increased for the physician and the biologist. Science is as unfeeling as it is indiscreet. Through it we know that our organization is so delicate and fragile that an invisible microbe, an unexpected gust of wind, a slight fluctuation of temperature, a violent mental shock, may in a few days ruin the masterpiece of creation, which resembles in its complexity and perishable character those ingenious and intricate clocks that mark the hours, and show the days of the week, the months, the seasons, the years, the rising of the sun and of the moon, but suffer, alas, so specially from one little defect—that of stopping permanently at the first jolt which they receive.

Another of the things which impressed me most deeply was the expression of beatific peace upon the corpse, in marked contrast to the spasms, struggles, and terrors of the death pangs. We are so accustomed to associate the facial expression with a particular feeling that it requires an effort for us to attribute the placid expression of the deceased to the final muscular relaxation; rather we tend to link up that immutable serenity with a corresponding condition of the conscience.

How supremely tragic seems this abandonment of the spirit and the unresisting surrender of our organs to all the disintegrating effects of cosmic forces! And what distressing indifference is that of nature as it casts away, like vile dross, the masterpiece of creation, the sublime cerebral mirror, in which it acquires consciousness of itself.

CHAPTER XVI

My return to study. I matriculate in drawing. My teachers of rhetoric and psychology. The impression produced by lessons in philosophy. An unfortunate prank. In search of foolish adventures.

A year of my life as a shoemaker's apprentice had passed when my father, satisfied with the educational experiment and considering me cured of my artistic madness, decided upon my return to my studies. I promised him sincerely to apply myself on condition that he should consent to enroll me in drawing, a subject perfectly compatible with classical culture and especially with the study of the physical and natural sciences. He finally yielded to my request, though not without scruples, and in order to ensure my regularity in the future, he engaged me as a shopboy in the barber shop of one Borruel, situated in the Plaza de Santo Domingo. If my recollections do not deceive me, I had to take that year psychology, sacred history, Latin, rhetoric and poetics.

As the reader will guess, as soon as classes started I undertook drawing with indefatigable enthusiasm. I soon passed from the details of physiognomy (eyes, noses, mouths) to whole heads and complete figures. I worked with such furious activity that before the end of three months I exhausted the school's collection of lithographic models. My teacher, Don León Abadías, surprised at such a strange case of pictorial eagerness, generously placed at my disposal his private collection of drawings, which he allowed me to take home in turn to work at during the winter evenings. My senses were enraptured and gratified by this work, in which I spent the days tirelessly, from dawn to dark ardently copying the noble lines of the Greek heroes and the beatific expression of the spiritual madonnas of Rafael and Murillo. It was the intoxication of the aesthetic instinct which at last quenched its thirst for the ideal in the pure stream of classic beauty.

My indefatigable pencil was never satisfied. When Don León had exhausted his portfolios, he promoted me to drawing from plaster casts and from nature, and finally he tried my skill at water colours. He was highly satisfied with my work, declaring more than once that he considered me the most brilliant pupil that had passed through his Academy. Such a flattering judgment filled me with noble pride. As was to be expected, when the examinations arrived my industry was rewarded with the report of excellent and a prize. Carried away by his generosity, my excellent master did more; he took the trouble to visit my father in Ayerbe to urge him enthusiastically that I should devote myself without swerving for a moment to the beautiful art of Apeles, in which he felt that brilliant triumphs awaited me. Led on by his enthusiasm, he was extreme in his praise of the neophyte; but all was in vain. It was impossible to persuade my father that there was anything more than a transient dilettantism in the artistic inclinations of his offspring.

In spite of my graphic mania, I studied rhetoric and poetics also with some profit, this subject being one which harmonized with my tastes and tendencies. The rhetorician, Don Cosme Blasco (brother of the illustrious writer Don Eusebio), a young master of gentle and polished speech, beneath which he concealed an energetic and robust character, was skilled in the fine art of making the subject interesting and the no less desirable one of stimulating the application of his pupils. He questioned everybody about the lesson, noted the answers every day, and arranged us on the benches according to their quality. I nearly always emerged creditably from the classes, but in spite of my desire to do so, I never succeeded in getting beyond the second or third place. The post of honour was always held by one of those students who combine with application and exceptional smartness a firm verbal retentiveness and recite by heart long passages in Latin or Spanish.[1] That wonderful gift which modern psychologists call spontaneous or organic memory, that capacity for retaining endless lists of disconnected words, that precious organic possession, the storehouse of the mind, the aid of attention and judgment, is just the quality in respect of which nature has been most miserly with me. My faculty of retention corresponds almost entirely with the logical or systematic memory, which is fed by attention and association, and works only on condition that a natural and logical relation is established between the new and old acquirements.

There is exemplified in me in an exaggerated fashion a characteristic or property of the resuscitation of ideas which has been carefully studied by Wund, James, and other psychologists, namely: that the recollection or memory image is not a mere copy of the perception, but is a new mental occurrence, produced by a synthesis which incorporates more or less related pre-existent elements.

I studied psychology, logic, and ethics with somewhat less profit, from lack of sufficient mental aptitude and from an invincible repugnance for all kinds of dogmatism. The teacher of this subject, Don Vicente Ventura, was a learned and zealous master, the brilliance of whose oratory was somewhat dimmed by his raucous and nasal voice. Suffused with deep religious feeling (which led him to prostrate himself for hours together in the cathedral, with his arms spread out in a cross and his soul in ecstasy), his words interpreted the rugged faith of the believer rather than the reasoned criticism of the philosopher. He was, above all, a panegyrist of religion and a pompous orator, making vibrant apostrophes of. apostolic indignation against materialist error and protestant impiety. A fervent admirer of scholasticism; for him there had lived only two great philosophic geniuses, Aristotle and Saint Thomas Aquinas. From time to time, swept away by the fire of his eloquence,

[1] Our model of diligent students was Arizón, who reached and never passed beyond the level of army surgeon. Never could we move him from the head of the class. What talents are wasted from lack of ambition!

he became so excited that he fairly wiped the floor with Locke, Condillac, and especially Rousseau and Voltaire. Knowing nothing of the lives, character, and behaviour of these philosophers, I often said to myself: "What can these gentlemen have done to Don Ventura that he should censure them so harshly?" And the worst of it was that, by dint of his abhorrence of the rationalists, he nearly made us sympathetic with him.

It would take too long and would be irrelevant to analyze here the states of conscience, which are not always sufficiently clear and definite, produced by such initiation into dogmatic psychology and elementary metaphysics. I will only remark that many things surprised me: first, that while in geometry, algebra, and physics every truth was founded firmly on reason and experience, in metaphysics and psychology these methods were looked upon with suspicion or conceded only secondary importance, the principle of authority and the allegations of emotion being adopted with blind confidence: second, that such transcendental and ultimate verities as the existence of God and the immortality of the soul, which ought to constitute unquestionable postulates of reason, like the axioms of mathematics, had to be skilfully defended with the subtilties and resources of the lawyer: third, that the same teacher of logic who prized so highly the application of the criteria of certainty to the problems of ordinary life, when he discussed later on the problems of metaphysics, took refuge without misgiving in the dicta—not always infallible and sometimes contradictory—of tradition and in the dogmatic affirmations of religious faith. Finally, I was exceedingly surprised by the multiplicity of schools of philosophy, an enlightening multiplicity which demonstrates either that human heads work differently, some regarding as error what others consider truth, or else that the sphere of religion and philosophy is almost entirely removed from the apprehension of the human understanding.

But we must give up these digressions, which are out

of place in an autobiography, and resume the thread of the story.

The session of 1868 proceeded and the examinations, from which I hoped to emerge moderately successfully, were approaching, when an unexpected event dashed my hopes.

One afternoon I was strolling along the road beside the town wall, not far from the Plaza de Santo Domingo, when I suddenly descried a wall which was freshly plastered and perfectly white. In those heroic times of my graphic mania, a clean surface, smooth and unadorned, constituted an irresistible temptation to pictorial efforts, and attracted me as a light attracts a night-flying moth. To see the wall, then, and to mark it with chalk and charcoal were matters of only a few moments. But that day the devil decided that I should forget myself so far as to portray some of my teachers, life size, and particularly my teacher of psychology and logic, Don Vicente Ventura, whose features, being exceedingly prominent, lent themselves admirably to caricature. With a pencil which was not at all flattering, I confess, I made conspicuous his one blind eye, his rather flat nose, and his broad, clean-shaven ecclesiastical [2] cheeks, which denounced from afar, by virtue of the intimate relation between idea and form, devotion to Thomism and loyalty to Don Carlos. When the sketch was finished, I stepped back from the wall to judge its effect. Several young people and some odd students happened to pass at that moment and the latter, seeing the figures and noticing the resemblance at once, burst out in chorus, "Look at the one-eyed Ventura!" And without there being any chance to avoid it, they began to throw stones at the caricature, accompanying their action with all sorts of broad jests and insults.

My evil star brought it about that just at this moment the original of the drawing should arrive and discover the ridiculous scene of the shooting in effigy. Overcome with

[2] In Spain, only priests and waiters were usually clean-shaven. (Translator's note.)

dread as I observed the fatal coincidence, I slipped away as inconspicuously as I could.

A very vigorous adherent of the principle of authority, Don Ventura burst out in righteous indignation when he saw himself mocked in effigy; he administered a severe reprimand to the boys and threatened to denounce them to the authorities if they did not tell him who was the author of the joke. He learned with sorrow that the author was the son of the doctor at Ayerbe, that is to say, the son of one of his most esteemed friends!

The exasperation of Don Ventura when he faced me in the classroom next day was inexpressible! He lost his habitual calm and broke out in a torrent of insulting epithets.

I was overwhelmed as I heard the formidable philippic. Stuttering with emotion, I did not manage to formulate a satisfactory excuse. I tried, however, to explain in timid phrases that it had not been my intention to annoy him in the slightest with that wretched caricature, which I had drawn thoughtlessly and as a mere pastime and especially that I had no part at all in the monstrous stoning. It was all in vain. Don Ventura maintained his implacable attitude. Choked with indignation and having no patience to listen to my excuses, he threw me violently out of the room.

When my father heard of what had happened he wrote to Don Ventura trying to placate him, but failed in the attempt. With great difficulty he secured my readmission to the class, where I was relegated, notwithstanding my sincere repentance, to the company of the irredeemable.

I was not disheartened in spite of everything. During the month of May I devoted myself earnestly to study, and the threshing-floors of Cáscaro and my good friends—the now famous Salillas among them—were witness to the long hours spent in poring over the "Psychology" of Monlau, in the task of extracting the essence hidden in the intricate concepts of *substance and accident, essence and existence, transcendence and immanence.* Many of the ideas eluded my weak comprehension, but I proposed to learn them by memory, according to the general custom, so as to pass the examination. I succeeded in this way, during the latter part of May, in having ready to be lighted a number of *fireworks,* that is to say a line of defence of words interconnected like a valencian string of rockets.[3]

Everything depended upon the examiner putting the priming at the beginning of the pyrotechnic contrivance and upon nervousness not wetting the powder for me. Unfortunately the powder got wet.

Hardly had I sat down upon the candidates' little stool when Don Ventura, whose dislike had not been diminshed in the least by my propriety and application during the preceeding months, raised himself majestically on the dais and delivered to the audience and to his fellow examiners these or similar words:

"Gentlemen: yielding to an indispensable duty of conscience, I must refrain from examining Señor Ramón. The hour of justice having arrived, I am anxious that no one be able to accuse me of being influenced by prejudice. Hence I entrust the examination to the proved rectitude of my colleagues in order that, free from all personal influence, they may grade as he deserves the most execrable pupil in the class, the one who, in his mad fury, did not hesitate to mock his master publicly and insolently, exposing the honourable gown of the professoriate to the jeers of scoundrels and the scoffing of the rabble."

I was struck dumb at hearing such hard words. I wished to withdraw from the examination and humbly indicated the fact to the Tribunal, stating: "I have studied the text attentively, but in the state in which I find myself I feel that I lack sufficient composure to answer the questions. Hence, I will abstain in turn, following the example of Don Ventura, and withdraw," "You do very wrongly," replied one of the examiners, with a sour and contemptuous look, "in distrusting the rectitude of the Tribunal, the impartiality and uprightness of which are far above your

[3] A series of rockets connected by a fuse.

malevolent insinuations. Sit down, and if you really know the subject you will be passed in spite of everything.''

I was so simple as to take the bait. To every question I answered something in accordance with the text, and, it appeared to me, considerably more than was required of my fellow students to obtain standing, especially considering the intense emotion which hindered me; but the examiners, as if in obedience to a countersign, led me into deep waters and metaphysical quibbles. And after more than half an hour of mortal anguish they finally upset me entirely. Then they dismissed me when they were satisfied.

Why should I go on? They wished to give me a lesson, and, in fact, I got one, profited by it, and never forgot it.

My state of mind was terrible! What was I to say when I went home? How was I to bear the just indignation of my parents? Yielding finally to a feeling of shame and discouragement, I made a foolish resolution, to go far, very far away, fleeing from my family and my masters. I desired ardently to live unknown among people whom I did not know and to be judged by my actions and not by my past record.

I communicated my design to some of my companions in misfortune. The project attracted them, and, with a combined capital of a few reals, we set out in search of adventures. Once on the way, we made various plans: some suggested that we should take positions as apprentices in some workshop or store; and finally some imprudently suggested that, until chance or Providence provided for our support, we should undertake pillaging and theft.

In the midst of these discussions and disputes we arrived at Vicien. Night was falling and, as we were beginning to be hungry, one of the party, called Javierre, had the salutary idea of visiting the local schoolmaster, who was his uncle, and was a good fellow and a strictly just man. Having agreed upon the plan, we solemnly entered the village, which we found bubbling with holiday excitement, with dancing and shouting in the square and maypoles in the streets. Pleased to see his nephew and his worthy companions, the very kindly master received us frankly and generously. We had a tremendous meal and slept ten hours at a stretch. Oh, the beautiful serenity of adolescence!

The next day, our spirits revived and our limbs rested, our ideas changed their direction, and the proposition most favoured by the group was the prudent one of returning to the abandoned fold. The sound sleep had scattered the romantic dreams, and the good digestion of the supper after dancing (in which some of the boys had engaged during the evening), had created in the company a healthy optimism which was propitious for repentance.

My specious sophistries were of no avail against those changeable fellows. They heard as if they were listening to rain, my supreme exhortations to honour their pledged word, and my enthusiastic evocation of the beautiful perspectives promised as by a free existence, rich in adventures. All preferred the certain flogging to the chimerical fortune, the dull past to the glorious future.

Finally I had to yield, and in the twilight of a sad day, which was to have been the first of an epic and triumphant exodus, I returned to Huesca, with the gloomy melancholy of the vanquished Don Quixote, with the bitter disillusion of Calicrates wounded before the beginning of the glorious battle.

CHAPTER XVII

Two inventions which caused me unspeakable amazement: the railway and photography. My initiation into anatomical studies. Macabre plundering. Memory of things and that of books. The dawn of love.

Observation of the attitude of the child confronted by the great inventions of science is bound to be instructive. This mental shock, besides revealing congenital intellectual tendencies, makes evident his true vocation.

The railway, which was then quite new in Spain, was the first of the things which astonished me. About the year 1865 or 1866 I had to travel to Huesca from the town of Sierra de Luna, where my family was living. I was accompanied by my paternal grandfather, a blonde highlander of seventy-five years, almost a giant, and remarkable for his agility and strength, who had been visiting his grandchildren and was returning to Larrés to settle down on the small holding whence he had come. As far as the first station (that of Almudévar), the journey was made on horseback. (It may be mentioned in parenthesis that I was then an expert equestrian.)

In order, however, to understand what follows it is desirable to explain an earlier event. Some months before, there happened, in the station at Tardienta, I think, a dreadful railway accident, in which many people were killed or injured.[1] It is unnecessary to say that the recollection of the catastrophe was continually in my mind, disturbing me very much. Thus, when the train appeared, I experienced mingled sensations of surprise and of fear. I should have been only too glad to return to the town. As a matter of fact, the appearance of the formidable machine was by no means reassuring. Imposing and threatening, there ad-

[1] This unfortunate occurrence took place on the very day when the line from Tardienta to Huesca was opened.

vanced before me a huge and hideous black mass of connecting rods, levers, gears, wheels, and cylinders. It seemed like an apocalyptical animal, a kind of colossal whale constructed of metal and coal. Its titanic lungs belched fire; its flanks emitted jets of boiling water; in its pantagruelic stomach burned mountains of soft coal; and the mighty snorts and screeches of the monster jarred my nerves and deafened my hearing. My unpleasant impression reached a climax when I caught sight of two stokers on the tender, covered with sweat and as black and ugly as demons, busy shovelling fuel into the wide fireplace. Then I looked at the tracks and my alarm increased still more as I observed the disproportion between the size of the locomotive and the flimsy, rusty, and disconnected rails, further weakened by rivets and mould marks. When the train passed over them, they seemed to tremble painfully, bending beneath the weight of the mass of metal. I lost my courage altogether.

Paralyzed with terror, I said to my grandfather: "I won't get onto it. I would rather walk." Without paying any attention to me, my colossal forebear stuffed me into a carriage whether I wished it or not. I burst into a cold sweat from terror. A smell of uncleanly and malodorous flesh offended my nostrils. I found myself jumbled together and, as it were, beseiged with portmanteaux, baskets, hens, rabbits, and coarse rustics and villagers.

Fortunately, my fright disappeared soon after the train started; the picture of the countryside served to distract my interest. Installed at the window, I watched with fascination the endless stream of gray villages, rachitic black poplar trees, telegraph poles, dusty carters, and yellow stubble fields. Finally, seeing how we progressed, I realized fully the advantages of that singular mode of locomotion. By the time we reached Vicien, my tranquility was completely restored.

Into this terror of the train, which will perhaps seem a little strange, there entered two elements—on the one hand, the unnerving recollection of the tragic derailment which had happened a few months before; and on the other, that instinctive and irresistible fear of the unknown when it presents itself with a terrifying aspect which is characteristic of children and savages. It is a case, as the psychologists say, of a primitive human instinct, which is modifiable, nevertheless, by the force of reason and of experience. Later on, when free from depressing emotions, I admired the wonderful creation of Watt and Stephenson and perceived all its enormous social import.

The impression produced by photography came later, I think in 1868, in the city of Huesca. It is true that a few years earlier I had come across an occasional itinerant photographer who practised the primitive method of Daguerre somewhat at a venture, equipped with a tent or booth, a box camera, and a huge lens. As is well known, the pictures were obtained on sheets of silver-plate, and exposures of several minutes were necessary. The daguerrotype, however, was quickly transformed into the admirable invention of photography on wet collodion. In this new method, the photogenic substances used were iodide and bromide of silver, spread over glass in a thin film. Twenty or thirty seconds in bright diffuse light were enough to produce a good plate. Portraiture was now quite possible. Besides, there had been secured the inestimable advantage of multiplication of the copies, since from one negative there could be made on paper as many positives as were desired.

Thanks to a friend who was on intimate terms with the photographers, I was able to penetrate the august mysteries of the dark room. The operators had equipped as a studio the vaults of the ruined church of Santa Teresa, near the station. It is superfluous to say with what lively curiosity I followed the manipulations necessary for the production of the photogenic layer and for the sensitization of the albumen-coated paper intended for the positive image.

All these operations astonished me unspeakably, but one of them, the development of the latent image by means of pyrogallic acid, positively stupified me. The thing seemed simply absurd. I did not understand how one could imagine that in the yellow film of silver bromide recently exposed in the camera there would be concealed the germ of a wonderful picture which was able to become visible under the action of a reducing agent. And then the extraordinary exactitude, the richness of detail in the photograph and that sort of analytical display with which the sun delights in reproducing the most difficult and complicated things, from the inextricable tangle of the forest to the simplest geometrical forms, without overlooking a leaf, a splinter, a cobble-stone, or a hair! And yet those unpretentious photographers performed such great miracles without the least emotion, entirely free and guiltless of all intellectual curiosity. From the answers to my eager inquiries, I gathered that the photographers were quite indifferent to the theory of the latent image. The important thing to them was to take many portraits and to take in still more money. They merely told me that the marvel of development was discovered by chance and that this most fortunate chance favoured first the famous Daguerre.

Accident! Still accident as the source of scientific knowledge right in the nineteenth century! Even now the world is full of enigmas, of hidden properties, of unknown forces. Consequently, science, far from being exhausted, invites everybody with inexhaustible veins of ore. Since, fortunately, we live in the dawn of man's knowledge of nature; since we are still surrounded with a dark cloud which is rent by human curiosity only here and there; and if, anyhow, scientific discovery is due no more to genius than to chance, then we can all be inventors. To do so, it is enough to play obstinately and persistently on one and the same number in this lottery. It is entirely a question of patience and perseverance.

While dreaming thus of photography, I cannot but record a sad reflection. What a great pity it is that we were born too soon! Those of us who are already old and are homesick for the golden days of childhood and adolescence,—what would we not give to possess to-day photographs of our boyhood and especially of our beloved parents in the full maturity of their strength and youth. What a delight it would be to gaze now upon the fresh beauty of our mothers, of whom, when we are over seventy, we recall so largely only the forms disfigured and faded by the sublime sacrifices of motherhood along with the injuries of time.

The summer of 1868 is associated in my memory with my initiation into anatomical studies.

I have already mentioned in an earlier chapter that throughout his career my father had been a skilful dissector and an ardent student of human anatomy. He used to say that his surgical successes were due more to the examination of bodies than to the reading of books.

It is important to recall, for the understanding of what follows, that those days were the golden age of artistic surgery, of precision and manual dexterity. The laurels won by Velpean and Nélaton in France, and by Argumosa and Toca in Spain were still fresh, and young physicians, expert in the subject matter of dissection, left the classrooms resolved to emulate with new operative feats the glory of such great masters. And it must be confessed that the undertaking was more difficult then than now. Formerly the heroes of the scalpel triumphed only when they had taken the trouble to scrutinize the most remote recesses of the organism.

At that time microbiology had not been born. Neither Pasteur nor Koch had made known their memorable discoveries, of such great value for the art of surgery. The guarantee of success depended then almost entirely upon the neatness and rapidity of the intervention and, especially, on the degree of clearness with which the complicated living mechanism was represented in the mind of the surgeon in the solemn moment of defloration of the virginity of the organs. The operator with a good foundation, educated in the amphitheatre, could foresee the course of the scalpel through the labyrinth of muscles, nerves, and bloodvessels with the same precision with which the artilleryman foresees the path of a projectile when he works out his equations.

After what I have just said, the reader will not find it surprising that my father decided to develop in me a taste for anatomy somewhat early. Relying, no doubt, upon the common aphorism, "He who strikes first strikes twice," he decided to inculcate the fundamental ideas of human osteology into his son immediately and vigorously.

"The study of the bones will seem to you dry and burdensome," he told me, "but you will find there, in compensation, an illuminating introduction to the knowledge of medicine. Almost all the commonplace doctors are such as a result of having had an insufficient elementary training. Internal pathology has not a little of the character of a contemplative science; like astronomy, it foresees eclipses which it cannot avoid; while external pathology, like a science of action and of control, ventures anything, changing and suspending at will the course of the organic processes. I should like to convince you thoroughly that your advantage and comfort depend upon being a surgeon rather than a physician. So far as the rewards are concerned there will always exist between the surgeon and the physician the same relation as between the diplomat and the military leader. He who triumphs by persuasion earns esteem not without envy, while he who triumphs in battle dominates even envy itself. Glory follows the latter quickly, the former may pursue it without ever overtaking it. It is a sad truth that man bows only before crimson glory! A little blood heightens the splendour of the success, stamping it with the hall-mark of popularity." [2]

By these arguments and others, which have escaped my memory, the scientific and social supremacy of surgery over medicine was demonstrated and the determination to initiate my anatomical education as soon as possible was justified. This was to commence with osteology, the basis

[2] Naturally, I am interpreting the substance of my father's reflections with full freedom as to the form, as I cannot remember his exact words after the lapse of fifty years.

and foundation of the whole medical edifice. Personally, I am convinced that the future dissector of Zaragoza, the professor of anatomy of Valencia, and the modest, but active and persistent investigator which I became later on were the fruit of these first lessons in osteology expounded in a barn. Perhaps it would interest the reader a little to know how we procured the scientific material for the new course of instruction. At the risk of being tedious, I shall enter into a few of the details.

To study the bones on paper, that is to say theoretically, would have been a didactic crime of which my master was incapable. He knew well enough that nature can be understood only by direct study, and that books are for the most part nothing but catalogues of names and classifications of facts.

But how to acquire the precious anatomical material? One moonlight night, master and pupil silently left the house and climbed the walls of the deserted cemetery. In a hollow in the plot of ground, we saw, tumbled in confusion and half buried in the grass, various skeletal remains derived, no doubt, from those wholesale exhumations or dispossessions which the living impose upon the dead from time to time under pretext of scarcity of space.

Deeply was I impressed by the finding and examination of these human relics! In the pallid gleam of the luminary of the night, those skulls half covered with fine gravel, and with irreverent thistles and nettles clambering over them seemed to me something like the hulk of a ship cast up on the shore. Restraining our emotions, and fearful of being surprised in our funereal task, we began the collection, picking out from that shoal of human shells the most complete and perfect and least weathered crania, ribs, pelves, and femurs.

As we climbed the wall of the cemetery, in leaving it, with our gruesome burden on our shoulders, fear made me hasten my steps. I seemed to hear in the rattling of the bones protests and imprecations from the defunct; each moment I feared that some ghost or sprite in suffering might intercept our steps and castigate the daring profaners of the dead.

Nothing happened, however. The shock of the supernatural, so appealing to and yet so feared by my morbid sensibilities, was entirely absent from that macabre episode, during which, to complete the commonplaceness of everything, there did not appear even the livid gleam of the will-o-the-wisp.

The checking-over and study of our gruesome spoils began at once. In this exodus across the stony human desert, our Moses was the monumental book of Lacaba, to which Cruveilhier was added later on; but it was really my father who led me to the promised land. Swept away by his irrepressible ardour in teaching, he devoted all his leisure hours to making me observe the most insignificant details in the conformation of the bones, developing in me, in the process, a quality little cultivated by the schoolmaster, namely the analytical sense, or rather the aptitude for noticing accidental differences and details in what is apparently ordinary and uniform. Nothing important remained unobserved in the internal or external morphology of each piece of the skeleton.

If things are looked at in their true light, my enthusiasm for anatomy formed one of the many evidences of my tendencies; for my artistic idiosyncracy, osteology constituted one more subject for pictures. Thirsting for the objective and the concrete, I seized eagerly the fragment of solid reality which it presented to me. Dry as they were, these facts were for me something more clear and definite than the dialectic of Don Ventura and the lucubrations of metaphysics. I felt a special delight, moreover, in taking apart and putting together again, piece by piece, the organic clock, and hoped some day to understand something of its intricate mechanism.

My father was greatly pleased as he observed my application. He saw at last that his son, although so much discredited by his mischievous escapades at the Institute of Huesca, was less idle and frivolous than he had believed; and in the optimistic forecast which every father likes to make of the future of his children, he thought that his offspring would not be reduced to vegetating sadly in a village. Why should he not eventually have to wear the honourable toga of the teacher?!

I remember still how great were his pride and pleasure—rather excusable in consideration of his double rôle of father and teacher—when he asked me to air my osteological knowledge before some professional friend, propounding such questions as: "What organs pass through the *sphenoidal foramen* and the *posterior foramen lacerum?* With what bones does the *orbital process* of the palatine articulate? At what point in the face is it possible to touch five bones with the point of a pin? How many muscles are inserted on the iliac crest and on the *linea aspera* of the femur?" These and a thousand other such questions I answered without hesitation, to the amusement of those present.

My father wondered, no doubt, that a boy who was considered—and such was the truth—to have a poor memory should have succeeded in retaining, after only two months of work, so many hundreds of difficult names and very many descriptive details regarding the connections of arteries, muscles, and nerves. "Bah!" he used to exclaim in a tone between severity and endearment, "your weakness of memory is the excuse with which you try to cover up your idleness." And in truth we were both in the right. As I have pointed out before, my memory was poor for miscellaneous words, for the dust of isolated concepts; but such mnemonic weakness was much diminished when the word and the idea were associated with some clear and vigorous visual perception. Besides, it is common knowledge, and is a fact well studied by the psychologists and educationists, that there is a tenacious association of verbal symbols and scientific concepts with the recollection of an object observed repeatedly and attentively.[3] The existence of exceptions seems doubtful; and I think that those who complain of an untrustworthy memory are mistaken in their method of learning. They read in books instead of reading in the objects themselves, they try to remember without taking the trouble to assimilate and reflect.

In order that my narrative may not be a mere record of monotonous antics of childhood or discussions of dry pedagogical problems, I am going to tell something now, by way of a sentimental interlude, about what the tender writer d'Amicis called in spiritual phraseology, the dawn of love, that is to say, that gentle and indefinable emotion which rises up in the early years of adolescence between young people of opposite sex.

I was approaching sixteen years of age at the time and lived in Ayerbe. My sisters Pabla and Jorja were in the habit of sewing and embroidering during the interminable winter evenings, sitting about the hearth with some intimate friends. One of the most regular attendants at our home circle was called Maria. She was fourteen and had sparkling black eyes, large and dreamy, glowing cheeks, light hazel hair, and those gentle curves of the body, perhaps somewhat overdeveloped for her age, which promised a splendid flowering in womanhood.

It was an insensible progression from curiosity to affection, passing through all the degrees of friendship. I soon noticed that meeting her was necessary for me, that her conversation gave me pleasure, that her absence disturbed and irritated me, and finally that I was seriously annoyed if I saw her accompanied by any other boy of the town. I delighted in showering a thousand attentions and trifling services upon her. I used to draw letters and ornamental

[3] Later on, when I read the modern books on psychology, I realized that I am what is called a visual. That which enters by my ears leaves but a fleeting trace, while that which comes through the eyes is impressed very firmly. Perhaps for this reason, in the field of art, I have been little interested in music or in oratory but, on the other hand, was always an ardent admirer of the play of light, of picturesque landscapes, and of all kinds of natural phenomena.

designs for her to embroider; presented her with sweetmeats and prints; lent her some book of poetry or sentimental novel, whenever I could; and praised her tastes, defending her opinion hotly in her little arguments with her friends. When the evening was over I rejoiced and took pride in accompanying her home.

My emotional condition, in sum, was one of sweet rapture, a sort of peaceful and ineffable beatitude, absolutely free from any sexual appetite. No improper thought ever crossed my mind. It is true that, although I was sixteen, the development of my sexual consciousness was somewhat retarded, as is usually the case in young people devoted to physical exercise.

It is unnecessary to say that I never went so far as to make an explicit declaration. Neither did I ever know for certain whether I succeeded in interesting her. Fear and timidity prevented me from finding out. Everyone knows that these incipient affections, which are essentially platonic, are afraid of verbal expression. It is such a tremendously serious thing to say "I love you!" For nothing in the world would I have risked so grave a confidence. Besides, a declaration involves the danger of a distressing outcome; perhaps it would bring about painful disillusionment. Restraint and indecision are preferable—they at least encourage hope!

Rarely does the dawn of love change into the noon of deep feeling and less often into satisfied passion. From puberty to young womanhood the girl is not disturbed by any serious occurrence; tranquil in her home, her emotional stability hardly involves any sacrifice; her life as a woman, for that matter, may follow the same smooth course. Quite the opposite is the case of the youth; the period between the ages of sixteen and twenty-one is associated with profound intellectual and emotional crises. He has to make a radical change in his environment, to go to the city to develop his career and carve out a future for himself; in consequence, his sensibilities are besieged by all sorts of temptations and incentives. How can one wonder that distractions and forgetfulness destroy affections which were established early!

That is what happened in my case; not because I was assailed by other loves, but rather through the dampening effect of absence. By degrees the image of the lovely girl faded from my memory. Besides, I seldom revisited Ayerbe after that time. I always liked to see her and talk to her, but I noticed that she had become too much of a woman. At last a certain strapping youth of the town, less timid and reserved than I, approached her parents and married her. To-day, she is a happy mother with many children and grandchildren.

CHAPTER XVIII

The September Revolution in Ayerbe. Destruction of the bells. The hatred of the town for the rural police. My professors of physics, mathematics, etc. I finally become reconciled to geometry and algebra, although too late. I obtain my bachelor's degree.

At the end of that summer we were surprised by the famous September revolution, an event which was to have such a great effect upon the intellectual and political life of Spain. Ayerbe, a town of six hundred inhabitants, known throughout upper Aragon for the liberalism of its people, could not remain indifferent to the national uprising. Thus, as soon as the telegraph brought the news of the battle of Alcolea, my compatriots rose also, proclaiming the "Progressive" creed and creating the indispensable *Junta revolucionaria,*[1] in imitation of the capitals.

I remember that it happened one beautiful autumn morning. From an early hour, the place lost its peaceful appearance; a strange disquietude seemed to take possession of the inhabitants, who formed groups in the square, discussing excitedly the bulletins from Huesca and Zaragoza. Incendiary revolutionary proclamations were read publicly and enthusiastic cheers were heard for Serrano, for Topete, and above all for Prim.[2]

Without understanding the significance of these events, I saw with surprise that, contrary to custom, the Civil Guards remained in their quarters, without interfering with the rioters, and that the rural police (*Guardia rural*), the terror of the peasantry, had disappeared, abandoning their equipment and uniforms, according to report. From nowhere, as if in obedience to a prearranged signal, there appeared upon all sides peasants armed with weapons of

1 Revolutionary committee. (Translator's note.)

2 Generals leading the revolution. (Translator's note.)

every sort and even with sickles and poniards. Certain individuals, who seemed to be in the secret of events, hurriedly organized from these people a batallion of volunteers, from the ranks of which was selected a garrison or permanent guard, which was installed in the palace of the Marquises of Ayerbe. In the window of the garrison company there blazed a red flag, with no emblem or coat of arms. Companies of townspeople, to which we boys and youths attached ourselves, marched through the streets to the strains of the municipal band, letting off steam with shouts of "Long live liberty! Down with the Bourbons! Death to the Conservatives!" With the fiery cadences of the hymn of Riego tirelessly played by the afore-mentioned band, there alternated wild cheers for the revolutionary leaders. A group of rebels tore down the portrait of Isabel II from the schools and burned it in the square amid the mockery and insults of the excited populace.

Then there took place an event which I have never been able to understand. In obedience to a certain calamitous decree of the provincial Revolutionary Junta, which ordered "that all the bells except those of the clocks, should be dismounted and sent to the National Mint," the revolutionary committee of Ayerbe took down the beautiful bells of the church and reduced them to fragments.

I confess that, notwithstanding my sympathy with the liberal movement and my taking as much satisfaction as anyone in these patriotic tumults, that act of useless vandalism brought me a shadow of regret. What positive benefit did the town receive from sending its bells to Madrid to be coined into a few handsful of small change? None whatever.

I was pained, especially, by the lack of artistic feeling in the town. How did the destroyers of those bells fail to realize that they were breaking up at the same time a living and very intimate part of their being, that they were renouncing cherished memories, that they were disowning things which could never be forgotten?

I do not know whether the pieces of bronze reached

Madrid, but I remember well that in a short time other bells had to be bought.

A few days after the events which I have been relating, the batallion of militia was organized more thoroughly, making use for this purpose of the stores of the Rural police and of a sufficient number of rifles which were contributed by ardent patriots. The moving spirits of that popular militia were Puego, Fontana, Nivela, and other old and consistent Progressives, whose democratic opinions had brought them deportations and persecutions without number in the ominous times of González Brabo.[3] It was due to these noble-minded patricians, as prudent as they were disinterested, that during the excitement and disorder of the early days there did not occur a single outrage; the members of the improvised militia gave vent to their hatred for reaction by devoting their attention to spectacular military manoeuvres and performing guard duty, organizing reserve corps, parading, and exercising.

Naturally, these parades and exercises stimulated our boyish enthusiasm, especially the manoeuvres of the squadron of sappers, in which a certain carpenter, an idealistic radical nicknamed *Carretillas,*[4] was conspicuous for his gallant and martial bearing. He had once been a member of the national militia, and had kept his brilliant tunic and huge helmet spotless so as to display them in the parades. His veteran's air and the brightly coloured uniform were objects of general admiration and envy. As was to be expected, the *Morrion*[5] of Carretillas took the fancy of the boys, who decided also to cap themselves with the venerable Progressive symbol; and so in a short time (I do not know upon whose initiative) most of us youngsters appeared decked out in a sort of high *ros,*[6] with no visor, a crown of red cloth, a cockade of the national colours, and dangling

[3] González Brabo, 1811–1871. Political leader in the reign of Isabel II and head of her government immediately preceding her deposition in 1868. (Translator's note.)

[4] "Wheelbarrows" or "push-carts."

[5] High military cap.

[6] Spanish shako.

ribbons upon which was blazoned the phrase "Long live Liberty!"

In Ayerbe, as in all the towns of Spain, the few cultured men who directed the revolutionary movement perhaps knew what it meant; but the people at large, and especially the proletariat understood nothing about its aims and scope. Almost everybody hoped that liberty would provide something which could be turned into an amelioration of the material conditions of life. It would be easy to recall events and remarks which prove the existence of this communistic desire, which is always latent in the hearts of the disinherited.

Here is a song which was very popular in Ayerbe at that time, and of which the clumsy lines are significant enough:

> The rural police thought
> that there would never end
> the collecting of eight reals [7]
> without knowing whence they came.

The following story, told to me by a friend in Ayerbe,[8] is also most eloquent. He asked one of the most enthusiastic patriots, hoarse with shouting, "Down with the Bourbons!"—"Do you know who the Bourbons are?" The man replied with an air of deep conviction, "What a question! The rural police of course!"

Why this hatred of the peasantry for the protectors of property? It is easily guessed. The rural police were detested on account of the excessive zeal with which they protected the interests of the landed bourgeoisie. These police molested and annoyed the poor villagers for the most insignificant reasons, imprisoning them or punishing them with heavy fines, without stopping to distinguish between

[7] The daily pay of the rural police—about 40 cents of American money—enough to live pretty well at that time, labourers earning about 4 reals. (Translator's note.)

[8] Many of these notes I owe to the kidness of my esteemed friend and fellow-student, Dr. Ricardo Monreal, the distinguished physician of Ayerbe, who has been so good as to supplement my hazy reminiscences with the rich stock of his recollections.

the professional thief and the poor fellow, goaded by misery, who gathered esparto grass in the thicket to make ropes for binding sheaves, or gathered a small load of whins and rosemary, or grazed a cow near the uncertain boundaries of an estate; trivial abuses which were generally practised and were mutually tolerated by all concerned as a venerable relic of patriarchal communism. Even we children felt this hatred for the brownish gray uniforms. Whenever they caught us in the act of scaling a wall or climbing a tree, even though it was in winter, the rural police either administered a terrific beating or entered a formal complaint, which was followed by the corresponding fine.

In spite of the enthusiasts for the so-called modern liberties and the stuck-up and hollow champions of individualism, who persist in ignoring the psychological abyss which separates the intellectual classes from the unhappy slaves of manual labour, the latter will always believe that liberty is synonymous with well-being. In vain is the day-labourer told that these two words signify different things, that liberty is only an instrument for the conquest of material happiness, which is not the exclusive heritage of the powerful; that if unemployment and misery come in spite of the free exercise of his faculties, he should resign himself to his fate, trusting in Providence and in the hope of a better life. To the poor, all these arguments are simple twaddle, if not murderous mockery.

Before terminating the narrative of my studies for the bachelor's degree, I must say a few words about my attitude towards such important sciences as physics, mathematics (geometry, trigonometry, and algebra), and natural history.

Whether it was that my head had become weary of frivolity and irregular behaviour and was beginning to settle down, or that the final courses of my secondary education fitted in better than Greek and Latin with my tastes and inclinations, it is certain that I paid more attention to them, especially to physics, chemistry, and natural history.

The teacher of the elementary course in physics and chemistry was Don Serafín Casas, a friend and fellow-student of my father. We liked his simple and clear way of expounding his subject, and I remember that, in consideration of our mathematical ignorance, he simplified greatly the lessons in equations and integrals. On the other hand, every law and every important property were demonstrated by conclusive experiments, which were for our ingenuous curiosity feats of supreme magic. With fascination and with attention ever more wide awake, we saw the strange and impressive apparatus set up on the table, especially the formidable electric machinery which was then the fashion.

I have already said how interesting I found physics, the science of miracles. Optics, electricity, and magnetism (which then fell into the general category of *imponderable* fluids), with their marvelous phenomena, held me spell-bound. Of course, the ideas acquired at that time were pretty elementary.

So carried away was I by my growing interest that, after I had already finished my course (1875 and 1877), I undertook to read the admirable Medical Physics of Wund and the Physiological Optics of the great Helmholtz. Such studies, besides satisfying imperative tendencies of my spirit, were necessary for me in order that I might master the theories of vision and of the microscope. In Wund's treatise, I studied with exceptional interest the doctrine of wave motions in the ether, a basic foundation of modern physics. As a matter of fact, I then missed very much a knowledge of mathematics, which I ought to have learned when I had the chance in the Institute at Huesca.

I had to do then what is necessary for all students who too late repent and become conscious of their ignorance. What was not assimilated at the right time and by degrees had to be acquired later on by unaided study, with all the inconveniences of haste and the lack of guidance. In my feverish and determined attack upon the science of numbers, I reached the point of immersing myself in differential and integral calculus, and with some humiliation, I found myself obliged to strengthen the foundations of my knowledge by returning to those modest and much thumbed manuals of geometry and trigonometry which I had read so carelessly in Huesca.

Unfortunately, the medical man has very few occasions for the use of calculus, except in some problems of the occulist and some questions of hydraulics (the determination of aberrations of refraction in the eye, the physical study of the circulation of the blood, etc.). Being essentially descriptive, the biological sciences deal almost exclusively with the qualitative, which escapes all quantitative determination. And only what is cultivated assiduously is known well.

However, the entire blame for ignorance of mathematics should not be laid upon the heedlessness or the inability of the pupils of the Institute. Some of the responsibility rests upon the masters. Many of these are such creatures of habit that they seem to be determined to instill into their pupils that the conceptions of geomery and algebra are merely useless speculations of idle geniuses, with no practical interest other than some vulgar applications to mercantile book-keeping, surveying, and architecture. Lacking interest themselves, they could not inspire their hearers. From these cold discourses, heart and enthusiasm were always absent.

In actual fact, I had no idea of the enormous importance of the science of calculus until I was twenty-three or twenty-four years old. I remember well how it came about. I wished to read the famous works of Laplace and, desiring to prepare myself to understand them, I decided, wisely, to consult some non-technical books on astronomy—among others, those of Flammarión which are so well known and popular and some by J. Fabre, the great observer of insects.

I liked the books of Flammarión very much, but they did not fully satisfy my thirst for understanding. They are infused with overflowing lyricism, unrestrained emotion, pompous descriptions, but few demonstrations. On the other hand the little manual of Fabre called "Le Ciel" was a brilliant revelation to me. Here also rhetoric blooms, used with discretion and restraint (it is well known that the "Prince of the Insects" was a sublime poet); but the phrases do not smother the ideas. In every page of the book there throbs the eager effort to initiate the reader into the essentials of geometrical methods, with the aid of which the tremendous laws of cosmography and astronomy were discovered.[9]

There, by that little book, which begins with the definition of a triangle and ends with the demonstration of the most sublime triumphs of astronomy, I was reconciled at last to the disdained geometry and the detested trigonometry. There I discovered with astonishment that the "science of space," with the aid of some instruments and the tracing of a few lines on paper, had successfully performed such feats as measuring the size and determining the exact shape of the earth, ascertaining the distance and the bulk of the moon, as well as those of the sun, determining the form of the orbits of the planets, etc. Also, coming down to more modest undertakings, it enabled us to find out the height and the breadth of a tower or of a mountain without climbing them, to ascertain the width of a river without fording it, to determine the position of a ship in mid ocean, etc., etc. In particular, the highly ingenious geometrical demonstration of the distance of the sun made by Hipparchus of Samos more than two thousand years ago filled me with undiluted admiration. It is true that trigonometry today provides us with much neater and more exact methods for the solution of this and other tremendous problems, but it is only fair to recognize that the Greek astronomer in

[9] Because of Fabre's marvellous skill in initiating young people to the study of the sciences, the minister Duruy, who knew him well, wished to appoint him tutor to the Prince Imperial. The "Hermit of Sérignan," however, declined, for he loved passionately life in the country and hated the formality and pretence surrounding the courtier.

revealing to us the sublime power of geometry, was one of those who opened up the way.

In conclusion, I came to realize a little late that the truths of mathematics, which dry and routine-ridden pedagogues consider—not without a certain aristocratic presumption—as a deductive structure (a chain of truths of which the first link grows out of the nature of the mind) erected *a priori,* independently of, and even with disdain for experience, are actually, on the contrary, inescapable truths imposed upon us by the objective world, something like the quintessence of the concepts derived from perception and scrupulously purified of non-essentials so that logical reasoning can manipulate them quickly and conveniently. Once I had recognized this, it no longer surprised me that the axioms and formulae of geometry and algebra correspond so exactly to external reality since, in the final analysis, they are derived from that reality.

But such illuminating truths penetrated my mind rather tardily, as has been said, when the fruit could no longer be copious or fertile. The whole universe, as well in the realm of the infinitely great as in the secrets of the infinitely little, is constructed in accordance with the formulae of a sage geometry and an admirable system of dynamics. But why had no teacher told me this though it is common and elementary knowledge?

Natural history I liked almost as much as physics, but it satisfied my intellectual appetite only imperfectly. I, who was enraptured with the contemplation of a bird's nest, who went into ecstasies over the flashing liveries of the beetles and the brilliant colour combinations of the butterflies and the birds, felt an absolute terror when I heard the strange and interminable nomenclature of animals and plants and the heavy downpour of classification.

Somewhat later, about the year 1874 or 1875, I became acquainted with the fundamental works of Lamarck, Spencer, and Darwin, and was able to taste the fruitful and elegant, though often inacceptable or exaggerated biogenetic hypotheses of Haeckel, the spirited professor of

Jena. Actually, the first refutation of Darwin's famous book, "The Origin of Species," which came into my hands was written by Cánovas del Castillo! It consisted of a certain open forum lecture, as eloquently written as it was weakly documented. It was sent to me from Madrid by one of the ardent admirers of the distinguished politician.

As a final conclusion to the story of the eventful period of my study for the baccalaureate, I may be permitted to transcribe here a few paragraphs from an article by Dr. R. Salillas, written upon the occasion of one of my modest academic triumphs. I have already mentioned that the first anthropological criminologist of Spain was one of my friends and classmates. He belonged to the congregation of the well-behaved and studious boys, but occasionally his natural restlessness and the spirit of adventure led him to take part in our escapades. In the following reflections, which were published many years ago in *El Liberal,* he sets down in addition some reminiscences which are not recorded in the present book.

REFLECTIONS OF DR. R. SALILLAS

The Island of Cajal.—The announcement of the publication of the autobiography of the distinguished histologist recalls to me vividly the period when I knew him.

And I remember it by a peculiar detail.

The boy of that time, of the time when we were in the second year of our course in the humanities (as it was formerly called) in the Institute at Huesca was not inconspicuous, unknown, or one of the crowd.

He had a personality which, if justly considered, corresponds with what can already be called his historical personality.

The panegyrists of Cajal, all of them famous, recognize that he has not had any master; that he has developed himself alone; that what he is is a manifestation of his own individual powers, of his strong will, and of his outstanding intellect.

He had no masters—nor did he want any, I would add.

That boy of surly appearance, not very sociable, who kept to himself whenever he could and who was always kept to himself by his attitude of reflective concentration, was to be classified among those characters which, according to Juan Huarte—another student of the University of Huesca—are called by the Italians *capricious* from their resemblance to the goats (*capra*), which live alone in the hills.

Cajal, at the period when I knew him, was not the pupil of any professor—and they treated him accordingly more than once!

The institute did not attract him with any appeal to his curiosity or any mental stimulus.

He went to classes, when he did go, as a result of self-conquest.

His inclination was very different.

When he followed his natural tendencies, he went out into the country, usually alone, sometimes with a very few friends, who followed but did not understand him; and whether his expeditions were long or short he always felt it irksome to have to return.

The first time that I earned a confidence from Cajal was when he read me a novel which he was writing and illustrating.

I do not know whether I admired him more as novelist or as artist.

That novel, for which at the time I had no comparisons, I should now classify among the *robinsonianas*:—a shipwreck, the escape on a log, the landing on a desert island, and the continuation of the adventure there, with the discovery of the flora, the fauna, and the savage inhabitants.

All this would not be anything extraordinary in the history of an autobiographer if one took into consideration that the making of verses and the writing of stories, dreaming, and drawing figures, even although much better than is generally the case, is, as Cajal himself has said, a kind of measles, an eruptive fever.

The important point is that the novel corresponds with the activities of its author, and that those activities, consistently manifested, lead to a valuable result.

Cajal was a novelist of action. He read us his novel and we acted it out together more than once.

The rushing water of an unimportant river, less important even than the Manzanares,[10] constituted the scene of the shipwreck.

In the little thickets of the Isuela, which is the stream referred to, at the hour of swimming there were seen some savages, smeared with mud from the bank, jumping and climbing about courageously and discharging the arrows from their bows with a certain amount of skill.

It was not a game, it was a dramatic performance.

Cajal believed and made us believe in the possibility of his novel being realized in actual life.

Little by little the novel, infiltering into our spirits and enslaving them, assumed the appearance of practicability, and then, with full cognizance of the dangers through which we should have to pass, the struggles with the elements, with wild beasts, and with men, we decided to undertake the adventure, but upon one determining condition—if we failed in our examinations, if we lost our year.

[10] The Manzanares is a small river which flows past the city of Madrid. (Translator's note.)

There were three of us.[11] I was the only one not compromised by the condition; but, full of anxiety, I took part in the preparations for the expedition, accompanied the participants when they set out, watched them go, and returned home filled with such distress as I do not remember experiencing on any other occasion.

Unable to conceal my feelings, I burst into a flood of tears of desperation, and alarmed my parents so much that I had to tell them between my sobs what had happened to my friends. My parents laughed while they heard it.

They came back, and their return contributed largely to the ultimate failure of the novel in real life.

But later, after many years during which I heard nothing of my classmate, when I learned what he was doing, when people were extolling his discoveries, I returned to my belief, and to a firm belief, that between that novel of "robinsonian" character and the reality of the scientific discoveries there had not been even a deviation from the plot.

Ganivet has said that the important thing is to keep the fire burning in the forge, and Cajal has said that the important thing is to have a guiding hypothesis. The important thing is to believe and to be able.

Cajal continued to believe in his island. He set sail, he found his bearings, and he arrived victoriously.

The island did exist!

In the central nervous organs, in the spinal cord and in the brain, is found in worth-while fashion the Island of Cajal.

[11] He refers to our running away to Zaragoza. Actually there were four members of the expedition, naturally four of the worst in the class.

CHAPTER XIX

I begin my medical training in Zaragoza. The Ebro and its poplar-lined promenades. My professors in the introductory course; Ballarín, Guallart, and Solano. I develop an interest in dissection under the tutelage of my father.

When I had completed the requirements for the bachelor's degree and gone through the ceremony of graduation, my father, more determined than ever to make a Galen of his son, accompanied me to Zaragoza and enrolled me in the course of the preparatory year. In order, moreover, that I should not be distracted by dissipation and bad company, he installed me as an attendant in the establishment of Don Mariano Bailo, a fellow countryman who was a friend and classmate of his, and who enjoyed an excellent reputation as a surgeon and was a man of strict principles.

The pleasure of seeing myself in a new city, and one which was populous and ennobled by great historical associations, was soon followed by sad disappointment. My friends from Huesca, the merry comrades of my glories and hardships, received me with the utmost indifference. Having gone ahead one or two years in their course, they had contracted new friendships, and for my desires to renew our former association they showed a disdain which cut me to the quick. It was my first disillusionment regarding friendship. For such coldness the blame was entirely my own. They had not severed themselves from me; it was I who had severed myself from them by being so backward in my course.

I consoled myself then in the way that I have always been in the habit of doing, as I have explained repeatedly, namely by bathing my soul in nature. The copious Ebro and its verdant and shady promenades [1] were there, offer-

[1] *Alamedas.* Promenades lined with black poplar trees. (Translator's note.)

ing a cheerful assuager to my disillusionment and promising me gentle delights in place of the vain effusions of companionship.

For one who is capable of appreciating its enchantment, the country is the sovereign soother of emotions, the unreplacable commutator of thoughts. "What do a blue sky and luxuriant vegetation add to our souls?" someone has asked. Nothing, in truth, for the proud man, the egotist, who, fed with his own ideas, lives always in himself; but much, very much for him who knows how to open his senses to the glories of the sunshine and the beauties of the countryside.

Besides these feelings, my artistic impulses and my budding interest in natural history also drew me to the picturesque banks of the Ebro at the time of which I am speaking. Among my irresistible tendencies is an extravagant desire to determine the courses of rivers and to discover their sources and tributaries, and the fact that this was the first river of considerable size which I had seen excited this hydrological curiosity in the highest degree. "Whence comes this formidable stream of water, I thought, the waves of which, after lapping the walls of the Pilar [2] quietly and gently seem to sing heroic hymns as they burst obstreperously through the stone bridge?"

Drawn by curiosity, I followed it upstream more than once as far as Alagón; at other times I went downstream to near Pina. I was stimulated also in my trips along the banks by the romantic hope of finding sylvan glades and idyllic wild-flower beds unprofaned by the footsteps of man.

But let us not wander from our subject. I expect that the reader will have had enough of these tiresome digressions, and it is time for me to tell something about my professors. These were the veteran Don Florencio Ballarín,

[2] The Cathedral of the *Virgen del Pilar*.—The great, ornate, new cathedral of Zaragoza, started in 1686 by Herrera. It contains the sacred pillar upon which the Virgin is supposed to have descended from heaven in 40 A.D.—"an event so strongly attested that Diego de Astorga, primate of Spain, on 17th. August 1720, excommunicated all who even questioned it." (Translator's note.)

professor of natural history; Don Marcelo Guallart, who taught physics, and Don Bruno Solano, an assistant temporarily charged with secondary instruction in chemistry.

I remember little about Don Marcelo Guallart. All I can say is that his lessons, learned and at the same time unpretentious, were rather monotonous, and that his class, which was not largely attended (it must not be forgotten that the *Gloriosa*[3] was still recent), merely filled the days full of spectacular and theatrical experiments.

My recollections of Ballarín and Solano stand out much more clearly and brightly, both of them having been masters who were worthy in every way of being remembered with enthusiasm.

Old Don Florencio Ballarín, a contemporary of Ferdinand VII, by whom he was persecuted for liberalism and also for disrespect to the august person of the monarch, was a learned teacher, endowed with a flexible imagination and a forceful diction. He was the first person whom I heard defend with true conviction the necessity of teaching objectively and with experiment, which is to-day so much talked about and so little practiced. He talked with the example before him, and thus his lessons in zoology and mineralogy were highly instructive to us, since they were given in the museum and in the botanical garden respectively.

What a pity it was that we did not come into the hands of Don Florencio when he was younger, when his powers were at their height! At the time to which we are referring, he was already seventy years old and suffered from that irritability and uncertainty of temper which is a distressing and almost inevitable defect of old age. I remember that in his corrections and punishments he often suffered from a lack of calmness and consideration. Errors in speech, furtive smiles, momentary distractions sufficed to put him beside himself; and filled with anger, he would overwhelm us with reproaches.

[3] The September revolution (1868).

One day he asked me to describe the arteries of the superior limbs. In timid and poorly-chosen words I replied, among other things, "that the brachial artery extends the length of the arm." "But good gracious," he interrupted indignantly, "*the length of!* One would think that you were a tailor taking the measure for sleeves!"

One of his excellent didactic methods which has been almost entirely abandoned nowadays, was from time to time to select a certain principle for discussion and to assign the defense of it to one student, whom his classmates questioned. When it came to my turn to be the questioner, I was overcome with nervousness. The subject was the mechanism of haematosis. The lecturer was my good friend Doctor Senac, now a learned army surgeon,[4] one of many whose great ability has been obscured by lack of ambition, who gave a fine discourse with ease and confidence. He defended the view, then much in vogue, that the venous blood was noxious to the organism on account of the carbon dioxide accumulated in it, of which it had to get rid in the lung. I, who had drunk from the same springs (Beclard's *Physiology*), asked him, or meant to ask, if it was not more probable that the harm was not in the excess of carbon dioxide, which is an entirely inoffensive gas, but rather in the absence of oxygen, which has been consumed in the capillaries in connection with the respiration of the tissues.

But this simple question was expressed with such clumsy and roundabout phraseology, and with such hesitancy and stammering that Ballarín, unable to endure me, ordered me harshly to be quiet, adding that I still preserved my rusticity. I was so simple that I did not understand the phrase nor, consequently, the mortifying intention.

Apart from these outbursts, however, Ballarín was a master whom we respected and venerated. Moreover, we were grateful to him because from time to time he graciously allowed us a day's holiday, and for a reason

[4] He died a few years ago. (Note in 3rd edition, 1923.)

which the reader would certainly have difficulty in guessing.

It was a matter of course! Whenever he arrived in the lecture room in a bad humour, with sunken jaws and an air of contrariety—and began the day's work mumbling thickly and unintelligibly the word, "Seño . . . res," we all mechanically picked up our hats and left the classroom, without any objection from the professor, who merely deplored his own absent-mindedness. The fact was that the good Don Florencio had left his teeth at home! Was this convenient forgetfulness, occurring in such a case of senile decay, voluntary or involuntary? That is a question which we were never able to settle.

It is a well-known fact that teachers, even those least subservient to routine, repeat phonographically every session certain phrases and examples which the students know and expect at definite places. This was so in the case of Ballarín, and among the stereotyped examples there was one famous one, which no student can have forgotten, to which he always referred when treating of the hardness of minerals.

"Gentlemen," he used to say, "the diamond corresponds with the number 7 in the scale of hardness; it is, then, the hardest substance known; but we must keep in mind that its resistance to scratching does not imply that it cannot be fractured. In fact the diamond itself is regrettably brittle. Here you have unimpeachable evidence of this lamentable property." And at that moment he would stretch out his hand over the desk to display a sparkling solitaire, marred by a star-shaped fracture in its centre. Then he would proceed to tell how, in a certain argument—I do not know whether scientific or political—being unable to persuade his opponent, he struck him a formidable blow on the head. The skull of his adversary however, was one of the things which should be rated 8 in the scale of hardness since it broke the precious diamond into a thousand pieces. At this point a general outburst of laughter was part of the ritual, which did not in the least disturb the equanimity of the good Ballarín.

Very different was the intellectual and didactic temperament of Don Bruno Solano. Eloquent, fiery, affable, not exempt from severity upon occasion, he made his class a temple where we heard, enraptured, the picturesque and interesting story of the loves and hates of different substances: the adventures of oxygen, a kind of Don Juan, a passionate and irresistible conqueror of the virginity of elements; the revenges of hydrogen, a jealous lover responsible for so much molecular widowhood; and the intrigues and mediations of heat and electricity, centenarian duennas capable of upsetting and divorcing even the closest and most stable molecular matrimonial bonds. Apart from these poetic extravagances which he did not abuse, however, Solano was a great teacher.

What pleasant, yea, angelic speech was his! What supreme skill he had in making comprehensible and delightful, by means of illuminating comparisons, the most difficult points or the most uninteresting and abstruse ideas! In this respect he resembled greatly the celebrated English physicist Tyndall, the great Echegaray, and the incomparable popularizer, A. Fabre.

I confess that when I visit Zaragoza, one of the things which sadden me most is the absence of my prematurely lost colleague.[5] His daily chats in the *Café Suizo,* where his friends and admirers met together, were a spiritual feast. His popularity was as great as it deserved to be. What has since come to be called *university extension* was one of many things which he initiated. He never kept his science for the privileged few who were officially enrolled, but spread it among the great public, creating bonds of interest and appreciation between the professor's chair and the workshop, between the laboratory and the factory. He was convinced that science should be linked up with life, to inspire and guide it. The exquisite sensibilities of artist and thinker, with which he was endowed, enabled him to perceive excellences even in the commonest things.

[5] Solano died young as the result of a surgical operation.

But Solano possessed in addition a magnificent literary gift. He was a writer who hardly wished to write! Testimony of his brilliant literary powers is given by those precious, and, alas, rare scientific and popular articles, by notes in the daily papers of Zaragoza, and especially by his most beautiful inaugural discourse upon the new directions of modern chemistry.

Returning, however, to my studies, I must state that, thanks to such splendid masters, I progressed fairly well, that is to say as well as was possible, in consideration of my still unripe judgment and my continual artistic divagations. Only once did I return to my old follies.

A certain chum from Huesca, called Herrera, an intelligent and rather quarrelsome fellow (blind in one eye as a result of one of his escapades), and a great admirer of my skill with the sling, begged me urgently to forget natural history for a day and to lend him my support in an encounter which was to take place in the threshing-floors of the suburb of La Magdalena, between students and garbage-pickers, or between "weaklings" and "noise-makers."

I had the weakness to listen to him and to fall into temptation. My sling did its duty. I cracked the crowns of a number of the enemy and contributed to the triumph of the "young gentlemen," in spite of the last minute reinforcements which the garbage-pickers received from their compatriots of the parish of San Pablo. Not feeling any elation in the victory, and being satiated with such childish behavior, I had the firmness not to backslide again. Everything has its own time, and that of childishness had passed. I was then nearly seventeen years old. My relative application permitted me to complete the preparatory course without mishap and to register in the first year of Medicine.

About that period (I think it was in 1870), my family moved to Zaragoza. My father, being anxious to provide a career for his sons, to supervise them from near at hand, and to free himself finally from the annoyances of rural medical practice, wrote certain examinations for physicians of the Provincial Medical Service.[6] Having secured an appointment he took up his residence in the Aragonese capital, where, soon after his arrival, the learned clinician Don Genaro Casas, who had been a fellow student and was now Dean of the Faculty of Medicine, gave him a temporary professorship of dissection.

Knowing my father's enthusiasm for anatomy and his pronounced vocation for teaching, the reader will easily guess the zeal and ardour which he put into the performance of his duties and his determination to make of his son a skilled dissector.

Here we were, then, both immersed in the subject. And with such a master who could shirk? Three years passed over us in that humble dissecting room, hidden away in the garden of the old hospital of Santa Engracia, as we took apart piece by piece the intricate mechanism of muscles, nerves, and blood vessels and checked up all the fine things that the anatomists told us. Before the imposing anatomical slab,[7] both brain and stomach protested at the beginning; but they soon became accustomed to it. Henceforth, I saw in the cadaver, not death, with its train of gloomy suggestions, but the marvellous workmanship of life.

As the method demands, in order not to get lost in the inextricable thicket of vessels and nerves, we used to work with the books open before us, guided by Cruveilhier and by Sappey. Our enthusiasm increased in proportion to the difficulties, and with a lavish expenditure of time (my father had then few patients) we devoted to our task all the leisure which was left to us by his practice, in my father's case, and by the study of other subjects in mine. Tireless himself, he would not allow fatigue in those about him.

Great was my profit from such a master and such a mode of learning; there is no teacher more zealous than he who studies in order to instruct. My pencil, which was formerly the cause of so much bitterness, at last found

[6] Physicians paid by the Government to serve in clinics for the poor. (Translator's note.)

[7] The marble top of the dissecting table.

grace in the eyes of my father, who now delighted in having me sketch whatever anatomical structures were revealed. What a satisfaction it was when, by dint of patience, we succeeded in freeing from its imbedding fat the diminutive ophthalmic ganglion with its delicate nerve rootlets, or examined in its hiding-place the complicated sphenopalatine ganglionic plexus, or when, at last, we triumphantly traced through the foramina in the petro-mastoid bone the slender petrosal nerves! With all this my sketch-books were enriched, giving an objective basis to my knowledge of the subject.

Gradually my anatomical water-colours grew into a very large portfolio, of which my father was quite proud. His enthusiasm went so far as seriously to plan the publication of an atlas of anatomy. Unfortunately, the backward state of the art of graphic reproduction in Zaragoza prevented the realization of the project.

In closing this chapter, I may add that, in view of my industry and of my relative skill in dissection, I was granted an appointment as assistant in dissection, at the end of my second year in medicine. This official position, flattering my self-esteem, accentuated still more my inclination to anatomy. It, moreover, enabled me to earn some fees by giving private lessons in practical anatomy.

CHAPTER XX

My professors of medicine. Don Manuel Daina and the prize for topographic anatomy. A singular method of examination. Our Dean, Don Genaro Casas. My controversial presumption. Short notes about some of the professors and some incidents which took place in their classes.

In spite of my periodical neglect of my work for art relaxations, I continued my course without mishaps, although without being permitted the luxury of excelling too much. To tell the truth, I studied attentively only anatomy and physiology; to the other subjects—medical and surgical pathology, therapeutics, hygiene, etc.—I devoted the attention strictly necessary to obtain a pass. To this a certain minister of the *Gloriosa* perhaps contributed somewhat since, out of his devotion to democratic equality, he reduced the results of examinations to two: pass and failure. I confess that I have never been able to see the educational advantage of the suppression of marks. At an age when laziness and heedlessness find so many opportunities to assail the will, what harm is there in stimulating emulation and even vanity itself? Let the miracle be done even if the devil does it. If there remains in the heart of the student any residue of unwholesome passion, life will soon look after doing away with it. The important thing is to add to the scientific inheritance acquired and to keep up the habit of work.

It will be said that for students with an inclination for academic distinctions there remained the prizes to be competed for. But not all industrious young men have the pretentiousness and boldness necessary for such competitions. I remember that the fear of seeming presumptuous and proud was the cause of most of the prizes in the faculty remaining unsought. It was certainly not from an absence of outstanding young men. Excluding myself, who could aspire only to the diploma in anatomical subjects, there were among my fellow-students a number of exceptional youths. I remember still Pablo Salinas, Victorino Sierra, Severo Cenarro, Simeón Pastor, Joaquín Gimeno, Pascual Senac, Andrés Martínez, José Rebullida and others. For my part, I tried my fortune only in *Topographic Anatomy and Operations,* the subject of which Don Manuel Daina was professor. Although the result was favourable, I lost the desire to try again. The incident is worth relating, however, to illustrate the fact that in cases of special preparation it may be harmful to study too much.

Don Manuel Daina had an absolute weakness for me. Misled by his excessive kindliness, he regarded me as the best of his pupils, and I measured up to such a flattering idea by doing my best in the performance of dissections, with which, as assistant dissector, I was officially entrusted. It will be understood, then, that when the session was over, Don Manuel urged me enthusiastically to compete for the prize, and that I prepared myself conscientiously in order to please him.

It is a well-known fact that in every academic program, besides the ordinary lessons, there are certain fundamental or merely difficult matters in connection with which the student has an opportunity to display his application and his retentiveness. My medical readers will remember that in the field of topographic anatomy these test subjects are the neck, the inguinal, the crural, and the perineal regions, and the popliteal fossa. Because of their difficulties and complexities, I had dissected them with care and drawn them more than once in my anatomical illustrations.

The examination arrived and I went up alone. I was assigned the inguinal ring and wrote about it at great length, ornamenting my description with a variety of diagrams and carrying my care of details so far as to indicate the dimensions in millimeters. While my paper was being read, I awaited proudly and confidently the verdict of the tribunal. From the anteroom I heard the judges disputing hotly. "What can be happening?" I asked myself in great alarm. Finally I learned that the jury had awarded me the prize. When they came out, Daina and his colleague embraced me and congratulated me, but Don Nicolás Montello (professor of surgical pathology) accosted me and said with a sour expression, "Understand that you are not fooling me. That is copied!"

In vain I tried respectfully to disabuse him of his error. In the opinion of the worthy Montello, it was impossible that a student should remember in millimeters the diameter of the inguinal canal. Fortunately, my master, Daina, who knew me well, defended me warmly. With his sensitive prudence, moreover, he forestalled the outburst of my anger, a passion to which at that time I was extraordinarily prone. Everything was arranged, but the incident contributed decisively to my desisting thenceforth from such competitions.

Don Manuel Daino deserves my affectionate recollections. Of winsome mien and friendly character, he enjoyed the respect and esteem which come to talent and equanimity when they are supported by a brilliant social standing. The same simplicity and elegance with which he dressed shone in his speech, which was correct, tranquil, persuasive, and shot through at times with rays of delicate irony. Don Manuel was perhaps the most *European* of our professors, probably the only one who had broadened his professional and scientific education by study abroad. He had been a pupil of the great surgical leaders in Paris. He used to hold us spellbound as he told of the operative feats of Nelaton and Velpeau, as well as of the unpardonable errors caused by superficial examination and by criminal eagerness to inflate the records of daring operations. Great was his worth as an operator, but his worth as a surgeon was greater still.

Don Manuel Daina tried out that session a very original system of grading. The day before the examinations, he surprised Cenarro and me with the following strange instructions: "I am convinced," he told us, "that no teacher, however industrious, knows his pupils so well as they do each other. Therefore, I have resolved to have you determine the grades. Here is the list. As I have a great deal of confidence in your rectitude and reliability, I approve beforehand of whatever you do."

We offered some timid excuses, but finally accepted the dangerous honour, promising—as was necessary—to keep the secret. That night Cenarro and I exchanged opinions as to the merits of our fellow-students, considering the ability, the industriousness and the regularity of attendance of each, and were able to draw up the reports with perfect unanimity. Among those whom we passed—we were, naturally, pretty lenient—I remember one Puego, a poor and industrious fellow, who had hardly been at classes at all on account of illness and whom the professor reckoned among those beyond redemption. Naturally, Cenarro and I began by awarding ourselves the rank of excellent.[1] Upon going over the list and observing the large proportion of passes and of changes of opinion Don Manuel was somewhat surprised, but he smiled good-naturedly and approved what we had done. Obviously, after such a report, examinations were a pure formality.

Another of the good teachers in the Aragonese Medical School was Don Genaro Casas, a friend and fellow-student of my father (both took their course in Barcelona). Short in stature and disfigured by a huge wen upon his forehead, he had a sickly and deformed appearance, which vanished as soon as he began to speak. For Don Genaro, Dean and almost creator of the Aragonese Medical School, besides being an eminent clinician and a model for zealous professors, had oratorical ability of the highest rank. He belonged to the select group of physicians who were also classical scholars and humanists, a class to-day almost entirely lost.

At that time, the medical schools were swayed by the vitalism of Barthez, which was inspired by Hippocratism, a doctrine of which Dr. Santero, then professor of clinical

[1] That year (1872) another minister of the revolution restored the grades of examination.

medicine in Madrid, was also an ardent partisan. It was natural that the teachers of the time—which we might call the *pre-bacterian era*—reacted with considerable heat against the materialistic and organistic tendencies of chemistry, histology, and later of bacteriology. But Don Genaro, though a confirmed vitalist, always knew how to do justice to the positive conquests of these sciences, the data of which he used to interpret very readily in the light of his organic spiritualism. I remember still the masterly exposition which he gave us of Virchow's *Cellular Pathology*, an essentially revolutionary book which appeared about that time. Naturally, Don Genaro accepted the facts, but he repudiated the conclusions drawn from them. It will be readily understood that the hesitation and partial acceptance of the learned professor did not please everybody; but even those of us who passed for more advanced and novelty-loving followed him with respect in his laudable efforts to reconcile the old and the new. We all revered and loved him, for his zeal as a teacher was as great as his ability and his kindness.

It is a fact that one day my old presumption tried the master's good will severely. I shall relate the incident—which I remember with sorrow to-day—to show how great were the rebelliousness of my character and the paternal tolerance of Don Genaro. I had read the above-mentioned *Cellular Pathology* of Virchow and some other books on pathological anatomy which were then in vogue, where the importance of the cell was defended by an inadequate objective analysis, as an autonomous living being, the exclusive actor in pathological events. Organic unity, so dear to vitalists and animists, emerged from the discussion completely defeated. Sickness was consequently something like a trivial frontier skirmish or a city riot, which the local powers should control automatically with little or no intervention from the central authorities, which latter were represented by the nervous system.

Insolent and over-confident after my somewhat ill-guided reading, I was annoyed at observing how Don Genaro placed a vitalistic interpretation upon all the cellular processes. In spite of my timidity and diffidence, the clash came at last. One day in class the master questioned me about inflammatory lesions and, after expounding the current descriptions, I had the boldness, in interpreting them, to oppose his vitalistic doctrine. With a fearlessnes at which I was surprised myself, I declared that hyperaemia and exudation are not defensive activities of the vital principle but merely effects of irritation and of the multiplication of the cells. "As I understand it," I added, "the central forces, if they really exist, take no part in the process, as is proved by the statement of Virchow that inflammation may occur in tissues lacking nerves and blood vessels."[2] Before my arrogance, my classmates looked at each other in stupefaction.

Don Genaro was not angry at my lack of respect; but rather showed himself glad to argue the matter with a pupil. By gentle phrases, he tried to persuade me "that the inflammatory act always represents a defensive reaction against noxious agents"; he pointed out that even in the bloodless tissues which I cited (cornea and cartilage) hyperaemia appeared, since fluid and globules of pus gathered about the lesion, and, finally, he added that the unquestionable purposiveness of the reactions under discussion, directed towards the elimination of the causes and the repair of the damage done, necessarily implied an immaterial principle capable of regulating and coördinating the organic activities. This principle could be nothing else than the vital force, the vegetative soul of the vitalistic school.

I, however, inspired by my recent reading, considered the vital principles of Barthez to be a myth concealing our ignorance (in which I was perfectly correct) and maintained my viewpoint obstinately, clinging rather disloyally to the literal sense of the words and declaring that I did not un-

[2] The reader will understand that, after the time which has passed, I cannot be certain of the exact terms of the polemic, but only of the arguments and of the spirit which stimulated them.

derstand how hyperaemia could develop where there were neither vessels nor blood (in cartilage and in the cornea).

In the end, I made a deplorable scene in the classroom and caused the excellent Don Genaro much distress. The latter met my father the following day and addressed him with these words, which I remember very clearly: "You have a son who is so stubborn that, when he believed he was right, he would not keep quiet even if the lives of his parents depended upon his silence."

The most serious thing about that disrespectful impertinence of mine was that, fundamentally, Don Genaro was right. Fortunately, regretting afterwards my lack of respect, I apologized sincerely to the master, and that outburst of a hot-headed youngster was forgiven by the fatherly Don Genaro. When some years afterwards, at the time when our faculty was changed from a provincial to a state one, our veteran professor obtained the chair of clinical medicine in honourable competition, no one was more sincerely pleased than I.

Somewhat less clearly do the distinguished figures of other masters appear in my memory. Outstanding among them was Don Pedro Cerrada, professor of general pathology, a conscientious clinician and thoughtful teacher, open-minded towards all the innovations of science. One remark of his I remember, as modest as it was prophetic: "I regret that I do not know enough chemistry, and I am too old to learn it. It is your task to study it, for therein lies the secret of many pathological processes."

Affectionate mention is merited also by Dr. Comín, professor of therapeutics, level-headed and admirably cultured, and a ready and elegant lecturer; Don Manuel Tornés, who was already very old at that time, a man endowed with admirable clinical discernment, and who was the venerated instructor in medical pathology; Don Jacinto Corralé, professor of anatomy, somewhat rough and outspoken, but punctilious in the performance of his duties and generous with his students; Eduardo Tornés, professor of forensic medicine (the son of Don Manuel), studious, winsome, and as gentlemanly as his father, from whom he inherited decorousness and seriousness of thought and of expression; Ferrer, the instructor in obstetrics, somewhat rapid and confused in his expositions, but an estimable clinician and a fine man; and, lastly, Valero, who occupied the chair of physiology, gifted with great vivacity in his speech and with notable pedagogical powers. All of them sowed useful seed in my mind, and to all I am cordially grateful. It was a great pity that the absence of laboratories and the inadequacy of the clinical material, partly sterilized their efforts.

To complete these notes on my professors, I shall relate a few anecdotes about the classes of Valero and of Ferrer.

Valero, our professor of physiology, was master of the difficult art of stimulating his pupils. He undertook to get the text-book (Beclard's physiology) thoroughly into our heads, and he succeeded in his task. To this end he questioned us all daily, choosing preferably the most difficult points. When the question tripped up one student, he went right round the class until he came to someone who could clear up the difficulty. Then he burst into praises of the fortunate one, who felt himself flattered and happy. In these discussions and honourable competitions there shone Cenarro, Pastor, Senad, Sierra, Rebullida, and especially Pablo Salinas, the more studious and brilliant of our classmates. The reason for all this is that pride, when wisely appealed to, works wonders. Naturally, no experiments were performed in that class, and so our rivalry produced only sterile and useless results.

Of Ferrer, our instructor in obstetrics, I have an amusing reminiscence. He reproved me one day—and with justice—for my irregular attendance at his class, rejecting indignantly the excuse which I offered, namely that my work in the dissecting room deprived me of the pleasure of listening to him assiduously. "Nevertheless," I added foolishly and vain-gloriously, "I study the lessons assigned every day and believe that I am reasonably up in the subject." "That we shall see right now," replied the teacher with annoyance, and, thinking to put me into difficulty, he asked me about the origin of the foetal membranes, a subject which he had developed with great enthusiasm. Seizing opportunity by the forelock, I solemnly approached the blackboard and, without becoming in the least excited, proceeded to spend more than half an hour drawing coloured diagrams to show the stages of the development of the blastoderm, the umbilical vesicle, the allantois, etc., explaining at the same time what the figures represented. I was truly epic!

The worthy Ferrer followed me with rapture. He had thought to humble me and had actually brought me resounding glory. The whole class applauded their fellow-student. My assurance and coolness in discoursing upon embryological subjects, which most of the students of obstetrics usually learn pretty badly, gave him such a high opinion of my studiousness that, after accepting my earlier excuses, he declared that I could count on passing the examinations with a record of "excellent" even if I did not attend the class any more. "The lecture which you have just given us deserved this standing and makes up for your negligence." I took advantage of his permission to the limit. Only from time to time did I appear at the class, as if I were conferring a favour.

The reader will have guessed that my brilliant triumph was the result of luck. On account of my interest in anatomy I had studied the development of the organs, and consequently the formation of the embryo, with considerable thoroughness. If my ingenuous instructor had tested me with other topics in the course, he would have discovered my utter ignorance.

My classmates, who knew me well, smiled at the credulity of the master and did me the favour of keeping the secret. For the rest, it is certain that in the long run we were all equal, for at that time the faculty had no obstetrical clinic, and to study *positions* and *presentations* without having been present at a delivery is like learning how to use a gun without having a gun.

CHAPTER XXI

I continue my studies without serious mishap. My manias for literature, gymnastics, and philosophy. My muscular prowess. The Venus de Milo. A duel with bare fists. Competitions in lifting weights. Incomprehensible caprice of a woman.

My tasks as a dissector and the ordinary amount of attention devoted to the later subjects of the course left me hours of leisure which I employed in gratifying my love of drawing and in other amusements. During these years (1871 to 1873) I developed three new manias—literature, gymnastics, and philosophy.

Let us consider briefly these sicknesses of youth.

Graphomania.—This was a typical example of contagion. There was rampant in Spain during the revolutionary period an epidemic of lyricism, which was aggravated by persistent inoculation from French romanticism. Upon the occasion of any political event, hymns and odes burst forth wholesale in the daily papers. The prosodists wrote in a lordly, noble and pretentious style (one will recall poor Bécquer, Donoso Cortés, Quadrado, and Castelar) and the poets composed strophes with musical cadences and sonorities. Among novelists, our idol was Victor Hugo; in the lyric genre, Espronceda or Zorrilla, and in oratory Castelar. Weak in the presence of the enslaving suggestive powers of our environment, many of us young men had severe attacks of the fashionable disease. As was to be feared, the sentimental temperaments, like mine, suffered worse ravages than the cool and utilitarian heads. I fell, then, into the temptation to make verses, to write legends and even novels. After a few years had passed, convalescence finally took place, and with it came bitter disillusionment. If I am not forgetting someone, from among my poetic classmates only Joaquin Jimeno continued to write, and became the editor of a political daily.[1] Jimeno, however, who afterwards came to be professor in the Faculty of Medicine, and an able and distinguished politician (he belonged to the *posibilista* party), had an excellent foundation in grammar and the humanities and exquisite literary taste, which I, unfortunately, lacked.

Why should I speak of my verses? They were a servile imitation of Lista, Arriaza, Bécquer, Zorrilla and Espronceda, especially of the last-mentioned, whose songs of the Pirate (*Canción del Pirata*), to Teresa (*Canto a Teresa*), The Cossack (*El canto del Cosaco*), etc., we young folk considered the supreme achievement in the lyric. Apart from the captivating music of the lines and the pomp and richness of the language, what most enraptured us in the poetry of the Estremenian bard was his boldly rebellious spirit, so like that of Lord Byron, as the Count of Toreno remarked with sanguinary significance.[2] Thanks to the good offices of my friend Jimeno, certain of the local newspapers generously published some of my poems, filled, as I realized later, with *ripios* [3] and commonplaces. I remember that of all my effusions, the one which had most success among my fellow students was a certain humorous ode written upon the occasion of a noisy student strike.[4]

A still greater influence upon my tastes was exercised by the scientific novels of Jules Verne, which were very popular at the time. So great was it that, in imitation of

[1] As a matter of fact there was another of my fellow-students, Fernández Brizuela, who continued to cultivate the muses with admirable success. This excellent friend, an indefatigable collector (he collected even the sketches and the poetic efforts of his fellow), died young after having practiced medicine for a number of years in Zaragoza.

[2] The Count of Toreno, a famous historian, engaged in a bitter polemic with Espronceda.

[3] Superfluous words inserted for the sole purpose of completing a line in poetry.

[4] Recently, one of my few surviving fellow students, Doctor Iraneta, showed me the humorous ode referred to, written to celebrate the firmness with which Dr. Valero's students of physiology persisted in our strike until we received full apology for certain vexatious remarks made by the professor in moments of anger. It was entitled "The Student Commune" and was written with such silliness that it does not deserve the honour of being printed.

"The Voyage to the Moon," "Five Weeks in a Balloon," "Round the World in Eighty Days," etc., I wrote a voluminous biological novel of a didactic character, in which were narrated the dramatic experiences of a certain traveller who, having arrived in some unexplained manner upon the planet Jupiter, met there monstrous animals, ten thousand times larger than man, although of essentially the same structure. In proportion with those living colossi, our explorer was only the size of a microbe and was therefore invisible. Armed with all sorts of scientific apparatus, the intrepid hero commenced his exploration by stealing into a cutaneous gland: he afterwards entered the blood, sailing on a red blood corpuscle; watched the epic struggles between leucocytes and parasites; observed the remarkable visual, acoustic, muscular and other functions, and finally arrived at the brain and discovered—think of it! there was nothing trivial about it!—the secret of thought and of the voluntary impulse. Numerous colored pictures, selected and adapted, naturally, from the histological books of the period (Henle, van Kempen, Kölliker, Frey, etc.), illustrated the text and showed in life-like fashion the exciting adventures of the hero, who, threatened more than once by the viscous tentacles of a leucocyte or of a vibratile corpuscle, freed himself from the danger by ingenious efforts. I am sorry that I have lost this little book, for it might perhaps have been transformed, in the light of the modern revelations of histology and bacteriology, into a delightful work of scientific popularization.[5] It was mislaid no doubt during my travels as an army surgeon.

Gymnastic Mania.—Brought up in small towns and hardened by the sun and open air, I was at eighteen a solid lad, agile and considerably stronger than the young men of the city. I prided myself upon being the strongest member of the class, in which I was entirely mistaken. Weary of

[5] Soon afterwards, the brilliant writer, D. Amalio Gimeno, the future professor at San Carlos (Madrid), published a novel on a somewhat similar subject called, if my memory is correct, "Adventures of a Red Blood Corpuscle."

PLATE 9

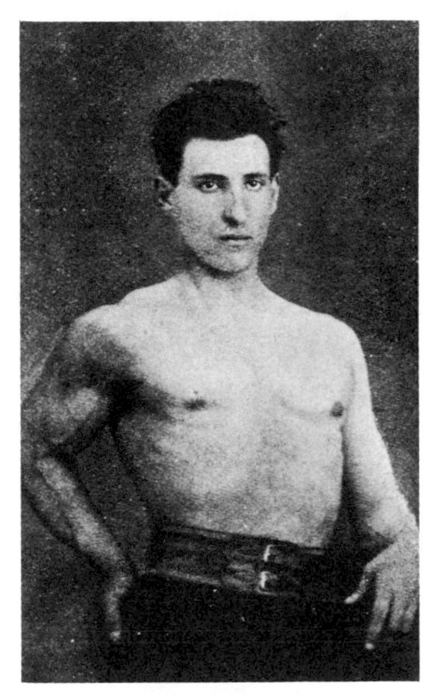

Fig. 16. The Author at Eighteen, four months after the onset of his gymnastic mania. Unfortunately, the almost monstrous muscular development attained in the year of violent exercises appears so weakened in the photograph that it is impossible to reproduce it by half-tone.

PLATE 10

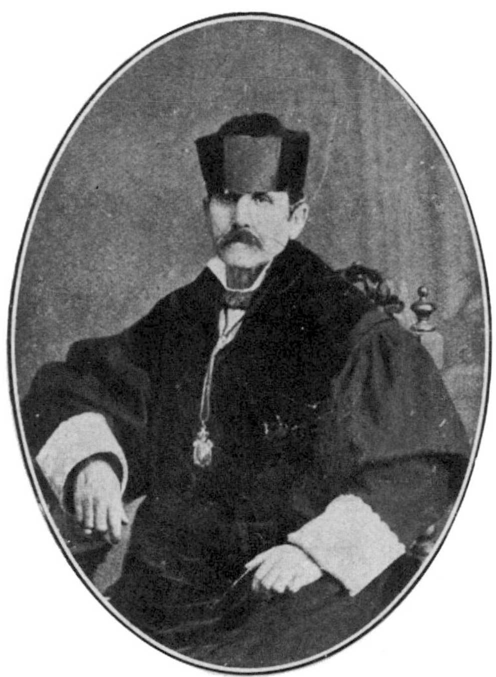

FIG. 17. DON JENARO CASAS. Dean of the Faculty of Medicine of Zaragoza and a close friend of my father.

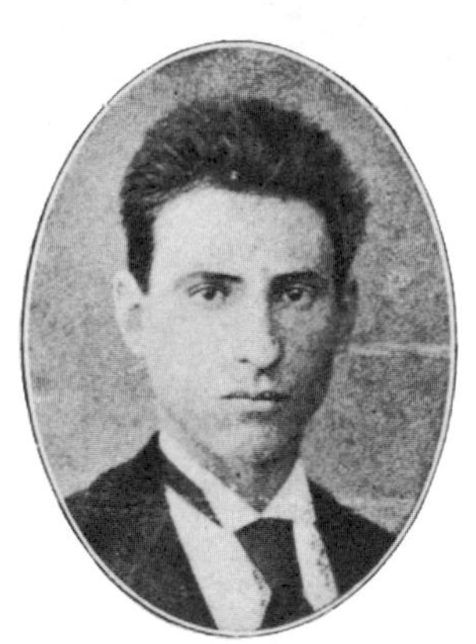

FIG. 18. THE AUTHOR AT THE BEGINNING OF HIS CAREER. Notice the sullen and unsociable expression.

my boasting, doubtless, a certain fellow student[6] of distinguished bearing, of medium height, lean faced and of few words, invited me to a contest with the wrists, a form of exercise which was much in vogue among the young men at that time. With great surprise and sorrow, I suffered the humiliation of defeat. I wanted to know how my rival had developed such tremendously strong muscles and he acknowledged frankly that the secret lay in the fact that for years he had enthusiastically cultivated gymnastics and fencing. "If strength comes from gymnastic exercises," I replied arrogantly, "continue to prepare, for in less than six months I shall beat you." A sceptical smile met my bravado. But I had an enormous vanity in these foolish boasts of physical strength, and the worthy Moriones did not know with whom he was dealing.

The following day, without saying anything to my father, I presented myself at the gymnasium of Poblador, which was then in the Plaza del Pilar. After some bargaining, we agreed to exchange lessons in muscular physiology (which he wanted to have in order to give his instruction something of a scientific tone) for lessons in physical development. Thanks to this arrangement, my father, who did not have to disburse a copper, was unaware that his son had negotiated one more distraction.

I began the task with extraordinary enthusiasm, working in the gymnasium two hours a day. Besides the regular exercises, I imposed upon myself a certain progressive programme, now adding more weight each day to the balls, now increasing the number of movements on the horizontal or parallel bars. I also vigorously cultivated high jumping and all kinds of swinging on the rings and the trapeze. Sustained by a determination which no one would have suspected in me, I not only fulfilled my promise to overcome my friend Moriones, but before the year was over I became the champion strong man of the gymnasium. Poblador

[6] My opponent was José Moriones, nephew of the general of that name, of chivalrous temperament and an excellent comrade. Like me, he entered the Army Medical Service, where he had a brilliant career.

was proud of his pupil and I was filled with enthusiasm at discovering how easily my muscles had responded to the stimulus of overwork.

In physical appearance I was not much of an Adonis. Broad shouldered and with monstrous pectoral muscles, I had a chest circumference exceeding 112 centimeters. When I walked, I showed that inelegance and rhythmic strut characteristic of the side-show Hercules. Like the paws of a beast, my hands unconsciously crushed those of my friends. A walking stick, which was transformed into a straw by my blunted sensibilities, had to be replaced by a formidable iron bar (it weighed sixteen pounds), which I painted to imitate an umbrella case. In sum, I was proud and even insolent with my coarse porter's figure and burned with eagerness to test my fists upon someone.

From that period of foolish and exaggerated cultivation of the biceps I retain two profitable lessons. The first is the conviction that excessive muscular development in young men leads almost inevitably to violence and bullying.[7] The ostentation of brute strength becomes a passion and a source of foolish presumption. One would have to be an angel to restrain in continual inactivity hypertrophic muscle fibres, anxious, as we might say, for employment and justification. Since there is no question of making use of them handling packages, one experiences a peculiar inclination to employ them upon the backs of one's fellows. The same thing happens with physical energy as with standing armies: the nation which has prepared the best instrument of war always winds up by trying it on the weaker or less well prepared nations.

The second lesson was the discovery, rather late, that physical exercise on the part of men devoted to study should be moderate and brief, without ever passing the stage of fatigue. It is a common phenomenon, but one which is rather overlooked by educators of the English school, that

[7] This observation does not apply to adult life. It is a well known fact that there are no people more peaceable in their social relations than gymnasts, pugilists, and boxers.

strenuous sports rapidly diminish the aptitude for intellectual work. When night comes, the brain, tired out by the excess of motor discharges—which seem to absorb the energies of the whole cerebral mechanism—falls upon books with the inertia of a paperweight. In such circumstances the structural differentiation of the central nervous system seems to be suspended or retarded; it might be said that the higher regions of the gray matter (the association areas) are repressed and, as it were, choked by the motor areas (the centres of projection). Such compensatory processes explain why most young people who excel in sports and other physical exercises (there are exceptions) have not much to say and have relatively poor and simple intellects.

I was on the point of becoming an incurable victim of athletic brutalization. Fortunately, however, the sickness acquired later in Cuba, weakening my blood and reducing my excessive muscular development, brought me a higher and more judicious appreciation of the value of strength.

The craving to display the strength of my arm led me more than once, against my naturally kindly disposition, to appear quarrelsome and even aggressive. I should like to mention a typical adventure, which portrays well not only the mental effects of my acrobatic and pugilistic mania, but also the state of mind of that ingenuously romantic and quixotic generation.

There lived in the Calle del Cinco de Marzo a certain very beautiful young lady with a sunny countenance, enhanced by great blue eyes. On account of the perfect classic lines of her figure and the dignified stateliness of her form, we called her the Venus de Milo. Various students used to frequent her street and gaze at her balcony without the innocent girl being aware, apparently, of the platonic cult of which she was the object.

More than real love, I felt for her the devotion and enthusiasm of the artist. She was the architype, the ideal beauty, the sublime model of a goddess, whom, if it had been possible, I would have translated on to canvas with almost religious veneration and devoted absorption. My feelings were so respectful and platonic that I never dared to write to her. My passion—if that singular sentimental condition can be so termed—was fully satisfied by looking at her on the balcony or in the street, or contemplating a certain photograph which an apprentice of the photographic establishment of Judez obtained for me as a result of bribery. Only once did I speak to her and then not with my face revealed, but disguised for Carnival, and taking advantage of a *fiesta* held in the bull ring. She seemed to me a modest and well-educated girl. Having heard her speak admiringly of the beauties of the Monastery of Piedra, I sent her by post a fine album of photographs of that admirable place, an album which I used to guard like an inestimable treasure. I did not even have the courage to inscribe the tribute to her.

One evening, according to my habit, I was passing through the Calle del Cinco de Marzo, making my formidable club ring noisily on the pavement, when there came to meet me a young man of my own age, massive, square, and strong. Without taking the trouble to introduce himself or making any pretences, this fellow forbade me categorically to walk along the street where dwelt the lady of both our thoughts, upon pain of receiving a tremendous beating. Such boldness flabbergasted my dignity as a bully. I was not acquainted with my rival, but observing his confidence, came to the conclusion that he must be a certain M———, a student in the engineering course, who by administering whippings had come to be the almost exclusive master of the situation concerning this girl.

If I had acceded to such a discourteous and humiliating request, not only my sense of honour would have protested, but also the millions of inactive muscle fibres which were eager to display their powers at little cost. Accordingly a duel with cudgels was arranged, to take place the same night in the woods of the Huerva. The high-sounding speeches exchanged by the two champions as we walked up the river bank in the direction of the field of honour were certainly as braggartly as they were laughable.

"What course are you in?" asked my adversary.

"I am in Medicine and expect to graduate next year."

"It is a pity that you are so advanced!"

"And you?" I asked in turn a similar question, with some loss of confidence.

"I am preparing for civil engineering and expect to enter this session."

"You will not lose so much," I replied, returning the repartee.

With these and other arrogant remarks we reached the field and removed our overcoats. In view of the inequality of the cudgels (I have said that mine was an iron bar), we agreed to depend upon our bare fists and whoever was knocked down first was to consider himself beaten. It was a kind of greco-roman struggle, as it is done today, though without so many useless ceremonials. We faced each other and, following the example, no doubt, of the English before the battle of Fontenoy, I exclaimed, "Give the first blow, sir!"

Neither backward nor lazy, my opponent struck me three or four staggering blows on the head which raised such lumps that I could not put on my hat afterwards. Fortunately, I had the advantage at that time of a head which was proof against blows and I sustained the formidable assault undaunted. When my turn came, after some thrusts to punish him, I closed upon him, lifted him up in the air and, whirling him round in my arms like an angry bear, awaited the surgical effects of the embrace. I did not have long to wait. My adversary's face turned livid, his bones creaked, and losing sensibility, he sank to the ground in an inert heap. As I gazed upon the effects of my barbarity, I suffered a terrible shock; I was afraid that I had choked him or at least had injured him seriously.

Fortunately, it was not so. Moved to sympathy and regretting my brutality, I attended to him solicitously and had the joy of seeing him come out of his daze and regain his breath. I helped him to rise and put on his coat; cleaned his clothes, soiled by the damp ground of the

Huerva, and his lips, which were reddened with blood; and since he walked with difficulty I offered him my arm and accompanied him home.

Before entering, my rival mumbled in a tone of sad resignation: "Since you have beaten me, I renounce my pretensions and you remain the master of the field."

"Not at all," I replied, making a great show of generosity and nobility. "We are disputing about the possession of something which has no real existence. Neither of us has made a declaration to the object of our anxious thoughts. Let us each write a letter to her and let her decide between us, if she cares to decide."

Seeing me so reasonable and disinterested he apologized for his former boasting, confessing to me that the girl had him bewitched. He was determined to marry her as soon as he had completed his course.

A few days afterwards, M., already recovered from his experience, returned to the street, greeted me in a friendly fashion and told me with an air of deep sorrow: "I have learned something terrible which has upset me extremely: Senorita X, whom we thought poor, has a dowry of fifty thousand dollars. Hence I must give up my courting with the deepest regret. If I write to her and she accepts my plea, will not everyone think that I am paying court to her from self-interest?"

"You are right," I replied in consternation. "We had better give up what is an impossible undertaking."

In actual fact we gave up thinking of the famous Venus de Milo.[8]

Such we were then! Will there be any among the youth of to-day who will not find our ingenuousness ridiculous or stupid?

[8] When I came back from America, I learned with surprise that the Venus de Milo, so much admired and sought after for her marvellous beauty, had not married, although she had extremely eligible suitors. Galloping consumption had carried her off in the flower of her youth. Her, who was a model of healthy and robust beauty and captivating grace! We must acknowledge that the microbes know how to choose!

M. and I finally became the best of friends. Admiring my muscular power greatly, he was anxious to know the secret of my strength, and when I told him of the gymnasium of Poblador, he went there full of enthusiasm. My one-time rival was transformed in his turn into a formidable athlete. Rather quiet, exceedingly formal and discreet, M. finished his engineering course brilliantly.[9]

At the risk of being wearisome I am going to mention briefly two other little examples of the vanity of muscular strength. My excuse is the devotion to what is called physical culture which is so fashionable now-a-days, and the growing cult of English sports.

The first occurrence took place in the town of Valpalmas, which I visited when I was twenty years old, upon a mission to collect some overdue debts for my father. I stayed at the house of an old friend of my family, Señor Choliz, a hospitable merchant, who showered me with attentions and courtesies. When my task was partly accomplished, I was invited to attend the festival which was commencing two days later. As is the general custom in Aragon, the projected sports consisted of foot-races, sack-races, climbing a greasy pole, performances by mountebanks, games of *la barra*[10] and *pelota,*[11] etc.

My interest in sports led me one morning to attend the graceful and manly game of *la barra,* which was carried on in the shelter of the high wall of the church; and when I was absorbed in the spectacle one of my companions said to me drawlingly: "These are not games for young gentlemen—for you dominoes, and billiards, are plenty, thank you!"

"You are mistaken," I replied. "There are gentlemen who are devoted to games of strength and who, with a little practice, could contend worthily with you."

[9] My friend who was called Alejandro Mendizábal, and who is now deceased, was one of the most prominent officers in the Engineering Corps. If he read these lines, how he would laugh at these youthful follies!

[10] Bar-throwing. (Translator's note.)

[11] Hand-ball. (Translator's note.)

"Bah!" continued the crafty fellow, "Using the baı requires hands less delicate than your worship's. Strength comes from digging and mowing." And seizing the heavy piece of iron he thrust it into my hands, exclaiming: "Come on, let us see how the weakling can manage!"

Stung to the quick, I grasped the weighty bar energetically, took up my position, and with a supreme effort hurled the projectile through the air. Great was the surprise of the scoffers! Contrary to all their expectations, I threw it farther than any of them.

" Good for the gentleman! What nerves he has!" exclaimed an onlooker.

The lusty and thickset lad who had been poking fun at me, however, did not give in. Instead, with a disdainful grin, he cried: "Bah! That is a matter of skill. Let us try something that needs real strength. I bet you cannot pick up a whole sack of wheat" (four fanegas).[12]

At this my pride as an athlete, restrained hitherto by consideration for my host and companions, overcame all barriers and in turn I dared to ask him: "What about you, who are making so much noise about it—how heavy a weight can you lift?"

"Well, when I'm not tired, seven *fanegas* don't bother me. But the strongest fellows in town can handle a *cahiz*" (eight fanegas).

"Come on then, and let us see which of us can manage that *cahiz* of wheat better."

The spectators formed a circle, the mayor came, and by common consent we proceeded to the establishment of a certain grain merchant in whose *patio* lay many sacks of wheat. I grasped a huge sack, which actually weighed the eight fanegas, took hold of the imposing mass with both arms, and with a powerful effort, the thin and pale-faced

12 A fanega is a measure of volume which differs in value in different parts of Spain. It is stated that in the Provinces of Huesca and Zaragoza the fanega equals 22.42 litres, a volume of wheat which would weigh about 37 pounds avoirdupois. Thus the *cahiz* would weigh somewhat less than 290 lbs. (Translator's note.)

little gentleman lifted the *cahiz.* I bore myself then as a man! The joker, on the other hand, lifted no more than the seven fanegas he had mentioned.

The amazement of the banterers was complete. In the eyes of those farm-hands, who were worshippers of brute strength, I acquired immediately sovereign prestige; and my triumph over my adversary was celebrated joyfully with a dance and collation in the open air. In the classical jota there took part proud maidens with whom I had run about as a boy and played at *pitos.*[13] Some of them threw me glances which seemed endearing.

The other gymnastic feat was of an acrobatic character. One night when the whole of my family came home late from the theatre, we discovered that the door key was lost so that we could not get into the house. It was Sunday, one o'clock in the morning and we had no hope of finding a locksmith. In a moment, I climbed up to the balconies of the first floor by clinging to the grilles of the *entresuelo:*[14] slipped daringly along the cornice of the facade; then opened the door from a balcony, entered the room, and opened the house door from inside. My intrepidity and coolness found grace that night in the eyes of my parents, who were observing my increasing enthusiasm for gymnastics with displeasure.

The cultivation of physical exercises, as the English educationists know well, retards markedly the unfolding of the sexual instincts in young people. In my case, in that happy period between nineteen and twenty-one years of age, the most charming girls were no more than pretty pictures or admirable sculptures. Besides, the adorable adolescents of former times, like those of to-day, perhaps from the lack of artistic instruction, did not use to distinguish between a robust and shapely torso, surmounted by broad shoulders and a stout neck, and the narrow chest of a lanky lordling. For them, masculine handsomeness is

[13] A game played by tossing a bone from the heel of a sheep or pig.

[14] In Spain the floor above the ground floor is called the entresuelo, and that above it in turn is called the principal or first floor. (Translator's note.)

expressed in the face, and after that in exceptional stature and in distinction of manners. Other things matter little.

Nevertheless, there are occasional exceptions, which can nearly always be attributed to literary suggestions. I may tell of a typical case of such influence, and one which was unique for me. With it I will bring to a close the wearisome record of my muscular vanity.

Accompanied by a friend, I was walking one festival day through the covered walk of the Paseo de Santa Engracia when I noticed that a very pretty young lady was looking at us persistently. Her great, shining, black eyes, her pink and white complexion, her shapely figure, sumptuously modelled according to the fashion of the time, drew the attention also of my companion, who was, indeed, a very handsome blonde youth of twenty. There was nothing to lead me to suspect that those incendiary and insistent glances were directed at my massive and ungainly carcass, but my friend, with a little humiliation, enlightened me.

"It is at you that she is looking," he said with a manner of deep conviction.

"You are mistaken," I replied. "It must be at you: your gallant figure has made one more conquest."

After several turns through the arcades, however, passing each time our insinuating heroine and her friends, I had no choice but to yield to the evidence. I followed her almost mechanically through the square and as far as her abode, on the threshold of which she took leave of her companions, but not without first casting me a shining and abundantly inspiring glance.

Having established informal courtship, a few months later I had the curiosity to inquire why, as between my attractive companion and my own common and powerful person, I had had the preference. And this was the reply, pronounced with delicious ingenuousness: "Because, on account of your athletic power and the breadth of your shoulders, you look like one of the famous and invincible knights of the Middle Ages. Besides your nose is almost exactly the same as that of Alfonso XII.''

''So that if Don Alfonso had been rather flat-nosed,'' I thought to myself, ''and if my chest had not been so broad, I should have remained without a sweetheart! Oh, the incomprehensible capriciousness of womankind!''

As this example shows, the measles of romanticism had spread even to the hearts of some young ladies of good family.

This—be it said in passing—was the one and only conquest which I owe to my muscles, although in collaboration, it must be acknowledged, with romantic serial novels and the nose of a monarch! But I should not assume the role of conqueror, since it was really I who was conquered, if such serious words can be applied to the transient amours of a stripling.

Mania for Philosophy.—After the gymnastic fad, by a compensatory reaction, I developed a craze for philosophy. One might say that the poor association cells of my brain, left behind by the excessive cultivation of the motor ones, asserted loudly their right to live. I gradually relaxed my silly athletic vanity, coming to realize at last that there are somewhat more respectable and desirable things than the display of brute strength. Even in the realm of individual competition, I finally came to consider it more laudable to overcome an adversary with reason than with blows. Thus I returned to my abandoned books of philosophy. To the tumbling of the acrobat there succeeded the pirouetting of the dialectician. In my eagerness to know how much the best thinkers had discovered about God, the soul, substance, knowledge, the universe, and life, I read almost all the works on metaphysics in the University library and some others lent me by friends. To tell the truth, this mania for reason was not a new thing in me, as has been seen in earlier chapters: it had already appeared when I was studying at the Institute; but after the Revolution (in 1871 to 1875) it had a dangerous recrudescence.

It seems to me that at that time this enthusiasm was

not entirely sincere; later on, no doubt, it became so. Then, however, rather than to meditate honestly upon such exalted matters, I desired to acquire the artifices of sophistry so as to astonish my friends. In this spirit of frivolous curiosity I read, without always understanding them, the works of Berkeley, Hume, Fichte, Kant, and Balmes. By good luck, those of Hegel, Krause, and Sanz del Río were not in the University Library. I craved radical and categorical theses. Consequently, I adopted *absolute idealism.* In truth, I was captivated by the gallant idealism of Berkeley and Fichte. It must not be forgotten that at that time I was a fervent and exaggerated adherent of the spiritual philosophy.

With an ardour worthy of a better cause, I pretended to demonstrate to my somewhat disconcerted comrades that the external world, the mysterious *noumenon* of Kant, does not exist, affirming resolutely that the *ego,* or rather my own ego, was the sole absolute and positive reality. Naturally, my friends Cenarro, Pastor, Senac, Sierra, and others, whom I vexed daily with my boring talk, objected to being considered phenomena, or creations of my autocratic *ego,* and protested energetically against my silly sophistries. At bottom, I was just as sure as they of the objectivity of the world; but I was seduced by the paradoxes and the tricks of dialectics.

It is unnecessary to remark that such childish charlatanism and juggling of ideas contributed very little to my spiritual development, unless one considers as positive profit a certain mental agility and somewhat of healthy scepticism. Nevertheless, this enthusiasm for philosophic studies, which acquired in later years a more serious character, while it did not exactly transform me into a thinker, contributed to producing in me a certain mental condition which is rather favourable to scientific investigation. This we shall consider in due course.

CHAPTER XXII

Newly graduated in medicine, I enlist in the Army Medical Corps. I join the army operating against the Carlists. The Spanish feeling of the Catalans. My transfer to the expeditionary force to Cuba. A conversation between two friends eager for strange adventures. Embarcation at Cadiz en route for Havana.

In June, 1873, at the age of twenty-one, I obtained the title of Licentiate in Medicine. My father wished to keep me with him for a time to study *descriptive and general anatomy* thoroughly, with the idea of writing upon the first competitive examinations which should be held for the filling of chairs in this subject; but the so-called *draft of Castelar,* that is the compulsory military service ordained by the celebrated tribune to meet the seriousness of the political condition, upset the paternal programme. Like all the able-bodied young men of that class I was, accordingly, made a soldier. I found myself obliged to sleep in the barracks, to eat in the mess-room, and to drill.

My life as a recruit did not last long. Examinations were announced for assistant physicians in the Army Medical Service and I decided to try them. If fortune should smile upon me and I should be appointed, instead of serving the Republic as a common soldier, I would serve her as an officer, with the rank of lieutenant.

With these hopes I applied for and obtained permission from my superiors to go to Madrid and take part in the tests. I studied hard for a few months and had the satisfaction of gaining an appointment, pleasantly surprising my family thereby. In the examinations, though I did not shine with great brilliance, I must have done not at all badly, since I was ranked sixth among a hundred candidates (for thirty-two positions). As a matter of fact, what lent me a certain prominence was the test in operative surgery, in which I described the anatomy of the leg minutely and methodically (it was a question of an amputation). On the other hand, in the remaining examinations I did not rise above the bounds of mediocrity.

Actually overwork with consequent loss of sleep was on the point of costing me failure. As a result of excessive study, I slept in on the day of the written examination and arrived at the Military Hospital (which then stood in the Calle de la Princesa) at eight o'clock in the morning, that is to say an hour after the examination began. On account of my absence, the tribunal had shut me out. It was a great triumph to secure entrance to the place of examination. By dint of entreaties I finally succeeded in melting the kindly Doctor Losada, one of the board of examiners. Once I was in the hall, more than fifteen minutes passed without anyone paying any attention to me or any of the candidates, who were all absorbed in their work, so much as making room for me to sit down and write. Devoured with impatience and determined in spite of everything, I procured a little bit of a table by squeezing in, snatched some sheets of paper from my nearest neighbour, and plunged into a dissertation on the etiology of cholera, the subject which had been assigned to us.

Hardly had I written two or three pages when the time was exhausted and the examination ended. Naturally my poor dissertation must have gained few or no marks.

Incidents of this kind have happened to me more than once in examinations, for among my defects perhaps the most serious was always the absolute lack of method and of measure in work.

After displaying myself in Zaragoza with my appointment as assistant physician in the Army Medical Service and flaunting my brilliant uniform before my envious comrades, I received orders to join the regiment of Burgos for operations in the province of Lérida.[1] This force, together with a batallion of chasseurs, a squadron of cuirassiers, and some batteries of field artillery, consisted of 1400

[1] My passport for joining the army of Cataluña is dated 3 September, 1873.

or 1600 men, under the command of the amiable and chivalrous Colonel Tomasetti.

Readers who have lived through those interesting and tumultuous days of the Revolution, when history was made every minute, will remember that, after the abdication of Don Amadeo of Savoy, and the unruliness and anarchy of the radical Republic, Castelar came into power. With a governmental sense which was lacking in his predecessors, he reëstablished military discipline with great severity, filled up the ranks of the disorganized army with his celebrated general levy, and, finally, restored the defunct Corps of Artillery.

Everything promised the beginning of an era of order and relative tranquility, the precursor of lasting peace. But first the Cuban insurrection had to be overcome and Carlism, which was becoming daily stronger and more threatening in the northern provinces, had to be put down.

To tell the truth, things had improved somewhat by the time I arrived in Cataluña. Already, one no longer heard the disgraceful "Let him dance!" with which the undisciplined soldiers used to insult their officers: now the superiors were obeyed, and an excellent spirit existed among the troops. The bands of Savalls, of Tristany, and of other rebel leaders, which had been engaged a few months before in all sorts of exactions and outrages, were retreating to a place of safety or were carefully avoiding contact with our troops.

Many liberal communities aided the activities of the flying squadrons, organizing local militias and inflicting an exemplary punishment more than once upon the Carlist hosts, as happened in Vimbodí. Our particular brigade had as its principal mission to prevent the sacking of the rich towns of the plain of Urgel and the frontier districts of the Province of Tarragona. This was the reason for continual marches and counter-marches from Lérida, our general headquarters, to Balaguer and Tremp; from Lérida to Tárrega; from Tárrega to Cervera; from Cervera to

Verdú or to Igualada; from Tárrega to Borjas and Vimbodí, etc.

In these comings and goings we passed about eight months without once meeting the enemy, in spite of pursuing him incessantly. I used to wonder greatly at the chronometrical exactitude with which our vanguard used to arrive at the villages occupied by the rebels just twelve hours after the latter had withdrawn. It seemed to be a game of blind-man's-buff. Obviously, in my position as physician and soldier I could not make any complaint. In eight months of war—more or less—I had no opportunity to hear the whistle of bullets or to treat a wounded man. The effects of some fall from a horse, indigestion, or an indulgence with the Venus of the cheap and vulgar, and there you have the full list.[2]

The criticism of that campaign I leave to the experts. I consider it indubitable that by preventing Carlist depredations in the prosperous Catalan cities we were fulfilling the main requirements. But my spirit, which craved strong emotions and warlike experiences, deplored the cautious peacefulness of the war.

[2] In connection with Venus, there was an event which cost me some annoyance: a certain captain who was married and had a family in Lérida, came to me one day for examination with unmistakable symptoms of recently acquired venereal disease. As this condition was common enough in that trying life in the field, it did not appear to me indiscreet to call things by their names. To my surprise, however, the officer suddenly changed countenance and became red with anger, exclaiming, "Take care, Doctor! I come from Lérida, and neither now nor for many years past have I had relations with any woman other than my wife. If that were true! The scoundrel!"

I understood the situation at once, and seeking a way of repairing or glossing over the *faux pas*, I replied: "Then it must be something else. Let us see: do you drink beer in excess?"

"A great deal; it is my favourite beverage."

"That changes the case. It is simply a urethral catarrh brought on by the elimination of hops, combined with the effects of cold. The indisposition is not serious."

When I left him pacified and prepared to follow an energetic treatment I drew a long breath. With my stratagem (at that time the irritating effect of beer passed for a fact) I had perhaps avoided a blood-stained drama; for the captain concerned had an extremently violent disposition and was jealous of his wife, whose reputation, it may be remarked in passing, was somewhat equivocal.

To-day, this cautiousness, reënacted a thousand times in our civil wars, causes me less surprise. It is a symptom of an incurable constitutional infirmity, characteristic of the Spanish people. Gracian declared: "The Spaniards are valiant, but slow." That is why the reconquest [3] was prolonged through seven centuries and our civil wars always last six or seven years. Happy are the countries in which diligence is one of the forms of patriotic honour! For every dynamic general, like Espartero, Cordoba, or Martínez Campos, we have reckoned by the dozen the sluggards who have worn the general's sash. O Saint Laziness, the patroness of our politicians and soldiers! If at least we had been able to spread our *disease of repose* to foreigners! But we must get on with our story.[4]

I have nothing of interest to tell of events during my stay in Cataluña. Those military promenades consolidated my physical education admirably and enabled me to study thoroughly the soul of the honourable Catalan *payés*.[5]

Although the army doctor was then entitled to ride, with the right, in consequence, to have baggage carried if he did not have a horse of his own, I preferred to make the stages on foot, chatting with the officers. On the long journeys, we took advantage of the mules to carry our equipment and especially the provisions collected by the practicante [6] and the male nurse; both of whom, it may be mentioned in passing, exercised an irresistible tyranny over me. They looked after my pay for me and guided me paternally in the thousand incidents and difficulties of military life. The orderly, a pleasant youth from Alicante, was a great prier

[3] The reconquest of Spain from the Moors by the Christians, commenced in the second decade of the eighth century by Don Pelayo of Asturias and completed in 1492 by Ferdinand and Isabel. (Translator's note.)

[4] While I am revising the third edition (Dec., 1922) Spain is bewailing once more the desperate sluggishness of our military action. We are incorrigible. We have been fighting in Melilla for a year and a half to recover, and that only in part, what was lost in two weeks of inexplicable mistakes and inconceivable lack of foresight. We have much to do yet.

[5] Catalan countryman. (Translator's note.)

[6] *Practicante.* The doctor's assistant who performs minor operations. (Translator's note.)

to smell out provisions. Even in villages recently sacked by the rebels, he knew how to get hold of a hidden chicken or to draw from its concealment some piece of *butifarra*.[7] As my two acolytes had sweethearts in almost all the towns, I often shared the fine gifts (pies, sweetmeats, handkerchiefs, socks, etc.) with which the poor girls thought to secure the flighty affection of their gallants. O youth, and how you beautify to the eyes of the old even the recollection of the most trivial incidents!

On one occasion I really believed that I was going to satisfy my desire for dramatic excitement by witnessing at last a formal act of war. My hopes were disappointed, however, although the operation undertaken turned out particularly distressing even for my exceptional powers as a pedestrian. This was what happened:

We were spending the night quietly in Tárrega, the delightful Capua of the Burgos regiment, when, before dawn, there sounded the reveille. We jumped up, thinking that, as usual, we would take the road to Agramunt or Verdú. Great was our disappointment. The day's march was a trying one, for it was more than fourteen leagues. It seems that during the night our colonel had received a despatch from the Captain General of Cataluña, ordering him to set march as soon as possible for el Bruch, where he was to escort a certain convoy which had left Barcelona for Berga, which was being closely blockaded by the Carlists at the time. We had, therefore, to proceed from Tárrega to Cervera, from Cervera to Calaf, from Calaf to Igualada, and from Igualada to el Bruch. After a few hours rest in the last-mentioned village, having joined the convoy, we arrived in the middle of the night at Manresa, where we slept. The soldiers were frightfully fatigued and our burden of sick and of stragglers was very large.

As for me, in spite of the fatigue and the distressing effects of a wretched pair of new boots, I had still sufficient spirit to admire from el Bruch the gigantic, ruddy masses

[7] A kind of sausage made in Cataluña. (Translator's note.)

of Montserrat, and to recall with the officers the famous rout of the French at the historic town. At last, on the following day we were joined by new forces and then continued our march by Sallent, where we slept, to the environs of Berga, where we pitched our tents. Throughout the journey, many precautions were adopted, as we feared that the Carlists might set an ambush or attack us in the gorges of the Llobregat. Dashing my hopes, however, the insurgents, aware perhaps of the considerable forces which escorted the convoy, raised the siege of the stronghold. I did not experience, then, any more warlike sensation than the bitter-sweet impression of a night in camp in the mountains surrounding Berga, apart from a severe catarrh brought on by the night dew. A few days later we returned to our headquarters in Tárrega.

During these military wanderings, I had an opportunity to become acquainted at close range with the Catalan character, and I retain pleasant and ineffaceable recollections of the people with whom I came into social contact. In Tárrega, in Cervera, in Balaguer, etc., we were received graciously, indeed with demonstrations of cordial good will. The allotment of billets upon our arrival was unnecessary; each man went to the house where he had lodged on previous occasions for he knew that the host would receive him amicably. I still have in mind my excellent host in Tárrega, a worthy cloth-merchant, the father of a number of fine and industrious children, who developed such a liking for me that he invited me to his table, presented me with game and sweets, and advanced me money when our pay was delayed. On one occasion, when I was ill and unable to join my company, he cared for me solicitously and, when I reached convalescence, was so generous as to provide me with money and a peasant's costume [8] for a rapid trip to Zaragoza to visit my family before my regiment returned.

In the houses where parties were held and even in the more modest families, the young ladies delighted in speak-

[8] The disguise as a peasant was necessary, for the Carlists often searched the train from Barcelona to Zaragoza and captured or even shot the officers.

ing Castilian [9] and were most eager to make our sojourn agreeable. They regarded Catalan as a domestic dialect, adequate only for expression of the feelings and emotions of the hearth. This sentiment of adherence to the army and love for Spain, moreover, was not confined to the little towns of the Valley of Urgel and of Priorato, which were grateful for our protection; it welled up spontaneously in all the Catalan provinces.

I shall always remember with gratitude the generous reception of my host at Sallent, a certain veteran physician who was the father of numerous progeny.

Seeing me soaked with rain, wearied by many hours on the march, and stiff with cold, my host's family received me graciously and heaped delicate attentions upon me. They kindled a fire, in spite of the lateness of the hour, prepared a delicious supper, and wrapped me in dry clothes while my uniform was drying before the blaze. Indeed one of the daughters of the doctor, pretty and fair as a *Gretchen,* made a deep impression upon me. If, instead of my spending one night in that peaceful home, my stay had been prolonged for a week, I should have fallen hopelessly in love. In a word, the amiable wife and daughters of my host, with their kindnesses and attentions which I could never pay back, made upon me the impression which the prodigal son must feel when he is restored to the bosom of his family.

The hard-working Catalans loved Spain and her soldiers in those days! Later on—I prefer not to know through whose fault—things seem to have changed.

While we were wandering about through the land of the Catalans in pursuit of the invisible and incoercible Carlists, there took place an event which was decisive for my future.

In April, 1874, I received orders transferring me to the expeditionary force in Cuba. At that time the separatist war in the Grand Antilles flared up again, causing the selection by lot from the Army Medical Service of the Peninsula of new personnel to compensate for casualties overseas. I

[9] The Catalan language is quite distinct from Castilian, which is the standard Spanish. (Translator's note.)

was one of those picked out by chance. Going to Cuba involved promotion to the next higher rank, that is to a captaincy (first assistant physician).

I took leave, then, regretfully of my fatherly hosts in Tárrega and Cervera, whom I was never to see again, as well as of the Burgos regiment, in which I left friends whom I shall never forget, among them my assistant and orderly.

To satisfy desires which had been nursed for a long time, I then paid a brief sight-seeing visit to Barcelona to gaze upon the sea, with which I was not yet acquainted (and upon which I was going to sail for eighteen days), to examine the ships in the port, and to climb up to the Castle of Montjuich. Thence I contemplated rapturously the superb panorama of the city, the plain sprinkled with factories and country houses, and the famous *Tibidabo,* crowned with pines. When my curiosity was satisfied, I returned to Zaragoza.

Instead of lamenting the result of the drawing of lots, I felt an inward satisfaction; I was going to cross the Atlantic, like the famous and heroic discoverers of the New World.

My eagerness to abandon the Peninsula and to see the world vexed my father greatly. He tried to dissuade me from the journey, advising me to apply for discharge. He depicted in the darkest colours the unhealthfulness of the island and the dangers of a campaign in which I should be exposed to the risk of an obscure death; he reminded me that my future was in the academic profession and not in the army; and finally he hinted at the fear that, on my return from Cuba, my knowledge of anatomy, which had been so laboriously acquired, would have evaporated, carrying with it to oblivion my lofty aspirations.

Always tenacious to my purposes, I put an end to his arguments by telling him that I should consider it a disgrace to desert my duty by applying for discharge from the service. "When the campaign is over it will be time to follow your counsel; for the present, my self-respect compels me to share the fate of my fellow army-physicians and to meet my debt of blood to my country."

To be perfectly sincere, I acknowledge now that, besides the austere sense of duty, I was drawn overseas by the bright visions of the novels which I had read, the irresistible craving for wandering in search of adventure, the longing to see for myself the people and the customs of foreign lands.

In this romantic eagerness—a thing of long standing in me, as the reader knows—I was always supported by some of my fellow students and, of course, by my brother Pedro, who was two years my junior. The latter, it may be remarked parenthetically, embarked upon an adventure of truly epic character. With a display of determination almost unbelievable in a boy of seventeen or eighteen, he discarded his student's gown and fled from home in company with a certain seductive adventurer. After embarking at Burdeos he eventually reached Uruguay where he passed through the most surprising experiences and dangerous episodes.[10] Contrary to all my father's predictions, his proper, impeccable, submissive and obedient son surpassed at one bound all the boasted wildness of his first born! I was left as it were humbled by my failure to do anything so great.

Among my classmates and friends, the one who shared most enthusiastically in my eagerness to see foreign lands was Cenarro. I remember that soon after graduation we were walking together one day along the paseo de los Ruiseñores,[11] talking of the future and, in a confidential

[10] There he filled the most varied offices: he was a soldier, a hero of the pampa, was wounded in several skirmishes and became the private secretary of a certain Indian chief who could not write, but who made up for it by being always ready to attack boldly. The prodigal returned to the home fireside eight or ten years later and, repenting of his conduct, settled down to work and finished his medical studies honourably. Today, become a clinician of repute, he is one of the professors in the Faculty of Medicine at Zaragoza. In due time we shall take note of his interesting and fertile investigations on the comparative histology of the nervous system.

[11] Promenade of the Nightingales.

mood, telling each other our inmost desires. The essence, if not the form, of our conversation was to this effect:

"I am extraordinarily enthusiastic," Cenarro told me, "about the army, and especially the Army Medical Service. That is the only career which can satisfy the most lively craving of my soul, which is to have a change of scene each day and to witness spectacles that are exotic and picturesque. An appointment in Puerto Rico, Cuba, Africa, or the Philippines would make me the happiest of men."

"I agree with you absolutely," I replied. "I too am tired of the monotony and routine of ordinary life. I am devoured by an insatiable thirst for freedom and for new emotional experiences. My ideal is America, and especially tropical America, that wonderland so highly praised by novelists and poets! Only there can life attain its full expansion and efflorescence. In our latitude even the plants seem ill-nourished and, as it were, fearful of the inevitable winter dormancy. A sumptuous orgy of forms and colours, the fauna of the tropics seems to have been imagined by a brilliant artist determined to surpass himself. What would I not give to abandon this desert and plunge into the inextricable jungle!"

My friend and I eventually satisfied our burning curiosity. A few years after the preceding dialogue, Cenarro, become an army surgeon, was living in Tangier, attached to the Spanish embassy. There he was able to study foreign customs and different races to his heart's content. As for me, before two years had passed I found myself shut up in that much admired West Indian jungle; in those shadowy glades, as sad and gloomy in reality as they are seductive and alluring in the affected descriptions of Bernardino and Saint Pierre. Those who have sung the praises of the tropical flora have merely overlooked one little detail: that that enchanting paradise is simply uninhabitable for the European.

But let us return to the narrative. When my father was once convinced that the resolution of his eldest son was unshakable, he tried to ameliorate my future position in the Antilles as much as possible. To this end, he procured for me letters of introduction to the Captain General and other important people in the island of Cuba. He hoped that, thanks to them, I should be assigned to some relatively healthy post, such as the garrison in Puerto Principe, Santiago, or Havana.

Provided with my letters, then, and having received my travelling allowance, I proceeded to Cadiz, whence the steamer España was to set sail en route for Puerto Rico and Cuba. There we were joined by several colleagues, including A. Sánchez Herrero,[12] who was accompanied by his wife, and Joaquín Vela, a congenial fellow countryman and almost a fellow student of mine, since he had graduated a year before I did.

The impression produced upon me by the "little silver cup" (Cadiz), with its white houses, its clean, straight streets intersecting at right angles, and swept by the sea breezes was excellent. Not so pleasant, however, was that produced by the people of Cadiz. Whether because of my air of a greenhorn, which invited ridicule, or because of the general custom of taking unscrupulous advantage of the stranger, the fact remains that during the two or three days which I spent in the Andalusian city, I had nothing but annoyances.

As soon as I left the station, I ran into a swarm of porters and urchins who would not listen to my protests, but immediately took possession of my belongings; and upon arrival at the hotel (I remember that it was the *Hotel del Telégrafo*), there arose a formidable row as to whether this one carried an umbrella, that one a hand bag, the other a stick, while the next imagined that he had heard himself ordered to look after the trunk, which a companion was already doing. It almost required force to pacify

[12] D. Abdón Sánchez Herrero abandoned his military career in Cuba and, by his talent and industry, eventually attained the chair of Medical Pathology in the University of Valladolid. Afterwards he occupied the same chair in Madrid, where he died prematurely.

the rabble, besides the distribution of a goodly handful of pesetas; and this was right in front of the representatives of the law, who took it all as a joke.

On the next day I went to some of the shops. I was amazed at the scandalous price of ordinary garments, all the stores asking me fifty reals for a hat which in Madrid would cost twenty-four. A friend who was more experienced than I explained the puzzle, informing me that the merchants of Cadiz were in league for the methodical and cruel despoiling of strangers, especially those from the Indies, raising the cost of clothing, hats and travelling equipment to double.[13] In the streets it was an expensive thing to ask the way of a bystander or a porter, for he at once extended his hand to be reimbursed for the service. So deeply seated in those people was the inconsiderate exploitation of strangers that even the bell-boys at the hotel charged a certain percentage for each traveller whom they accompanied to shops, cafés, or places of amusement. These I abstained from attending, remembering the gifts which the women of Cadiz gave to Alfieri.[14]

To conclude the account of this tiresome trickery, I will mention what happened as I was embarking. I engaged a boat in the harbour to board the steamer and when we had gone about half way the boatman stopped short, laid down the oars, and said that as there was such a violent east wind I should, according to the tariff, pay him double in advance. When this took place, there was hardly half an hour until the liner was to set sail. Exasperated by the cynicism of the boatman and sick of pilfering and fraud, I threw myself at the cheat, and seizing him by the throat, shouted, "You will row with all your might or I will break your neck this minute." Fortunately, when he felt the harsh caresses of my fists, the rascal softened, resuming his work vigorously and murmuring that it had

[13] If my memory does not deceive me, the combine of the merchants was called in the slang of the city the Society of the *guiris*. It is unnecessary to say that the people living near the city escaped their fraud.

[14] Count Vittorio Alfieri, 1749–1803, an important Italian dramatic poet.

all been only a joke. The terrible east wind had vanished in a twinkling.

I suppose that things will have changed greatly since that distant time and that the local authorities will have been sufficiently jealous for the good name of the city and the safeguarding of its sacred economic interests to have taken steps to eradicate such excesses. For these things, small as they seem, are of transcendental importance for the prosperity of a commercial centre. As for me, I was so well chastened that never, not even after having passed several times in later Andalusian journeys near the home of Columela, have I felt any inclination to revisit it. There are abuses which are never forgotten.[15]

I was not surprised when I heard, some years later, that almost the whole of the commercial and maritime activity of Cadiz had been absorbed by Barcelona, the ships, either native or foreign, which made that city a port of call being very few.

[15] These judgments are not to be interpreted as an expression of ill will towards a city which I do not know. I learned later from the testimony of many friends that life in Cadiz, when one resides there, is delightful. The courtesy and generosity of the men and especially the fascination of the women are incomparable. I was not surprised then by the homage of submission, love, and admiration which Dr. Federico Rubio paid some years later, in his delightful book, ''La mujer gaditana'' (The Woman of Cadiz), to the seductive daughters of Cadiz, who were the joy, the ornament, and the grace of pagan Rome two thousand years ago.

CHAPTER XXIII

Arrival at Havana. I am assigned to the field hospital of "Vista Hermosa." I soon become ill with malaria. I make use of my enforced idleness to learn English. My suffering becomes worse and I am granted leave to convalesce in Puerto Principe. After the commencement of my recovery, I am assigned to the infirmary of San Isidro on the "Trocha del Este" (East Road). The life at *La Trocha.* My ingenuous quixoticness leads me to correct administrative abuses, with the sole result that I am prosecuted by the Commander of the forces.

The crossing to Puerto Rico and Cuba was made with a smooth sea and in splendid spirits. At that time the *Compañía Trasatlántica* of Comillas provided good comforts and amusements were not lacking on board, besides play and gossip, the useful recourse of all voyages. I have never been much interested, however, in mischievous tales and tattle. During the day, I concentrated my attention on the magnificent spectacle of the sea: the flight of the gulls, the pursuit of the sharks, the leaping of the flying fish, and those creatures like floating flowers of delicate and gelatinous aspect which are called medusae, siphonophores, etc. When night came, I engulfed myself in the contemplation of that sky, the constellations of which changed as we approached the equator. Even in the black swell (the *black sea* of Homer, a phrase which Magnus used to deny that the Greeks knew the colour blue) were fascinating surprises. On calm nights it was not confined to copying passively the lights of the firmament, but glowed with deep and mysterious resplendence. My childish curiosity was fascinated by following the phosphorescent wake produced by swarms of noctilucas, excited by the formidable disturbance of the propeller. As may be seen, the sensation of floating between two infinites caused me no fear. I still had fresh in my mind what I had read of the evolutionists, who regard the sea as the cradle of life, and the rhythm of the waves evoked in me the panting heart-throbs of the mother fervently embracing her children. It is true that I had not so far seen the goddess Thetis in her murderous outbreaks.

Towards the sixteenth day of the voyage, there appeared very early in the morning the city of San Juan de Puerto Rico, with its imposing fortress and its white houses arranged on picturesque terraces. Impatient to tread the soil discovered by Columbus, I took advantage of the stopping of the steamer to wander through the city and its immediate environs, where I saw with wonder some examples of the tropical flora. At last, we resumed the voyage and two days later arrived in Havana.

Wondrous and unforgettable is the panorama of the populous Cuban city seen from afar. At the left, as one enters the harbour, towers the imposing bulk of the *Castillo del Morro* bristling with cannon and comparable in appearance and position to that of Montjuich; and at the right, spreading in endless series, are houses, palaces, and villas separated by the most beautiful gardens where graceful palm trees rise. Finally, once one is inside the harbour, a kind of semilunar bay bordered by innumerable coves and headlands, one sees the port, fronting the business area; while in the background rise several green hills, the slopes of which are sprinkled with picturesque suburbs.

It would be inopportune for me to stop to describe the beauties of Havana and the fertile regions round it, which are already sufficiently well known. No more does it enter into my calculations to describe minutely my impressions as a traveller. I will only say that the first great American city which I visited seemed to me to be merely a continuation of Andalusia. In fact, the speech, soft and variegated with pleasant lisping,[1] is Andalusian; the houses (built with a lower and an upper floor), with their enchanting patios and gardens, are Andalusian; and the spirit of the Creole,

[1] In Cuba, as in Andalusia, the soft *c* and the *z*, which in Castile are pronounced *th*, are given approximately the sound of the letter *s*. (Translator's note.)

sensitive and visionary, but languid and indolent, is Andalusian too.

It was perhaps a serious mistake for the economic prosperity of Spanish America that from the first use was not made for colonizing of the strong racial material in our northern parts, which is industrious, thrifty, and highly prolific, instead of drawing preferentially on the people of Andalusia and Estremadura, who are intelligent, generous, and capable of all sorts of heroism, as history shows, but have less aptitude for the profitable struggles of commerce and industry.

As to my impressions in seeing the sights of the capital of the Antilles, I will confine myself to saying that everything attracted my curiosity and in everything I found reason for surprise and basis for instruction. The strange mixture of races in the streets; the richness of the parks where, besides strange flowers and gigantic century plants, there grew the lofty royal palm; the delicious fruits of the country, like the banana, the coconut, the mango, and the pineapple; the luxuriant trees with evergreen leaves, festooned with Spanish moss or climbing lianas; a sky now blue, now gray, ready to burst into a torrential shower; and up above that abounding nature, which seems to chant a hymn to the joy of living, the fatherly sun beating straight down like molten lead upon our heads.

When something is ardently coveted, the reality usually mocks the hope. I was not disappointed, however. In the presence of the living reality, the descriptions in books retained their fascination. I lived as in a dream, and as if under a sort of spell.

In some connections, nevertheless, I suffered disillusion; for example, in the famous virgin forests, so celebrated by the romantic poets. In response to my repeated questions, the people of the country pointed out the jungle to me, but the impression made by this was insignificant. Instead of woods a thousand years old, never profaned by the foot of man, I found a common thicket with scattered shrubs and small cedars and mahogany-trees growing in disorderly fashion. I consoled myself up to a certain point with the reflection that the necessities of colonization had involved the clearing of the primaeval forest. What a pity it was not to have arrived four centuries earlier, when Columbus and his company trod upon such sublimely virgin strands!

With the animal life also I was disappointed. The native animals were becoming scarce and those which I did see were far from impressive. Not a jaguar, not so much as a single rattlesnake! In my wanderings through the outskirts of the city, I could discover only the all too common cosmopolitan sparrow, a bird imported from Spain; some crows and thrushes, and a certain tiny and not at all showy little bird called *vigirita* by the countryfolk. (In allusion, no doubt, to the weakness and delicacy of this little bird, our soldiers called the creoles *vigiritas,* and especially the *mambises* or insurgents; on the other hand, we people from Spain were called sparrows and big-footed.) Only in cages could I admire the many-coloured parrot and some exquisite specimens of humming birds from Peru.

I was vexed likewise by the total extinction of the native race, of which traces perhaps remain in the country people of the present day. In its place, assigned to the rudest labour, appeared the negro race and its various mixtures of which the longshoremen of the wharf were outstanding examples. As for the creoles, they impressed me as pale hothouse plants living indolently and parasitically at the expense of the sap of the Africans and mulattos. Occasionally, nevertheless, I met individuals of active and robust type among the creoles; but for the most part, and excepting some unusual natures, the white race seemed to me incapable of withstanding the ardours and dangers of the tropical climate. The white man degenerates rapidly there. I refer, naturally, to the European engaged in agricultural labour and exposed, in consequence, to a multitude of parasites, of which the mosquitoes are often carriers (malaria, yellow fever, etc.). Naturally, the Cuban or the peninsular Spaniard who is confined to the city and engaged in business or professional work which does not involve muscular exertion or exposure in the open air resists much better the enervating effects of the climate; but, even so, his vigour is maintained only by repeated admixtures of European blood.

By reason of this perfect adaptation to sedentary life, the Cuban woman not only has preserved the racial type better than the men, but has refined her delicate femininity, acquiring, as well in her spiritual as in her physical characters, sweetness and gentleness such as are exceptional or unknown in the beauties of Europe. When they speak they sing and when they look they caress. This explains why most of our overseas leaders and generals fell into the nets of these languid and fascinating beauties.

In such explorations and enjoyment of novelties about a month passed. The period of acclimatization being over, it then became necessary to distribute the medical officers recently arrived from the Peninsula. For this purpose, we were assembled one day in the quarantine station and told of the vacancies. There were places for regimental physicians in the active columns, for instructors on duty in the city hospitals, and, finally, for directors of field infirmaries.

If the reader recalls the foolishly quixotic character of the author of this book, he will readily deduce that I would be assigned to one of the worst positions. This was, in fact, the case. Inspired by feelings of justice and self-sacrifice, for which I got no thanks, I refrained from presenting my letters of recommendation. I wished to undergo my fate, or rather the fate which my colleagues did not wish to undergo; the latter, somewhat more practical and untroubled by my scruples, moving heaven and earth to procure the hospital appointments, which were absolute sinecures, or failing them, those of regimental physician. For the fools and those without influence there were reserved the infirmaries in the jungle and on the trochas, isolated stations where supplies were obtained with difficulty, and which were extraordinarily unhealthful.

Obviously, the regimental physician in the field also

underwent grave dangers; but he had at least the advantage of drawing his pay regularly. He knew, moreover, that after some days of marching through the jungle he could return to the capital of the district to recuperate, repair damage, and take part in the pleasures of social life.

The reader will readily guess that the infirmary which I was to direct was one of the most dangerous and isolated; that of Vista Hermosa, hidden away in the midst of the jungle in the district of Puerto Principe, in the middle of a region devastated and depopulated by the war.

A few days after the distribution of allocations, the steamer which was to convey us to Nuevitas set sail, bearing several physicians going to the central department and a considerable body of fresh troops to make up for casualties. An armoured train conveyed us in a few hours from Nuevitas through the uninhabited jungle to the capital of the Camagüey. I lodged at the famous White Horse Inn, where my friends Vela and Sánchez Herrero also put up. At last, after a few days rest, I arrived at my destination, taking advantage of the visit of a flying column conveying rations to the infirmary of Vista Hermosa.

It was while we were still on the march, during a halt of the column, and under the roof of an abandoned station, that I had the first word of the imminent advent of the Bourbon monarchy. I had been invited to have coffee with some leaders and officers, when a certain Aragonese major surprised me with the question, fired at short range: "You, who have just arrived from Spain, what is the news of the conspiracy which is supposed to proclaim Don Alfonso?"

"I believe," I mumbled, "that the conservative Republic of Castelar deserves the confidence of the Army."

"I see clearly, fellow-countryman, that you have been living out of the world. What! Do you not know that the whole army, without exception, is Alphonsist, and that some day, in spite of the resistance of the politicasters, the Republic will fall?"

PLATE 11

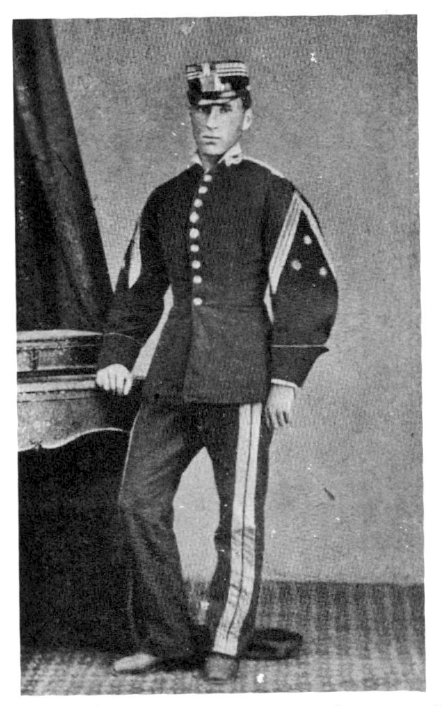

Fig. 19. Portrait as an Army-physician when About to Embark for Cuba.

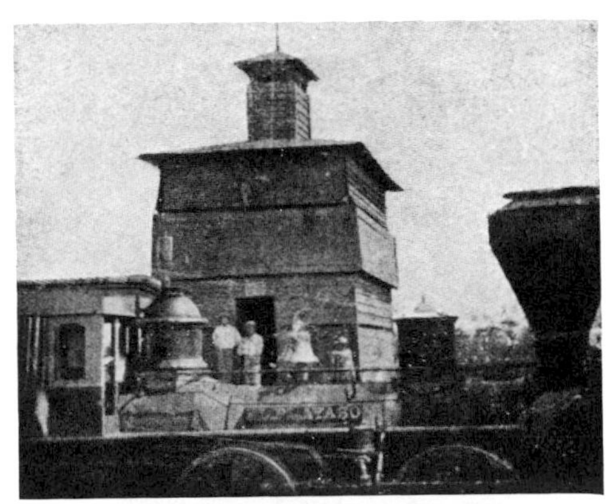

Fig. 20. A Fort of the Infirmary of San Isidro, on the *Trocha del Este*. The photograph, which I took by the collodion method, shows primarily the locomotive of the American type, with an enormous funnel-shaped smoke stack.

PLATE 12

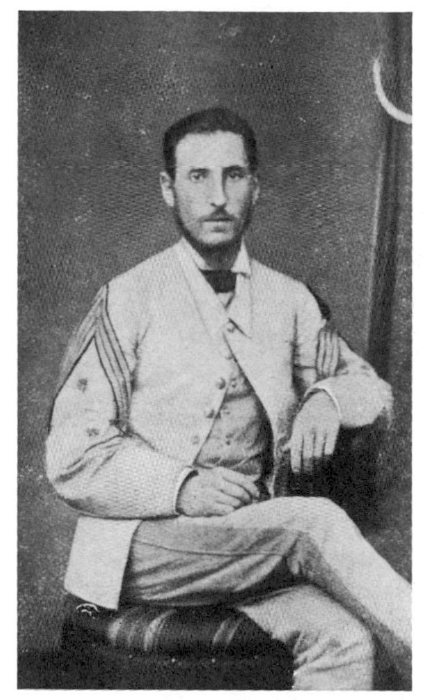

FIG. 21. PHOTOGRAPH OF THE AUTHOR TAKEN IN PUERTO PRÍNCIPE after convalescing from the malaria contracted in Vista Hermosa.

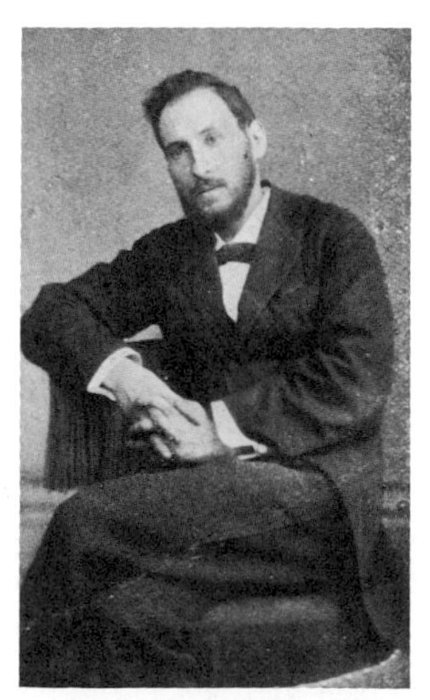

FIG. 22. THE AUTHOR in 1877, after his return to Spain, and still showing traces of the malarial cachexia.

Full of amazement, I glanced interrogatively at the Colonel, the commander of the force, expecting to see in his expression some sign of disapproval, or at least of disagreement. Quite the contrary. I soon found out that what my fellow-countryman had said was the everyday gossip of officialdom and that the army in Cuba, like that of the Peninsula, had passed over *en masse* to the Alphonsist camp.

In vain Castelar, with his political prudence and his wisely conservative principles, worked to consolidate the Republic on a permanent basis, the ideal of the Revolution; the rememberance of lack of discipline in the army and of the disgraceful scenes at Cartagena [2] had entirely alienated republican feeling from the hearts of the army and of the middle classes. The coup d'état of Pavía [3] was at hand.

Then there rose in my memory certain occurrences which I had witnessed in Cataluña, concerning the significance of which I had not stopped to think. When our column was passing the night in some important town, the officers who were frequenters of the café or the casino separated into two groups: the principal body, with the Colonel at the head, gathered about one or several adjoining tables whispering, so as not to be heard by the others; while a certain small contingent, made up of junior and senior officers who had been appointed by the Republic, formed a group apart. Here was, then, the peculiar situation of the republican officers (whose number diminished continually) in an actual Republic acting as if they were ashamed of the source of their appointment, and being treated disdainfully and almost with hostility by their monarchist colleagues.

Events soon made good the predictions of the major. It is well known that shortly afterwards (December 29,

[2] Several mutinies in the army.

[3] The setting of Alphonso XII upon the Spanish throne. (Translator's notes.)

1874) there occurred the military uprising at Sagunto and the proclamation of Don Alfonso XII.

The encampment at Vista Hermosa was a small community spread over the slopes of a gentle elevation, encompassed by extensive jungles. On the highest eminence rose a solid square fort, built of heavy logs and pierced with loopholes. In it was stationed a company (somewhat diminished by sickness) under the command of a captain. A short distance away was established the hospital, an enormous wooden barrack, roofed with palm thatch and having room for about two hundred beds. At the corners, facing the jungle, projected two stout towers, reinforced with a parapet of logs. In the shelter of the fort and of the infirmary, which were the only buildings of any importance, were spread out the shops and some miserable huts belonging to Chinese and negroes. In the outskirts was a clearing, kept free from trees, the exuberant overgrowth of which had to be cut down frequently to keep it from invading the barracks [4] with its powerful increase and, at the same time, facilitating surprise by the enemy.

Once a month, the rations necessary for the hospital and the garrison were sent to us from Puerto Principe, use being made for this purpose of the movements of bodies of active troops. In the intervening periods, we were absolutely cut off from the world, it being dangerous to venture further than a kilometer into the woods, lest the insurgents should be lying in wait for us. Shots were exchanged almost every day between them and the sentries.

At that time the infirmary placed under my care housed more than two hundred patients, almost all cases of malaria or dysentery, derived from the flying columns on service in the Camagüey.

I slept close to my patients, in the great barrack, in a little room separated from the rest by a partition of boards. Besides a bed and a table, my apartment contained, in picturesque confusion, muskets of soldiers who

[4] Dwelling for the negro workers, not a military barrack. (Translator's note.)

had died, cartridge boxes and equipment of all kinds, boxes of biscuits and sugar, and jars of medicines—especially sulphate of quinine, the patron saint of victims of malaria in tropical countries. With crates and empty tin cans I fitted up a photographic laboratory in one corner and erected the book-case for my meagre library.

At first, in spite of the fatigue and the depressing effects of looking after so many sick men, I got along very well, spending my leisure time pleasantly enough in reading, drawing, and photography. Fortunately, as I have said before, I have endured the absence of social life quite well, thanks to the noble vice of making pictures and to my love of reading.

But against microbes neither the seduction of art nor flights of the imagination are any protection. My spirits kept up well but at the same time my body weakened. Nor were the rations, which consisted of bread, biscuits, rice and coffee, the most adequate to create good blood. In vain I tried to tone up my system by adding to the menu from day to day a banana or coconut, stolen at some time or other by some marauding negro from an abandoned plantation.

Finally, my resistance weakened and I succumbed to malaria. Clouds of mosquitoes surrounded us. Besides *Anopheles claviger,* the ordinary carrier of the malarial protozoön, the almost invisible *gegén* tormented us, along with an innumerable army of fleas, cockroaches, and ants. The wave of parasitic life swept over our couches, raided our provisions, and enveloped us from every side.

How terrible is ignorance! If we had known then that the exclusive vehicle of malaria is the mosquito, Spain would have saved thousands of unhappy soldiers struck down by this disease in Cuba or in the Peninsula. Who could have suspected it? To avoid, or to check significantly the wholesale slaughter it would have been sufficient to protect our beds with simple mosquito nets or to clear out the mosquito larvae from the ponds in the neighbourhood.

Taking heroic doses of quinine sulphate helped little. One soon improved, but after a few days the attack recurred. This was daily in my case, because, no doubt, of very frequent reinoculations with the plasmodium. At the same time I had lost my appetite and my strength; my spleen hypertrophied; my colour became yellowish; I walked with an effort, and anaemia, the terrible malarial anaemia, set in with all its train of alarming symptoms. Finally, I was prostrated and unable to wait upon the patients. A foolish assistant supplied for me; everything was a mess. As a crowning misfortune, I developed dysentery in addition to malaria.

How admirable is the optimism of youth! My life was as seriously threatened as those of the poor dysenteric, tuberculous, and malarial soldiers who were dying all about me, and yet I had such confidence in the strength of my constitution that, whenever the symptoms were mitigated somewhat, I took advantage of my forced rest to learn English, to which end I had procured in Havana a considerable number of American books and illustrations, as well as the indispensable Ollendorf.[5] I believed firmly that whenever I should be able to get away from the influence of those miasmas (at that time the miasmas of the swamps were supposed to be the cause of malaria), I should rapidly regain my health. I am certain that my simple faith in the *vis medicatrix* saved me.

During these months there took place in Vista Hermosa a certain surprise attack which revealed to us the strength of mind and determination of my patients. It was about dawn when we were wakened by a tumult of voices and shots. I leaped from my bed, dressed hastily, and found that a party of the enemy, ambushed in the neighbouring jungle, was trying to take us by surprise. In fact one could see among the trees a confusion of cavalrymen and foot soldiers, mostly negroes and mulattoes. As it was discovered in time, the commander of our settlement

[5] A method for learning English.

quickly took defensive measures and, full of concern for me, offered me asylum in the fort.

"Don't worry," I told him. "If the insurgents attack the hospital, we shall be able to defend ourselves; and in any case my duty is to remain with the patients."

All this happened in a moment. The febrile attack had overtaken me and I was in a state of almost delirious excitement. Nevertheless, I seized a gun, picked up some cartridges, and ran through the wards inviting those who were not too seriously ill to join in the defence. Most of them, even those prostrated with fever, got up on their beds and took down their Remingtons. Those who were able to get on to their feet concentrated themselves in the bastions of the barrack; those who could not knelt in their beds, pointed their guns through the windows and took aim at the enemy. There was a volley in reply to the fire of the insurgents.

The rebels, finding us thus forewarned, retired without attempting to repeat the exploit at Cascorro, another settlement like ours, where a few weeks previously they had surprised and massacred the garrison and the patients.

Once more my mad desire for warlike experiences was fortunately frustrated. In my enthusiasm I often forgot that my task was not to fight but to cure the suffering. It is obvious that a foolish eagerness for notoriety, for vainglory, pursued me even in my sick-bed.

My illness, as I have mentioned, went from bad to worse; in view of which I applied to the Inspector of Health at Puerto Principe for a month's leave. Although with difficulties and arguments about the length of time (there being no one to take my place), it was finally granted. After I reached the capital of the Camagüey, suitable treatment and, more than anything, the cessation of new infections, relieved me greatly. The photograph reproduced here gives an insufficient idea of the emaciated and angular appearance of my face, even at the time of greatest improvement. Actually, I had fallen into that state of organic decay known as malarial cachexia, which was to drag on for many years and of the distant repercussions of which upon my health I am still the victim.

In consideration of my relative convalescence, the head of the Department of Health, Dr. Grau, attached me to the group of physicians on duty at the Military Hospital in Puerto Principe, where I mixed with friends from the Peninsula and had the pleasure of knowing Dr. Ledesma,[6] who was already outstanding as a most skilful surgeon.

I remained in the city for a month and a half. This was the pleasantest period of my stay in Cuba. Every afternoon there met in the *Café del Caballo Blanco* (White Horse Café) a group of comrades, including Joaquín Vela and Martín Visié, an excellent friend and a fellow student. In spite of my wanderings through cafés, casinos, and private assemblies I had the force of character to resist the four great vices of our officialdom: tobacco, gin, gambling, and women. It is true that I was not in condition for such amusements.

Alcoholism especially made havoc in the army. Of brandy and of gin, more even than of yellow fever, could it be said that they were the best allies of the insurgents. Smoking the most expensive cigars, and drinking all the gin and rum they liked, it was not strange that many junior and senior officers decayed both physically and morally. Besides, their pay being withheld, they were in economic straits.

I also struggled with difficulties of this kind although for reasons beyond my control. During the four months of my residence in the island, I had received only my first pay as captain (125 gold pesos). In vain I sent the certificates for my salary to Havana each month. The penury of the doctors in infirmaries was not due only to the classic lack of system in the Spanish administration; it was owing also to the defalcation of a certain Villaluenga, pharmacist in the Military Hospital at Havana and Paymaster

[6] Dr. Ledesma, the famous head of the Army Medical Service, became physician to the Royal Household, as is well known, through his merits in his profession.

General of the Medical Corps, who absconded to the United States with ninety thousand pesos and a strumpet.

In the distribution of pay there was an irritating lack of equity. The military physicians on service in the capitals received their salaries punctually; those with the army were usually somewhat delayed, although they could make use of the resort of drawing advances from the regimental coffers or of pledging their earned pay in commercial houses; but we poor fellows who served on the military roads or in the field infirmaries were dependent on the avariciousness of the office of the Paymaster General in Havana, and, lacking friendly relations with the merchants in the cities, were frequently forsaken.

This was my experience. When I had explained my precarious situation to Dr. Grau, he had the kindness to negotiate a loan (125 pesos) among my colleagues, to be repaid, as was just, from my back pay. In these wretched circumstances my request for assistance was excusable. Yet I learned with surprise, through my friend Visié that that collection for the benefit of a colleague had produced deep annoyance. "What sort of man is this," they said, "that has just come to the Island and asks for alms to live? Let him call upon credit like other people. Let him waken up and look out for himself, and give up his nun-like scruples.[7]

As a matter of fact, I was never very far-seeing, and

[7] They had such broad and lively ones that they collected the same pay three or four times in different shops. But it is better not to speak of certain financial arrangements. It is only fair to record, in exculpation of the sharp dealers, that the disorder of the administration reached a peak at that time, justifying to some extent irregularities which would have seemed intolerable in normal times and would have called for rigorous treatment.

That some idea may be formed of the extent of the administrative corruption, these words may be transcribed from the report of General Jovellar to the Minister for the Colonies (January 13, 1874): "The immorality in all branches of the administration, without excepting that of Justice, is the most corrupt in the world. It would be necessary to discharge at least three quarters of the magistrates, judges, and employees of the civil administration as well as military extortioners." Moreover, if we must believe those who know the underlying causes of the recent disaster of Annual (1921), our administrative incompetence is still as bad. We never learn.

on that occasion my colleagues tarnished a good action with an injustice. They forgot that I had spent four months in an uninhabited country, and during three of them had been seriously ill! My credit! What merchant in Puerto Principe would have lent his money to a poor, unknown devil with a ghostly face, and probably condemned to die very shortly in some remote corner on the military roads? That contemptuous commiseration was a hard but necessary lesson, which I never forgot. I vowed then that in future I would never ask anyone to lend me a single cent, and to this day I have fulfilled my resolution faithfully and strictly.

The death of the medical director of the infirmary of San Isidro on the East Road (*trocha del Este*) put an end to my temporary position as professor on duty in Puerto Principe. Without considering that there were available other assistant physicians more recently arrived than I, or thinking of the fact that my health was still far from being established, Dr. Grau appointed me to replace my late colleague, who had indeed taken the place in his turn of another doctor who had also fallen in the fulfilment of his duty.

I accepted the new charge without protest, although, as a matter of fact, it gave me little pleasure to take my place in the queue for death with my unfortunate predecessors.

The infirmary of San Isidro was one of the several field hospitals near the East Military Road, which commenced in Bagá, a little settlement on the broad bay of Nuevitas. Situated in a low and marshy region, it presented, if possible, even more unhealthful conditions than Vista Hermosa, over which its only advantage was the greater facility of communication and of procuring supplies. For between San Isidro and San Miguel de Nuevitas, the principal city on the road, not far from Bagá, there ran daily a military train or *plataforma,* as we called it. To protect the field hospital, a vast shed with room for three hundred patients, there was erected a strong, square fort, intended for the garrison. Some poor huts, inhabited by washerwomen and negro labourers, completed the little settlement, which was absolutely dependent on San Miguel for the necessaries of life and for all other commercial relations.

My fate showed itself adverse in arranging this new position. The hygienic deficiencies of San Isidro were certified, on the one hand, by the garrison, two thirds of which were nearly always ill, and on the other, by the remarkable fact that this spot—a vast plain crossed by swamps—had been chosen as a place of correction for drunken and dissipated officers. One or two months of exile in San Isidro was considered a drastic treatment sufficient to subdue the most incorrigible rebels. It was said, and not without reason, that when the gentle sentence had been carried out, the turbulent officers tasted the sweetest of peace: some being dead; the rest lying helpless on the sick-bed.

Soon after my arrival, I was able to witness the efficacy of that place of expiation. A certain drunken and quarrelsome captain had just died, and two officers whose terms had recently been completed were preparing with weak steps and languishing mien to take their places on the train to freedom. To replace them, there arrived a few days later a certain captain of the Headquarters Staff who was half crazy, but very clever, and with whom, indeed, I had vigorous philosophical discussions, and three officers from different parts of the service who were accused of promoting scandals and committing inexcusable excesses in cafés and other places of amusement. They were cheerful and talkative fellows. Listening to their stories of their prowess the time passed pleasantly. Such dramatic amorous conquests! So many ingenious tricks to circumvent the detested vigilance of husbands and fathers! Such infallible stratagems against the coffers of the money-lenders!

The distressing thing was that such entertaining chats soon stopped. One or two weeks later, almost all those arrogant Lovelaces succumbed to fever. And when the hour of their longed-for liberation struck, they rose from their couches determined not to remain in San Isidro one minute more. Two of them were carried to the train on stretchers. I remember that when they bade me adieu, they looked at me with pity such as the ransomed of Argel [8] must have shown for the captive without hope.

Such was the peaceful and salubrious retreat with which Dr. Grau honoured me in recognition of unquestionable qualifications. I did not complain and I do not complain today. After all, in the long run, somebody had to get the worst of it.

It may not be out of the way to explain to the reader the meaning of the defensive system of the military roads (*trochas militares*).

The *trochas* of Cuba were highways bordered by strong palisades, with or without barbed wire entanglements to reinforce them, and defended by a blockhouse at every five hundred metres, where small detachments of soldiers were on guard. Every thousand metres or more there was erected a wooden fort, where a company, or a part of one, was stationed. Here and there were settlements; and in them the line was guarded by military bodies of some importance, under the protection of which were sheltered hospitals and magazines.

The so-called East Road or Bagá Road, although it was not completed, extended from north to south about fifty-two kilometres, took in three or four field hospitals, and kept several thousand soldiers shut up in enervating immobility. The road from Júcaro to Morón, which was much more extensive, kept inactive eight or ten thousand, who had to be renewed every three or four months. There were times at San Isidro when three quarters of the garrisons of the military line were confined in hospitals, cramming them so that the blockhouses and forts remained almost abandoned and at the mercy of the enemy.

In theory the plan—a childish one enough—seemed well

[8] A moorish stronghold where Christian prisoners of war were held for ransom. Cervantes was confined there for five years. (Translator's note.)

worked out. Our military tacticians must have reasoned somewhat like this: the Great Antilla has the shape of a sausage, with two central constrictions dividing the land into three main parts; that of *las Villas,* the Western department, rich and prosperous, the tranquility of which it was very important to ensure; the Central department, or that of *Camagüey,* where the insurrection always had determined participants; and, finally, the Eastern (Bayamo, Holguín, Santiago, etc.), where the rebellion reached its full height. "If we cut the island from North to South," our consummate strategists must have thought, "through the aforementioned constrictions, by means of stockades and forts, those regions will be converted into perfectly water-tight compartments. Once they are finished, the roads will keep the prosperous department of Las Villas, the fount of such rich resources, from the revolutionary fever; and in this way a relatively small army can clear out the rebels methodically from each of the separate compartments in succession." Not a thought did those generals give to the unhealthfulness of the country or to the debilitating effects of inactivity.

The repeated misfortunes of the campaign proved that the fortified roads were a most serious error both hygenic and military. Perhaps that from Júcaro to Morón served some useful purpose at first, when the revolutionary companies attained only slender proportions or consisted of soldiers of little experience; but later the disadvantages greatly surpassed the very questionable benefits. Everybody could see—and it is established in the declarations of General Portillo and the reports to the government of Captain General Concha—that those impregnable Chinese walls were tactically ineffective. The insurgents crossed them with impunity (there will be recalled for example, among other celebrated sallies, that of the Júcaro road, carried out by Máximo Gómez in 1874 to spread the flame of the rebellion to Las Villas); they immobilized uselessly a large army which would have been highly efficient in active pursuit; they augmented unspeakably the casualties from sickness, especially during the rainy season (many forts were erected in swamps and marshes!); and finally, they used up fabulous sums in operations of grading, fortifying, constructing stockades and maintaining hospitals and depots for stores and medical supplies. And this just when the economic afflictions of the Mother Country, almost destitute of credit and bled by two tremendous wars in the Peninsula, were overwhelming.

By the time, later on, when, having been taught by bitter experience, we abandoned the military roads, they had cost over 20,000 victims.[9]

It is amazing and infuriating to recognize the blindness and obstinacy of our generals and governors, and the incredible insensibility with which at all periods they have squandered the blood of the people! How distressing it is to think of the complete irresponsibility which our blundering generals and our egotistical ministers have enjoyed!

In mentioning these matters after the occurrence of the colonial catastrophe,[10] it is difficult to resist the temptation to examine into the causes of so many reverses and to recall the tremendous blunders of our overseas policy. It is sad to realize that the characteristic of Spanish statesmen was always obstinately to ignore the lessons of history. Our politicians always lived in the present, intent upon the conflict of the moment, without giving the least thought to the future. Neither the tragic lessons of the emancipation of America nor two exhausting campaigns in Cuba, nor yet the advice of the few clear-sighted

[9] From the rather incomplete statistics concerning that campaign which were published, it appears that about 58,000 soldiers and officers died by sickness alone. Adding to this number that of 16,000, which was the reckoning of the soldiers returned to the Peninsula as cripples in the campaign (and of whom a great many succumbed in their home towns or in the hospitals of the Peninsula), we obtain a total of 74,000 casualties by illness, almost all fatal. And we are not counting in that number those who fell in battle, nor the prisoners and the missing, who numbered thousands.

[10] The loss of the Spanish colonies in the Spanish-American War, 1898. (Translator's note).

political men we have had, such as Aranda, Prim, and Pi y Margall, made any impression upon the untamed egotism of our alternating oligarchies.

With a lack of prudence incomprehensible in men of outstanding ability, men like Castelar and Cánovas thought that Cuba—that Cuba which hated us, and of which the independence, desired by the whole of America, was inevitable—was worth the sacrifice of Spain. The effective phrase of the famous Conservative statesman, "to the last man and the last peseta," has passed into history as an eloquent testimonial of how in Spain it is possible to reach the pinnacle of power without knowing at first hand the causes of our discords (to my knowledge, no Spanish ruler of that time visited Cuba or North America) or possessing the wisdom and foresight needed to safeguard the essential interests of the country. Other nations were much more skilful in such conflicts. Remember that Portugal and Holland preserved their colonies in spite of the greed of greater powers. How depressing it is to realize that the timely adjustment of our political standards with regard to the government of our Asiatic and American possessions would have maintained intact the glorious patrimony of our ancestors!

To rectify our management, we did not need to invent anything new. All we had to do was to imitate England, the unsurpassed master of the arts of politics, which is always attentive to the lessons of actuality. From the separatist war of the United States she extracted the great principle of autonomy, thanks to the sincere and generous application of which the movement for secession ceased in her colonies, which, in spite of political differences, we see today more closely united than ever in spirit and affection to the Mother Country.[11] Meanwhile, our political evo-

[11] While these lines were being written, in 1916, Canada, India, Australia, South Africa, etc., felt as their own the war between England and Germany, and, displaying an admirable racial patriotism, were sending military contingents to the scene of the struggle. Here is the fruit of political generosity, which is nothing else, in fact, but the highest and most clear-sighted practicality! (Note to the second edition.)

lution in respect of colonial government consisted of passing from a tutorial rule to an assimilative one. And when, compelled by circumstances, we planned to dictate reforms in Cuba, the only thing we thought of was to set up a colourless pretence of administrative and political autonomy, that is to say, one of those half measures, devoid of generosity or magnanimity, hateful alike to the Creoles and the Peninsulars, which resolute temperaments, in their hatred for the central government, always reject as intolerable farces. It is well known that the Cubans rose in rebellion when they realized the insignificance of the projected reform.

If, at least, at the end of the first Cuban war—which, like all civil conflicts, terminated in a compromise—we had kept honestly our solemn promises; if, instead of carrying subtle formulae to the Court, our rulers had ratified legally the conditions of the peace of Zanjón, as Martínez Campos offered to do, we should perhaps have avoided the second separatist war and with it the disastrous clash with the United States! We fell because we did not know how to be generous and just.

But with these gloomy digressions I am losing sight of my subject and failing to fulfil my promise. Let us return, then, to San Isidro.

My medical work at San Isidro was very heavy, since there were more than three hundred patients. Fortunately, there was little variation or difficulty in the pathology of the cases: small-pox (which made havoc among the negroes), chronic ulcers, dysentery, and malaria.

But while the professional duties, although heavy, did not call for a great deal of mental exertion, the maintenance of the hospital on the other hand did very seriously. In San Isidro,[12] a large proportion of the employees used to defraud the State, from the commander of the of the garrison down to the male nurses and cooks. As

[12] I have reason to believe that the same thing happened in many other hospitals and that no importance was attached to it.

was to be expected, the Quixote that I had within me rebelled upon noticing such ignoble abuses and I launched myself resolutely into the struggle, just when my health broke down again seriously.

The method which the dishonest members of the staff employed to live parasitically at the expense of the administration was as follows. On two or three occasions the patients for whom fowl had been prescribed complained to me of the insipidness and the washed-out appearance of the portions served. Surprised at the complaint, I determined to ascertain at any cost why the birds in the henrun had lost their fine flavour so quickly. I chanced one day to be walking through the outskirts of the settlement when I came upon a well-stocked poultry yard belonging to the cook of the hospital. This discovery was like a ray of light to me, and piecing the facts together and following the clues, I finally solved the problem, besides uncovering many other abuses carried on through the complicity of the cook and nurses for the benefit also of the commander and officers of the garrison.

The mysterious disappearance of the fowls was brought about in two ways. First, by agreement with the cook, the patients received as good helpings of chicken pieces from which the broth had previously been extracted, and which were thus despoiled of their substance. Second, the male nurses charged up in the book of prescriptions and diets, which I signed each day, a certain number of extra portions. Thanks to such a commonplace scheme the nurses and officers ate chicken at every meal, and even had some left over to populate the corral of the cook, a big negro who was as deceitful as he was insolent.

A comparison of the diet lists before and after they were sent to San Miguel by the male nurse (made by memory, so as not to excite suspicion) established the actuality of the abuse and showed me besides that, by employment of the convenient method of making additions to the lists, practically all the meat, eggs, sherry, and beer consumed by the officers and male nurses came out of the budget of the hospital.

When I indignantly confronted the cook and male nurses, the actual authors of the fraud, there took place the following scene, which they faced with surprising cynicism, as if they had nothing to fear. In reply to my urgent questions, they declared that sharp practice, if such a venial irregularity could be so termed, was the customary thing at the infirmary; that, thanks to his prudent tolerance, my predecessor had been able to live at peace with the officers, and besides to save almost the whole of his salary; and, finally, that I had better give up my trouble-making and foolishness and conform to the established administrative practices. And this occurred when, stricken anew with malaria, I was parsimoniously laying out my last cents and negotiating for a loan against one delayed instalment of my pay with a certain merchant of San Miguel, so as not to have to have recourse to the hospital kitchen!

Still, if this "absentmindedness" had been due to necessity, I should have calmed my scruples; but I knew definitely that the senior and junior officers, were in prompt receipt of what was due them. As for the cook and the male nurses, they carried on a nefarious traffic with the fruits of their dishonesty.

In this way there came about inevitably a clash with the major. In a private conference I censured his unethical procedure; I explained to him that for me it was a matter of conscience to eliminate such irregularities, since the responsibility for the administration of the hospital rested upon my shoulders; and I added finally that I was determined to correct the abuses radically.

The major became very angry, reproaching me and even making fun of what he called my mischievous tattling, but he did not try to cover up the facts. Perhaps he considered me incapable of bringing order into the administration of the hospital. However, when, a few days later, the senior and junior officers found themselves without free extras and learned that the requisition books of the hospital were checked daily, there was a violent reaction. There was at once commenced a campaign of petty annoyances and insidious trifles against me; I was cut by everyone; everything possible, in fact, was done to undermine the moral strength of a sick man. Needless to say, the cook and male nurses could see, and not without satisfaction, how the disease was rapidly wasting away my physique. A more suspicious person than I would have feared poisoning. Fortunately, I was able to preserve an incurable optimism.

Among the irritations with which the major tried to annoy me was one that almost raised a serious personal conflict between us. On nights of alarm (which were no rarities at San Isidro), he wished to put two of his horses into the hospital, beside the patients, so as to protect them from plunderers. In justification of this caprice, he alleged that there was not room for them within the fortifications at his residence and that the infirmary was the safest place to keep them. I repeatedly objected to such an insanitary suggestion, which he renewed several times, and finally the major gave it up, but snarlingly. All pretence of friendliness now being abandoned, he thought, no doubt, that he need not pay any attention to my scruples; and one night, when I was in bed with a high fever, I heard the horses led into the ward, bringing with them an insufferable smell of the stable. I dressed hurriedly and came out almost staggering to confront the grooms, whom I drove out vigorously, compelling them to take out the animals. Meanwhile the commander, being informed of the occurrence, came in a fury, exclaiming in an angry voice "Who are you to disobey me? I am the representative of the supreme authority here and it is your duty to respect my orders without question!" "I beg your pardon," I replied, "within these walls there is no authority higher than mine. The responsibility for the treatment and care of the patients rests upon me and I cannot conscientiously consent to the ward being turned into a filthy stable in deference to your caprice."

Blind with wrath and oblivious of the fact that he was facing a very sick man, he impetuously assumed a threatening attitude. I put myself upon the defensive, ready to return blow for blow. The fever put my brain in a whirl and for a moment I saw everything red. Fortunately the officers, somewhat more discreet than their major, saw the absurdity of the situation and separated and pacified us.

As was to be expected, the commander drew up an indictment against me for insubordination and threats against my superior. Proceedings were instituted. Documents piled up like foam. My superior in the hierarchy declared that he would not stop until he had sent me to prison. For the carrying out of his threats he trusted largely in a certain uncle of his, Brigadier X, who was then resident in Santiago and who was very influential in the Captain General's office. Eventually, however, what was to be expected happened. When, as a result of my declarations and denunciations, the authorities in Puerto Principe became acquainted with the scandalous grafting and the abuses of authority condoned or committed by the military head of San Isidro, everybody, including the famous general upon whom his nephew placed so much reliance, hastened to bury the matter in oblivion. Nobody, then, made any further reference to the proceedings against me, and an opportune change of command for reasons of health —we were all more or less invalids there—finally reestablished peace in San Isidro.

At any rate, I succeeded in my undertaking to purify the hospital administration so far as possible. Thenceforward, irregularities, maladversions, and sharp practices, if they still existed, were reduced to a tolerable minimum.

How heartbreaking it is for a patriotic spirit to see after forty-nine years that a great proportion of our soldiers, government employees, and even men in high political positions continue to plunder the State! It is a fact that to many Spaniards the State is a pure abstraction, an empty figment of the mind. To defraud it is to defraud nobody. What a strange paradox to believe that one is robbing nobody when one is robbing everybody! Gone is the religious feeling which in olden days put some restraint even upon inveterate greed, and we have not been able to replace it with patroitism, the strong and moralizing religion of powerful nations.

CHAPTER XXIV

My amusements in San Isidro. The dances of the negroes and the harp of the Savoyard. My illness becomes more severe and my application for a temporary relief from my post is refused. I ask for complete discharge. Thanks to the abandonment of the *Trocha* I finally get away from my location. A month in the hospital of San Miguel.

The time I spent in San Isidro seems, as I look back upon it, dim and shadowy as if I saw it through a thick mist. My position became more wretched every day. Most of my time was spent in bed without any comfort or attention, so to speak—other than those lavished by an assistant (he of the cheating) who cordially detested me. In spite of quinine, tannin, and opium (for dysentery), any relief I obtained was transient and short lived; the improvement which I hoped for so eagerly seemed to hold off indefinitely, mocking my expectations. For the first time, I began to doubt the powers of resistance of my system. During the gloomy hours when I dragged myself from my couch and was able to breathe the open air and watch the activities of the people, how enviously I looked at the robust health of the negroes, the ignorant labourers of the Trocha! At times that surge of life and overflowing happiness seemed to me almost like an insult.

Those Africans, brought to Cuba in slave ships, taught us a lesson in patience and resignation. Far from feeling homesick for their distant birthplace, they celebrated their festivals merrily and noisily, with hilarious jollifications and savage songs. It is a fact that the negro is almost immune to malaria.

The dancing of the groups of negroes was a strange and fascinating spectacle. While some couples, half-naked, danced incessantly beneath a burning sun, other primitive blacks marked the time by beating huge drums made from tree trunks. From time to time, a wild, shrill voice intoned a simple melody, perhaps a translation of some old chant learned in the forests of Africa. By frequent repetition there were engraved indelibly upon my memory the lines:

"I it was who killed the alligator,
Alligator. . . .
Alligator. . . .
I it was who killed the alligator."

This went on continuously for eight or ten hours, a chorus of savage shouts saluting the singer at the end of each stanza.

Those African dancers had muscles of steel. The sweat ran down their ebony skins in rivers and the sun glanced from the sculptured muscles of their bodies with metallic reflections. Far from wearing out their fierce excitement, this terrific exertion seemed to stimulate them. With some couples the *crescendo* of pirouettes, contorsions, and erotic movements reached an absolute frenzy. It is certain that no European could have stood one half of that excessively violent exercise.

Among our relaxations at San Isidro there were also harp concerts. But this requires that we turn back for certain explanations.

At that time, the Island of Cuba was a yawning abyss swallowing up soldiers; and as the voluntary enlistment for overseas service was increasingly deficient, the recruiting officers of the Peninsula resorted to all sorts of stratagems, even the most repulsive and infamous. To this end, recruiting agents did not scruple to frequent gaming-houses and taverns and, when a suitable stage of intoxication had been reached, to enlist not only all the vagrants and degenerates but also any young foreigners who fell into their clutches. Thus there came to Cuba some Savoyards, unfortunate artists who at that time used to wander through Spain singing the hymn of Garibaldi to the accompaniment of the harp.

One of these wretched Italians landed in the infirmary of San Isidro. He was suffering from hepatitis and dropsy, and his jaundiced face showed, besides, the indelible stamp of chronic malaria. I do not know how he had contrived, throughout his unlucky wanderings about the Island, to keep his precious musical instrument, beside which he used to sleep in the infirmary, fearful that it might be taken from him. This musical soldier was an obliging and good-natured fellow, and when the fever left him, he entertained us with open air concerts. By accommodating us he gained not only our gratitude, but also a few pesos which he saved towards his longed-for repatriation.

I seem to see him still in the moonlight, his face yellow, his expression downcast and sad, his abdomen dropsical—a morbid touch which gave him an aspect tragically grotesque. Placed in the centre of the group of listeners, resting his body against the trunk of a tree, he would produce with precision and feeling which our hunger for music transformed into something sublime, romances of Rossini and Donnizetti, Neapolitan songs, and airs of Savoy transfused with gentle melancholy.

I have already stated that my illness tended to grow worse. In the six or seven months which I spent at San Isidro I experienced only fleeting moments of relief. My liver and my spleen became alarmingly distended and the terrible dropsy set in. In vain I begged my medical chief, Doctor Grau, for temporary leave of absence. "There is no one to take your place," he always replied. "Hold on as long as you can; and whenever I receive a new draft of physicians, I shall make an effort to relieve you."

My hopes began to wither before that passive resistance, which had all the appearance of pitiless abandonment, and I finally came to the conclusion that if I was to save my life, it was absolutely necessary to remove myself with all possible speed from the effects of that unhealthful atmosphere.

But how was I to do so? In my desperate situation, I saw only one remedy: to ask for my final discharge on account of ill health, thus renouncing a military career and returning to the Peninsula. Consequently, I submitted a petition to the Captain-General through the health authorities at Puerto Principe; but when I was anxiously awaiting the reply, I was informed by a friend that in the capital of Camagüey they were refusing to transmit my application. My inhuman chief, Doctor Grau, doubtless thought that my worn-out system could carry on for a few months longer.

I owe my life to a certain chivalrous brigadier whose name, with unintentional ingratitude, I have forgotten. I have already explained that, as a defensive measure, the *trochas* had fallen into discredit, although nobody was willing to shoulder the responsibility of suppressing them. At the instance of the Captain-General, a tour of inspection of these lines of fortification was ultimately made, and the brigadier to whom I have referred, whose task it was to visit the road of Bagá or of the East, where I was stationed, was impressed so forcibly by what he saw of the bad condition of the soldiers and the tremendous number of patients who were rendered permanently unfit for service, that he ordered the forts to be dismantled and the garrisons withdrawn at once. Sympathizing with my condition and learning that my application for discharge had been held up, perhaps intentionally, in the district capital, he took upon himself the task of seeing it through personally, promising me, moreover, that he would hasten the action of the Captain-General as much as possible.

When the *Trocha del Bagá* was abandoned, the patients were distributed to various hospitals, especially to that of San Miguel, where I went to reside, this time not as medical director, but as one of the many clinical cases.

There, in a poorly and scantily furnished pavilion assigned to sick officers, I had another opportunity to experience the hopeless inefficiency of official charity. Even in the best organized charitable institutions, the sufferer often feels himself more or less abandoned; he always lacks that tender and watchful solicitude of which only the mother and the wife possess the secret. Obviously there is no lack of sisters of charity or male nurses, but through habit these worthy people soon acquire a depressing insensibility to other people's suffering. Besides, the sick person desires privileges; he would like to be the centre of general preoccupation; and he wants to find, in a word, fresh susceptibilities and affections which are not yet dulled by the daily struggle against pain. But that is almost impossible, as it is also impossible for the distressing incidents of sickness to adjust themselves to administrative routine.

For my part, accustomed to pretty poor attention in San Isidro, I bore my emotional solitude with relative resignation. Not so my immediate neighbours, among whom, was a certain lieutenant colonel of a violent disposition, who swore and worked himself into a passion when the sisters of charity did not respond immediately to his distressing shouts. In his annoyance, this officer—ill with advanced tuberculosis and other things—began in his madness to call with revolver shots. The first time we heard the volley, we certainly all thought that he had committed suicide or had wounded some hospital attendant who was too forgetful or lazy. I endeavoured to calm him and, so far as my physical condition permitted, attended at his bedside to assuage his consuming thirst and administer his medicines.

After a few weeks, I improved sufficiently to leave the hospital and proceed to Puerto Principe. Thanks to my beneficent brigadier, my new application had had the desired effect. In order, however, to obtain my final discharge as unfit for service, it was an essential requisite that I undergo a medical examination. This was done, then, in Puerto Principe, the result being a report of acute malarial cachexia, incompatible with any military service.

This formality complied with, and notification received that the Captain-General consented to the issuing of the discharge,[1] I set out for Havana, where I was to receive my back pay, obtain my passport, and await the steamer.

[1] The preliminary order for the final discharge was issued with the date May 15, 1875. The passport is dated May 21, 1875; and states that, since I am ill, my transportation to the Peninsula is in charge of the military Administration.

Being unfit for service, I was entitled to free transportation, but my economic difficulties were serious. Eight or nine instalments of my pay were due me. On account of the administrative orgy going on, I ran the risk of having to pass several months in Havana collecting what was owing to me, just when my condition demanded as quick a return home as possible.

In order to avoid such a serious eventuality, I had the foresight to write to my father a month previously. In the letter I depicted honestly my distressing situation and asked him to send me some money. Having received a draft from him, I was able more tranquilly to go about negotiating with the paymaster for the receipt of my back pay. At first he refused to pay me on the pretext that the appropriation for the last quarter had not yet been put through; but by dint of supplications and importunities I finally succeeded in collecting my dues—not, however, without leaving in the clutches of the greedy functionary between forty and fifty per cent of their amount. Nevertheless, without counting my father's money, I collected about six hundred pesos, with which I wiped out some small debts and acquired what I needed for the voyage home. Oh, our inveterate administrative abuses, and how dearly poor Spain has paid for them, always impoverished, always bleeding, and always forgiving and forgetting!

CHAPTER XXV

My removal to Havana, where I have a recurrence of my illness. My voyage home in the steamer *España*. Bodies of soldiers thrown into the sea. Transatlantic card-sharps. Love and malaria. My return to the study of anatomy.

A few days before the steamer sailed, and when I already had my passport and the ticket for the voyage, I suffered an acute attack of dysentery. Shipwreck in sight of port! How I was consumed with anxiety as I saw myself prostrated anew, with no friends to wait upon me and just at the longed-for moment of liberation!

At length Providence took pity upon me, and taking advantage impatiently of a slight amelioration, I embarked hurriedly on the steamer *España,* which was sailing en route for Santander. Along with me, many soldiers unfit for service also left the Island. The wretched fellows were sick like me; but, less well cared for, they travelled third class, herded together in crowded quarters and subjected to a diet inadequate or not sufficiently nourishing. It gave me satisfaction to attend to them, procuring for them the medicines which they needed, and encouraging their hopes. Several of these miserable creatures died during the crossing. What a heart-rending spectacle it was to watch the casting of the remains to the sea at dawn! On the other hand, some more fortunate invalids improved visibly. The purity of the air and the absence of new infections both contributed to their improvement, but the most efficacious agents were those two supreme spiritual tonics: the hope of soon seeing their native land and the joy of returning to the bosoms of their families.

I was one of those who improved rapidly in the pure sea air. By the time I reached Santander, I was a new man; I had a good appetite, my fever was gone, and I was strong enough to wander about through the highland city.

I was saved! There remained only a certain distressing emaciation and the straw-coloured pallor of anaemia.

After painting a picture of such heart-rending gloom, it will be well to add a pleasant touch. Our country has always been the fertile producer of organized roguery and of the picaresque. If Quevedo came back to life, he could still write his most witty and joyous ballads. In this respect we have not yet degenerated. The reader will easily guess that in a Spanish transatlantic liner, where all the social classes are brought together, there could not be absent, besides daughters of joy and typical examples of professional swindlers and extortionate office-holders, some genuine representatives of that cheating characteristic of the Spanish rogue so perfectly portrayed by our writers of the golden age. It fell to my lot to share a stateroom with one of these professional gamblers, who had no other occupation or source of livelihood than that of coming and going continually between Spain and Cuba, in order, working together with others of his trade and by the most polite methods, to empty the pockets of wealthy "*Indianos,*"[1] merchants with savings, and generals and high officials with fat profits.

Our elegant gamester always travelled first class, flashed enormous solitaires on his fingers, wore a showy chain on his watch, and dressed with that pretentious and vulgar ostentation characteristic of the low class man grown rich. From the first day, he pretended to be very sympathetic with my misfortune; and desiring to protect me and to provide amusement suitable for my rank, invited me in friendly fashion to join a game of "banker," wherein, thanks to the skill of my generous patron, I was absolutely sure to gain.

"I never deal," he told me, boasting of his restraint; "I confine myself to placing only small sums on a card. Only when I know several of the cards after four or five hands by the designs on the backs—and that is my secret—do I stake amounts of importance, and I always win."

[1] A Spaniard returning wealthy to the mother country from America.

As I shook my head incredulously, he added;

"Don't be a baby! When you see me back a card heavily, go in with me with all you have. You are sure to win three or four thousand pesos at a sitting."

Needless to say, my crafty counsellor was wasting his time pitifully. Apart from the distrust which I have always felt towards people who wished to patronize me without knowing definitely whether I deserved their patronage, I have never had the fever for gambling. Nor have I ever felt what Virgil called by the much-abused phrase: *auri sacra fames.* To me it appears that the affairs of life proceed and resolve themselves according to an inexorable logic, absolutely independent of any mystical influence.

I thought, and moreover, I still think, that there is only one rational and certain source of economic prosperity, hard work fertilized by the cultivation of the mind. Far from sympathizing with the loser in play, I regard him as a thwarted swindler, or as a covetous loafer. His honesty almost always ends when he loses his last cent.

I had soon reason to congratulate myself upon my distrust. Several rich merchants, who had been invited like me to bet on the same cards as the above-mentioned crook, were stripped clean. The wretches had lost in a few sessions of play twenty years of honourable work and stringent economy. For one of them we even had to pay for the boat to take him ashore. The poor fellow had lost fifteen or twenty thousand dollars, the capital with which he had expected to establish himself in his home town and provide for the happiness of his family.

I must have reached Santander about June 16, 1875. A swarm of ragged women surrounded us, quarrelling over our baggage. The scenery of the province of Santander delighted me, its luxuriant vegetation impressing me as comparable only to that of Cuba. From what I was told by various people, I learned with profound disillusionment that Spain possessed only a narrow zone of climate like that of other parts of Europe: between the Cantabrian coast and the range bordering the high Castilian tablelands. The rest—a lofty plateau burned up during five months of the year—is a place of expiation which can be inhabited only by farmers who are hardened by excessive work and simple food.[2]

On the way to Madrid, I visited Burgos, and admired its marvellous cathedral and its interesting monasteries of *las Huelgas* and *la Cartuja.* Then, after resting for a few days in the capital, I had at last the unspeakable joy of returning to Zaragoza and embracing my parents and my brother and sister. They found me yellow and emaciated, with an unhealthy appearance which distressed them. What would they have said if they had seen me two months previously?

Although I did not recover my former vigour nor succeed in getting rid entirely of the malarial anaemia, I became much stronger in the air of my native land with nourishing food and the unreplacable care of a mother. From time to time the fever returned, but quinine was now more efficacious.

When I had improved, then, so far as possible, it became necessary to think of the future. I had to reshape my life, directing it once more towards its old course. My father, who was always active in my behalf, kept urging upon me that a professional career was the ideal most in

[2] Later (in 1876, I think) I took a short trip into the south of France with a former chum (the son of Sr. Choliz of Valpalmas), who was receiving a commercial education in Oloron. We crossed the border at Sumport and visited Pierrefitte, Oloron, and Pau. My surprise when I saw the extraordinary richness of the French soil was indescribable. When I observed the luxuriant wheat fields in which a man could hide standing upright; the meadows, green and succulent even in August; the orchards and gardens flourishing without irrigation; the comfort and prosperity of the peasants, whose neat and comfortable dwellings contrast so strongly with the decay and poverty of those inhabited by our farmers; the proximity and richness of populous towns and cities, etc., I had for the first time the melancholy vision of the physical causes of the age-old weakness of Spain. Only then did I begin to understand her chequered history, and her innumerable misfortunes, and to see an explanation for her utter inability to fight, either in the realm of arms or in that of scientific, industrial, and commercial intercourse, with the rich and populous France and the other European nations which enjoy great geographic and climatic advantages.

accord with my training and tastes, since my inclination for clinical work left a good deal to be desired. My health, moreover, being rather poor, did not permit the physical effort which is required for the service of an urban clientele, among whom the young doctor must inevitably gain experience with patients living on the fourth floor and in garrets.

In connection with my sickly appearance and by way of a bitter-sweet interlude, I may relate the first of my sad experiences of love affairs. Shortly before I joined the army, I paid court to a certain young orphan lady, who was agreeable and well educated. The letters from her which I received during the campaigns in Cataluña and Cuba were a sweet comfort to me.

Upon returning to Spain, I immediately visited my sweetheart, who lived with her uncle, her only remaining relative. She received me well but without the effusiveness and joy which I expected after nearly three years of friendship and such a long absence. At succeeding meetings her reserve and coldness increased disquietingly.

Naturally, in my condition as an invalid and as a physician without patients, I was far enough from being what is called a good match. Through my ill-fated voyage overseas, I had lost both my health and my career. Hence it was necessary for me to open up a new path for myself through life. And that would be a long story.

I was consequently assailed by tormenting doubts as to the true state of the affections of my sweetheart. Was it aversion, indifference, or affection which was real but restrained by the dictates of good breeding? Did she perchance have some other suitor?

In order to dispel my uncertainty once and for all, I resolved to perform a decisive experiment. Words may be deceitful, but expressions always tell the truth. My plan was disrespectful and imprudent. It consisted of determining the reaction of my betrothed upon the receipt of a furtive kiss. Knowing her excessive modesty, the test was invested with qualities of extreme seriousness.

I recognized that a kiss leaves a good deal to be desired as a reagent of love, and especially in the case of unexpected and purely epidermal kisses, impressed upon the cheeks. In this connection I recall the ingenious anatomical classification given by a certain French medical man, who valued the sentimental worth of the kiss according to the following scale: cutaneo-cutaneous kisses, mucoso-cutaneous kisses, and mucoso-mucosal kisses. I did not consider it prudent to commence with number three of the scale, but with number one. Nevertheless, I carried out the test with unspeakable bashfulness and timidity, naturally, since it was the first kiss that I had ever given to a woman, despite the fact that I was over twenty-four years old.

On a certain day, then, after a languid and spiritless conversation, the tragic moment arrived. When I was saying good-bye, I gathered together all my courage, approached my always severe sweetheart, and brusquely imprinted upon her face the projected osculation.

My betrothed suddenly turned pale, uttered a cry of indignation, and quickly drew back her head. Offended modesty coloured her cheeks, and (what was highly significant for me) she wore an expression of instinctive repugnance, almost of loathing. In an altered voice she exclaimed; "Never did I think that you would offend me in such a way! Neither my education nor my own beliefs will allow me to tolerate such sinful liberties; and even if they did not prohibit it, prudence would do so, for there are men so ungentlemanly that they are capable of telling the weaknesses and compliances of their fiancées to the loungers in the café."

I was annihilated by such cruel words. I mumbled some phrases of apology, offered my hand automatically, took one melancholy look at the place where I had spent so many happy hours, passed through the door and never returned. What would have been the use?

The test had given a conclusive result. For that woman I was a poor invalid and—who would have thought it?—a villain besides. I consider it justifiable and laudable that a virtuous and well brought up young lady should repulse overexpressive advances of a thoughtless lover, but what hurt me most was that a lady should consider me so little of a gentleman. There are certain misdemeanours which can be suspected only when the image of the lover hardly has any place in the feminine heart. Moreover, a damsel who was discreet but in love would have found more gentle and indulgent arguments with which to correct the excesses of an over-impetuous fiancé. Later I learned from a third person that my fiancée was completely disillusioned. Pity rather than love bound her to her betrothed. My personality displeased her and she distrusted my health, which was considerably weakened. We must agree that the prospect of premature widowhood in the midst of poverty has little attraction. And the woman, when she follows the instinct of her kind, is always right.

Thus it is seen how the organism of the malaria contracted in the service of my country deprived me first of my health and then of my betrothed. Fortunately, not all women are so prudent and far-sighted. There are always angelic creatures with a vocation to be sisters of charity who, instead of rejecting a pale face and sunken eyes, ask themselves if it would not be possible and even ethically beautiful to restore broken health by dint of tenderness and maternal care and to return a man to society. And frequently they succeed.

The disappointment was great but not incurable, fortunately. I soon came to the conclusion that betrothals were not for me. My problem, like the problem of Spain, according to Costa, was of the school and the pantry—and of the apothecary's shop in my case. The important things first of all were to regain my lost physical strength, to study hard, and to carve out a career for myself. This could be accomplished only by following the road mapped out by my father. The rest would come to me as I did so

Accordingly, I resumed my attendance at the amphitheatre, renewed my acquaintance with my abandoned books of anatomy and histology, and began to prepare myself for the competitive examinations for professorships.

While I was doing this, thanks to the good friendship of Dr. Don Jenaro Casas, I was appointed by the *Joint Commission on Medical Studies* to a temporary assistantship in anatomy, with annual compensation of 1000 pesetas.[3] Two years later (April 28, 1877), when the Faculty of Medicine of Zaragoza acquired official rank, I received the appointment of *temporary auxiliary professor,* a position which at that time (the Faculty was in process of reorganization) involved a great deal of work, on account of the numerous vacant chairs. There were occasions when I had to conduct three classes in a day. From these appointments and the proceeds of some private tutoring in anatomy, I earned sufficient not to be entirely dependent on my family.

I cherished lofty ambitions. Although I was struggling with an excessively shy and retiring disposition, I aspired to be something, to emerge triumphantly from the plane of mediocrity and to collaborate, if my powers permitted, in the great work of scientific investigation. Resolute in this patriotic desire—which all my colleagues considered pure insanity if not presumptuous pretentiousness—I worked to attain the modest living and the uninterrupted leisure indispensable for the projects I had at heart. This *aurea mediocritas* was involved for me at that time in the honourable gown of the schoolmaster.

[3] At that time the Faculty of Medicine at Zaragoza, which did not yet have official standing, was supported jointly by the province and the city. A commission of city councilors and provincial deputies directed the studies and issued the diplomas. My appointment is dated November 10, 1875.

CHAPTER XXVI

Having decided upon an academic career, I graduate as doctor and prepare for examinations for professorships. Initiation into microscopic studies. Failure, as expected, in my first examinations. The defects of my intellectual and social education. These corrected in part, I finally succeed, obtaining the chair of descriptive anatomy in the University of Valencia.[1]

Nothing worth relating happened in 1876 and 1877. I remained in Zaragoza studying anatomy and embryology, and in my spare time assisting my father in the exacting service at the Hospital, supplying for him in the periods on duty and taking charge of the treatment of some of his private surgical patients.

My aspirations to an academic appointment (which were prompted continually by my father rather than felt spontaneously) obliged me to take a doctor's degree. It would have been wise to register officially in Madrid for the three courses standing in which was then compulsory for the attainment of the coveted hood of doctorate (history of medicine, chemical analysis, and normal and pathological histology). My sojourn for a year in the capital would have brought definite and inestimable advantages: I should have been personally acquainted with some of my future judges; I should have attended examination ceremonies so as to master the technical and polemical aspect of such disputations; and, finally, I should have acquired, so far as was possible for my nature, which was so brusque and shy, that veneer of pleasing ease and urbane courtesy which do so much to sell positive merit. My father, however, fearful, no doubt, that my artistic tendencies might flare up again if they were removed from his vigilance—and perhaps he was right—determined to enrol me in these courses extra-

[1] From this chapter on, the text was written much later than what has gone before, in the years 1916 and 1917, during the terrible European war.

murally, keeping me in Zaragoza. For the study of chemical analysis he entrusted me to the direction of Don Ramón Ríos, a very illustrious pharmacist, who was at that time at the head of a very highly regarded factory of chemical products. As for the history of medicine and normal and pathological histology, I was to assimilate these by self-tuition, studying the text books, since there was nobody in the Aragonese capital who could teach me them.

When the month of June came around and I was ready to undergo the tests in Madrid, I suffered two disagreeable surprises: all the fund of analytical knowledge which I had laboriously acquired in the laboratory of Dr. Ríos turned out to be useless, because, as those who studied in those days will remember, the worthy Rioz, professor of that subject in the Faculty of Pharmacy, required from medical candidates, with a consideration which contained a good deal of disdain, only a brief set of four or five questions, in each of which he included merely some examples of analysis of mineral waters, the composition of urine, milk, and blood—typical examples which everybody learned by heart in order to get through. It transpired that labour had been wasted also in the assiduous study of the history of medicine, following a certain French treatise which was the official text. My fellow students in Madrid, who were in the secret, disillusioned me greatly by informing me that the prescribed work was useless since Dr. Santero required almost exclusively what was set forth in a certain booklet, unknown to me, called *Prolegomenos clinicos*, in the pages of which the celebrated professor of San Carlos [2] eloquently developed a system of medical philosophy and gave free rein to his fervent passion for Hippocrates and hippocratism. Only Dr. Maestre de San Juan, the professor of histology, adhered faithfully to the announcement of his course, examining according to the text and the official programmes.

Consequently, I had no choice but to cram in three or four days of feverish work Dr. Rioz's elegant descriptions

[2] The hospital and medical school in Madrid. (Translator's note.)

of analysis and Dr. Santero's fiery and enthusiastic vitalistic assertions. It was only by great good luck that I came through the ordeal with no worse consequences than a horrible headache and a certain bitter aversion for the ill named freedom of teaching, thanks to which it frequently happens—now as then—that the independent student, relying upon the promise of the official curriculum, is ignorant of the subject matter explained by the professor and that the latter omits, sometimes, with admirable assurance, topics which, according to the regulations, it is his duty to expound.

Inspired by some beautiful microscopic preparations which Dr. Maestre de San Juan and his assistants (Dr. López García among others) were so kind as to show me, and anxious besides to learn general anatomy as thoroughly as possible since it is the indispensable complement of descriptive anatomy, I resolved to set up a microscopic laboratory upon my return to Zaragoza. Thanks to the never-failing kindness of Don Aureliano Maestre, I passed easily in histology, but I had never seen preparations made nor was I capable of carrying out the simplest microscopic examination. Moreover, what was worse, there was no one in Zaragoza at that time who could orientate me in the realms of the infinitely small. Besides, the Faculty of Medicine, in which I was an assistant and auxiliary, was very short of equipment. Only in the laboratory of physiology was there a fairly good microscope. With this veteran instrument, thanks to the good friendship of Dr. Borao,[3] who was then assistant in physiology, I admired for the first time the amazing spectacle of the circulation of the blood. This highly suggestive demonstration I have already discussed elsewhere.[4] Here I will say only that it contributed predominantly to my development of a love for microscopy.

[3] This amiable fellow student, son of the rector of the University of Zaragoza, Don Jerónimo Borao, died very young.

[4] Cajal: "Reglas y consejos sobre investigación biológica," 5th edition, pp. 105–106.

When I had selected an attic as a laboratory for my attempts at microtechnique and gathered together a few reagents, I lacked only a good microscope. The slender remnants of my pay in Cuba were not sufficient to buy one. Fortunately, during my last visit to the capital I had learned that in the Calle del León, number 25, on the ground floor (I have not forgotten it yet!) there lived a certain dealer in medical instruments, Don Francisco Chenel, who supplied upon the instalment plan excellent microscopes by Nachet and Verick, a French make which was then much in vogue. I accordingly opened a correspondence with this merchant and arranged the terms; they consisted in the payment in four instalments of 140 dollars, the price of a good model of Verick instrument with its accessories. The magnifying power of the lenses (which included a water immersion objective) reached to over 800 diameters. A little later, I purchased from the same dealer a Ranvier microtome, a *tournette* or turn-table and many other conveniences for microscopy. All this was provided by my modest salary as assistant and the meagre returns from private tutoring in anatomy; but the financial foundation of my laboratory and library was my economies in Cuba. Thus it appears that the diseases acquired in the great Antille turned out in the long run to my advantage. I am certain that, if it had not been for them, I should not have saved a cent during my residence overseas, and, consequently, should not have had available the necessary resources for my scientific education.

It was essential also to procure books and periodicals devoted to microscopy. I had few of the former, since I did not read German, the language in which the best treatises upon anatomy and histology were published. Only in French versions was I able to read the *General Anatomy* of Henle, and the classic treatise on *Histology and Histochemistry* of Frey. Van Kempen and Robin, excellent French books, likewise served me as guides. For practical work, I was able to consult Beale's *Microscopio en Medicina,* his *Protoplasma y vida,* and Latteux' well-known *Manual técnico.* As for scientific periodicals, the shortness of my funds compelled me to confine myself to subscribing to some English archives (*The Quarterly Journal of Microscopical Science*) and a French monthly review edited by E. Pelletan (*Journal de micrographie*). Of Spanish works, I had that of Dr. Maestre de San Juan, very full of facts but very difficult to read.

As is evident from what I have said, I began to work alone, without teachers, and with not very abundant equipment; but to everything I applied my ingenuous enthusiasm and my strength of will. The essential thing for me was to mould my brain, to reorganize it with a view to specialization, to adapt it strictly, in the end, to the tasks of the laboratory.

Naturally, during my honeymoon with the microscope I did nothing but satisfy my curiosity without method, examining things superficially. There was presented to me a marvelous field for exploration, full of the most delightful surprises. With the attitude of a fascinated spectator I examined the blood corpuscles, the epithelial cells, the muscle fibres, nerve fibres, etc., pausing here and there to draw or photograph the more captivating scenes in the life of the infinitely small.

The demonstrations being so easy, I was excessively surprised by the almost total absence of objective curiosity on the part of our professors, who spent their time talking to us at great length about healthy and diseased cells without making the slightest effort to become acquainted by sight with those transcendental and mysterious protagonists of life and suffering. What am I saying!—Many, perhaps the majority of the professors in those days, despised the microscope, considering it even prejudicial to the progress of Biology! In the opinion of our academic reactionists, the marvellous descriptions of cells and of invisible parasites were pure fantasy. I remember that at that period a certain professor in Madrid, who was never willing to muddle his mind by looking through the ocular of a magnifying instrument, characterized microscopic anatomy as *celestial anatomy.*[5] The phrase, which became popular, portrays well the mental attitude of that generation of teachers.

Doubtless there were noble exceptions. In any case, however, it is important to realize that even the rare masters who made use of the instrument of Jansen and believed in its revelations lacked that robust faith and that intellectual unrest which lead to checking the descriptions of scientists personally and with diligence. Perhaps they regarded histological technique as a very difficult discipline. Testimony of such indifference and lack of enthusiasm touching investigations which have since revolutionized science and revealed immense horizons to physiology and pathology, is given by a curious story of A. Kölliker,[6] the famous German histologist, who visited Madrid in the year 1849.

I was beginning, as I have said, to decipher delightedly the admirable book of the intimate and microscopic organization of the human body, when there were announced in the Gazette vacancies in the chairs of descriptive and general anatomy in Granada and Zaragoza. The notice upset me, for I was far from being ready to take part in the arduous contest of the examinations. As has been pointed out in earlier paragraphs, before entering the lists I should have liked to attend contests of this kind, to find out the tastes of

[5] Useless anatomy, from the phrase "musica celestial." (Translator's note.)

[6] A. Kölliker: *Erinnerungen aus meinem Leben*, Leipzig, 1892. In a letter to his family included in this book he describes the Museum of Natural Sciences, which was then (1849) installed in the Custom House (the present Ministry of Finance), and adds: "I must tell you an anecdote about the director, Graelis. There is displayed in his laboratory a splendid French microscope and, when I asked him if he had investigated anything with it, he replied that he had not yet had an opportunity to apply it to his scientific work as he did not understand its manipulation. He asked me to make some demonstration with the instrument. I proceeded, along with a friend (M. Witich) to show him the corpuscles of the human blood and the striated muscle fibres, before which spectacle he manifested childish delight and thanked us warmly.

If the illustrious German scientist had visited our Faculties of Medicine and Sciences twenty years later he might have found just as much neglect and apathy. The imposing microscopes of Ross or Hartnak reposed immaculate in their mahogany cases, serving no other purpose than to excite in vain the curiosity of the students or the ingenuous admiration of simpletons.

the public and of the judges, in fine, to determine the criterion by which are estimated the exact values quotable in the university market. My progenitor, however, like all fathers, had considerable illusions about the merits and capacities of his son and was immovable. I had no choice, then, but to obey him. So with little hope and, as the saying is, trying to pluck up heart, I went to those examinations in which nine or ten candidates, some of them really brilliant, struggled with all their strength for three posts.

During the exercises, my well-founded misgivings were fully confirmed. They made manifest, as I expected, that in classical descriptive anatomy and methods of dissection I showed up as well as the best. Honesty compels me to acknowledge, however, that in certain respects I showed at the same time lamentable deficiencies: overlooking bases of interpretation drawn from comparative anatomy, ontogeny, or phylogeny; ignorance of certain minutiae and side lights upon histological technique brought into fashion by Dr. Maestre de San Juan and the recent book of Ranvier, with which I was unacquainted; and, finally, neglect of all those speculations of an ornamental character, the highly prized flowers of thought which ennoble arid questions of anatomy and elevate discussion and render it agreeable.

This was not all, however. On that occasion I revealed, besides, defects of intellectual and social education unsuspected by my father. I was handicapped especially by my ignorance of the forms of courtesy employed in academic contests; the impression I made was dulled by exaggerated excitability, due, doubtless, to my natural timidity, but above all to my being unaccustomed to speaking before select and critical audiences; and, finally, I was caused to fail by my plain and uncultured style and even, I believe, by the most outstanding of my good qualities—the total absence of pedantry and pompousness in exposition. Among those polished youths, educated in the classic rhetorical style of our athenaeums, directness of thinking and simplicity of expression sounded rustic and vulgar. In my provincial candour, I was astonished at the grace and elegance with which some candidates of eloquence made pleasure excursions through the vast field of evolutionary or vitalistic doctrine, or, changing their register, proclaimed, à propos of nothing and filled with evangelical unction, the existence of God and of the soul in connection with a description of the form of the calcaneum or of the ileocaecal appendix.

However, resuming my narrative, I may add that only in two points did I attract considerable attention from the audience and the jury: in my coloured drawings on the blackboard on the day of the discourse, and in the copious details with which I adorned the few questions on descriptive anatomy which were asked me in the first session (most of the subjects had reference to histological technique and general questions, in which I was very weak). As for the practical examination, upon which my father based such great hopes, it was, as usual, pure comedy. There was chosen, in fact, a most simple dissection, the preparation of some articular ligaments. From this test we all emerged equal.

In my failure, which I felt most keenly because of the disappointment and disillusion which it was going to cause my father and teacher, I was consoled somewhat by the knowledge that I received a vote for one of the chairs and that I owed this vote to a teacher so learned, upright, severe, and conscientious as Dr. Martínez y Molina, who was called with reason *the pearl of San Carlos.*[7]

After more than a year had passed (1879), competitive examinations were announced for the vacant chair in Granada. Conscious of my defects, I had endeavoured to overcome them so far as possible. I perfected myself in histological technique, using as guide the admirable book entitled *Manuel technique d'histologie,* written by Ranvier, the illustrious professor at the Collège de France; I learned

[7] Long afterwards I was told that Dr. Martínez y Molina, the only judge who discovered any merit in the humble and unknown provincial, kept my coloured drawings of bone tissue and the process of ossification for a long time for use as demonstrations in his lectures. I was so timid and diffident at that time that I did not even dare to visit him to thank him for his generous and stimulating notice.

to translate scientific German; I acquired and studied conscientiously various German works on descriptive, general, and comparative anatomy; I posted myself in the modern theories of evolution, of which the standard-bearers at the time were the great Darwin, Häckel, and Huxley; I extended considerably my knowledge of embryology; and, finally, I adorned myself with some of those speculative niceties which, as I could see, won over audiences and examining boards, perhaps more than they should. Thus, for the first time in my life, I determined to be somewhat knowing, and to sacrifice to the graces.

I was tranquil and hopeful, busy giving the final touches to my intense anatomical preparations, when a friend stopped me one day, and blurted out:

"I want to give you a piece of advice. Do not go up for the approaching examinations for the chair at Granada."

"Why not"?

"Because your time has not yet come. Leave it for later and everything will turn out as you desire."

"But—"

"Take notice, my boy, that the examining board which has just been appointed has been selected for the express purpose of making Aramendia professor, as Dr. Calleja, the invariable arranger of medical juries, has a great admiration for his talents."

"But Aramendia has always prepared for examinations in medical pathology and has never concerned himself with anatomy!"

"Quite true; but there is no prospect of a vacancy in pathology for several years. His powerful patrons wish to make him professor at once; and since, for the present, the only open door is descriptive anatomy, they will take that. Come! Know for once how to be at least submissive and reasonable, and avoid increasing the number of your enemies with your imprudences. If you give way, you will win the favour of all-powerful personages, upon whose goodwill your future depends—."

"Thank you for your advice, but I cannot follow it. If I gave up the examination, my father would be furious and I should have no choice but to bury myself in some little town. Besides, after several years of assiduous preparation in anatomy, would it not be shameful to fail to take advantage of the first opportunity which presents itself to justify my pretensions? Important as it may be to obtain the desired appointment, it is still more so to demonstrate to the judges and the public that I have increased my knowledge and that, having been made conscious of my defects, I have been able, if not to correct them entirely, at least to diminish them somewhat, triumphing over myself."

"Then you will never be a professor, or you will become one very late, when you are gray-haired!"

"If cowardice and abdication are the price, I shall never be one."

I was soon able to test the correctness of the warning. In fact, the tribunal, with some exceptions, was made up of friends and supporters of the man who at that time exercised complete and irrestible control over the allotment of medical professorships. In excuse of the personage referred to, I must, nevertheless, state that Aramendia had been a brilliant student of his, that he was adorned by great endowments of character and ability, and, besides, that to assure the triumph of the inexperienced anatomist, there was exerted all the influence of Dr. Fernández de la Vega, professor of anatomy in Zaragoza, who was a relative of the illustrious president of the tribunal and a fellow student and close friend of the candidate alluded to.

At the appointed time,[8] the examinations took place. In them I had the good fortune to make evident the progress resulting from my application. My knowledge of histology brought me moments of brilliant display and the study of the German books and periodicals, which were unknown to my competitors, none of whom understood that language,

[8] In 1880.

lent to my work a tinge of erudition and up-to-dateness which was exceedingly pleasing.

There was only one opponent who withstood my assaults and turned them aside with the greatest ease, if not by the superiority of his anatomical preparation (which was by no means ordinary), by the clarity and acuteness of his understanding and the incomparable beauty of his diction. I refer to the illustrious and too soon departed master, Don Federico Olóriz, who, already in that, his first contest, displayed the extent of his worth and showed what could be looked for from the future professor in the Faculty of Medicine at Madrid.

On that occasion, Don Federico, who took part in the argumentation with me, attacked me vigorously, believing perhaps that I was the only serious adversary with whom he had to deal. And when, chatting amicably in the corridors of San Carlos, I apprised him of his error, naming the fortunate official candidate, he laughed at what he called my unpleasant Aragonese joking.

"But he is no more than a bright young man who displays very clearly his inexperience in anatomical studies and in the art of dissection!"

"Well, this improvised anatomist will be professor in Granada and you, with all your knowledge and ability, will have to resign yourself to the humble rôle of his assistant or else to change your course entirely."

"Absurd!"

The absurdity, however, came to pass. The friends of the president once more gave proof of the inviolability of his discipline and poor Olóriz, the wonder of the listeners and of the judges, had to content himself with third place in a group of three (I gained the second).

With all this, I do not wish to indicate that the preferred candidate was a poor professor. The dictator of San Carlos was not in the habit of favouring incompetents. I have already indicated that Aramendia was a young man of great brilliance and application and that, if he had really intended to, he would have become an excellent teacher of anatomy. In this competition, he lacked sufficient theoretical preparation and a vocation for the scalpel. So, when an opportunity presented itself, he transferred to a chair of clinical pathology in Zaragoza, where he turned out, as was to be expected, to be a good teacher of clinical medicine. Later, with the applause of many—including my own very sincere approbation—he rose by competitive examination, to a chair of clinical pathology in San Carlos.

I think it was in 1879 that, as a result of examinations, I was appointed Director of Anatomical Museums in the Faculty of Medicine at Zaragoza. Of those competitions, in which there took part, among other young men, a certain very brilliant student from the School of Valencia—a most passionate follower indeed of Darwin and Häckel—I wish to recall only one fact which illustrates the great sympathy, with which my fellow countrymen and my teachers favoured me. When the last test was over, the two Zaragozan professors voted determinedly for the Valencian candidate; and all the three professors from elsewhere, who had just gained their chairs by competition and had therefore minds clear of petty jealousies, accorded their suffrage to me. To these upright men, one of whom was Don Francisco Criado y Aguilar, who was afterwards professor in the Faculty of Medicine in Madrid,[9] I owe eternal gratitude. It is a fact that, among many other serious defects, I have always had an utter incapacity for adulation of the powerful.

After four years had passed (1883), there were announced two new vacancies to be filled in turn by competitive examination; the chair in Madrid, made vacant by the

[9] That result was decisive for my career. If any of the outside judges who had the kindness to support me had listened to the rancorous voices of certain Aragonese professors, my life would have followed a different channel; for my father, considerably disappointed by my downfall in Madrid, had determined, in case of another failure, to turn me into a practicing physician. And he would certainly have accomplished it, although he would not have been able to make me abandon my chosen pursuit of microscopic investigation.

decease of the noble and cultured doctor Martínez Molina, and that in Valencia, unoccupied owing to the death of Dr. Navarro. Modest and humble as always in my aspirations, I entered only the contest for Valencia; with better judgment, Olóriz applied for both positions.

On that occasion there was demonstrated once more the truth of the common adage: "From the excess of the evil springs the remedy." The scandal produced by the injustice done to Olóriz or me in the previous examinations for the chair at Granada (1880) had repercussions between the University and the Government. Hence, Sr. Gamazo, who was then Minister of Education,[10] was determined to avoid new abuses and appointed, or brought about the appointment of a tribunal the competence and independence of which were above any suspicion. The presidency of the new board of examiners was assigned to Dr. Encinas, who, with the outspoken frankness which was habitual to him, told the minister: "No tricks will avail where I am in charge. Upon the word of a gentleman, I promise here and now that either the selection will be unanimous or none will be made. And this will be true both for the professorship in Madrid and for that in Valencia."

And so it came about.

Thanks to the impartiality of this tribunal, upon which none of the previous judges had a place, Olóriz and I, provincials unprovided with protectors, at last attained the honour of University professorships. As we had expected, the brilliant disciple of the School of Granada triumphed over his competitors by unanimous vote of the judges; and the same tribunal, except for the president, who, on account of illness, was replaced by the great Letamendi, had also the kindness to select me, *nemine discrepante,* for the chair of Anatomy of the Faculty of Medicine in Valencia. I had always had a fervent respect for the very brilliant Catalan master; but from that time there were added to a simple

[10] Ministro de Fomento. This minister had charge of Education, Public Works, Agriculture, Commerce, etc. (Translator's note.)

intellectual admiration my warm and loyal homage of affection and gratitude.[11]

[11] When those examinations were over, I formed a close friendship with the famous professor of general pathology at San Carlos, going almost daily to his house, where he had set up a laboratory of microscopy and bacteriology. Letamendi was anxious to illustrate with photomicrographs his work *Curso de Patología general,* which was then in preparation, and I offered to make some examples and to teach the master's assistants how to prepare ultra-rapid bromide-gelatine plates, which were then almost unknown. What a delightful time I spent close to that man, whose brilliantly witty and acute mind shed the brightest of light upon the most abstruse problems and who, when he did not convince (he was, unfortunately, extraordinarily given to paradox), at least knew how to make one think!

CHAPTER XXVII

I fall ill with a serious affection of the lungs. Depression and hopelessness during my convalescence in Panticosa. The restoration of my health in San Juan de la Peña. Photography as pabulum for my thwarted artistic tastes. I marry and enter upon the cares of family life, which do not impede at all the progress of my studies. The mistaken prognostications of my parents and friends in regard to my wedding. My first scientific efforts.

The desire to combine in a single chapter everything connected with my failures and successes as a competitor in examinations has led me to change the chronological order of my narrative. Consequently, I must now reascend the stream of my recollections and mention some events which took place in the period between 1878 and 1883, the date of my taking possession of the chair of anatomy in Valencia.

In the year 1878, I was sitting one night in the garden of the Café de la Iberia with my dear friend Don Francisco Ledesma—a talented lawyer, who was at that time captain of the Military Administrative Staff—playing a strenuous game of chess. When I was deeply absorbed in the consideration of a move, I was suddenly attacked by a pulmonary haemorrhage. I covered up the occurrence as well as I could so as not to alarm my friend and continued the game to its conclusion; then returned home anxiously, the haemorrhage ceasing almost entirely on the way. I said nothing to my family, ate very little supper, avoided all conversation at table, and went to bed immediately afterwards. In a short time I was seized by a formidable haemorrhage: the blood, red and foaming, ascended with a rush from my lung to my mouth, threatening to choke me. I called my father, who was visibly alarmed and prescribed for me the treatment usual in such cases.

The pallor and progressive emaciation which he had noticed in his son for some months back, together with the effects of the malaria, never completely eradicated, had led him to make a serious diagnosis. Naturally, my father was careful to conceal his dismal prognostications, but I easily divined them through his careful interrogation and his artificially encouraging words.

A physician, besides, rarely deludes himself about his own condition. The symptoms of the terrible disease which I had read in books were too fresh in my memory, as were the sad images of unfortunate soldiers who, after their repatriation, died in the hospitals or in their own homes, victims of the tuberculosis which came as an aftermath of the treacherous malaria. In addition, my external appearance could leave no doubt: the high fever following the haemorrhagic seizure, the dyspnoea, the persistent cough, the perspiration, the emaciation—all the features of my illness coincided, point for point, with those deplorably exact descriptions in the text-books of pathology. What would I not have given then to efface the scientific knowledge which I had acquired! What agony to be a physician and a patient at the same time!

The fact is that I fell into a state of depression and despair such as I had never known even in the most serious of my experiences of sickness during my stay in Cuba. My discouragement was also contributed to, no doubt, by the somewhat vivid and rankling recollection of my downfall in Madrid.

It was impossible for me to eradicate from my mind the distressing idea of death. It clung to my overwrought sensibilities with an obstinacy which defeated *a priori* the best design therapeutic and hygienic campaigns. I considered my career at an end, my destiny fulfilled, my idea of contributing to the common heritage of Spanish culture a pure chimaera.

I realized bitterly that the extravagant romanticism which I had acquired during my adolescence from my foolish perusal of Chateaubriand, Lamartine, Victor Hugo,

Lord Byron, and Espronceda had poisoned my mind. Because of it, I had consumed in trivialities all the rich patrimony of constitutional energy inherited from my elders. In my desperation, I became a misanthrope and got to the point of despising the most holy and venerable things.

Two months later, nevertheless, I was able to leave my bed, but without joy and without illusions. "This is a respite," I said to myself, "not a resurrection. New attacks will come, and with them the inevitable *dénouement!*"

Only religion could have consoled me. Unfortunately my faith had been profoundly shaken by my reading of books on philosophy. It is true that two great principles had been saved from the wreck: the existence of the immortal soul and that of a supreme being who ruled the world and life. But the sort of stoicism after the model of Epictetus and Marcus Aurelius which I then professed (if I really professed any philosophy) did not transcend the world of the mind and the sphere of the will. The vital instinct, which is essentially egoistic, rebelled against the practical consequences of a philosophic conception which makes happiness depend upon serene resignation to destiny and blind obedience to natural laws.

'I admit," I reflected, "that the old, especially if philosophical, die impassive and resigned; death comes at its appointed time, when the primal purpose of life has been fulfilled and a modest place has been made in the luminous temple of the spirit." Through this consideration, I understood quite well how Epicurus, when he was old and tormented with a urinary calculus, should rise above his tortures and write to his friend Idomeneus these words in which noble and consoling pride shines forth: "I write these lines to you and your friends as I bring to a close the last happy day of my life. I am troubled with strangury and dysentery in unsurpassable degree, but I can confront it all with a joy of mind due to remembrance of our past discussions."[1]

[1] Translation of A. E. Taylor in "Epicurus." The Spanish version ends with the phrase *discoveries and ratiocinations,* to which the next sentence refers. (Translator's note.)

Where were my discoveries to console me? How is he to accept death with resignation who, having never really lived, leaves no trace of himself either in books or in hearts? This idea of the irremediable uselessness of my existence plunged me into the utmost anguish.

Calmer and more courageous than I, my father conceived hopes of a cure as soon as he noticed the first slight signs of improvement in my malady. To establish and increase the betterment, he sent me, as soon as summer came, to the baths at Panticosa, which were so highly regarded. He wished me to stay for a month or two when I had taken the waters, accompanied by my sister, gathering strength in the fine air on the summit of the famous Monte Pano, that is at San Juan de la Peña, where there is a half-ruined convent, inhabited by shepherds and surrounded with age-old forests. The programme, as we shall see, was carried out to the letter.

In Panticosa I began to recover somewhat from my dejection. Nevertheless, I experienced from time to time acute attacks of blackest gloom in Leopardi's manner.[2] The sentimentalism of my adolescence sprang up again dangerously at that time. Sometimes I wrote verses filled with foolish and impious apostrophes; at other times, inspired with almost suicidal thoughts, I climbed, halting and feverish, to the peaks nearest the baths and sank myself deep in the contemplation of that blue sky, almost black as a result of the clarity of that pure air, where soon, I thought, my wandering soul would have to lose itself forever. I remember that one afternoon, seized with a fit of gloomy melancholy, I scaled a lofty crest, which I reached breathless and almost fainting, and reclining upon a stone, I conceived the plan of letting myself die with my face to the stars, far from men and with no other witnesses than the eagles nor other shroud than the approaching snow of autumn. What madness!

But that poetic and romantic death which I craved (or pretended to crave, through pure morbid diletantism; for

[2] An Italian poet of the early nineteenth century whose works are steeped in gloom. 1798–1837. (Translator's note.)

really I cannot now analyze clearly those nebulous states of consciousness) never arrived. A strange thing, moreover, was that the more atrocities I committed, the less serious I found my condition. My system of treatment consisted of doing everything contrary to the advice of the doctors. Nevertheless, contrary to my expectations, after some weeks the bringing up of blood ceased; the fever diminished; my general condition improved; and finally my lungs and my muscles, which were subjected to barbaric tests, functioned better and better. It was demonstrated that one does not die when one thinks to do so. When least expected, the horse which we considered contemptible and weak turns out more spirited than the rider, to whom it usually gives eloquent lessons in discretion and prudence. Little by little the conviction that I should live found its way into my heart and mind.

Besides the unquestionable improvement, the suggestive and admirable spectacle of the tranquility of the consumptives contributed not a little to giving me courage. It is well known that bravery and courage are essentially contagious. None of those tubercular patients, most of them young like myself, acknowledged their disease; rather, they declared intrepidly that they suffered from simple catarrhs or from stomach trouble. Some said that they came to the baths not from any need but purely from gratitude toward the miraculous water; words of confidence which sounded bitterly ironical when one looked at the livid circles round the sunken eyes and the feverish roses in the cheeks. Even those confined to bed mostly seemed satisfied, appearing to cherish a firm belief that they would soon be cured. It is true that they were not physicians!

I remember in this connection the response of a very charming young lady from Cervera, whom I knew through having been several times billeted in her house when I was in Cataluña. Surprised at seeing the ravages which the treacherous disease had wrought in her beautiful face, I asked her, rather indiscreetly, how she was.

"I—very well, thank goodness," she replied. "Fortunately, there is nothing the matter with me. I have come to this watering place to accompany my father, who is troubled with a chronic catarrh. I am so well, that within two months I expect to marry L." (a very honourable proprietor of the neighbourhood).

A few months later I learned that the brave girl, who had thought her wedding so near, had died of consumption. And women have a power of resistance to the disease which we men lack. Instinct gives them incredible strength. They know or guess that beauty is the radiance of health and conceal with exquisite modesty, and sometimes with the most subtle artifices, their innermost sufferings.

The affability of the consumptives, and especially the quiet courage of the patient from Cervera, finally made me ashamed. I determined from that time not to be ill. Autocratically imposing itself over my lungs, my brain decreed that all was unjustified apprehension. The meticulous details of the regimen, the prescriptions of the works on hygiene and the pharmacopeia were over for me. In my contempt for therapeusis, I stopped entirely the drinking of the famous nitrogenated water and resumed an absolutely normal life. It was true that my lungs grumbled somewhat and that my heart persisted in beating faster than it should; but I vowed that I would pay no attention to them. Let them do as they liked! And I took up drawing, photography, conversation, and walking as if I had before me a prospect of endless life and activity.

When I returned from the baths and passed through Jaca to install myself and my sister in the new monastery of San Juan de la Peña I was very cheerful and had all the indications of real convalescence. The peace and picturesqueness of the place, a nutritious diet of meat and milk, daily rambles through the surrounding forest, interesting visits to the ancient monastery of la Cueva,[3] where the former kings of Aragon sleep their eternal sleep, excursions to take photographs in the region about the mountain and

[3] The Cave or Grotto.

the neighbouring village of Santa Cruz de la Serós, etc., finally brought me not only confidence that I should live but also physical strength and mental tranquility. Here I was, then, restored to the current of existence, with its anxieties and its struggles. My time had not yet come!

The sun, the open air, silence, and art are great physicians. The first two are tonics for the body, the last two still the vibrations of sorrow, free us from our own ideas, which are sometimes more virulent than the worst of microbes, and guide our sensibilities towards the world about us, the fount of the purest and most refreshing pleasures. Besides, coming back to my own case, my sister Paula turned out to be an ideal nurse!

I consider that photography, of which I was then an ardent amateur, helped very efficaciously to distract and calm me. It obliged me to take continual exercise and, by offering me the daily solution of artistic problems, it flavoured the monotony of my retreat with the pleasure of difficulties overcome and with the contemplation of the beautiful pictures of varied and picturesque scenery.

This enthusiasm for the art of Daguerre had been born some years before, as I have already described, in the heroic epoch of collodion, and its cultivation formed a happy compensation destined to satisfy the pictorial tendencies which had been conclusively defrauded as a result of the change in my professional course. For only the photographic lens can satisfy the hunger for plastic beauty of those who do not enjoy the leisure necessary for the methodical exercise of the brush and the palette.

Later, after I was married, I carried my cultivation of the art of photography to the point of becoming a manufacturer of gelatine-bromide plates, and passed my nights in a barn pouring sensitive emulsions in the red glow of a lantern, in the face of the wonder of curious neighbours, who took me for a goblin or a necromancer. This new occupation, so different from my devotion to anatomy, was the result of the insistent demands of professional photographers. Ultrarapid gelatine-bromide plates, which were manufactured at that time by the firm of Monckoven, and which were certainly exceedingly expensive, were then almost unknown in Spain. I had read the formula for the sensitive emulsion in a recent book and set out to manufacture it in order to satisfy my enthusiasm for instantaneous photography, a purpose unattainable with the troublesome procedure of wet collodion. I had the good luck to hit the mark at once in the essential manipulations and even to improve the formula for the emulsion; and my successful snapshots of incidents in the bull ring, and especially one of the presidential box crowded with beautiful young ladies (the occasion was a charity bull fight, patronized and presided over by the aristocracy of Aragon), created a furore, being passed round the photographic studios and exciting the amateurs. My rapid plates pleased the people so much that many desired to try them.

Thus, without wishing it, I found myself obliged to manufacture emulsions for the photographers both in the capital and elsewhere, hurriedly installing a work room in the barn of my house and turning my wife into an assistant. If I had been in touch with an intelligent partner and had possessed a little capital at that time, an extremely important and perfectly viable industry would have been created in Spain; for in my experiments I had come across a method of preparing an emulsion more sensitive than those known till then and therefore very easily protected from the inevitable foreign competition. Unfortunately, absorbed in my anatomical studies and the preparation for my examinations, I abandoned that rich vein which presented itself to me so unexpectedly.

Begging the reader's pardon for the foregoing digression on photography, I will conclude the account of my illness by adding that I returned to Zaragoza in October with almost flourishing health and devoted myself more enthusiastically than ever to the dissecting room and to histological studies.

At the end of 1879 when, my sickness forgotten, I succeeded in obtaining the appointment of Director of the Anatomical Museum, I determined to marry, contrary to the advice of my parents and friends, who presaged a disaster. For an impenitent dreamer, a despiser of filthy lucre and of all social prejudices, it is obvious that my marriage had necessarily to be a love match.

I became acquainted with my future wife in the following way: As I returned from a walk through Torrero one afternoon, I met a young woman of modest demeanour, accompanied by her mother. Her rosy and smiling face resembled that of the madonnas of Rafael and, even better, a certain German coloured print representing Marguerite in *Faust*, which I had admired greatly. I was attracted, no doubt, by the sweetness and gentleness of her features, the slender beauty of her figure, her great green eyes framed with long lashes, and the luxuriance of her fair hair; but I was seduced most of all by a certain air of child-like innocence and melancholy resignation emanating from her whole person. I followed the exquisite unknown as far as her home; I ascertained that she had lost her father—a minor officeholder—and that she was an honourable, unassuming, and industrious girl; and I became her suitor. Some time later, the counsels of my family being powerless to dissuade me, I married—not without studying thoroughly the psychology of my fiancée, which turned out to be, as I hoped, the complement of my own.

My resolution, according to the comments of acquaintances in clubs and cafés, was unanimously considered to be madness. Certainly, looking at the step from the economic viewpoint, it might have led to ruin. Courage was needed, in fact, to set up a household when my whole income amounted to a salary of twenty-five dollars a month and eight or ten more, at most, gathered from tutoring in anatomy and histology. It was for this reason that the wedding was celebrated almost secretly; I did not wish to trouble relatives or friends with proceedings which concerned me alone.

I remember that a certain acquaintance, surprised at seeing me enter with such lack of hesitation and such in-

PLATE 13

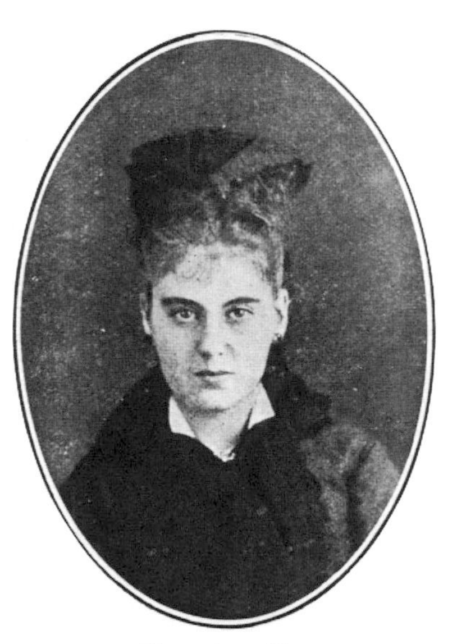

FIG. 23. PORTRAIT OF MY FIANCÉE A YEAR BEFORE SHE BECAME MY WIFE. This photograph, altered by time, gives little idea of the physiognomic characteristics of the original. At the risk of grave indiscretion, I reproduce it here, for my helpmate, with her abnegation and modesty, her love for her husband and children, and her spirit of heroic economy, made possible the persistent and obscure labor of the writer. (The exotic and horrible feminine hat was unknown at that time.)

trepidity into the ranks of fathers of families, exclaimed: "Poor Ramón is lost for good! Farewell to study, science, and lofty ambitions!"

The auguries were of the worst. My father foretold my death in a short time; my friends gave me up as having finally failed.

In principle my censors were right. It is unquestionable that, in most cases, feminine vanity together with the requirements and exacting cares of the home monopolize for financial support the whole of the mental activity of the husband, upon whom is imposed the well known *primum vivere* with all its desolating prosaicness. In affairs of this kind, however, it is more necessary than in the lessons of general experience to take special note of the individual conditions, tendencies, and innermost feelings. Besides, we often forget that in conjugal associations, besides economic factors, people are also activated by decisive ethical and sentimental considerations, under the influence of which there are produced unlooked for and almost always happy metamorphoses of the physical and spiritual personalities of the spouses. As a result of these changes and of the consequent integration of activities, the conjugal association constitutes a superior entity, capable of creating mental and economic values which are entirely new or are barely latent in the individuals combined.

From their not having taken these factors into account, the prophesies of my friends turned out entirely wrong. Physically, I improved visibly so that everyone recognized that I had never been so well since my return from Cuba. My wife, with an abnegation and tenderness more than maternal, devoted herself to caring for me and establishing my health upon a firm basis. As for my abandonment of study and of all lofty ambition, which was so positively foretold, it will suffice to remark that a few years later, when I had already two children, I published my first scientific contributions and gained the chair of anatomy at Valencia by competitive examination.

It is an essential condition for peace and harmony in

married life that the wife should accept willingly the ideal of life pursued by the husband. The happiness of the home, and the noblest ambitions are lost therefore, when, as we often see, the wife sets herself up as the spiritual director of the family and organizes according to her own ideas the programme of the activities and aspirations of her mate. Upon this head, I must confess that I have never had any cause for complaint.

Far from lamenting the almost entire diversion of my income to the dissipations and vanities of dress, the theatre, or domestic luxury, as has happened to many followers of science or art in Spain,[4] I found in my helpmate only assistance to pay for and satisfy my pursuits and to continue my career. There was no money, then, for fine clothes, theatres, carriages, or summer holidays, but there was enough for books, periodicals, and laboratory equipment. Moreover, although these eulogies seem strange and even out of place from my pen,[5] I take pleasure in declaring that, in spite of a beauty which seemed to invite her to shine and to display herself in visits, promenades, and receptions, my wife condemned herself joyfully to obscurity, remained simple in her tastes, and without other aspirations than peaceful pleasure, good order in the administration of the home, and the happiness of her husband and children. That my choice had been a good one, considering my character and tendencies, was quickly recognized by my parents, especially by my mother, who developed a sincere affection for her daughter-in-law, with whom she had in common so many domestic virtues and so many similarities of taste and character.

[4] I refer to this particularly in my book *Reglas y consejos sobre la investigación biológica*, 5th ed., p. 154 et seq.

[5] I should be unjust if, out of mistaken discretion, I should fail to say that during my first years as a professor only the unsurpassable self-abnegation of my wife made my scientific work possible. So much so that a certain highly talented lady used to say: "Half of Cajal is his wife."

PART TWO

THE STORY OF MY SCIENTIFIC WORK

CHAPTER I

My first attempts at investigation. Monographs on inflammation and on the nerve endings. Knowledge of myself and of men of science. I attain confidence in my modest aptitudes.

Without entirely passing over events foreign to my scientific work (I take into consideration that I am not writing exclusively for specialists, but for a cultured public of varied interests), the second part of this book will be the story of my laboratory work. I consider that it is not without interest to narrate how I conceived and realized the rather chimerical idea of building up histology in Spain in spite of the indifference, when there was not actual hostility, of the intellectual atmosphere.

I believe that I have already mentioned that during the last years of my residence in Zaragoza, when I was director of the Anatomical Museum and had married, I set up in my own house a modest laboratory of microscopy with the double purpose of giving lessons to students for the doctorate and of improving my histological technique. There, in a mean building in the *Calle del Hospital,* I commenced to try out my investigative powers, drawing my inspiration mainly from the wise counsels of Ranvier's *Tratado de Técnica Histológica.*

As may be imagined, my first efforts (two in number, published in Zaragoza in pamphlet form) were pretty weak.

The first of them, entitled: *Experimental observations on inflammation in the mesentery, the cornea, and cartilage,* appeared in 1880, illustrated with lithographs which I executed myself,[1] lacking resources to pay an artist. A

[1] In order to illustrate my pamphlets economically, I made a practical study of the manipulation of the lithographic pencil and burin. All my publications from Zaragoza and Barcelona (1880 to 1890) contain lithographs engraved by my own hands. I was so much taken with this method of reproduction that I went so far as to apply photography to the art of lithography, and secured acceptable results. The Zaragozans of my time will perhaps

heated discussion was going on at the time among anatomo-pathologists as to the essential mechanism of inflammation and especially the interesting problem of the origin of the pus cells. Wishing to form my own opinion on the subject, I studied the debated question experimentally, repeating and analyzing carefully the famous experiments of Cohnheim upon the inflamed mesentery of the curarized frog. Unfortunately, I was then largely under the influence of the ideas of Duval, Hayem, and other French histologists (who denied that the white corpuscles pass through the walls of the blood vessels) and was led to a conciliatory or compromising solution, erroneous, as are almost all intermediate opinions in science.

Overlooking the conclusions, this pamphlet contains a considerable number of new details regarding the modifications of the cells of the inflamed tissues (cornea, cartilage, and mesentery); the phagocytic power of the platelets of the blood is pointed out in it for the first time; the alterations of the inter-cellular cement of the epithelium of the peritoneum, of the capillaries, etc., are extensively studied; small new points which, like everything else which I gave to the press in those days, passed absolutely unnoticed by the scientific world. Indeed, it could not be otherwise, since I wrote in Spanish, a language absolutely unknown to investigators, and had timid editions of one hundred copies printed, which were rapidly exhausted in gifts to people whose interests were foreign to the subject. After all, nothing very important was lost in the forgetting of these small contributions. In fact, in connection with these timid efforts at research, a discouraging remark by some of the professors came to my ears: "Who is Cajal, that he should judge the foreign scientists?" So deep in the vitals of our race had taken root the conviction of our sad and utter incapacity for the cultivation of science!

remember a special number of the newspaper commemorative of the granting of a concession for a railway from Zaragoza to Canfranc, some of the drawings in which, made in pen and ink by Pradilla and other outstanding Aragonese artists, were reproduced photolithographically by me. It was, I believe, the first time that photography was applied to engraving in Spain.

More substantial, and of more strictly objective character, was my second publication, which also was issued in Zaragoza, under the title of *Microscopic observations upon the nerve endings in voluntary muscles,* and was illustrated by two lithographic plates coloured by hand. In this monograph the manner of termination of the nerve fibres upon the striated muscles of amphibians, as revealed by the methods then in vogue (gold chloride and ordinary silver nitrate), were examined, the descriptions of Krause and Ranvier, then much discussed, being confirmed in principle. As a positive contribution to the knowledge of the subject there were described in this pamphlet certain new types[2] of terminal arborization of nerve fibres (four varieties); an interesting improvement of Cohnheim's silver nitrate method was explained (previous treatment of the muscles with water containing acetic acid); the employment of gold toning to reinforce the images obtained with silver was suggested;[3] and, finally, there was described the first application to the tissue of the peripheral nervous system of ammoniacal silver nitrate, a reagent which in course of time was to become, in the hands of Fajerstajn and others, the basis of valuable methods of impregnation of the nerve fibres and cells.

Despite the mediocrity of the results, these attempts at research work were highly instructive to me. They led me to a knowledge of myself and a knowledge of the psychology of scientists.

It is obvious that, with much boldness and presumption, I attributed to myself, *a priori,* some aptitude for scientific investigation. My only excuses are my youth and, especi-

[2] These types were later regarded as the fruit of the personal investigations of Dogiel, professor at Saint Petersburg, who, naturally, was unacquainted with my work. See Dogiel: "Methylenblautinction der motorischen Nervenendigungen in dem Muskel der Amphibien und Reptilien," *Arch. f. Mikr. Anat.,* Bd. XXXV, 1890. Cuccati also unconsciously confirms some of my descriptions: *Intern. Monatsch. f. Anat. u. Physiol.,* Bd. X, 1888.

[3] Reinforcing and toning with gold chloride is now regularly used in silver impregnations (method of Bielschowsky and its variants, reduced silver nitrate, procedures of Achúcarro, Río Hortega, Da Fano, etc). No one knows who was the first to advise this improvement of the coloration.

ally, the psychological fact that without a certain lack of modesty nobody accomplishes anything important. Anyway, as I adventured in the objective examination of biological problems, my faith in myself increased, for it seemed to me that the presupposed qualities were confirmed *a posteriori,* among the most outstanding being patience bordering upon obstinacy in the mastering of histological methods, dexterity and skill in replacing expensive experimental arrangements with simple and improvised contrivances, indefatigable persistence and enthusiasm for the observation of facts, and, finally, best of all, open-mindedness for sudden changes of opinion and correction of errors and preconceived ideas; all of these qualities are naturally of secondary rank, but adequate for the work undertaken. Besides, in this work, which my colleagues and friends considered wearisome, I found the most fascinating of amusements. When I was eagerly occupied at the eye piece, the winter evenings passed rapidly, without my missing theatres or social gatherings. I remember that once I spent twenty hours continuously at the microscope watching the movements of a sluggish leucocyte in its laborious efforts to escape from a blood capillary.

However, as I said before, I became acquainted not only with myself but also with men of science; for nothing enables one to penetrate more deeply into the minds of other investigators than critically to compare their personal interpretations with the actual facts, following from close at hand the plan of action and the steps employed by them to overcome the obstacles and snares with which nature seems to defend herself against human curiosity. In this careful comparison of the model and the copy, there are revealed the intellectual lucidity, the solid culture, the technical difficulties, and sometimes the brilliant findings of genius; but there appear also the prejudices, carelessnesses, and equivocations of the man of science. Once they are discovered, these little mistakes are very useful in that they possess the virtue of jolting the diffidence and inertia of the beginner. From the general checking up of books by comparison with the objects, I came to the conclusion at that time that scientists—except in the rare cases of really great minds—are men like everybody else, without any advantage other than that of having prepared themselves adequately for investigation under the direction of illustrious teachers and in the lukewarm greenhouse of the scientific schools.

The most valuable fruit, however, of the aforementioned efforts at experimentation was the profound conviction that living nature, far from being drained and exhausted, keeps back from all of us, great and small, immeasurable stretches of unknown territory; and that, even in the regions apparently most worked over, there remain still many unknown things to be cleared up.

My enthusiasm, however, did not reach to the point of forgetting the difficulties of the undertaking and failing to recognize my poor preparation for embarking upon it. In spite of my youthful presumption, I soon realized some of my defects: it was urgent that I should extend and bring up to date my knowledge of physics and other natural sciences; that I should avoid the seductions of theorizing and the fascination of my own hypotheses; that I should restrain the natural tendency to premature publication, to the precipitate interpretation of facts without previously exhausting and carefully weighing all the possibilities; and, above all, that I should increase my knowledge of the literature sufficiently to obviate the bitter delusion of taking for ones own harvest the fruit of another's labour.

The correction of this last deficiency, which worried me very seriously—the Spanish universities being both then and now very deficient in respect of collections of foreign periodicals—demanded new pecuniary sacrifices. I added to the list of my subscriptions two more: the *Journal de l'Anatomie et de la Physiologie,* published in Paris by Professor Robin, which summarized the discoveries of French microscopists, and the *Archiv für mikroskopische Anatomie und Entwicklungsgeschichte,* a very fine publication illustrated with admirable coloured lithographs and directed by the illustrious W. Waldeyer, of Berlin, in which the most valuable contributions of the German, Russian, and Scandinavian histologists and embryologists saw the light.

I understood also that, besides foreign text-books, I must acquire those monumental monographs built up by up-to-date and accurate bibliography and written by famous savants or by groups of accredited investigators. The model at that time of this class of extensive treatises, invaluable for the devotee of the laboratory, was the *Handbuch der Lehre den Geweben* of Professor Stricker, each of his chapters being placed in charge of a renowned specialist. To this category of extensive monographs belonged also the excellent books of Ranvier entitled, *Leçons sur le Système nerveux* (two volumes) and *Leçons d'Anatomie générale,* as also the well documented treatises of Schwalbe upon the nervous system (*Lehrbuch der Neurologie*) and the sense organs (*Anatomie der Sinnesorgane*).

When, at the end of 1883, I prepared to transfer myself to Valencia, my family had been increased to the extent of two children and another was about to be born. It was thus demonstrated that, contrary to the expectations of my friends, the children of the flesh did not smother the children of the mind. If each newborn child brings a loaf of bread under his arm, as the old saying has it, each paper published brought not only the noble satisfaction of the mind but also the material bread for existence. These latter gave me the reputation of being studious and hard working—the only merits acknowledgment of which is not withheld, because they do not excite envy—and contributed to sustaining and raising the credit of my modest Academy of Anatomy and Histology. Eventually, along with my later books, they won me valuable sympathy and approval in Madrid.

CHAPTER II

My removal to Valencia. My rambles through the city and its surroundings. The orators of the Valencian Athenaeum. The cholera epidemic of 1885 and the prophylactic inoculations of Doctor Ferrán. Entrusted by the committee at Zaragoza with the study of anticholera vaccination, I give a lecture in the Aragonese capital and the committee rewards my labour by publishing my studies and presenting me with a magnificent microscope. Results of my investigations on cholera. I publish a book on histology. The wonders of this science and my transports of scientific lyricism.

At the beginning of January, 1884, I removed to Valencia and took possession of the chair of Anatomy. I lodged temporarily with my family at a hotel situated upon the Market Square, near the famous *Lonja de la Seda.*[1] Later, after buying the necessary furniture, we installed ourselves in a modest house in the *Calle de las Avellanas* (Hazelnut Street), where there was a large room suitable for a laboratory. A few days later a daughter was born.

Faithful to my creed that things are more interesting than people, I devoted a few days to exploring the attractions of the city. I visited the magnificent cathedral; climbed the Miguelete[2] to admire the luxuriance and extensiveness of the *huertas*[3] on the outskirts and the silver ribbon of the Mediterranean in the distance; I examined the suburbs of the city and the enchanting little towns of Cabañal, Godella, Burjasot, etc. I visited the port of *El Grao,*[4] the customary promenade of the townspeople of Valencia on holidays, and finally, overflowing with artistic and archaeological enthusiasm, I tackled the ruins of the Roman theatre at Sagunto.

1 The silk exchange, described as one of the best remaining specimens of civil architecture of the Middle Ages. (Translator's note.)

2 The famous tower of the ancient cathedral. (Translator's note.)

3 *Huertas.* Market gardens.

4 The sea-port of Valencia.

I found myself in a country new to me, with a most genial climate, in the fields of which flourished the century plant and the orange tree, and among the people of which dwelt courtesy, culture, and intelligence. Hence is Valencia called the Athens of Spain.

I was cordially received in the Faculty of Medicine. The rector at that time was the distinguished surgeon Ferrer Viñerta, who had a brusque disposition, vehement and autocratic, but good-natured and benevolent at the bottom. Shining lights among the academic staff were masters of such prestige as Campá, Gimeno, Ferrer y Julve, Peregrín Casanova, Gómez Reig, Orts, Magraner, Machi, Crous y Casellas, Moliner, etc. I felt quite at home in that circle of excellent colleagues. With their southern quickness of perception they realized at once that the new member of the staff was not going to usurp anybody's privileges either in the academic sphere or in that of professional practice, but would live quietly but independently engaged in his favourite studies.

In order to divert myself somewhat from the pursuit of microscopy, which absorbed and almost deformed all my faculties by allowing them to function in the one direction alone, I became a member of the *Casino de la Agricultura,* a club for smart people, where I came into contact with a circle of cultured and highly agreeable persons. From time to time, as a rest from chat and discussion, I took part in the noble game of chess, and had the honour to play against the champion of Valencia, Sr. Rosello. This was my only vice (I have never drunk or smoked). Later on I shall tell how I extricated myself from the grip of a game which absorbed to excess my modest mental powers. In it no money is put up, as its panegyrists say, but something more is staked; one's brain, the most valuable capital that one has.

For the same reason I joined the *Valencian Athenaeum,* a scientific and literary society similar to that in Madrid, where there gathered at that time the most select and brilliant of the young intellectuals of the Levantine region, in an unpretentious meeting place in the *Plaza de Mirasol*.[5]

This literary and political atmosphere did me a great deal of good, preventing in my brain those dreadful compensatory atrophies of professional specialization by reason of which every day we see sorrowfully outstanding mathematicians, physicists, chemists, and naturalists discoursing foolishly and at random whenever they are drawn away from their habitual studies and compelled to talk about philosophy, art, or the social sciences.

I have already referred to the unpretentiousness of my home. I should like to add that I confined myself, conscientiously and systematically, to economic mediocrity so that I could dispose as I wished of all the time which was left free by my official teaching. Convinced that a balanced budget is an essential condition for domestic peace and for the mental tranquility indispensable for scientific labour, I determined to live within the fifty-two dollars a month to which my professional salary amounted (3,500 pesetas per annum). However, as a laboratory in full activity consumes almost as much as a family, I had to seek, as usual, for some source of additional income, not in medical practice, as was the usual custom, but in the extension of my pedagogical function. Hence, I organized in Valencia, with still greater success than in Zaragoza, a practical course in normal and pathological histology, which was attended by a good many physicians who were working extramurally for the doctorate, and by some doctors desirous of extending their knowledge of histology and bacteriology; this last being a science which was then rising promisingly upon the horizon under the impulse of the discoveries of the genius of Pasteur and Koch. As a matter of fact, one of my students was the high-spirited, cultured, and active Jesuit, P. Vicent, who, as in the case of most of the ecclesiastical polemicists, sought in science only decisive arguments in support of his fixed beliefs.

[5] The author lists with comments the names of many of his colleagues and acquaintances. (Translator's note.)

With the additional income, I not only avoided the dreaded deficit but supported my laboratory comfortably and, in addition, procured scientific apparatus of the utmost use; for example, an automatic microtome by Reichert, which did me the greatest service. Up to that time I had used no other microtome than a common barber's razor (the primitive microtome by Ranvier which I possessed had more drawbacks than advantages), in the use of which I had certainly acquired considerable skill, but with which it was impossible to secure regularly thin sections of any size.

The cholera of 1885, which made such ravages in Valencia and its environs, compelled me temporarily to abandon the cells and to fix my attention on *Bacillus comma,* the insidious causative organism of the desolating epidemic (recently discovered by Koch in India). I have remarked in preceding pages that upon the scientific horizon there was dawning a new world, *microbiology,* dedicated to the study of microbes or bacteria (microscopic fungi which are the agents of infection) and of the mechanism of their pathogenic action upon man and animals. The very recent and surprising conquests of Pasteur and Chaveau in France, and of Koch, Cohn, Löffler, etc., in Germany attracted lively interest among microscopists, many of whom deserted the old histological field founded by Schwann and Virchow to open up shop in the almost virgin territory of the invisible enemies of life. I also was dazzled by the new scientific star which illuminated with unexpected clearness the dark problems of medicine, and for some months I yielded to the seductions of the world of infinitely small beings. I made broths, stained microbes, and ordered the construction of incubators and sterilizers to culture them. When I had mastered these manipulations, I sought and obtained in the cholera hospitals the famous bacillus of Koch and devoted myself to testing the form of its colonies in gelatine and agar-agar, with the other biological characteristics, rich in diagnostic value, indicated by the illustrious German bacteriologist.

These were days of intense excitement. The population, decimated by the calamity, lived in terror, though never (be it said to the honour of Valencia) did it lose its serenity. The hospitals, especially that of San Pablo, overflowed with cholera cases. I remember that in my own street (*calle de Colón*) there were several deaths from the disease. In my family, fortunately, the germ did not gain a foothold, in spite of visiting some infected person and using water from a well which was probably contaminated.

As usual, contradiction and doubt held sway among the doctors. The older Galens, suspicious of any novelty, clung in theory to the doctrine of miasmas and in practice to the inevitable laudanum of Sydenham. The believers in microbes, mostly young men, recommended boiling the drinking water and taking no food or drink which had not been subjected to adequate preliminary cooking. I attribute to the use of boiled water and other hygienic precautions the immunity of my family despite my keeping in my home laboratory excrement from cholera cases and cultures of the organism in gelatine and broths.

When the epidemic was at its height (July 2, 1885) my fourth child was born.

In the midst of the general alarm there appeared in Valencia Doctor Ferrán, a celebrated physician from Tortosa, preaching through the mouths of eloquent friends and admirers the new gospel of the anticholera vaccine. After a number of laboratory experiments on guinea pigs and courageous and self-sacrificing autoinoculations, he believed that he had found a culture of the bacillus which, when inoculated into man, immunized him with certainty against the virulent microbe entering by the buccal passage.

The medical profession, excited by the announcement of the vaccine referred to, discussed the subject vehemently in academies and athenaeums, in the technical reviews, and even in the daily newspapers. As ever, there appeared in the debate that insuperable dualism of old and young, of the conservatives and the lovers of novelty. In the eyes of the first, the vaccine was a deplorable scientific error, if not a money-making scheme of the worst kind; the second waxed enthusiastic over the initiative of the Tortosa physician, whose talents and industry they exalted to the clouds. Finally, certain ardent devotees of Ferrán carried their zeal for health to the point of organizing a committete or society for the purposes of propaganda, of manufacturing the vaccine on a large scale, of procuring from the Government and from the authorities the right to try out the new immunization, and, once the permission was obtained, to carry it out systematically in all the provinces affected.

I was urged insistently to join the committee referred to, but declined humbly the honour of collaborating in the common efforts; I wished to preserve my independence of judgment and to remain free from any suspicion of mercenary motives.

Few of us preserved the serenity of mind necessary to form judgments during that upsurging of passionate feelings in which interests fought more bitterly than ideas. My doing the right thing at the time is not something of which I can be specially proud; there is nothing easier than to find the right path when our thoughts are inspired among the serene heights of patriotism and the will keeps itself clear of any illegitimate cupidity. The best reward for my conduct I receive today as I see that, in spite of the years that have passed, I can still maintain, *mutatis mutandis,* my points of view of those days in both scientific and moral spheres.

The circumstances that I lived in Valencia and that I was engaged in microscopy caused me to be designated by the Provincial Government of Zaragoza, along with Dr. Lite, the official delegate, to study the epidemic disease raging in the Levantine region (there was still argument as to whether it was or was not cholera) and to issue a statement upon the true value of the prophylaxis.

Having collected the necessary data, that summer I travelled to Zaragoza (July, 1885), and expounded the results of my studies and experiments before the governing body in the presence of a large audience. My conclusions definitely confirmed as cholera the character of the epidemic, which by that time had spread through a large part of Spain; they attributed the responsibility for the infection to the bacillus of Koch, as a matter of great probability; they cast doubt upon the so-called experimental cholera in rabbits and guinea pigs, in which animals injection of the microbe produced only local inflammatory phenomena or septicemias which differ considerably from the cholera syndrome in man; and with regard to the principal point, namely prophylaxis, I declared myself not to be favourably inclined towards the procedure of Ferrán, though admitting that it was entitled to scientific study (pure cultures of the bacillus injected under the skin are harmless) but without building up very high expectations as to its efficacy.

My attempts at prophylaxis in animals showed me that the problem of immunization was somewhat more difficult than was thought. As Ferrán claimed, subcutaneous injections of cultures of the bacillus actually produced in the guinea pig a certain resistance to later and stronger doses of the virulent microbe inoculated in the same way; but since the *Bacillus comma* of Koch has no pathogenic action when introduced into the intestine of that rodent, it was impossible to obtain a decisive and conclusive test of the efficacy of the injection. To attain such a demonstration, it would be necessary to find a mammal which could be infected with cholera through the mouth and which would become refractory to intestinal infection as a result of previous subcutaneous inoculation of pure cultures of the virulent or attenuated bacillus. Unfortunately, such an animal, which would be suitable for the elucidation of the prophylactic problem, was not then known.

At the end of September of that year, according to my promise to the provincial government of Zaragoza, I had ready an extensive monograph entitled *Estudios sobre el microbio virgula del cólera y las inoculaciones profilácticas* (Studies on the rod microbe of cholera and prophylactic inoculations), Zaragoza, 1885. The booklet, which was printed at the expense of the said governing body, was illustrated with eight lithographs, which I executed myself, some of them being reproduced in colour.

It is unnecessary to point out that such a monograph, published as the outcome of an official mission, and without the facilities necessary for the work, does not contain any new facts of importance. It represents primarily the fruit of a work of confirmation and contrasts with the memorable and at that time quite new discoveries of Koch and the fine contributions of Hueppe, van Ermergen, Nicati and Riesch, Ferrán, etc. Nevertheless, as is usually the case with a minute and careful study, its pages contain some original descriptive details and certain theoretical considerations not without value.

Among other trifles that were original, there appeared the technical details of a practical and simple method for staining the *Bacillus comma* and another designed for colouring and making permanent mounts of its colonies in gelatine, agar, etc. (These were cited and confirmed later by van Ermergen.)

On the scientific side, I added: (*a*) a detailed comparative study of the microbes of waters and excrements which possess, like the bacillus, the property of liquefying gelatine; (*b*) the demonstration (independently of Pfeiffer) that the microbe of Koch, thought not highly pathogenic in subcutaneous injection, is extremely virulent within the peritoneum of the guinea pig; (*c*) the most important point, the experimental proof of the formation of antibodies, that is to say, of the possibility of protecting animals from the toxic effects of the most virulent bacillus by previously injecting hypodermically a certain quantity of a culture which has been killed by heat.[6]

On the theoretical side, my memoir contained some considerations worthy of attention, since they were brought

[6] Almost all authors attribute to two American bacteriologists, D. E. Salmon and Theobald Smith ("*On a new method of producing immunity from contagious diseases,*" Proc. Biol. Soc. Washington, Feb. 22, 1886), the honour of having proved the possibility of vaccinating animals by the inoculation of dead cultures. It is perhaps legitimate to recall that demonstration of this was first made public by me in September, 1885. At that time also Ferrán

forward afterwards by famous bacteriologists in appraising the theoretical foundations and practical value of the vaccines of Ferrán, Haffkine, Kölle, and others. "It seems difficult to see," I said, "how the mere hypodermic inoculation in man of a pure culture of bacilli, which are incapable of migrating towards the intestine, or, consequently, of producing any disturbance comparable to cholera, can have the power completely to sterilize the digestive tube, an organ continuous with the external world and the sole terrain in which the organism of that disease flourishes and develops its formidable pathogenicity." Many years later, Metchnikoff, the great investigator of the Pasteur Institute in Paris, expressed a similar opinion. I shall not mention here, because of their merely critical and circumstantial character, certain other observations of considerable bacteriological importance.[7]

Needless to say, all these modest theoretical-experimental contributions passed unnoticed by bacteriologists. Those were times of considerable difficulty for Spaniards devoted to research. We had to fight against the universal belief in our lack of culture and in our radical indifference towards the great biological problems. It was admitted that Spain might have produced some artist of genius, some long-haired poet, and gesticulating dancers of both sexes; but the supposition that a real man of science could arise within her was considered absurd. Perhaps the disdain with which savants then treated us was contributed to in some degree by the clumsy and selfish attitude adopted by Ferrán towards the foreigners sent to investigate his cholera prophylaxis (his unyielding determination in keep-

and Pauli announced that they had solved the same problem; but as they did not state in 1885 how their vaccine was prepared, divulging this only later in the *Compt. Rend. de l'Acad. des Sciences* (session of Jan. 18, 1886), my priority can not be in the least doubt.

[7] One of these points was the subject also of a separate publication in *La Crónica Médica*, Valencia, Dec. 20, 1885.

Among the various authors who have unwittingly confirmed these studies there may be cited for example, Podwyssowsky (Centralblatt f. path. Anat., etc., 1893), who describes and draws the same things eight years later, with the same interpretation.

ing secret the method of preparation of his vaccine will be recalled) and the flagrant errors of the Tortosan doctor in connection with the morphology and multiplication of the bacillus of Koch.

All the same, though my work had no echo in the laboratories of Paris and Berlin—and little was lost thereby—it brought me, on the other hand, a material and spiritual reward of the utmost value for my career. The provincial government of Zaragoza was pleased by the zeal and disinterestedness with which I laboured to serve it and decided to recompense my industry by presenting me with a magnificent Zeiss microscope. Upon the receipt of that unlooked for acknowledgment, my satisfaction and happiness knew no bounds. Beside such a splendid *Statif,* with a profusion of objectives, among them the famous 1.18 homogeneous immersion, which was then the last word in magnifying optics, my poor Verick microscope seemed like a rickety door bolt. It gives me pleasure to recognize that, through such a thoughtful gift, the enlightened Aragonese body coöperated most effectively in my scientific labour from that time forward, since it placed me on a level technically with the best equipped foreign microscopists, enabling me to attack the delicate problems of the structure of the cells and the mechanism of their multiplication without misgivings and with the requisite efficiency.

I have already mentioned that the investigation upon cholera which I have been describing led me to have a taste for bacteriology and for the study of pathological problems. Many times I have asked myself if it would not have been better for my mental and economic future to have yielded to the fashionable tendency and, following the example of many others, to have abandoned definitely the cell for the microbe. Certainly there was no lack of incentives and reasons to justify a change of attitude. The path of histology condemned me absolutely to poverty, in recompense for which, if I should be successful, the only prospect to invite me was the cold praise or the lukewarm and critical respect of two or three dozen savants, who would be rather more inclined to competition than to panegyrics; while the path of bacteriology, being less frequented at that time and being bordered by almost virgin territory, promised to the fortunate investigator inexhaustible economic rewards, conspicuous popularity, and perhaps glorious adoration. Before me, as living examples and outstanding objects for emulation, were those benefactors of humanity represented first by the names of Pasteur, Koch, and Lister, and later by those of Behring, Roux, Ehrlich, Löfler, Schaudin, Grassi, Metchnikoff, etc.

Nevertheless, influenced by my own inclinations and especially by motives of an economic nature, I finally chose the cautious path of histology, the way of tranquil enjoyments. I knew well that I should never be able to drive through such a narrow path in a luxurious carriage; but I should feel myself happy in contemplating the captivating spectacle of minute life in my forgotten corner and listening, entranced, from the ocular of the microscope, to the hum of the restless beehive which we all have within us. As for the economic reason referred to, it was nothing else than the expensiveness of bacteriological work.

Histology is a modest and inexpensive science. A microscope having been acquired, the cost comes down to that of replacing a number of not very costly reagents and procuring from time to time some frog, salamander, or rabbit. Bacteriology, however, is a luxurious science. Its cultivation requires a whole Noah's Ark of propitiatory victims. Every experiment undertaken to determine the pathogenic power of an organism or the action of toxins or vaccines requires a whole hecatomb of rabbits, guinea pigs, and sometimes sheep and horses. In addition to this, there is the expenditure which the care and treatment of so many experimental animals costs, as well as that of gas necessary for the maintenance of autoclaves and ovens for sterilization and incubation.

Such was the rather prosaic and mundane consideration which obliged me to remain true to the religion of the cell and to bid a sorrowful farewell to the microbe, which I deigned to salute only occasionally in connection with some special analysis or test for verification, suffused by that respectful regard, not free from envy, with which we salute a millionaire friend from whom our poverty separates us irremediably.

When I returned to Valencia, then, in October 1885, I continued to devote myself enthusiastically to the examination of the living tissues. The fruit of that labour, which continued through two or three years (1885–1888) was a series of communications on comparative histology, devoted to the structure of cartilage, the crystalline lens, and especially the muscle fibres of insects and some vertebrates. I should be guilty of ingratitude and forgetfulness if I did not acknowledge at this time that in connection with the nomenclature and systematic relationships of the insects and other animals studied (amphibians, reptiles, etc.) I received invaluable assistance from the illustrious naturalist Boscá, then Director of the Botanic Garden at Valencia; from my excellent friend Arévalo Vaca, professor of natural history; and from Dr. Guillén, the distinguished medical naturalist.

I busied myself also at that time with the publication of an extensive work on histology and microscopic technique which appeared in separate parts. The printing was in charge of the enterprising Valencian publisher Don Pascual Aguilar, who did not stint on the cost and had the first fascicle (devoted to technique and general principles) ready in May, 1884.

A variety of motives inspired me in this undertaking: the desire to collect together all the more or less original observations which I had gathered in the broad field of histology; the advisability of disciplining my vagrant curiosity by fitting it to the rigid frame of a programme drawn up beforehand; and, above all, the patriotic desire that there should see the light in our country an anatomical treatise which, instead of devoting itself to a modest reflection of European science, should, so far as possible, develop its own viewpoint based upon personal investigation. I felt ashamed and sad at the realization that the few books on anatomy and histology thitherto published in Spain which were not translations lacked original illustrations and presented exclusively descriptions copied in servile fashion from foreign works.

The years 1884 to 1885 were devoted enthusiastically to this work. When completed, it comprised 203 woodcuts made from my preparations by an excellent Valencian artist and contained 692 pages of small print. The first edition was soon exhausted, so that, contrary to my expectations, a second had to be printed in 1893, when I had removed to the University of Barcelona. The publisher, Aguilar, as I understand, made a good thing out of it.

While I am talking about my publications of those times, I must not overlook certain popular articles on histology which appeared under the title "The marvels of histology" in *La Clínica,* a professional weekly published in Zaragoza under the direction of my classmate and friend Don Joaquín Gimeno Vizarra. Some of these articles, overflowing with fantasy and ingenuous lyricism, were afterwards reproduced and amplified in the *Crónica de Ciencias Médicas de Valencia.* They were signed *Doctor Bacteria,* the dreadful pseudonym which I used for my philosophic-scientific temerities and my semiserious critiques.

Apart from the style, which was inspired by the exuberant and verbose manner of the great Castelar—the Castelar style without Castelar!—I entertained in the little writings referred to the worthy purpose of calling the attention of wide awake physicians to the ineffablé enchantment of the almost unknown world of cells and microbes and to the very great importance of studying it objectively and directly.

As I write these sheets, I have the articles before me. The reader will pardon the vanity of my old age if I declare that now, after thirty-nine years have passed, I find some solace in reading these impetuous scientific-literary effusions. Leaving to one side the exaggerations in thought and the incorrectnesses in form, there ascends from them something like a comforting aroma of youthful confidence and robust faith in social and scientific progress. I also find attractive a feeling of curiosity newly satisfied and a passionate ardour for the study of the arcana of life which we should seek in vain today in the early writings of the cautious, unexcitable, circumspect, and money-loving young intellectuals.

As a sample of my style in those days and of the philosophic-biological ideas which attracted me, I am going to transcribe a few paragraphs from the aforementioned articles in *La Clínica.*

Among the captivating spectacles which the microscope presents, I enumerated:

"Amoeboid or protoplasmic contraction, which enables the wandering leucocyte to open a breach in the vascular wall and desert the blood for the surrounding regions, like a prisoner who files through the grating of his cell; the tracheal and laryngeal fields, sown with vibrating cilia which wave, in virtue of hidden stimuli, like a field of grain before the wintry blast; the tireless lashing of the spermatozoön as it hastens breathlessly towards the ovum, the loadstone of its affections; the nerve cell, the highest caste of organic elements, with its giant arms stretched out, like the tentacles of an octopus, to the provinces on the frontiers of the external world, to watch for the constant ambushes of physico-chemical forces; the ovum, with its simple and severe architecture guarding the secret of organic form, its protoplasm resembling the nebula, where there whirl about in embryo innumerable worlds which will emerge in future cycles; the geometrical architecture of the muscle fibre (a sort of highly complicated Voltaic battery) where, as in a locomotive engine, heat is transformed into mechanical energy; the gland cell which, in a simple way, fabricates the ferments of the living chemical laboratory, generously consuming its own substance for the benefit of the other elements, its brothers; the fat cells, models of domestic economy, which, in preparation for future famines, store up the surplus foodstuffs from the feast of life to utilize them when the organs go on strike and in the great nutritive conflicts. All these phenomena, so varied, so marvellously coördinated, draw us with an irresistible attraction and the contemplation of them inundates our spirits with the purest and most lofty of satisfactions."

To see the protagonists of such surprising phenomena close at hand, and to become confidentially intimate with them, I added: "Come with us to the laboratory of microscopy. There, upon the stage of the microscope, tear up the petal of a flower without consideration for its beauty or its perfume; then take a fragment of animal tissue; tear it apart without respect, although its contractile fibres pulsate and tremble at the touch of the needles. Afterwards, look diligently through the window of the ocular and—a remarkable fact, a stupendous discovery—the leaf of the plant and the tissue of the animal will reveal to you in every part the same structure: a sort of honeycomb built up of little cells and more little cells, separated by a small amount of interstitial cement, and harbouring in its cavities not the honey of the bee but the honey of life, in the form of an albuminoid material, semisolid and granular, in the bosom of which is enclosed a tiny corpuscle, the nucleus.

"Now examine a drop of saliva, a little of the epithelium which covers your tongue, a drop of your blood, the mould upon decomposing organic substances, etc.—and always the same architecture appears: cells and more cells, more or less modified, repeating themselves monotonously, with wearisome uniformity.

"This uniformity in the composition of organic tissues, liquid as well as solid, in the muscle as well as in the nerve, in the stem as well as in the flower; this precise repetition of the same melodic theme forms the primordial truth of histology; the basic fact upon which is founded the grandiose and transcendental *cellular theory* of Schwann and Virchow."

Later I expound the physiological aspect of such a supreme conception and, taking into account the danger in which such facts seem to place individual unity, I ask myself: "Can it be that within our organic edifice there dwell innumerable inhabitants which palpitate feverishly, with impulses of spontaneous activity, without our taking any notice of them? And our much talked of psychological unity? What has become of thought and consciousness in this audacious transformation of man into a colony of polyps? It is certain that millions of autonomous organisms populate our bodies, the eternal and faithful companions of glories and of toils, of which the joys and sorrows are our own; and certain also that the existence of entities so close to us passes unperceived by the ego; but this phenomenon has an easy and obvious explanation if we consider that man feels and thinks by means of his nerve cells and that the *not I,* the true external world, already begins for him at the frontiers of the cerebral convolutions."[8] (In this lies hidden in obscure and embryonic form the hypothesis afterwards formulated by Durand de Gross and Forel concerning the existence of multiple medullary and ganglionic consciousnesses, unknown to the ego, which would represent the privileged and autocratic consciousness of the brain cells.)

Influenced largely by the ideas of Haeckel and Huxley and by Claude Bernard's not very fortunate theory of the *plasson*[9] I declared myself a believer in principle in spontaneous generation, in spite of the experiments of Pasteur, which I considered conclusive only in so far as they bore upon the origin of existing life.

In another article, I announce, perhaps for the first time, a conception which since has had learned and authoritative exponents in Germany: that of an intercellular competition and struggle within the body.

"Who will dare to deny that there exists a severe rivalry in the race among the spermatozoa so that, in order to ac-

[8] Naturally, such rather daring considerations do not clarify in the least the secret of the unity of consciousness. And what is more serious is that, notwithstanding the efforts of physiology, psychophysics, comparative psychology, and classical philosophy, the wall remains and always will remain impenetrable.

[9] The protoplasm of a non-nucleate cell.

complish the supreme act of fertilization, they hasten towards the ovum in a dense crowd? Only one of them, the strongest or the most fortunate, will survive the destruction which is inevitable for its more sluggish companions. It alone will rend the mysterious veil of the vitelline membrane and, losing its degrading tail, unite itself at last in sublime conjugation which the female nucleus. From this kiss of love will arise the innumerable progeny of the cells of the organism. But only that privileged spermatozoön will attain the supreme reward of perpetuating the race and conserving and transmitting, like a new vestal virgin, the sacred fire of life.''

I then pointed out the rigorous competition for nourishment among the cells of a single tissue, the homeric struggles carried on among the semi-asphyxiated elements of inflamed regions or those of the elements threatened by the invasion of tumors. Finally, independently of Metchnikoff (and many years before him), I spoke of ''the reactions of the cells against the animal or vegetable germs which swarm through the atmosphere and penetrate into the organism; of the incessant war carried on between the small and the great; between the visible and the invisible, etc.''

However, to lessen the crudeness of this depressing truth (the universal struggle), I add that ''Thus, as in every civilized nation the vital competition is done away with or greatly attenuated by the division of labour which makes the citizens have common interests and aspirations, so also in the organic state, thanks to the foresight of the nerve cells, to the allotment of functional rôles, and finally to the suppression of idleness and of excessive individual liberty, etc., the struggle disappears or is moderated, appearing only when the communal nourishment (of organs or cells) is seriously threatened from either internal or external causes.''

In another passage I laid emphasis, in agreement with many biologists and philosophers whom I had not read, upon the fact that nature is concerned only with the life of the species. ''A single life, however great it may be, even though ennobled by the fires of genius, signifies nothing in the eyes of Nature. That a whole town should succumb; that entire races should be annihilated in the struggle for existence; that zoological species formerly powerful should be sacrificed in the barbarous battle matters little to the controlling principle of the organic world.—The essential thing is to win the conflict, to reach the goal which is the final objective of organic evolution."

What is this ultimate aim, if it exists? A profound mystery!

In another article, I console myself for the inscrutability of the tremendous arcanum and of the inexorable sanction of individual death by proclaiming the eternity and continuity of protoplasm, that is to say of the substance which after me, and with a great wealth of details, Weismann called the germ plasm.

"Let us console ourselves with the consideration that if the cell and the individual succumb, the human species, and above all the protoplasm are imperishable. The accidental dies, but the essential, that is the *life* lives on. Comparing the organic world with a tree of which the trunk is the original protoplasm, of which the branches and leaves represent all the species produced later by differentiation and improvement, what does it matter that some twigs are broken off by the storm if the trunk and the basic protoplasm persist with unabated vigour, giving promise of shoots of ever greater beauty and luxuriance? Critically speaking, there are not progenitors and progeny, there are no independent individuals, alive or dead, but only one single *substance*, protoplasm, which fills the world with its creations, which grows and ramifies and moulds itself temporarily into ephemeral individuals, but which never dies. In our being there moves still that ancient protoplasm of the *archiplast* (that is to say, the first cell which appeared in the cosmos), the point of departure, perhaps, of the whole of organic evolution." It is a gloomy consolation to die as a sacrifice to the survival of the species!

(There is a curious correspondence between this pseudo-pantheistic doctrine and some of the later lucubrations of Weismann, Dantec, and others.)

"This protoplasm filled both space and time with its creations; it crawled in the caterpillar, dressed itself with rainbow colours in the plant, adorned itself with the crown of intelligence in the mammal. It began unconscious and ended conscious. It was the slave and plaything of the cosmic forces and it ended as the driver of nature and the autocrat of creation." (There will be noticed also remarkable agreement with the well-known ideas of Schopenhauer, Hartmann, Spencer, etc., whom I had not yet read. Can it be that some résumé of the philosophy of the unconscious published up till then had reached me? I do not remember it.)

"Whither is life going?" I ask in another passage of the same audacious article. Who knows? But then I thought it probable that evolution tended to produce forms ever more perfect, more progressive, although I had no very clear view of the concept of perfection.

"Has it reached its limit and exhausted its fecundity in the human organism or is it keeping in its portfolio plans for still higher organisms, for beings infinitely more intelligent and understanding, who are destined to rend the veil which covers first causes and to do away with all the laborious polemics of scientists and philosophers?" (Who can not see here in outline the theory of the superman which was later upheld by Nietzsche?)

"Who knows?"—I continued.—"Perhaps this demigod, protoplasm, will also die on that sad, apocalyptic day when the torch of the sun is quenched, when the embers in the heart of our globe become cold and there remain upon its crust only funerary debris and barren ashes! Day of horror, solitude filled with anguish, night of utter darkness, that in which, with the light of the Universe, the light of thought is extinguished! But no! This is impossible! When our miserable planet is worn out and frigid old age has consumed the fire at its heart, and the earth becomes a glacial and unproductive desert, and the red and dying sun threatens to overwhelm us with everlasting darkness—organic protoplasm will have attained the culmination of its work. Then the king of Creation will abandon forever the humble cradle which rocked his infancy, will boldly attack other worlds, and will solemnly take possession of the Universe!"

It is easily seen that I had not read Clausius or made the acquaintance of the fateful predictions of thermodynamics! In comparison with my ingenuous optimism, that of Metchnikoff is very modest when, in a later book (*Studies upon human nature*), he merely promises to the human species that, when the neurons shall have learned better to defend themselves against phagocytes and intestinal toxins, it will have a tranquil old age, peaceful and exquisitely attuned to the idea of death! Preceding by many years the much talked of fantasies of Wells, I gave as the fundamental purpose of evolution, the eternity of life and the invasion and conquest of the mature stars so as to provide a worthy residence for the semidivine superman. *Excusez du peu!*

Fortunately, I was not long in getting over these cloying flights of imagination, in which, nevertheless, there was latent, from time to time, some thought that, if adequately developed and documented, and kept clear of useless rhetoric, might have constituted the germ of a serious book on natural philosophy.

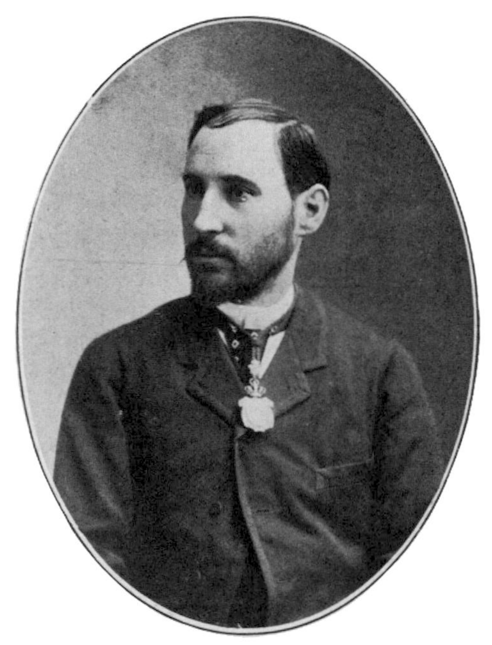

FIG. 24. THE AUTHOR IN 1884, when recently transferred to the chair of Anatomy in Valencia.

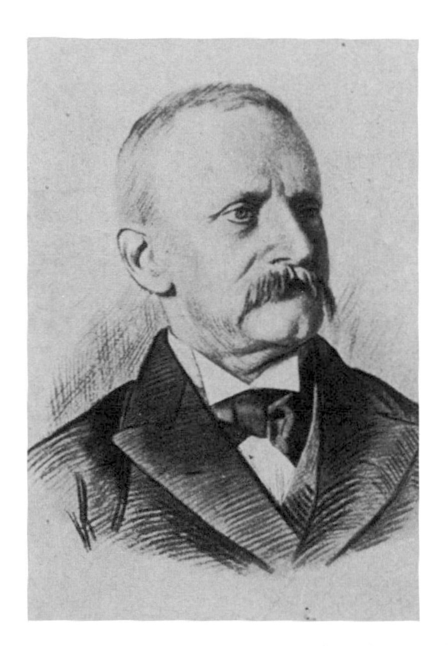

FIG. 25. DR. W. KRAUSE. Professor in the University of Göttingen and the first scientist to encourage the author in his efforts as an investigator.

CHAPTER III

I decide to publish my work abroad. Invitation from Professor W. Krause, of Göttingen, to contribute to his periodical. Work on epithelium and the muscle fibre. My first explorations in the nervous system. Difficulties encountered. Good qualities of the method of Golgi and the excessive nationalism of scientists. My amusements in Valencia: the excursions of the *Gaster-Club* and the marvels of suggestion and hypnotism.

Although the fruit of my inquiries up to then had been paltry enough, I was overtaken by a longing desire to export it to the foreign market. Such an enterprise seemed to me actually indispensable for the purposes of my scientific education. Only in contest with the strong does one acquire strength. The same thing happens with the nerve cells as with troops: trained exclusively for civil wars or in expectation of revolts of the rabble, they will have difficulty in facing a foreign army organized technically and prepared mentally for war on a large scale, that is to say for international conflicts. Besides, the severe criticism of foreigners is absolutely necessary for us; it wounds the flesh rudely and harshly, like a chisel on the marble but it models and beautifies the intellectual statue; and, while it shows up our defects without any consideration, it brings us at the same time the positive knowledge of our powers.

Realizing these facts, I took advantage of the first opportunity which presented itself to contribute to German periodicals, then, as now, the ones which were most widely read and most authoritative. A celebrated histologist of the University of Göttingen, Dr. W. Krause, was my introducer into the scientific world. Under the title of *Internationale Monatschrift für Anatomie und Physiologie* this professor published a monthly review in which there appeared communications in French, English, Italian, and German. He had read some little paper of mine and, being somewhat short of original materials, he benevolently invited me to contribute, offering to pay for all the chromolithographs required and to recompense me with fifty copies. Delighted by the invitation, I hastened to comply with his wishes and sent him from Valencia, with an interval of two years between them, two monographs written in mediocre French and illustrated with a profusion of drawings.

I should be guilty of ingratitude if I did not recall here that Dr. Krause, then professor of histology in Göttingen and now [1] in Berlin, inspired me greatly with his advice and aided me with his letters full of valuable bibliographic references. In his kindness, he went so far as to lend or present to me copies of old papers which it was difficult or impossible to acquire in the German market. I wish to take advantage of this occasion to offer to my old master and generous mentor the expression of my heart-felt gratitude and sincere affection. Later on, in connection with a visit to Germany, I shall have occasion to speak farther of the distinguished investigator.

The first of the communications mentioned was entitled *Contribution a l'étude des cellules anastomosées des épithéliums pavimenteux,* the second, which appeared in 1885, *Observations sur la texture des fibres musculaires des pattes et des ailes des insectes.* The collection and preparation of the material for the latter (an extensive monograph with four large lithographic plates) cost me about two years, during which I examined numerous orders and species of insects. My communication contained numerous original observations but, unfortunately, if it demonstrated zeal and industry in the observation and description of the facts, it was not so fortunate in their interpretation.

There was current in histology at that time one of those diagrammatic conceptions which temporarily fascinate the mind and influence young workers decisively in their inquiries and opinions. I refer to the reticular theory of

[1] He died, like many of the older scientists, during the mournful years of the terrible European war.

Heitzmann and Carnoy, which was applied very ingeniously to the constitution of the striated substance of muscles by Carnoy himself, the author of the famous *Cellular Biology,* and afterwards by the Englishman, Melland, and the Belgian, van Gehuchten. Impressed by the ability of these scientists and by the prestige of the theory, I had the weakness to regard the contractile substance, as they did, as a tiny lattice of delicate fibres (the *preexistent filaments* seen in preparations with acids and with gold chloride) united transversely by the net postulated at the level of the line of Krause. As for the primitive fibrils, they were supposed to be the result of post mortem coagulation. Later on I changed this opinion, which was vigorously criticised by Rollet, Kölliker, and others, who declared rightly that the so-called artifacts could be observed even in the living muscles of certain insects.

I insist upon these details because I wish to warn young men against the invincible attraction of theories which simplify and unify seductively. Ruled by the theory, we who were active in histology then saw networks everywhere. What captivated us specially was that this speculation identified the complex structural substratum of the striated fibre with the simple reticulum or fibrillar framework of all protoplasm. Whatever the cell might be, amoeba or contractile corpuscle, the physiological basis or rather the active factor, was always represented by the network or elementary skeleton.

From these illusions no histologist is free, least of all the beginner. We fall into the trap all the more readily when the simple schemes stimulate and appeal to tendencies deeply rooted in our minds, the congenital inclination to economy of mental effort and the almost irresistible propensity to regard as true what satisfies our aesthetic sensibility by appearing in agreeable and harmonious architectural forms. As always, reason is silent before beauty. The case of Phryne[2] repeats itself continually. Neverthe-

[2] Greek hetaira who, when placed on trail, won an acquittal by displaying her extraordinary beauty to the judges.

less, no error is useless so long as we are attended by a sincere purpose of emendation; and being convinced that enduring fame accompanies only the truth, I wished to be correct at any price. Hence, later on, I reacted vigorously against those theoretical conceptions, under which reality is lost or distorted.

In my systematic explorations through the realms of microscopic anatomy, there came the turn of the nervous system, that masterpiece of life. I examined it eagerly in various animals, guided by the books of Meynert, Hugenin, Luys, Schwalbe, and above all the incomparable works of Ranvier, of whose ingenious technique I made use with conscientious determination.

It is important to remember that the technical resources of those times were quite inadequate for attacking the great and alluring problem effectively. Colouring agents capable of staining selectively the processes of the nerve cells so that they could be followed with some certainty across the formidable tangle of the gray matter were as yet unknown.

It is true that since the time of Meynert the method of thin serial sections treated with carmine or haematoxylin had been practised with some success, and to this was added, by that time the method of Weigert for staining the myelinated fibres; but, unfortunately, the best preparations revealed only the protoplasmic bodies of the nerve cells with their nuclei and a little, very little, of the beginning or initial course of the dendritic processes and nerve fibres. Somewhat more helpful for revealing cellular morphology, was the procedure of mechanical dissociation brought into fashion by Deiters, Schülze, and Ranvier. This isolation of the elements was usually accomplished by means of needles upon slides, following maceration of the nervous feltwork in weak solutions of bichromate of potash. In the case of nerves, such a method produced very clear images, especially if, following the example of Ranvier, Shieffer-decker, Segall, etc., it was combined with the impregnating action of silver nitrate or Osmic acid—either before or afterwards, according to the circumstances. Applied, however, to the analysis of ganglia, of the retina, of the spinal cord, or of the brain, the delicate operation of freeing the cells from their matrix of cement substance and of disentangling and spreading out their branching processes with needles was an undertaking for a Benedictine.

What a delight it was when, by dint of much patience, we succeeded in isolating completely a neuroglia element, with its typical spider-like form, or a colossal motor neuron from the spinal cord, its robust dendrites and axis cylinder free and well separated! What a triumph to capture, in fortunate dissociations of the spinal ganglia, the bifurcation of the single process or to clear from its neuroglial bramble thicket a cortical pyramid, that is, the noble and enigmatic cell of thought! These modest successes as dissectors filled us with ingenuous pride and heart-felt delectation. The worst of it was that such a rather childish display of technical virtuosity was incapable of satisfying our eagerness to elucidate the inscrutable arcanum of the organization of the brain. Our feverish curiosity was eluded whenever we referred to the difficult question of the origin and termination of the nerve fibres within the centres and to the no less fundamental and urgent one of the intimate connections between the cells. Nobody could answer this simple question: How is the nervous impulse transmitted from a sensory fibre to a motor one? Certainly, there was no lack of hypotheses; but all of them were without sufficient objective basis.

Nevertheless, in spite of the weakness of our methods of analysis, the problem attracted us irresistibly. We saw that an exact knowledge of the structure of the brain was of supreme interest for the building up of a rational psychology. To know the brain, we said, is equivalent to acertaining the material course of thought and will, to discovering the intimate history of life in its perpetual duel with external forces; a history summarized, and in a way engraved in the defensive neuronal coördinations of the reflex, of instinct, and of the association of ideas.

Unfortunately, we lacked a weapon sufficiently powerful

to pierce the impenetrable thicket of the gray matter, that constellation of unknowns, as it was called, in his brilliant phraseology, by Letamendi.

In spite of all this, my pessimism was exaggerated, as we are about to see. Obviously, the *desideratum* referred to was and is even today an unattainable ideal, but some progress towards it could be made by taking advantage of the technique of the time. As a matter of fact, the instrument of revelation already existed; only I, isolated in my corner, was not acquainted with it, nor had it yet become known to any extent among scientists, in spite of having been made public in the years 1880 and 1885. It was discovered by C. Golgi, the famous histologist of Pavia, through the favour of chance, the muse who inspires great discoveries. In his staining experiments, this savant noticed that the protoplasm of the nerve cells, which is so refractory to artificial staining, possesses the valuable attribute of attracting strongly a precipitate of silver chromate when this precipitate is produced right within the thickness of the pieces of tissue. The *modus operandi,* which is of the simplest, consists essentially of impregnating fragments of gray matter for several days in solutions of potassium bichromate (or of Müller's fluid), or better still, in a mixture of bichromate and 1 per cent osmic acid solution, and treating them afterwards with dilute solutions (0.75 per cent) of crystalline silver nitrate. In this way there is formed a deposit of silver bichromate which, by a happy peculiarity that has not yet been explained, picks out certain nerve cells to the absolute exclusion of the others. When one examines the preparation, the granules of the gray matter appear coloured brownish black even to their finest branchlets, which stand out with unsurpassable clarity upon a transparent yellow background, formed by the elements which are not impregnated. Thanks to such a valuable reaction, Golgi succeeded during several years of labour in clarifying not a few points of importance in the morphology of the nerve cells and processes. As I have already mentioned, however, the admirable method of Golgi was then (1887–1888) unknown to the immense majority of neurologists or was undervalued by those who had the requisite information about it. Ranvier's book, my technical bible of those days, devoted to it only a few lines of description written so as to discourage interest. It is abundantly clear that the French savant had not tried it. Naturally, those, like myself, who relied upon Ranvier thought that the said method was not worth bothering about. The Germans manifested a similar disdain.

I owe to L. Simarro, the famous psychiatrist and neurologist of Valencia, the unforgetable favour of having been shown the first good preparations made by the method of chromate of silver which I ever saw, and of his having called my attention to the exceptional importance of the book of the Italian scientist devoted to the examination of the finer structure of the gray matter.[3] The circumstance is worthy of being set down because, besides being of decisive importance in my career, it demonstrates once again the vivifying and stimulating power of things seen, that is, of the direct perception of the object, as compared with the very weak, not to say ineffectual influence of the same things when they reach the mind through the cold and second hand descriptions in books.

In the year 1887 I was appointed judge for the examinations for professorships in descriptive anatomy. Anxious to take advantage of my stay in Madrid to inform myself of the latest advances in science, I got into communication with those in the capital who cultivated microscopic studies. Among other instructive visits, I may mention one to the Museum of Natural History, where I became acquainted with the very unassuming but learned naturalist, Don Ignacio Bolívar. Another was devoted to the histological laboratory at San Carlos, directed by the worthy Dr. Maestre, whose assistant, Dr. López García, showed me the latest technical novelties of Ranvier, of whom he had been a most devoted and creditable pupil. There was also a visit paid

[3] Golgi: *Sulla fina Anatomia degli organi centrali del sistema nervoso.* Milano, 1885.

to an unofficial *Biological Institute,* established in the Calle de la Gorguera, in which several young physicians were working, among them Dr. Federico Rubio and especially Don Luis Simarro, who had recently arrived from Paris and had embarked on the noble undertaking of promoting among us a taste for research. Finally, I spent some time in the private laboratory of this distinguished Valencian neurologist, who, being devoted to the professional specialty of mental diseases, was engaged in analysing the changes in the nervous system (with the aid, it is true, of a very extensive neurological library), trying out patiently and carefully all the new technical methods which appeared abroad.

It was there, in the house of Dr. Simarro, situated at number 41, Calle del Arco de Santa María, that for the first time I had an opportunity to admire excellent preparations by the method of Weigert-Pal and, particularly, as already mentioned, those famous sections of the brain impregnated by the silver method of the savant of Pavia.

I expressed in former paragraphs the surprise which I experienced upon seeing with my own eyes the wonderful revelatory powers of the chrome-silver reaction and the absence of any excitement in the scientific world aroused by its discovery. How can one explain such strange indifference? Today, when I am better acquainted with the psychology of scientific men, I find it very natural. In France, as in Germany—and more in the latter than in the former —a severe scholastic discipline holds sway. Out of respect for the master, no pupil is wont to use methods of investigation which he has not learned from him. As for the great investigators, they would consider themselves dishonoured if they worked with the methods of others. The two great passions of the man of science are pride and patriotism. They work, no doubt, from love of the truth, but they labour still more in behalf of their personal prestige or of the intellectual supremacy of their country. A soldier of the mind, the investigator defends his native land with the microscope, the balance, the retort, or the telescope. Whence, far from accepting with gratification and interest the advances accomplished in foreign countries, he receives them grudgingly, as if they brought him insufferable humiliation;—unless the invention should be of such magnitude and such extreme industrial importance that to ignore it would constitute a sin against patriotism. How many times in my already long career have I suffered from the discouraging effects of such pettiness! Later on, nevertheless, I shall have occasion to praise scientists who, as honourable exceptions, feel pleasure in heightening, by works of confirmation or amplification, foreign merit which has been overlooked or ignored. But how rare are such noble characters!

On my return to Valencia, I decided to employ the method of Golgi on a large scale and to study it with all the patience of which I was capable. Innumerable tests by Bartual and myself in many parts of the central nervous system and many species of animals convinced us that the new method of analysis had before it a brilliant future, especially if there could be found some way of overcoming its highly capricious and uncertain character.[4] The procuring of a good preparation constituted a delightful surprise and gave rise to jubilant hopes.

Up to that time, our preparations of the cerebrum, the cerebellum, the spinal cord, etc., confirmed fully the discoveries of the celebrated histologist of Pavia, but nothing new of any importance arose out of them. I did not, however, lose faith in the method on that account. I was fully convinced that, in order to make a significant advance in the knowledge of the structure of the nerve centres, it was absolutely necessary to make use of procedures capable of

[4] It was due, no doubt, to these inconstancies of chrome-silver impregnation that Simarro, the introducer of the methods and discoveries of Golgi into Spain, abandoned his efforts in discouragement. In a letter to me in 1889 he said: "I received your last publication on the structure of the spinal cord, which seems to me an important work but not *convincing*, because of the method of Golgi, which, even in your hands, who have perfected it so much, is a method which *suggests* rather than demonstrates." Unfortunately, Simarro, who was endowed with great talent, lacked perseverence, the virtue of the less brilliant.

showing the most delicate rootlets of the nerve fibres vigorously and selectively coloured upon a clear background. It is well known that the gray matter is formed by something like a very dense felt of excessively fine threads; and for following these filaments thin sections or completely stained preparations are worthless. What is required for this purpsoe is very intense reactions which, nevertheless, permit the use of very thick almost macroscopic sections (the processes from nerve cells are sometimes many millimeters or even centimeters long), the transparency of which, in spite of their unusual thickness, is made possible by the exclusive colouration of some few cells or fibres which stand out in the midst of extensive masses of cells that are uncoloured. Only thus does the undertaking to follow a nervous conductor from its origin to its termination become possible.

In any case, we were now in possession of the required instrument. It remained only to determine carefully the conditions of the chrome-silver reaction, and to regulate it so as to adapt it to each particular case. And if the brain and other adult central organs of man and other vertebrates are too complex to permit of scrutinizing their structural plan by the method referred to, why not apply the method systematically to lower vertebrates or to the early stages of ontogenetic development, in which the nervous system should present a simple and, so to speak, diagrammatic organization?

Such was the programme of work which I laid out for myself. It was commenced in Valencia, but only after I had removed to Barcelona was it completed, with a perseverance, an enthusiasm, and a success which surpassed my expectations. Of this, however, I shall treat at the proper time.

My time during my residence in the Valencian capital (the years 1884–1887) was not devoted entirely to hard and feverish labour in the laboratory. The artistic and philosophic furrows of my brain were also employed. It was necessary to allot to each cell its rations and to each reasonable instinct a convenient opportunity for exercise. In the guise of relaxing agents for neurons in danger of hardening from disuse, I developed two kinds of amusement: picture-taking excursions and the experimental study of hypnotism, a budding science which at that time was attracting the curiosity of and inspiring a passionate interest in the minds of the public.

I shall not say much about the excursions, the narrative of which could be of interest only to the few survivors of those agreeable and health-giving trips. I shall recall merely that a group of fellow members of the *Casino de la Agricultura* organized a gastronomic-recreative society labelled humourously the *Gaster-Club*. The purposes of this gathering of congenial people were simply to make Sunday excursions to the most attractive and picturesque regions of the kingdom of Valencia; to take photographs of interesting scenes and landscapes; to give specially intensive play, from time to time, to muscles and lungs by walking among the carob trees, palms, pines, and rose-bay trees; and, finally, to enjoy the tasty and famous Valencian *paella*.[5] The constitution, which I drew up, prohibited, as a heinous and abominable thing, whatever savoured of politics, religion, or philosophy, with their inevitable derivatives, heated controversies, disturbances of digestion, and straining of cordial friendship. Discussions were permitted only about science and art, and those in simple and easily comprehensible terms. We had declared war without quarter upon emphatic statement and declamation.

Thus from *paella* to *paella,* and always in pleasant and agreeable company, we visited all the attractive corners of the Levantine region: Sagunto, Castellón, Játiba, Sueca, Cullera, the Desert of Las Palmas, Burjasot, La Albufera, Gandía, the mountain ranges of Monduber and Espadán, etc., passed in succession before the lens of my kodak, being embalmed in prints which we few survivors of that genera-

[5] A dish composed of rice, chicken, and other ingredients. (Translator's note.)

tion preserve with pious care as mementos of the youth to which we long to return.

As for the other distraction referred to, it had a more scientific flavour and consisted in the experimental confirmation on a large scale of the very famous experiments on artificial somnambulism and phenomena of suggestion carried out in France by Charcot, Liébeault, Bernheim, Beaunis, etc. These investigations in morbid psychology undertaken in other countries by famous scientists, accustomed to exact observation, made a tremendous impression. Thanks to them, many of the stupendous marvels related by Mesmer and exhibited pompously by the theatrical magnetizers finally received naturalization papers in science. A new science, the direct heir of mediaeval witchcraft, had appeared.

It must be acknowledged that, despite three centuries of true science, the love of the marvellous still possesses a deep root system in the human mind. Even yet we are too superstitious. Thousands of years of blind faith in the supernatural seem to have created in the brain something like a *religious centre.* Almost completely absent in some people, and fallen into atrophy in others, it persists powerfully in the majority. However much of a free thinker he may be, who has not heard tolling at some time those mystic bells of Ys [6] of which Renan speaks, or felt springing up again vigorously the belief in genii, fairies, and ghosts?

At this time, however, we were not concerned with supernatural manifestations, but with surprising and considerably discussed activities, or, if it is preferred, anomalies of cerebral energy.

To study these methodically, several friends, some of them members of the *Casino de la Agricultura,* organized a *Committee for Psychological Investigation.* We inaugurated our inquiries with the search for and capture of

[6] Ys or Is, a legendary Breton city engulfed by the sea in the fourth or fifth century. The sound of the bell is supposed still to rise from the waves at times. The legend forms the basis for the libretto of Lalo's opera "Le Roi d'Ys." (Translator's note.)

suitable subjects. Through my house, converted for the purpose into a club house, there streamed the most remarkable kinds of hysterics, neurasthenics, maniacs, and even accredited spiritualistic mediums. In a short time we gathered together a voluminous collection of interesting records. Much to our astonishment, we had to confirm nearly all those stupendous phenomena which had been described by the savants, especially those pointed out by Bernheim of Nancy. It would be idle to mention the results obtained in detail. There was nothing new or specially interesting, especially now, when so many masterly treatises concerning studies of this kind have been published.

I shall mention only the experiments in hypnosis upon individuals who were healthy and apparently free from any neurotic taint (some of them lawyers, physicians, etc.). The indispensable degree of lethargy and passivity having been attained, there were produced at the command of the hypnotizer both during sleep and after awakening, catalepsy and analgesia; congestions and haemorrhages by suggestion; positive and negative hallucinations of all sorts (visual, acoustic, and tactile); total or partial amnesia; the calling up of forgotten or almost forgotten memory images; multiple personality; the eclipse or inversion of the most inveterate feelings; and finally the total abolition of free will, that is of the critical faculty and the power of conscious selection of motor reactions. Even actions most repugnant to the disposition, or most contrary to morality and decency were carried out of necessity, as by the decree of fate. One subject adjusted his life strictly for a whole week to a special programme full of extravagant and illogical actions suggested when in the hynotized condition.

Turning suggestion to the therapeutic field, I succeeded in performing prodigies which would be envied by the most skilful of the miracle-workers. I may cite: the radical transformation of the emotional condition of patients (an almost instantaneous step from sadness to joy); the restoration of appetite in hysteroepileptics who would not eat and were extremely emaciated; the cure by a simple command, of diverse kinds of chronic paralysis of a hysterical nature; the sudden cessation of attacks of hysteria with loss of consciousness; the complete forgetting of painful and distressing occurrences; the total abolition of the pains of childbirth in normal women;[7] and, finally, surgical anaesthesia, etc.

The fame of certain wonderful cures accomplished in cases of hysteria and neurasthenia spread rapidly through the city. Crowds of unbalanced people, and even those completely mad flocked to consult me. That would have been a fine opportunity to create for myself a lucrative practice if my disposition and tastes had been suitable. However, having satisfied my curiosity, I dismissed my patients, to whom, naturally, I did not choose to send any bills: I was sufficiently recompensed if they lent themselves docilely to my experiments.

During those epic inquiries in morbid psychology the only things which persistently resisted me were those extraordinary phenomena bordering upon spiritualism, namely: vision through opaque bodies, sensory transposition, mental suggestion, telepathy, etc., stupendous marvels which are affirmed seriously by Ochorowicz, Lombroso, Rochas, Zöllner, Richet, R. Gibier, Flammarión, Myers, etc.

Were these failures, perhaps, because they were impossible? I believe so today. The adherents of Allan Kardek and the believers in radiant cerebral energy will perchance say that I was unfortunate. Nevertheless, I put the best of will into my observations and spared neither cost nor effort to procure subjects endowed with the most transcendental qualities. But it was enough for me to attend a séance of divination, mental suggestion, double sight, communication with spirits, demoniac possession, etc., for all the marvellous powers of the mediums or of the hysterical priers into the unseen to vanish like vapour in the light of the simplest criticism. The amazing thing in those sessions was not the subjects, but the incredible in-

[7] A case of this kind was published afterwards in Barcelona in the *Gaceta Médica Catalana,* August 15, 1885.

genuousness of the audience, who took as manifestations of the supernatural certain nervous phenomena of the mediums (particularly autosuggestion), or the mere coincidence of facts, or the effects of mental habit, or, finally, the easy and well known artifice of Cumberlandism, which was afterwards so much exhibited in the theatres.

In sum, and passing over here the incredible marvels attributed to certain mediums, I must say that the above-described experiments concerning suggestion caused me mingled sentiments of surprise and disillusionment: surprise at recognizing the reality of phenomena of cerebral automatism deemed thitherto tricks and deceptions of circus magicians; and sad disillusionment by the consideration that the human brain, which is so highly lauded, the "masterpiece of creation" suffers from the enormous defect of suggestibility; a defect as a result of which even the most outstanding intelligence may, upon occasion, be converted by the activity of skilful suggesters, conscious or unconscious (orators, policitians, warriors, apostles, etc.), into the humble and passive instrument of deliria, ambitions, and greed.[8]

[8] Notwithstanding the scientific apparatus with which they were observed, I regard with suspicion the supernatural phenomena related by W. Crookes, Zöllner, Flammarión, Lombroso, W. James, Luciani, etc., who were deceived by Eusepia Paladino and other mediums no less cunning. These downfalls of minds which have shown in the realm of science that they possess critical faculties of the first rank teach us how dangerous it is to approach the study of the phenomena of communication through mediums—which lend themselves so readily to fraud and swindling—with a prejudice in favour of the possibility of communication of the dead with the living. Whenever such a *state of belief* is lacking, the ingenious devices of the mediums are discovered even by the least sagacious observers. I could quote most eloquent examples of this. Later on, I shall cite a typical case, which I observed in Madrid with all the precautions of the most scientific analysis.

CHAPTER IV

My transfer to the chair of histology in Barcelona. My new colleagues on the Faculty. The group in the Café de Pelayo. My investigations upon the nervous system lead to interesting results. My excessive scientific fecundity during 1888 obliges me to publish a Review of Microscopy. The laws of the morphology and connection of nerve cells. I cure myself finally of the vice of chess.

In the middle of the year 1887 the plan of medical instruction was reorganized. The subject of normal and pathological histology, which appeared in the prescription for the doctorate, and which was taught by Dr. Maestre de San Juan, was incorporated in the requirements for the licentiate. Considering my interests, it was natural that I should take advantage of the reform by applying for one of the new professorships created—an easy thing after all, since the new legal arrangements treated anatomy as a discipline related, in respect of transfers and competitive examinations, to the subject just set up.

The vacant chairs in Barcelona and Zaragoza, having fallen to me as a result of the examinations, I hesitated some time in making my choice. My first inclination was to the Aragonese capital. Towards it I was drawn by the love of my native district, recollections of my youth, and affection for my family. Over these sentiments, however, there prevailed considerations of a frankly utilitarian nature. For a man dedicated to one idea and resolved to devote his whole activity to it, great cities are preferable to small ones. In the latter, people know each other too intimately. The human animal threatens us too closely for us to live in holy peace. Grudges and even quarrels break out every day and one's time is spent in propitiating one's friends and combating one's enemies. It is important to realize, besides, that at that time, on account of the presence of two or three unbalanced characters, the faculty of my venerated *Alma Mater* burned with passions and antagonisms unbecoming to the decorum of the academic gown. Unfortunately, there is no lack of malevolent spirits in the great university communities; but here the effects of the human toxins, being diluted by distance, are lost or attenuated significantly.

Fearful, then, that my energies would be dissipated in rude and annoying friction, I finally resolved, contrary to the advice of my family, to move to the City of the Counts.[1] My calculations were justified, for in Barcelona I found not only the peaceful atmosphere indispensable for my work, but also facilities unobtainable in Zaragoza for organizing a well equipped laboratory and for publishing pamphlets illustrated with lithographs and engravings. It was in the first years which I spent in the City of the Counts that the most important of my scientific communications were published.

Anxious, as ever, not to disturb the balance between income and expenditures, I installed myself modestly in an inexpensive house in the *Calle de la Riera Alta,* near the Hospital of Santa Cruz, where the Faculty of Medicine was housed in those days. Later, when I could count upon other emoluments (the fees paid by some physicians who wished to extend their knowledge of histology and bacteriology in my laboratory), I removed to the *Calle del Bruch,* to a new and relatively luxurious house. There I had at my disposal a beautiful room in which to set up the laboratory and a garden adjoining which was very convenient for keeping the animals used for experimentation.

Among other young men of ability who received instruction in microscopy there were Durán y Ventosa, son of the ex-minister Durán y Bas; Pi y Gilbert who made a brilliant showing in examinations for professorships in histology and published some work in my *Revista;* Gil Saltor,[2] the future professor of histology in Zaragoza and of external

1 Barcelona.

2 He died a few years after becoming professor of surgery in Barcelona.

pathology in Barcelona, who was too soon taken from us; Bofill, who became in the course of time an excellent naturalist; Sala Pons, who in after years published some interesting investigations upon the structure of the brain of birds, the spinal cord of amphibians, etc.

As the proverbial courtesy of the Catalans is well known, it is superfluous to say that I found in my colleagues of the Faculty an attitude of consideration and respect. The Catalan is reputed to be somewhat brusque and excessively reserved with strangers but is adorned with two very fine qualities: he feels and practices whole-heartedly the double virtue of industry and economy; and, perhaps as a result of this, he avoids squabbling and meddling and respects religiously the time of other people.

With many of my colleagues [3] I developed bonds of sincere regard and I recall a number of them with admiration. It was a shame that so brilliant a group of masters had to perform their duties in the ancient and ruinous Hospital of Santa Cruz, where, if there was no lack of patients and opportunities, yet the space for class rooms and laboratories, indispensable for clinical instruction, was not available. For my own part, everything possible was done to enable me to organize the teaching of microscopy. Thanks to the generosity of Dr. Rull, I procured a relatively spacious room for preparation and demonstrations in histology and bacteriology, besides a good Zeiss microscope and some sterilizers and incubators. Dealing with few but very industrious and serious students, I was able, despite the small size of the laboratory, to give a practical course rather more thorough than that given at present in Madrid, where the seething crowd of four hundred students disturbs the good order of the class room and sterilizes the best planned pedagogical efforts.

Still a novice in pathological anatomy, I determined to acquire first-hand knowledge of this branch of medicine, performing autopsies and initiating myself into the secrets

[3] A paragraph about the professors at Barcelona is omitted here. (Translator's note.)

of experimental pathology. Fortunately, there were plenty of subjects in the Hospital of Santa Cruz. I spent several hours every day in the dissecting room and collected tumors, examined areas of infection, and cultured bacteria. Almost all the figures in connection with inflammation, degenerations, tumors, and infections in the first edition of my *Manual de Anatomía patológica general* (Barcelona, 1889–1890) are drawings of preparations which I made from that rich necroscopic material, to which there were added some tumors and infections contributed by professors in other hospitals or by the municipal veterinaries. The carrying on of these studies and the writing of the book refered to were the principal tasks of the year 1887 and the earlier part of 1888.

I have remarked elsewhere that the laboratory man, separated from politics and professional practice and not a frequenter of casinos and theatres, requires the invigorating atmosphere of the club to keep him from intellectual isolation or from falling into eccentricity. It is necessary that something of what is going on in the world should reach him after being simplified and elaborated by other minds. It is idle to point out that if such meetings are to be pleasant and educative they must include diverse temperaments and specialists in different fields. Only the rich, that is, those who are purely capitalists, and people of evil character are to be carefully excluded; for if the latter cause unpleasantnesses, the former, with their crude arguments which never rise above the earth, demagnetize those with high ideals. The well organized group presupposes a judicious distribution of the roles. One will discuss politics at table, another business; one will comment lightly and pleasantly upon local or national events, another will wax enthusiastic over literature or art; someone will cultivate the comic note; even the serious voice of a jealous defender of the social order and of the well known partnership between church and state will be heard from time to time; but for the laboratory man the most useful and inspiring fellow members will be his colleagues in other faculties, who can discuss without pedantry the latest advances in their respective sciences.

While it did not entirely fulfill this ideal, the circle at the *Café de Pelayo* (afterwards removed to the *Pajarera* in the *Plaza de Cataluña*), to which I was introduced in the early months of 1887, turned out to be singularly agreeable and profitable to me. There was a preponderance of professors of the Faculty of Sciences, which was an advantage; but the membership included also politicians, writers, physicians; and men of affairs.[4]

I consider excessively egoistic that ancient saying, of which Cicero disapproved, that one should love as if one had to hate; but I regard it as prudent for the safeguarding of one's sacred liberty not to push friendly intercourse to the extreme of that sticky intimacy which wastes our time, intrudes in domestic affairs, and restrains one's tastes and impulses. In this discreet reserve, however, I made an exception in favour of Victorino García de la Cruz, professor of chemistry, one of the most regular and agreeable of those who used to meet in the club referred to. While his philosophic ideas did not always harmonize with mine, we agreed in many tastes and inclinations; a similar disinterestedness in money; the same interest in art and, lacking it, in photography; and finally, an equal enthusiasm for original investigation and for the intellectual renaissance of Spain.

[4] One of these was Pablo Calvell, a lawyer and manufacturer, who was endowed with a genius for delicate satire and was fertile in witty and apt remarks. I regard the following yarn as the best I have ever heard. A group of companions were saying good-bye at the station to the shrewd Romero Robledo, among them the deputy, Sol y Ortega, and Pablo Calvell. When it came to the final hand-shakes, the famous republican leader felt in his pocket for a card. Then he exclaimed: "Never mind! I have none but it does not matter. I am so well known that if you need anything from me it will suffice to write on the envelope: *Sol, Barcelona,* and the letter will reach me."

His sly companion, who had been annoyed by the pompousness of Sol y Ortega made the same gesture and exclaimed: "What a coincidence! I have no cards either! Fortunately I am a prominent personage too. If you ever do me the honour of writing to me, address me simply *Pau, The Milky Way,* and the letter will reach me!" (Translator's note; *Pau* is a familiar diminutive for *Pablo,* while *Sol* means *Sun.*)

During several years of intimacy, Victorino was the sole confidant of my projects. I told him every day about the state of my labours, the obstacles which held me back, and my dearest hopes and illusions. At first he listened to me with surprise, almost with incredulity. While he was a sincere patriot, hopelessness had taken possession of his spirit and paralyzed his strength. Finally, however, my preaching produced a kind of contagion in him, and, following my example, he ended by seeking in the field of physics, which he always cultivated ardently, some subject for study which would be inexpensive and so would be accessible to the limited means which he had at his disposal. In after years, recalling my encouraging exhortations, he used to say that without my stimulus his interesting discoveries on the laws of turbid liquids and cloudy gases and other scientific accomplishments of definite value would never have appeared. In the course of these memoirs, we shall see frequent confirmation of the dictum of Cisneros: "Brother Example is the best preacher." Poor Victorino! He died while still young, after attaining well-founded fame.

Resuming the narrative of my labours, when my preparatory studies in pathological anatomy were well advanced, I resumed my investigations on the nervous system with unusual ardour. The method of Golgi began to be productive in my hands.

The year 1888 arrived, my greatest year, my year of fortune. For during this year, which rises in my memory with the rosy hues of dawn, there emerged at last those interesting discoveries so eagerly hoped and longed for. Had it not been for them, I should have vegetated sadly in a provincial university without passing in the scientific order beyond the category of more or less estimable delvers after details. As a result of them I attained the enjoyment of the sour flattery of celebrity; my humble surname, pronounced in the German manner (Cayal), crossed the frontiers; and my ideas, made known among scientific men, were discussed hotly. From that time on, the trench of science had one more recognized digger.

How did it happen? The reader will, I hope, forgive me if I devote a few remarks and explanations here to an occurrence so decisive for my career. I declare, in the first place, that the *new truth,* laboriously sought and so elusive during two years of vain efforts, rose up suddenly in my mind like a revelation. The laws governing the morphology and connections of the nerve cells in the gray matter, which became patent first in my studies of the cerebellum, were confirmed in all the organs which I successively explored. I may be permitted to formulate them at once:

1. The collateral and terminal ramifications of every axis cylinder [5] end in the gray matter, not in a diffuse network as maintained by Gerlach and Golgi, and most other neurologists, but by free arborizations arranged in a variety of ways (pericellular, baskets or nests, climbing branches, etc.).

2. These ramifications are applied very closely to the bodies and dendrites of the nerve cells, a contact or articulation being established between the receptive protoplasm and the ultimate axonic branchlets.

From the anatomical laws stated spring two physiological corollaries:

3. Since the final rootlets of the axis cylinders are applied closely to the bodies and dendrites of the neurons,[6] it must be admitted that the cell bodies and their protoplasmic processes enter into the chain of conduction, that is to say, that they receive and propagate the nervous impulse, contrary to the opinion of Golgi, according to whom these parts of the cell perform a merely nutritive rôle.

4. The continuity of substance between cell and cell being excluded, the view that the nerve impulse is transmitted by contact, as in the junctions of electric conductors,

[5] The axis cylinder, or axon, is the fibre which conducts the nerve impulse away from the cell body. A nerve is a bundle of many such fibres. (Translator's note.)

[6] The neuron is one complete nerve element, the architectural unit of the nervous system, and typically comprises a cell body, one or more dendrites, *i.e.,* processes which conduct towards the cell body, and an axon. (Translator's note.)

or by an induction effect, as in induction coils, becomes inescapable.

The laws mentioned, a purely inductive outcome of the structural analysis of the cerebellum, were afterwards confirmed in all the nervous structures examined (retina, olfactory bulb, sensory and sympathetic ganglia, cerebrum, spinal cord, medulla oblongata, etc.). Later studies by myself and by others (Kölliker, Retzius, van Gehuchten, His, Edinger, v. Lenhossék, Athias, Lugaro, P. Ramón, Cl. Sala, etc.) revealed that these structural and physiological standards apply equally, without modification, to the nervous system of vertebrates and to that of invertebrates. As happens with all legitimate conceptions, mine become more thoroughly established and gained progressively in dignity as the circle of confirmatory studies was extended.

However, in my eagerness to condense the essentials of the results obtained in brief propositions, I have not replied as yet to the question formulated in preceding paragraphs.

How were these laws discovered? Why did my work, after being confined for two years to the modest confirmation of the accomplishments of Deiters, Ranvier, Krause, Kölliker, and, especially, Golgi, suddenly acquire surprising originality and broad importance?

I wish to be frank with the reader. To my successes of those days there contributed, without doubt, some improvements of the chrome silver method, particularly the modification designated the *procedure of double impregnation;* but the principal thing, the really efficacious cause, was—who would have thought it?—*the application to the solution of the problem of the gray matter of the dictates of the most ordinary common sense.* Instead of taking the bull by the horns, as the saying is, I permitted myself some strategic subterfuges. This demands explanation.

I have already pointed out in the previous chapter and repeated a moment ago that the great enigma in the organization of the brain was the way in which the nervous ramifications ended and in which the neurons were mutually connected. Repeating a simile already used, it was a case of finding out how the roots and branches of these trees in the gray matter terminate, in that forest so dense that, by a refinement of complexity, there are no spaces in it, so that the trunks, branches, and leaves touch everywhere.

Two methods come to mind for investigating adequately the true form of the elements in this inextricable thicket. The most natural and simple apparently, but really the most difficult, consists of exploring the full-grown forest intrepidly, clearing the ground of shrubs and parasitic plants, and eventually isolating each species of tree, as well from its parasites as from its relatives. Such was the approach employed in neurology by most authors from the time of Stilling, Deiters, and Schültze (mechanical and chemical dissociation) to that of Weigert and Golgi, in which the isolation of each form of cell or of each fibre is procured optically, that is by the disappearance or absence of colour of the majority of the interlacing elements in the gray matter. Such tactics, however, to which Golgi and Weigert owed important discoveries, are inappropriate for the elucidation of the problem proposed, by reason of the enormous length and extraordinary luxuriance of the nervous ramifications, which inevitably appear mutilated and almost indecipherable in each section.

The second path open to reason is what, in biological terms, is designated the ontogenetic or embryological method. Since the full grown forest turns out to be impenetrable and indefinable, why not revert to the study of the young wood, in the nursery stage, as we might say? Such was the very simple idea which inspired my repeated trials of the silver method upon embryos of birds and mammals. If the stage of development is well chosen, or, more specifically, if the method is applied before the appearance of the myelin sheaths upon the axons (these forming an almost insuperable obstacle to the reaction), the nerve cells, which are still relatively small, stand out complete in each section; the terminal ramifications of the axis cylinder are depicted with the utmost clearness and perfectly free; the pericellular nests, that is the interneuronal articulations, appear simple, gradually acquiring intricacy and extension; in sum, the fundamental plan of the histological composition of the gray matter rises before our eyes with admirable clarity and precision. As a crowning piece of good fortune, the chrome silver reaction, which is so incomplete and uncertain in the adult, gives in embryos splendid colourations, singularly extensive and constant.

How is it, one may ask, that scientists did not hit upon so obvious a step? Certainly the idea must have occurred to many. In after years I learned that Golgi himself had already applied his method to embryos and young animals and obtained some excellent results; but he did not persist in his efforts, perhaps not thinking that he could progress by such a path in the elucidation of the problem of the structure of the centres. So little importance did he evidently attach to such experiments that in his greatest work, already cited, the observations described have reference exclusively to the adult nervous system of man and mammals. In any case, my easy success proves once more that ideas do not show themselves productive with those who suggest them or apply them for the first time, but with those persevering workers who feel them strongly and put all their faith and love in their efficacy. From this point of view, it may be affirmed that scientific accomplishments are creations of the will and rewards of ardour.

Realizing that I had discovered a rich field, I proceeded to take advantage of it, dedicating myself to work, no longer merely with earnestness, but with fury. In proportion as new facts appeared in my preparations, ideas boiled up and jostled each other in my mind. A fever for publication devoured me. In order to make known my thoughts, I made use chiefly of a certain professional medical review, the *Gaceta Médica Catalana.* The tide of ideas and impatience for publication rising rapidly, however, this outlet became too narrow for me. I was much annoyed by the slowness of the press and the lateness of the dates of appearance. To extricate myself once and for all from such fetters, I decided to publish upon my own account a new review, the

Revista trimestral de Histología normal y patológica. The first number saw the light in May, 1888, and the second appeared in the month of August of the same year. Naturally, all the articles, six in number, sprang from my own pen. From my hands emerged also the six lithographic plates which were included. Financial considerations obliged me not to print more than sixty copies altogether at the time and these were distributed almost entirely among foreign scientists.

Needless to say the vortex of publication entirely swallowed up my income, both ordinary and supplementary. Before that desolating cyclone of expenditure, my poor wife, taken up with caring for and watching five little demons (during the first year of my residence in Barcelona, another son was born to me), determined to get along without a servant. She divined do doubt that there was maturing in my brain something unusual and of decisive importance for the future of the family, and, discreetly and self-sacrificingly, avoided any suggestion of rivalry or competition between the children of the flesh and the creatures of the mind.

As a distraction for the reader, who, I suppose, will be surfeited with the foregoing lucubrations, I should like to tell here how I freed myself from a tenacious and inveterate vice, the game of chess, which seriously menaced my evenings.

Knowing my fondness for the noble game of Ruy López y Philidor, various members of the *Casino Militar* invited me to join it.

I was weak enough to do so; I made my debut with varying success, measuring myself against players of considerable skill; and soon my skill increased and with it the morbid eagerness to overcome my adversaries. In my foolish vanity, I reached the point of playing four games simultaneously, against separate combatants, besides numerous onlookers who discussed at length the consequences of every move. There was one game that lasted two or three days. In my desire to shine at all costs and my confidence in my rather good visual memory, I even played without looking at the board.

Needless to say, I acquired as many books on the aristocratic pastime as I could lay my hands on and I even fell into the folly of sending solutions of problems to foreign illustrated papers. Carried away by the growing passion, I found my sleep broken by dreams and nightmares, in which pawns, knights, queens, and bishops were jumbled together in a frenzied dance. After being defeated the evening before in one or several games, it often happened that I wakened with a sudden start in the early hours of the morning, with my brain burning and in a whirl, breaking out in phrases of irritation and despair and exclaiming: "I am a fool! I had a checkmate at the fourth move and did not see it." In fact, putting the board on the table, I proved with sorrow the delayed clairvoyance of my *unconscious mind,* which had been working within me during the few hours of repose.

This could not continue. The almost permanent fatigue and cerebral congestion weakened me. If one does not lose money in playing chess, one loses time and brain energy, which are worth infinitely more, and one's will is turned aside and runs through the wrong channels. In my opinion, far from exercising the intelligence, as many claim, chess warps it and wears it out. Conscious of the danger of my position, I trembled before the distressing prospect of becoming converted into one of those amorphous types, sedentary and corpulent, who grow old unproductively and insensibly, seated at a card table or a chess table, without arousing any sincere affection or exciting, when the inevitable apoplexy or the terrible uraemia comes, more than a feeling of cold and formal commiseration. "To bad about Pérez! He was a good player! We shall have to look about for someone to take his place."—For the player at a club or casino is no more than a table leg, something like the common picture which occupies a place in the room simply to balance the others.

But how was I to cure myself thoroughly? Feeling myself incapable of an inexorable, "I do not play any more," the possession of a will of iron; constantly excited by the eagerness for revenge, the evil genius of every player; the only supreme remedy which occurred to me was the *similia similibus* of the homeopathists: to study the works upon chess thoroughly and reproduce the most celebrated plays; and besides to discipline my rather sensitive nerves, augmenting the imaginative and reflex tension to the utmost. It was indispensable, also, to abandon my usual style of play, with consistently romantic and audacious attacks, and stick to the rules of the most cautious prudence.

In this way, expending my whole inhibitory capacity in the undertaking, I finally attained my desired end. This consisted, as the reader will have guessed, in flattering and lulling to sleep my insatiable self-love by defeating my skilful and cunning competitors for a whole week. Having demonstrated my superiority, eventually or by chance, the devil of pride smiled and was satisfied. Fearful of a relapse, I abandoned my place in the casino and did not move a pawn again for more than twenty-five years. Thanks to my psychological stratagem, I emancipated my modest intellect, which had been sequestrated by such stupid and sterile competitions, and was now able to devote it, fully and without distraction, to the noble worship of science.

CHAPTER V

Some details about my publications of 1888. The "basket endings" of the cerebellum, the axons of the "granules," and the mossy and climbing fibres. Decisive value of these discoveries for the solution of the problem of intercellular connections. "Reticular theory" of Gerlach and Golgi. The brilliant observations of His and Forel. Confirmation in the retina and the optic lobe of the "laws of connection" induced from the analysis of the cerebellum. Structural plan of the spinal cord. Verification of the manner of termination in the centres of the afferent and sensory nerves. Other works of less importance.

As I have indicated in the foregoing chapter, in abbreviated form, the more general conclusions of my studies upon the nerve centres during the years 1888–1889, it may be permissible for me now to enter into an exposition, as simple and clear as possible, of the more interesting discoveries. These discoveries have reference to the cerebellum of birds and mammals, the retina, the spinal cord, and the optic lobe of birds.

Cerebellum.—My studies upon the structure of this nerve centre began in young and adult birds and those upon the cerebellum of mammals came soon after. Two memoirs and some preliminary notices were devoted to this fertile theme in 1888 and 1889.

In the first, published in May, 1888, there are already established the principal facts upon which are based the anatomo-physiological laws enumerated in the preceding chapter. In substance: in connection with the analysis of the axons of the small stellate cells of the molecular layer of the cerebellum, there is described for the first time the true manner of ending of the nerve fibres in the gray matter, a problem concerning which we possessed only hypotheses. This interesting observation, which was confirmed afterwards by numerous authors (Kölliker, van Gehuchten, Retzius, Edinger, v. Lenhossék, Athias, etc.), is represented in Fig. 26, *c,* which depicts the cerebellum of mammals. This shows how the axis cylinders of the small stellate cells in question soon take up a direction transverse to the cerebellar convolution, describing an arc and giving off numerous collateral branches characterized by progressive thickening. Finally both the end of the main fibre and its numerous descending processes break up into terminal fringes or tufts applied closely to the bodies of the cells of Purkinje, about which they form a kind of complicated nests or baskets.

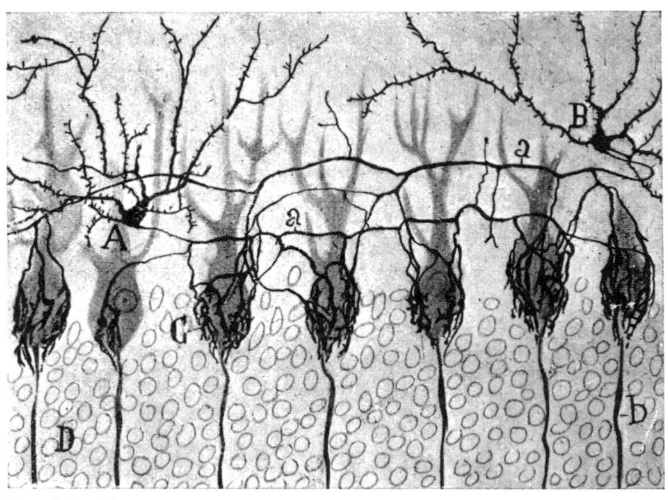

FIG. 26. TRANSVERSE SECTION OF A CEREBELLAR LAMELLA. Semidiagrammatic. *A* and *B,* stellate cells of the molecular layer (basket cells), of which the axon (*a*) produces terminal nests about the cells of Purkinje (*C*): *b,* axon of the Purkinje cell.

Also worthy of mention on account of its theoretical value is the presence in the granule layer of a special type of centripetal fibre, christened with the name *mossy fibre,* which exhibits, both at its ultimate ending and in its collateral branches (Fig. 27, *a*), bunches or rosettes of short tuberous appendages ending freely. Later observations of mine brought out the fact that such excrescences articulate directly with the claw-like arborizations of the granule cells, arborizations which also were described for the first time, it may be mentioned in passing, in the communication referred to.

Finally, in the work cited the attention of scientists is called to the existence round the dendrites of the Purkinje cells and, in general, round all such protoplasmic processes, of a sort, of down of very fine short appendages (peri-

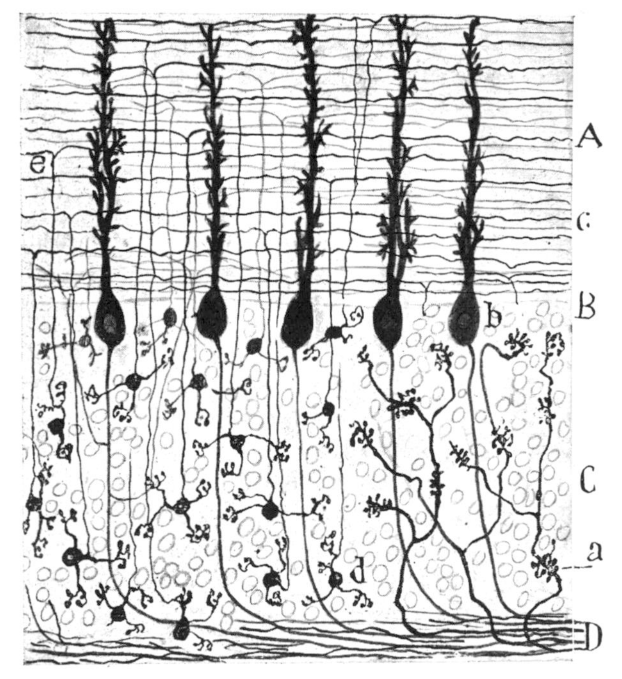

FIG. 27. LONGITUDINAL SECTION OF A CEREBELLAR CONVOLUTION. *A*, molecular layer; *B*, layer of Purkinje cells; *C*, granular layer; *D*, white matter; *a*, tuft of a mossy fibre; *b*, body of a Purkinje cell; *c*, parallel fibres; *d*, granule cell with its ascending axon; *e*, division of this axon. (Semidiagrammatic.)

dendritic spines), which were observed and studied afterwards by many authors.

The second communication relative to the cerebellum, published in August, 1888, contains two outstanding facts:

(*a*) The discovery of the exceedingly delicate axon of

the granule cell[1] (the very small cells of the second layer of the cerebellar cortex), which, as is shown in Fig. 27, *c, d,* ascends to the molecular layer (the outer layer), where, at levels which differ for every cell, it divides at a right angle, forming two very slender branches running in opposite directions (Fig. 27, *e*). These very long processes, which I designated *parallel fibres* because of their parallel courses in the same direction as the cerebellar convolution, and thus perpendicular to the system of branches of the Purkinje cells, appear in enormous numbers, fill up all the interstices in the molecular zone, and after a long, continuous trajectory, end in the extremities of each lamina. So general is their occurrence and so uniform their disposition that they are found with practically the same characters throughout the vertebrate series, from the fish to man. Thus they constitute an important factor in the cerebellum.

(*b*) The other fortunate finding was that of the climbing fibres (Fig. 28, *n*). These robust conductors arise in the centres of the pontine region of the brain; invade the white core of the cerebellar lamella; cross the granule layer without branching; afterwards attain the level of the cells of Purkinje; and finally run over the bodies and principal outgrowths of these elements, to which they adapt themselves closely. When they reach the level of the first branches of the dendritic trunks of the Purkinje cells, they break up into twining parallel networks which ascend along the protoplasmic branches, to the contours of which they apply themselves like ivy or lianas to the trunks of trees (Fig. 28).

This fortunate discovery, one of the most beautiful which fate vouchsafed to me in that fertile epoch, formed the final proof of the transmission of *nerve impulses by contact.* As such it was recognized by outstanding scientists

[1] Golgi had already succeeded in differentiating among the processes of the granule a finer fibre or axon, but he did not manage to colour more than its initial portion and believed that it broke up immediately into a diffuse interstitial net.

when, in after years, they confirmed my description of the mossy and climbing fibres.

Looking back over the work of the three-year period from 1891 to 1894, I might add some other discoveries of less importance concerning the cerebellar cortex. To assist the reader who is not very familiar with such material, a

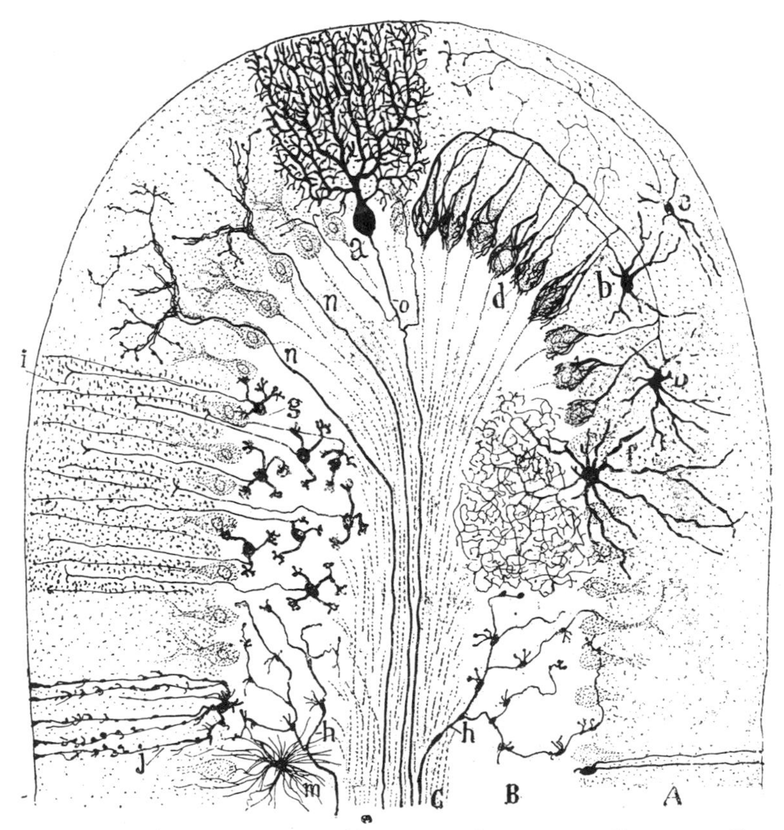

FIG. 28. SEMIDIAGRAMMATIC TRANSVERSE SECTION OF A CEREBELLAR CONVOLUTION OF A MAMMAL. *A*, molecular layer; *B*, granular layer; *C*, layer of white matter; *a*, Purkinje cell with its dendrites spread out in the plane of section; *b*, small stellate cells of the molecular layer; *d*, descending terminal arborizations embracing the cells of Purkinje; *e*, superficial stellate cell; *f*, large stellate cell of the granule layer; *g*, granules with their ascending axons bifurcating at *i*; *h*, mossy fibres; *j*, tufted neuroglia cell; *n*, climbing fibres; *m*, neuroglia cell of the granule layer.

figure is reproduced here in which is represented diagrammatically the state of our knowledge of the cerebellum after my observations of 1888 and 1889. This schema (Fig. 28) was constructed to illustrate some lectures which I gave later (1894) before the *Academia de Ciencias Médicas de Cataluña.* Of the unexpected success of these lessons, which were at once translated into French, English, and German, I shall have something to say later on.

The conclusions of my investigations concerning the cerebellum contradicted completely the ideas current at that time regarding the minute anatomy of the gray matter. Obviously my views were too revolutionary to be readily accepted. By this time, however, I nourished the certainty that I was not mistaken; for actually, the laws which I enunciated were the simple expression of the facts, without any mixture of the subjective. It was not now a case of one hypothesis more, but of a legitimate induction with all the guarantees of certainty which could be desired, as distinguished histologists and neurologists later recognized. I had been too well punished by the error which I had committed in my temerarious interpretation of the structure of muscle tissue to proceed lightly or to allow myself to be led astray by a mere theoretical conception, whether my own or that of someone else.

In order that the reader may readily follow the course of my researches and may excuse the polemical tone of some of my future writings, it is advisable to explain briefly at this point the opinions which were then current among scientists regarding the intimate constitution of gray matter.

Two main hypotheses disputed the battle field of science: that of the network, defended by nearly all neurologists; and that of free endings, which had been timidly suggested by two lone workers, His and Forel, without rousing any echo in the schools.

The network hypothesis was a formidable enemy. The reader will notice that here also, as in the case of the striated muscle fibre, the preconception of a reticulum was in our way; however, on this occasion the supposed diffuse net was not intracellular but intercellular. Originated by Gerlach and afterwards supported by Meynert and other celebrated neurologists, in an epoch when methodological penury was an excuse for flights of the imagination, the reticular theory at last received from Golgi a new and attractive structural form and even a certain appearance of being founded upon observed facts.

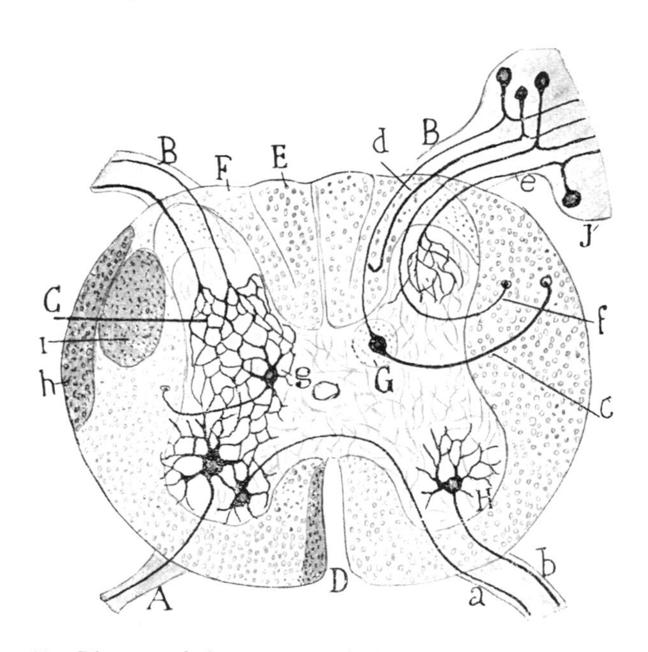

FIG. 29. Diagram of the structure of the gray matter of the spinal cord according to the authors of the pre-Golgi epoch. *A*, anterior root; *B*, posterior root; *C*, interstitial net of the gray matter: *D*, anterior sulcus; *E*, column of Goll; *F*, column of Burdach; *G*, column of Clarke; *H*, motor cell; *I*, crossed pyramidal tract; *J*, sensory ganglion.

For the savant of Pavia, the gray matter formed the place of meeting and fusion of all the afferent and efferent fibres of the nerve centres, as well as of the axons of the intrinsic association elements. To this reticulum, which was continuous and immensely rich in fibres, the following factors contributed: (1) The terminal ramifications of the sensory axis-cylinders, or those simply afferent from other nerve centres; (2) the collateral branches of the axons of certain large elements, designated by Golgi *motor cells* (the large pyramidal cells of the cerebral cortex, the Purkinje cells of the cerebellum, etc.) and which I christened, so as not to commit myself as to their physiology, *elements with long axons;* and (3) the terminal arborizations of the axis-cylinders of other nerve cells, arbitrarily considered *sensory* by Golgi, which I termed *cells with short axons.*

In contrast with Gerlach, according to whom the ultimate terminations of the dendritic branches of the neurons also entered into the formation of the diffuse reticulum, Golgi reduced the components of the latter to the axonic ramifications. In order that the reader who is not familiar with matters of this kind may be able to understand easily the reticular hypotheses of Gerlach and of Golgi, the manner in which these two savants conceived the anatomo-physiological connections to be established between motor and sensory roots of the spinal cord is represented schematically in Fig. 29, *c,* and Fig. 33, I, *c.*

I have already pointed out that the suggestive power of certain formulae which are extremely diagrammatic depends upon their convenience. The hypothesis of the network once being accepted, nothing is easier than the objective study of a group of neurons or of the behaviour of the terminations of a bundle of fibres; the whole matter is reduced to taking for granted that the final axonic branchlets, after several dichotomies, are lost or disappear in the aforesaid interstitial network; in that sort of unfathomable physiological sea, into which, on the one hand, were supposed to pour the streams arriving from the sense organs, and from which, on the other hand, the motor or centrifugal conductors were supposed to spring like rivers originating in mountain lakes. This was admirably convenient, since it did away with all need for the analytical effort involved in determining in each case the course through the gray matter followed by the nervous impulse. It has rightly been said that the reticular hypothesis, by dint of pretending to explain everything easily and simply, explains absolutely nothing; and, what is more serious, it hinders and almost makes superfluous future inquiries regarding the intimate organization of the centres. Only by dint of evasions, irrelevances, and subterfuges could this conception (which, moreover, was upheld almost exclusively by Golgi and his immediate disciples) be adapted to the exigencies of physiology, where the doctrines of reflexes, instinctive actions, functional localization in the cerebrum, etc., demand imperiously the recognition of perfectly circumscribed paths or channels of conduction through the cerebrospinal axis.

Against the network theory there fought, as has already been said, only two observers of high standing, His and Forel, who, announced (1887) with reservations and restraint which were excusable in view of the paucity of precise facts of observation, the possibility that the processes of the nerve cells terminate freely in the gray matter. A natural corollary of this view was the transmission of nervous impulses by contact. Thus, in view of the impossibility of discovering recognizable anastomoses within the gray matter, Forel suggested that probably the processes of the nerve cells touch each other like the foliage in a wood. As for the illustrious professor at Leipzig, proceeding by generalization (1886) he conjectured that since the nervous arborizations of the motor end plate (already well known) end freely, as everyone knew, entering into contact with the striated material, it was logical to postulate a similar terminal arrangement for the conductors which spread and ramify within the cerebro-spinal centre.

In discussing this matter, however, His and Forel did not go beyond the sphere of hypothesis. It was impossible, without descending to the plane of structural analysis, to refute Golgi, who brought against the cautious theoretical statements of those scientists an elaborate account of conscientious observations. To settle the question definitely it was necessary to demonstrate clearly, precisely, and indisputably the final ramifications of the central nerve fibres, which no one had seen, and to determine besides which parts of the cells made the imagined contact. For to admit vaguely the fact of mediate transmission or articulation between the neurons without indicating precisely between which processes of the cells it occurs is almost as conveniently dangerous as the handy reticular theory. Let us suppose, for example, as seems to be deducible from what Forel had shown, that the aforesaid contact is of a diffuse nature, taking place between dendrites belonging to neighbouring neurons, or between branches of different axons, or, finally, between dendrites and terminal axonic branchlets. The inevitable and fatal result of such an assumption would be that the paths of nerve impulses must be indeterminate, and essentially, that the reticular theory is resurrected in a new form, a species of protoplasmic pantheism as pleasing to those who disdain observation as it is contrary to the postulates of embryology, physiology, and pathological anatomy. To affirm that everything communicates with everything else is equivalent to declaring the absolute unsearchability of the organ of the soul.

My work consisted just in providing an objective basis for the brilliant but vague suggestions of His and Forel. With the fortunate discovery of the basket endings and of the climbing fibres, I showed that contact does not exist between dendrites alone, nor between branches of the nerve fibres, but between the latter on the one hand, and the bodies and dendritic processes of the neurons, on the other; that, in fact, a cell often forms connections with branches of fibres coming from diverse sources and that, reciprocally, each axon may make contact, by means of collateral and terminal branches, with different types of neurons; notwithstanding which, there exist in the gray matter definitely delimited conduction paths, in agreement with the requirements of neurophysiology and neuropathology.

I have already remarked that legitimate conceptions are characterized by gaining strength rather than losing ground in the light of new observations. This was the case with the law of transmission by contact when it was submitted to the test of the structural analysis of the retina and the optic centres.

Retina.—It was in the retina of birds that this work of assaying was initiated. It would be useless and inopportune after the foregoing discussion to enter into descriptive details here, and it will suffice to mention a few of the new facts brought out in the paper on that subject.

(*a*) It was shown that the rods and cones terminate freely at the level of the external plexiform layer, articulating with the external tuft of the bipolar cells (Fig. 30).

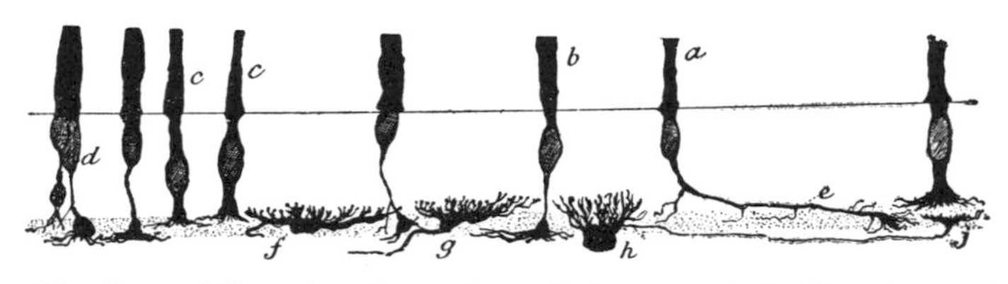

FIG. 30. Zone of the external granules and the external plexiform layer of the retina of the bird. *a, b, d,* varieties of cones; *e,* rods; *h,* horizontal cells.

(*b*) Under the external plexiform layer some special elements were discovered with brush-like form, provided with ascending dendrites spread out in that layer (Fig. 30 *h*).

(c) Centrifugal retinal fibres were found, this is a special category of fibres in the optic nerve which cross the internal plexiform zone and end by a free, varicose arborization among the spongioblasts. This interesting fact, which has served as a basis for the theory of the *nervo-nervorum* of Duval, among other fertile conceptions, was confirmed by Dogiel, who had previously denied it (Fig. 32, *b, c, d, e*).

(*d*) Landolt's club in the bipolar cells of birds, and the collaterals of their axons (Fig. 31, *A*) were discovered simultaneously with their observation by Dogiel.

(*e*) Many new forms of spongioblasts (nerve cells without axons) were described.

(f) Several layers of nervous arborization were demonstrated in the internal plexiform zone, showing that at these levels the dendrites of the ganglion cells come into relation

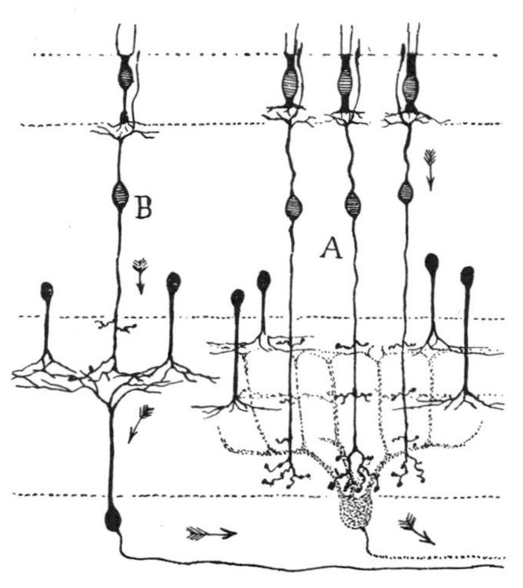

FIG. 31. Diagram showing the connections among the various neurons of the retina of the bird and the course of the nerve-impulse. *A*, bipolar cells.

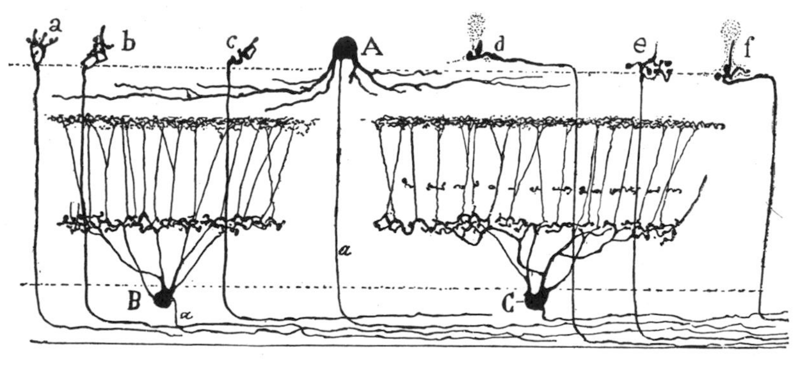

FIG. 32. Some types of ganglion cells (*B*, *C*) in the retina of the bird: *b*, *d*, *e*, *f*, terminal arborizations of centrifugal fibres; *A*, displaced ganglion cell.

with the axons and collaterals of the bipolar cells by contact and not through a diffuse net, as Tartuferi had described in the retina of mammals (Fig. 31 *A*, *B*).

(*g*) Many morphological details about the fibres of Müller in the birds were discussed.

Figures 30, 31, and 32 show diagrammatically the most essential of my discoveries in the retina. There should be noticed, especially, how the three series of neurons (rods and cones, bipolar cells, and ganglionic cells) are connected in two concentric planes.

Muscle Spindles.—Of some importance for muscular physiology is another little paper which appeared in the same number of the *Revista de Histología,* entitled *Terminaciones nerviosas en los husos musculares de la rana* (Nerve endings in the muscle spindles of the frog).

In this communication, which was based upon revelations of the methylene blue method of Ehrlich, it was pointed out:

(*a*) That in the spindles of Kühne in amphibians and reptiles (small muscle fibres which have a specific nervous termination, apparently sensory, but then of uncertain significance) there exist two kinds of nervous arborizations: one, already known, continuous with thick fibres; another (or others), undescribed, which is finer.

(*b*) Since the small arborization is identical with ordinary motor end plates, and the larger or specific one resembles the "musculo-tendinous organs" of Golgi, the former were considered motor, the latter sensory. The excitation of this terminal apparatus during contraction of the muscle would arouse in the brain a perception of the state of contraction of the muscle (muscle-sense of the physiologists).

Similar facts were later announced by Ruffini, Hubert and de Witt, Dogiel, Sherrington, and others, who followed my physiological interpretation, though unknowingly.

Two other articles of somewhat less importance were also published in 1888. These were devoted respectively to the structure of the muscle fibres of the heart and to that of the nerve fibres of the cerebral electric organ of the torpedo.

This completes the publications of 1888.

Spinal Cord.—During the year 1889 my activity continued with unabated vigour and diligence, applying itself to various neurological problems, but concentrating particularly upon the study of the spinal cord in birds and mammals.

In attacking this question, of which I knew the obscurity well from experience in explaining the organization of the spinal axis in my anatomical lectures, I was actuated first of all by the aim to elucidate so far as possible the difficult problem of the ending of the posterior or sensory roots. Although, in view of the outcome of my investigations of the cerebellum, it was presumable that similar arborizations would also follow the *law of pericellular contact,* it was essential to confirm this agreement *de visu,* to ascertain with precision the actual course of the sensory fibres through the gray matter, and to single out, finally, the neurons with which they connected.

Before giving a detailed account of my observations, it will not be superfluous to remind the reader briefly of the state of our knowledge of the organization of the spinal cord in the eighties.

It is true that physiological experiments and the data gathered from pathological anatomy, both human and comparative, with the assistance of the method of secondary degeneration (Waller, Türk, Charcot, Bouchard, Löwenthal, Münzer) or that of atrophy (Gudden and Forel), had succeeded in establishing the motor or sensory character of many nerves, in localizing in a broad way the nuclei of origin of the centrifugal and of termination of the centripetal ones, and, finally, in differentiating, within the thickness of the columns of nerve fibres, separate paths or systems of fibres of identical function (the pyramidal tract for voluntary movements, the ascending cerebellar tract, the bundle of Goll, formed by central sensory fibres, etc.). For its part, macro-microscopic analysis had gained some positive successes, delimiting in the gray matter, besides those large areas called the anterior and posterior horns, certain regions of distinctive structure, such as the motor cell groups of the ventral horn, Clarke's column, the substance of Rolando, the white, or anterior, and gray, or posterior commissures, etc. It was known likewise, or rather it was divined—for there was no trustworthy demonstration of the fact—that the fibres of the white matter were continuations of the axons of neurons situated in the gray matter which, after a more or less extensive longitudinal course, returned into the horns, across which they formed bundles in different directions, spreading finally into a diffuse and tangled plexus.

Concerning the principal points, however, in the histology of the spinal cord, that is regarding the problem of the origin and termination of the fibres entering from the longitudinal columns, the genesis of the commissures, and, finally, the ultimate fate of the exogenous or sensory fibres, neurologists merely hazarded conjectures which were frequently confused, sometimes contradictory, and in any case beyond the reach of proof. In truth, the histology of this nervous organ presented only one important datum which was solidly established; the true origin of the anterior roots. From the time, then already remote, of Deiters, Clarke, and Kölliker it had been obvious that the great multipolar nerve cells of the anterior horn projected forwards large axis cylinders which, crossing the antero-lateral column, emerged from the cord to make up the anterior roots and distribute themselves finally to the voluntary muscles.

For this poverty of exact anatomical knowledge, needless to say, it was the methods of investigation that were responsible, these being quite inadequate for a successful attack upon the problem. For example, the method of secondary degeneration already cited, or Gudden's and Forel's method of atrophy, while they permitted the picking out of the situation and course of certain nervous pathways in the white matter, showed themselves incapable of indicating definitely their origin and termination in the gray matter; and as for the histological methods of Weigert or of osmic acid, which are able, as is well known, to present the myelinated fibres intensely and selectively stained, they met an insuperable barrier in the mischance that precisely the most interesting segments of the nerve fibres, that is to say the segment nearest the cell and its terminal ramification, lack the myelin sheath (which is what holds the colour), and consequently are inaccessible.

The enterprise could be undertaken with some hope of success only by the method of Golgi, which stains precisely those unmyelinated segments of the nervous protoplasm. Only through the exceptional powers of revelation of the chrome-silver reaction was it possible to hope for a little light in that chaos of contradictory opinions. However, as has already been stated, this precious resource had not been applied by any histologist, or had been applied in the adult cord where the black reaction is most uncertain and where, besides, the great distances covered by the processes of the cells and the structural complexity of the gray matter sterilize all efforts at analysis.

In fig. 29, based upon the most authoritative neurological texts of the time, I reproduce a diagram of the structure of the cord. Within the gray matter is seen a diffuse network (*c*, *g*) in which are supposed to fuse, according to Gerlach, the ends of the dendrites and the arborizations of the posterior or sensory roots. In Golgi's opinion, as I have already said, the net is composed exclusively of the terminations of the nerve.

Observe that the axons of the largest neurons in the cord are supposed, by conjecture, to be continuous with the fibres of the white matter (Fig. 29, *g*); but as such conductors are very few as compared with the tremendous number of coarse and fine fibres revealed by the method of Weigert within the thickness of the gray matter, the majority of the nerve fibres proceeding from the white matter remain without known connections.

At the level of the anterior root will be noticed entering it the axons of giant cells of the anterior horn; but the error is committed of granting the existence of crossed motor axons (Fig. 29, *a*).

In the region of Clarke's column, Fig. 29 shows, in agreement with an opinion very generally held (Freud, Edinger, Schiefferdecker, Lenhossék, etc.), certain spherical or fusiform corpuscles, lacking dendrites but having two axonic processes, one continuous with the posterior root, the other directed towards the lateral column, where it would help to form the ascending cerebellar tract (Fig. 29, *G* and *C*).

The gelatinous substance of Rolando would contain only neuroglia with a varying quantity of nerve fibres.

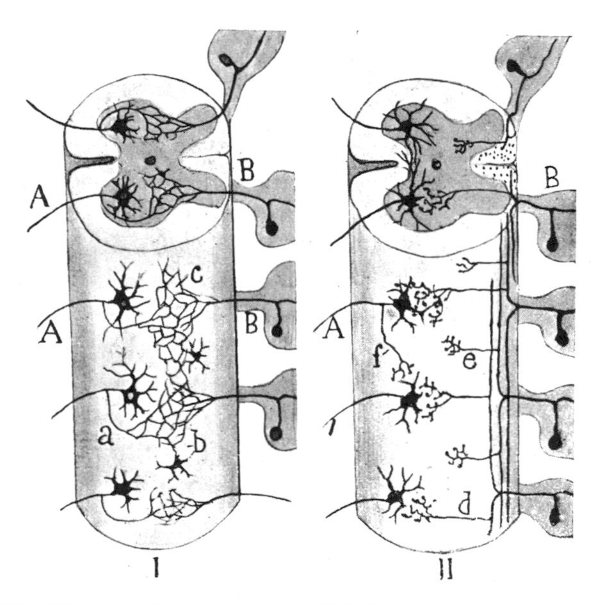

FIG. 33. Diagrams for comparison of Golgi's conception of the sensory-motor connections in the spinal cord (1) with the result of my investigations (11). *A*, anterior roots; *B*, posterior roots; *a*, collateral of a motor root; *b*, cell with a short axon which Golgi believed to take part in the formation of the net; *c*, diffuse interstitial network; *d*, one of my long collaterals in contact with the motor cell; *e*, short collateral.

Finally, the fibres of the posterior root coming from the sensory ganglion are indicated as behaving in very diverse ways: one bundle of fibres, as has been said already, was supposed to ramify and lose itself in the thickness of the gray matter, entering into the continuous net of Gerlach or of Golgi (Fig. 29, *B*); another fascicle, without branching in the gray matter, was supposed to bend sharply to ascend in the column of Burdach (*d*); while some fibres, finally, were considered to reach the commissures or the substance of the anterior horn.

This, I repeat, was one of very many interpretations, perhaps the simplest, for the structural formula varied under the pen of each writer. For myself, I can state that in the decade of 1877 to 1887, I suffered many headaches from the effort to extract something clear from the descriptions of scientific authorities, as to the composition and course of the sensory roots. I preserve still a note book dated 1877 in which I have recorded and drawn in several colours (to help in the critical times of my examinations for professorships) three perfectly irreconcilable schemes, taken from the current neurological texts. Baffled and lost in that *mare magnum* of fibres and cells, I frequently despaired of my modest powers of understanding. How capricious is fate! Who would have said then that, as time went by, it would be my lot to contribute to the partial disentangling of the spinal skein!

This was due simply, as already mentioned, to the fortunate event of applying the method of Golgi to the study of the spinal cord in embryos of birds and mammals. It would be idle, after the above explanation, to enter into the details of my researches, which the curious reader will find in the text of my books and monographs on the subject. Here I shall limit myself to enumerating the most important conclusions of my communications of 1889 and 1890:

1. The collaterals of the white matter were described in detail. These are branches which spring at right angles from the longitudinal fibres in all the white columns, enter horizontally into the horns of the gray matter, and end there by free, thickened, varicose ramifications applied intimately to the contours of the bodies and dendrites of the neurons. (Figs. 34, *e, f* and 35, *H*.)

2. The composition of the commissures was elucidated (Fig. 34, *f, i, a*).

3. In connection with the termination of the axons, there

was established a rational classification of the neurons in the gray matter, namely: motor or radicular cells, funicular or tract cells, and commissural cells, according to whether their respective processes left the cord, entered the white columns of the same side, or crossed over to enter those of the opposite side (Fig. 34, *j*, *m*, *n*).

4. Bifurcation of fibres into ascending and descending branches was demonstrated (Fig. 36).

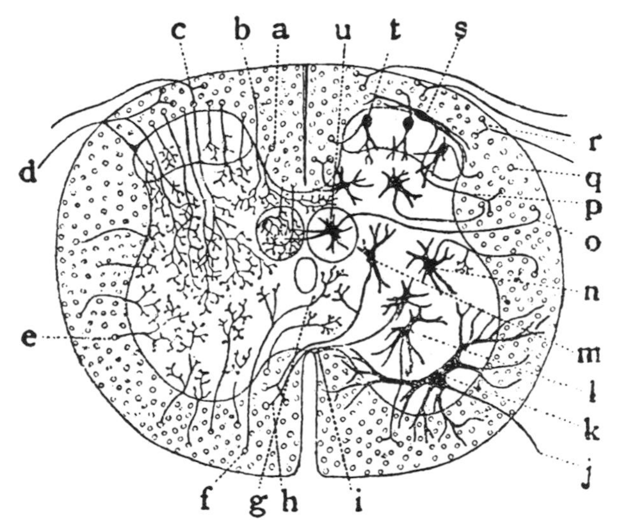

FIG. 34. Diagram of the arrangement of the nerve cells of the spinal cord and collateral fibres of the white matter; *a*, crossed collateral of the posterior commissure; *b*, collateral of the posterior horn; *c*, long collateral of the posterior column; *f*, collaterals of the anterior commissure; *j*, motor root fibre; *k*, motor cell; *m*, commissural cell; *n*, tract cell; *r*, sensory root fibre; *u*, column of Clarke. (This figure is a copy of one of the wall plates used in my lectures in 1894.)

5. The existence was established of fibres which sent branches into different columns, a fact vaguely hinted by Golgi but not recognized, until I rediscovered it.

6. The substance of Rolando was shown to contain very numerous small neurons giving rise to short correlation fibres.

7. The true terminal arrangement of the sensory fibres was demonstrated in both birds and mammals. It is shown diagrammatically in Fig. 33, *II*.

8. The neuroglia (supporting) cells were shown to be derived from the lining layer of the central canal.

9. The unipolar sensory cells in the spinal ganglia were shown to pass through a bipolar stage in development, in which they resemble the corresponding cells in lower animals.

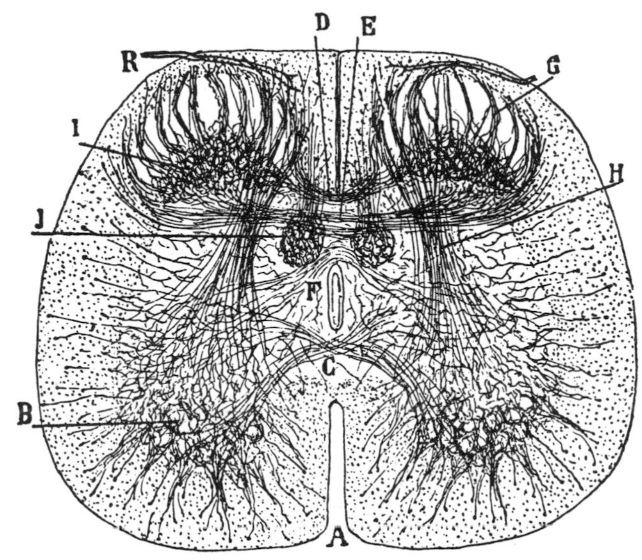

FIG. 35. GENERAL APPEARANCE OF THE COLLATERALS IN A TRANSVERSE SECTION OF THE SPINAL CORD. *B*, plexus of collaterals of the anterior horn; *C*, anterior commissure of collaterals, *E*, crossed collaterals of the posterior commissure; *G*, collaterals for the posterior horn; *H*, long or sensory-motor collaterals; *J*, plexus of collaterals in the column of Clarke. (All these fibres were regarded as main axon terminals before the appearance of my work, and the existence of their final arborization was unknown.)

Apart from their constructive value, the foregoing observations regarding the spinal cord display a certain critical ability. They are important both for what they deny and for what they affirm. When the prejudice against the method of Golgi was dissipated, thanks to the preaching of Kölliker and of myself, many investigators, including Kölliker, van Gehuchten, Edinger, v. Lenhossek, Azoulay, Lugaro, etc., explored this nervous organ in embryos and young animals and agreed unanimously in the final rejection of definite assumptions which were based on incomplete observations. Such were: the crossed motor roots (Fig. 29, *a*), the sensory fibres continuous with neurons of Clarke's column (Fig. 29, *g*), the posterior root fibres which

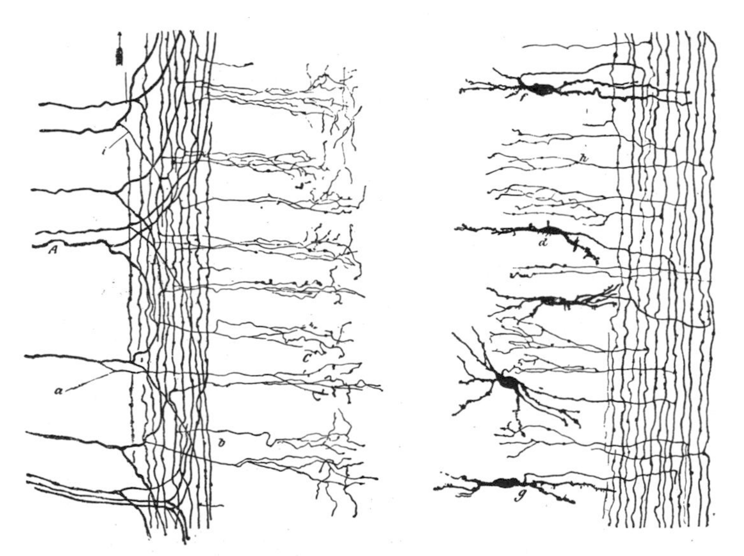

FIG. 36. LONGITUDINAL SECTION OF THE POSTERIOR AND LATERAL COLUMNS OF THE SPINAL CORD to show the arrangement of the posterior roots and the origin of the collaterals. *A*, sensory root. (Notice the bifurcation of the posterior or sensory roots, which was unknown to the scientific world.)

did not divide and were continuous with fibres in the column of Burdach (Fig. 29, *d*), etc.

The Optic Lobe of Birds.—We have just seen how the sensory nerve fibres end in the spinal cord. Do the centripetal sensory fibres behave in the same way, that is to say those coming from the retina, the olfactory bulb, the acoustic nerve, etc.? The question had theoretical interest of the first order. The exploration of the optic centres, then, was required in order to see whether the law of contact by means of free pericellular observations is fulfilled by them also.

Of all the nerve centres, the most suitable for this investigation, on account of its being singularly susceptible to the revelations of the chrome-silver reaction, is the optic lobe of bird embryos and of birds a few days old (chick embryos from the sixteenth day on, birds recently hatched, etc.). The position within this organ of the optic fibres, or conductors from the retina, was quite well known, thanks to the studies of Stieda, Bellonci, and other authors. Such fibres make up a superficial zone, under which they form a concentric plexus, in the meshes of which appear the receptive neurons.

Apart from the demonstration of the manner of ending of the optic fibres, the monograph referred to contains numerous morphological and structural facts of positive value. It is unnecessary to mention them all here. The reader who is interested in such matters will require to consult my memoirs of 1889 or the translation published two years later in the Internationale Monatschrift of Dr. Krause. I will cite only the points with some physiological value. These were:

(*a*) the demonstration that the fibres of the optic nerve end in the outer zones of the lobe by complicated, free, varicose arborizations, which connect by contact with the receptive processes of numerous more deeply situated cells;

(*b*) the discovery of a great number of morphological types of neurons.

Valuable contributions on the anatomy of the optic lobe of birds were made afterwards by Kölliker, van Gehuchten, and especially my brother, who devoted several important communications to the subject as we shall notice later. In brief, these works confirm the fundamental conclusions drawn from my observations, namely; that also in the sensory centres afferent impulses are propagated by contact from the centripetal or retinal fibres to the dendrites and cell bodies of the central neurons.

The intensive work in my laboratory in 1889 enabled me to gather a few other interesting new facts in other sense organs and even in non-nervous tissues.

Among these sallies beyond my chosen realms, one worthy of mention was *Nuevas aplicaciones del método de coloración de Golgi.* In this it was shown that each olfactory cell in the nasal mucous membrane is continuous with a single fibre of the olfactory nerve, refuting finally the supposed ramifications of these fibres mentioned by Ranvier and Castronuovo. The existence within the protoplasm of salivary gland cells of delicate ramifications continuous with the secretory ducts was proved. The bile capillaries in the livers of various vertebrates were described independently of Kupffer. Also it was proved that the sympathetic nerve fibres end freely on the gland cells.

Another of the modest communications referred to was published in a professional review, *La Medicina Práctica.* It contains an attempt at theoretical interpretation of the mass of morphological facts collected in the previous monographs. In this Golgi's grouping of all nerve cells into motor and sensory types (types I and II) was replaced by the terms *long-axon cells* and *short-axon cells.* The bipolar, or sensory cells (olfactory, retinal, and spinal ganglion) were classed as a special category of neurons, laying the foundation for the theory of dynamic polarization later set up by van Gehuchten and me, and afterwards replaced by the theory of axipetal polarization today generally held. The receptive function of the dendrites was maintained. A hypothesis relating the manner of branching of the axons to the number and form of the elements to which they run was formulated, etc.

CHAPTER VI

The excessive reservedness of scientists towards my publications. To prevent distrust, I decided to demonstrate my preparations before the German Anatomical Society. In Berlin I make the personal acquaintance of the famous histologists Albrecht Kölliker, His, Waldeyer, and other Teutonic scientists. My visit to the histological laboratory of W. Krause in Göttingen. A short trip through the north of Italy. Personal impressions of the German scientists.

It is natural that every author should aspire to the approval, and if possible the applause, of his public; and mine, consisting of a limited number of specialists, was found abroad, scattered through a few German, French, Italian, Swiss, English, and Scandinavian universities. In order to feel that inner satisfaction which is our principal reward in research and to continue working with enthusiasm, it was necessary for me to win over unprejudiced and intelligent scientists. It would have been foolish to hope for unanimous applause. How was I to convince investigators long since devoted to the defence of erroneous facts or gratuitous hypotheses? I had to allow for the fact that my ideas were bound to arouse the opposition of the *reticularists,* and particularly of the school of Golgi; and although my publications of that period contributed largely to making known the methods and the positive accomplishments of the Pavia professor, the good will of scientists is usually so paradoxical that they are more pleased by the defence of an obvious error which has become wide-spread than by the establishment of a new fact.

In the realm of the spirit as in that of material things, the law of inertia is the great obstacle which has to be overcome.

Meanwhile I lived in a state of restlessness and suspicion. I was a little alarmed by the silence maintained by the authors to whom I had sent complimentary copies of my Review during the latter half of the year 1888 and the first half of 1889. Several works upon the structure of the nervous system which I received in the latter year either did not mention me or did so contemptuously, as it were in passing, and without attributing any importance to my opinions.[1] From consulting the German periodicals I gathered the impression that most of the histologists had not read my papers. It is true that Spanish is a tongue unknown to scientists.

I wished, however, to persuade them at all costs. I rebelled against the idea of passing for deluded or being considered a pretender. I resorted to two methods for gaining the confidence of impartial authors: the first was to translate my chief neurological papers into French, publishing them in the most authoritative German periodicals; the second was to demonstrate my best preparations to the scientific men personally and thus to establish the legitimacy of my views.

The translations were begun in 1889 and continued in 1890 and the following years. The *Internationale Monatschrift für Anatomie und Physiologie* of my friend Dr. W. Krause inserted two memoirs: one devoted to the structure of the cerebellum and the other to the study of the optic lobe in birds. In both were included a few new facts besides those which had appeared in the *Revista trimestral;* for I usually continue working in the laboratory even while

[1] Even in 1890, M. von Lenhossék, Professor in Basel, in a memoir devoted to the study of the posterior roots of the spinal cord, made the following reservations concerning my conclusions: "It is very surprising that so fundamental a fact—he refers to the bifurcation of the sensory roots—should not have been discovered by anyone in spite of the cord having been explored for fifty years in all directions and by all methods. When, as in the case of the spinal ganglia, a Y-division of the nerve fibres certainly exists, the fact is perfectly susceptible to proof, as the observations of Ranvier, Stannius, Kuttner, etc., show."

Soon afterwards Lenhossék surrendered to the evidence, becoming a convinced supporter of my ideas, which he illustrated with interesting discoveries in divers regions of the nervous system. Scientists of such nobility of character as the Hungarian neurologist are not numerous, however. See Lenhossék, *Hinterwurzel und Hinterstrange.* Mittheilung aus dem Anat. Inst. im Vesalianum, Basel, 1890.

I am correcting the proofs. Professor Carl v. Bardeleben, of Jena, with whom I established correspondence, condescended also to give cordial hospitality in his then recently commenced *Anatomischer Anzeiger* to my communications upon the retina of birds and the minute structure of the spinal cord.

The translations mentioned made known the most essential of my scientific contributions; but these alone, although illustrated by plates copied from nature with scrupulous care, would not have gained me many adherents. The latter came as a result of the employment of the second step mentioned—direct objective demonstration. Nothing convinces like things actually seen, especially when they are clear and positive.

To this end I applied for membership in the German Anatomical Society, to which belonged anatomists, histologists, and embryologists of many nations, especially of the German confederation and of Austria-Hungary. This association met each year in a different university city. During the sessions, the members discussed current anatomical problems; demonstrated, in support of their views, the gross and microscopic preparations which they had procured; explained the details of the methods used; in fine, pointed out to the lovers of investigation the fertile directions and the veins recently opened up for scientific exploitation. Finally, concurrently with the work of the congress, the manufacturers showed the recent developments in instruments for observation and experiment.

International scientific congresses have been much abused since then. Nevertheless, the meetings of specialists offer undeniable advantages to lovers of the laboratory. In them, methods are exhibited and the acquaintance of scientific men is made. It is a great thing to see for oneself the best analytical results from a method in the hands of its inventor; but intellectual and friendly exchange with the inventors is worth still more. It is good tactics to cultivate the friendship and assure for oneself the goodwill of those with whom, as a result of similar tastes, one will have to converse and perhaps contend in noble and amicable controversy. Only friendly intercourse moderates and softens the churlish attitudes of chauvinism; thanks to it, emulators and rivals belonging to different countries attain mutual understanding and esteem, acquiring in the end full realization that they are collaborators and colleagues in a great and common task, full of difficulties and of dark secrets.

The above mentioned anatomical society was holding its meetings that year, 1889, in the University of Berlin during the first fortnight in October. Having obtained the permission of the rector to take part in the proceedings of the Congress, I gathered together for the purpose all my scanty savings and set out, full of hope, for the capital of the German Empire. On the way, I paid instructive visits to the university cities of Lyons and Geneva and also to Frankfurt-am-Main, a town which lacks a university but has scientists of the highest order. There I made the acquaintance of the celebrated neurologist Carl Weigert, the originator of valuable methods for staining nervous tissue; of Edinger, the greatest authority on comparative neurology; and, finally, of Ehrlich, the inventor of the staining method which bears his name, who, later on, was to obtain the Nobel prize as the reward of his great discoveries in the domains of bacteriology and serotherapy.

It is unnecessary to say that my colleagues at the congress accorded me a courteous reception. There was in it an element of surprise and expectant curiosity. It was a shock for them, no doubt, to meet a Spaniard who cultivated science and had of his own volition entered upon the paths of research. At the conclusion of the reading of papers, to which, on account of my impatience, I devoted little attention, there came the demonstrations.

From an early hour I was installed in the laboratory devoted to this purpose, where numerous microscopes shone upon large tables before broad windows. I unpacked my preparations; I requisitioned two or three of the magnifying instruments besides my own excellent Zeiss model, which I had brought as a precaution; I focussed them upon the sections which showed the most important facts regarding the structure of the cerebellum, the retina, and the spinal cord, and, finally, I began to explain to the curious in bad French what my preparations contained. Some histologists surrounded me, but only a few, for, as happens in such competitions, each member of the congress was looking after his own affairs; after all, it is natural that one should prefer demonstrating his own work to examining that of someone else.[2]

Among those who showed most interest in my demonstration I should mention His, Schwalbe, Retzius, Waldeyer, and especially Kölliker. As was to be expected, these savants, then world celebrities, began their examination with more scepticism than curiosity. Undoubtedly, they expected a fiasco. However, when there had been paraded before their eyes in a procession of irreproachable images of the utmost clearness, the axons of the granules of the cerebellum, the pericellular basket-endings, the mossy and climbing fibres, the bifurcations and ascending and descending branches of the sensory roots, the long and short collaterals of the columns of white matter, the terminations of the retinal fibres in the optic lobe, etc., the supercilious frowns disappeared. Finally, the prejudice against the

[2] Perhaps the reader would be interested in a transcription of some comments upon my demonstrations at Berlin, taken from the lecture of the celebrated neurologist van Gehuchten, delivered in 1913, upon the occasion of the solemn festival held at Louvain to mark the twenty-fifth year of his professorship.

"The facts described by Cajal in his first publications were so extraordinary that the histologists of the time—fortunately I did not belong to the number—received them with the greatest scepticism. The distrust was such that, at the anatomical congress held in Berlin in 1889, Cajal, who afterwards became the great histologist of Madrid, found himself alone, exciting around him only smiles of incredulity. I can still see him taking aside Kölliker, who was then the unquestioned master of German histology, and drawing him into a corner of the demonstration hall to show him under the microscope his admirable preparations, and to convince him at the same time of the reality of the facts which he claimed to have discovered. The demonstration was so decisive that a few months later the Würzburg histologist confirmed all the facts stated by Cajal." (See Le Nevraxe: Livre Jubilaire, Vols. XIV and XV, 1913.)

PLATE 15

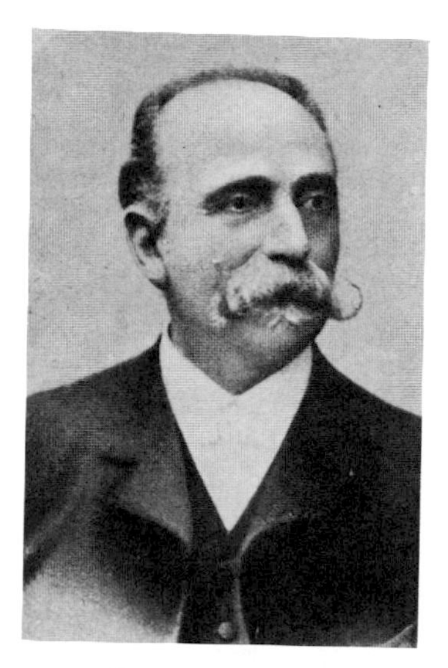

FIG. 37. PROFESSOR C. GOLGI, OF THE UNIVERSITY OF PAVIA.

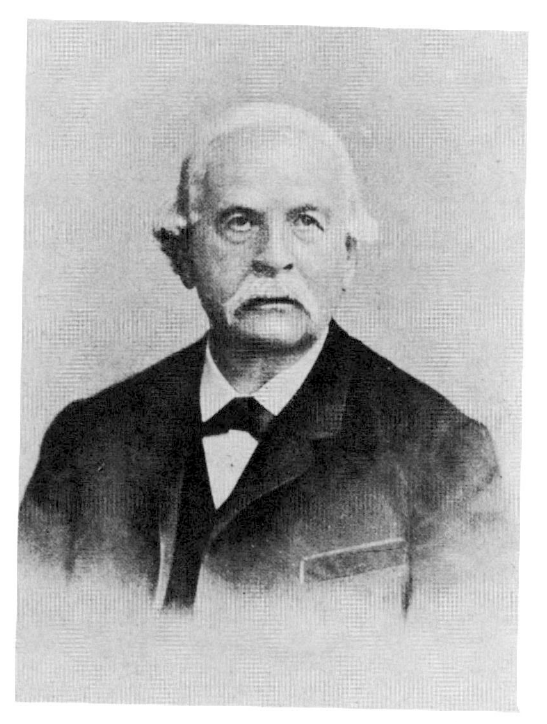

FIG. 38. DR. ALBRECHT KÖLLIKER, Professor in the University of Würzburg.

PLATE 16

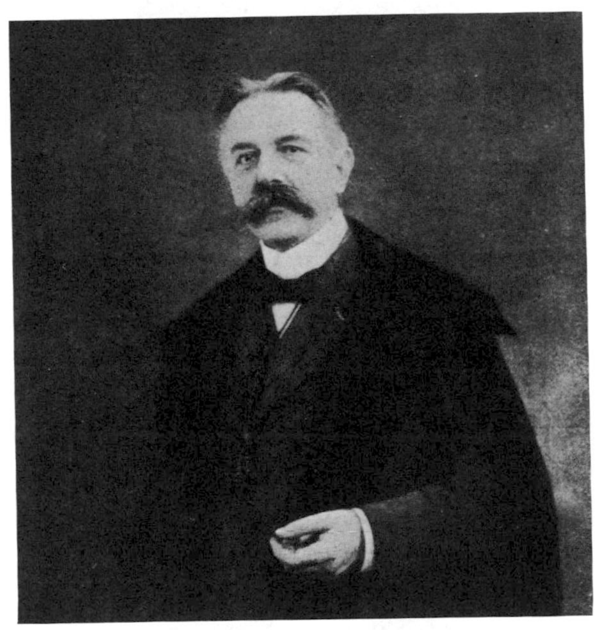

FIG. 39. DR. A. VAN GEHUCHTEN, Professor in the University of Louvain.

humble Spanish anatomist vanished and warm and sincere congratulations burst forth.

They besieged me with questions about the technical conditions by virtue of which such preparations had been obtained. "We have tried the method of Golgi repeatedly," they told me, "and all we have got are disappointments and failures." Then I explained to them in clumsy French, minutely and patiently, all the little secrets of the manipulations of the chrome-silver process; I pointed out the ages and conditions of the embryos and animals which were most favourable for procuring good preparations and indicated the practical rules which tended to lessen so far as possible the capriciousness of the method.

The most interested of my hearers was A. Kölliker, the venerable patriarch of German histology. At the end of the session he took me in a splendid carriage to the luxurious hotel where he was staying; entertained me at dinner; presented me afterwards to the most important histologists and embryologists of Germany, and, finally, made every effort to render my sojourn in the Prussian capital agreeable.

"The results that you have obtained are so beautiful," he said to me, "that I intend to undertake a series of confirmatory studies immediately, adopting your technique. I have discovered you, and I wish to make my discovery known in Germany." [3]

In actual fact, during 1890 and the succeeding years, there appeared in various German *Archives*, and especially in the *Zeitschrift f. wissenschaftliche Zoologie*—of which Dr. Kölliker was director—a series of magnificent monographs on the cerebellum, the spinal cord, the medulla oblongata, the optic lobe, etc. In them, my modest scientific conquests were not only confirmed, as he had promised, but

[3] In a letter received soon after my return to Barcelona, Kölliker repeats the promise: "Vous avez un grand mérite," he told me, "d'avoir employé le procédé du chromate d'argent rapide dans les jeunes animaux et dans les embryons. Ainsi ne manquerai-je de faire ressortir vos admirables travaux, en me réjuissant que le premier histologue que l'Espagne a produit soit un homme aussi distingué que vous et tout a fait a l'hauteur de la science." (Würzburg, November 16, 1889.)

were extended and perfected remarkably, besides being embellished with ingenious physiological interpretations.

I am very deeply grateful to the distinguished master of Würzburg. There is no doubt that the truth would have made itself clear eventually. Nevertheless, it was due to the great authority of Kölliker that my ideas were rapidly disseminated and appreciated by the scientific world. A noble exception among great investigators, Kölliker united a great talent for observation, aided by indefatigable industry, with enchanting modesty, and exceptional rectitude and calmness of judgment. It was to the great Bavarian master that I alluded particularly when, in earlier chapters, while deploring the intolerable egotism and vanity of certain men of science, I declared that there were others most learned and at the same time upright, impartial, and honourable.

So little did he sacrifice at the altar of haughty self-importance that, although he had been a supporter of the reticular theory, he abandoned it completely, adapting himself with the flexibility of a young man to the new conceptions of contact and of the morphological independence of the neurons. In his friendliness for me, he carried his goodwill so far as to learn Spanish in order to read my earliest communications. Later on, his noble modesty reached its culmination in his personally translating for his *Zeitschrift. f. wissenschaftliche Zoologie* the text of a work of mine on the hippocampus, etc. For all this and for many other proofs of friendship, borne witness to in letters and publications, I preserve an ineffaceable recollection of and profound gratitude towards the glorious master.

At the meeting in Berlin I had the honour also of having discussions with the illustrious Gustav Retzius, Professor of Anatomy at Stockholm, one of the most sagacious, industrious, and conscientious investigators whom I have known; with W. His, the great embryologist of Leipzig, to whom I referred in the previous chapter; with Waldeyer, the venerated master of German anatomy and histology, professor in the University of Berlin; with van Gehuchten, the young and already brilliant professor from the University of Louvain, with whom I had already corresponded in connection with our studies upon muscle fibres; and finally with Schwalbe, C. Bardeleben, and other anatomists of renown. Of some of these, who were afterwards converted into generous supporters of my ideas, I shall speak in the next chapter.

On my way back from Berlin, I made a stop at the little town of Göttingen, where I had the pleasure of meeting personally my friend Dr. W. Krause. With him I spent three or four delightful days. He showed me the most important things in the city, especially the museums and laboratories of the university; he presented me to one of his colleagues who was a great collector of pictures and admirer of Spanish painting (he was enchanted with what he claimed to be a Velasquez that he possessed, which was, however, a decidedly doubtful one), who entertained us with a sumptuous banquet; and, finally, he took me to his official laboratory, which was set up, it is true, in an unpretentious dwelling house, and in which there were working a few pupils surrounded by materials and instruments by no means luxurious, but adequate. Needless to say, I was anxious to show Dr. Krause my preparations and even presented some to him. Those connected with the retina, a subject to which he was devoting himself particularly, interested him greatly.

In our conversations at table we exchanged observations about the organization of our respective universities. It filled me with astonishment to learn that professors were chosen almost freely, without competitive examinations. The absence of a uniform plan of teaching also shocked me, as did what resembled the systematic abandonment of that spirit of unity and centralization, so highly regarded in Spain as a result of the servile imitation of the French university organization. Each science had its own quarters which received the name of institute, and included the lecture room, the laboratory for the professor and his students, the library, etc. There were no examinations except at the end of the course. Finally, the professors, classified into the categories of *Privatdozent*, *professor extraordinary* (*ausserordentlicher Professor*), and *regular professor* (*ordentlicher Professor*), instead of being engaged according to a uniform scale of salaries, were paid by the state and the city on the basis of their merits, besides receiving in addition honoraria from their pupils.

Suppression of examinations, university autonomy, remuneration from the students, appointment without competitive examination and often by a sort of contract! Here was a series of reforms which, if applied to Spain, the classical country of routine and favouritism, would have reduced us before ten years had passed to a state of savagery. It is with reason that Paulsen has said that every country has the university system that it requires, that is, the best possible in view of the condition of social ethics.

After this pause in a peaceful little German university, which was as fertile in great savants as it was free from intrigues and ambitions, I proceeded on my homeward way. I paid flying visits to picturesque Lucerne and the poetic Lake of the Four Cantons; crossed the Alps through the St. Gotthard Pass, regretting deeply that the state of my finances would not permit me to loiter in contemplation of those incomparable panoramas, and finally passed through the north of Italy, particularly the famous university cities of Turin, Pavia, and Genoa.

In Turin I had the pleasure of making the personal acquaintance of the distinguished Italian histologist Julio Bizzozero and the no less famous professor Angelo Mosso. I remember that their respective class rooms and laboratories were established in an ancient convent, in very unsuitable quarters. I wished to ascertain what resources the university had and what were the salaries of the professors, and I met with two surprises: first, that the Italian professor, though his value was so high, earned little more than ours (the salary limit for the oldest was 10,000 liras) while his annual production, didactic and scientific, was infinitely superior; and second, that, inspired by lofty motives

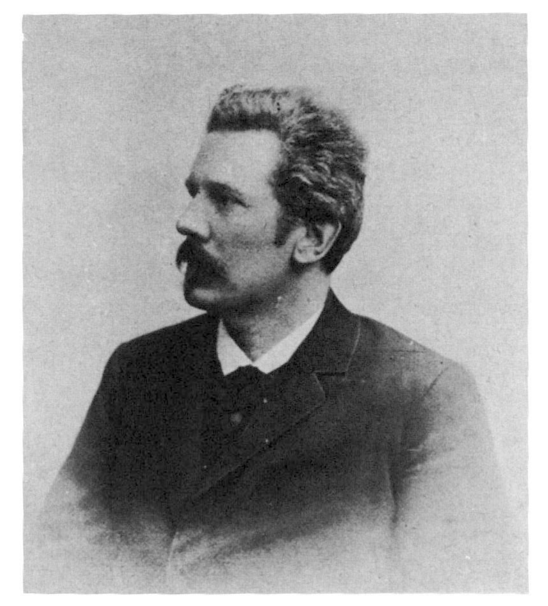

FIG. 40. DR. G. RETZIUS. Professor of Anatomy in the University of Stockholm.

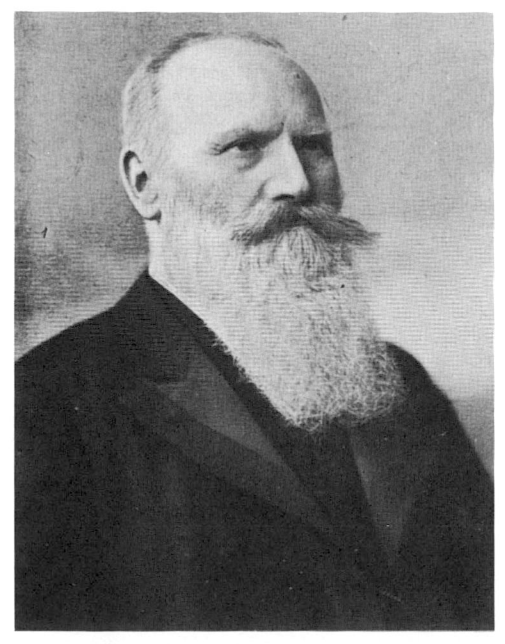

FIG. 41. DR. WALDEYER, Professor of Anatomy in the Faculty of Medicine at Berlin.

of patriotism and love of science, the governing bodies of the people (corresponding with our civic and provincial governments) and wealthy individuals would add to the meagre appropriations destined for equipment in the state budget, rich gifts in support of scientific experiments. A board of trustees composed of important individuals and of representatives of the authorities used to administer these supplementary funds according to the needs of each subject and each professor.

Here was a mode of procedure which will be stupifying to our municipal and provincial governments, which are so satisfied with uncultural and unpatriotic corporate provincialism. Apart from their high educational and cultural value, the university and other official institutions bring to the city at the same time great prestige and not inconsiderable profit. Even if not from community of purpose and love of science, yet through pride and easily understood emulation, these governing bodies ought to hasten to the aid of the state by providing the money for extension of teaching, for improving that which already exists, and, finally, for nurturing the spirit of investigation. But could these truths, clear and simple as they are, penetrate either into the thick heads of our ediles or into the no less solid ivory of the brains of our potentates?

I did not have the pleasure of finding the illustrious Professor Camilo Golgi in Pavia. He was in Rome, whither he was taken at certain times of the year by his responsibilities as a senator. We may note in passing that in Italy it is customary for the most renowned men of learning to receive, among other rewards, investiture as members of the Upper Chamber. The absence of the master disappointed me very greatly. I am perfectly certain that, if I could have shown him my preparations and expressed to him at the same time my admiration for him, future polemics and vexations misunderstandings would have been avoided.

Finally, after a flying visit to Genoa, where I was very well received by the professor of anatomy, I went back to Marseilles and returned to Barcelona.

From this rapid survey of the foreign universities, I drew the firm conviction that the cultural superiority of Germany, France, and Italy depended not upon the educational institutions but upon the *men*. As I have already stated, the material resources at the disposal of worthy men of learning appeared to me little better than in our country, and in some cases markedly worse. One often meets in Germany a Privatdozent who has great discoveries to his credit and who, nevertheless, is restricted for many years to remuneration which our assistants would disdain. But there is another fact of even greater significance: relatively often (this phenomenon occurs in England also) the university calls to its bosom investigators of genius who have developed independently, in isolated localities, with a garret as a laboratory, and with no other resources than the modest economies of a town physician.

It is obvious then, that in the northern countries, apart from the form of educational organization, there exists a widespread and deeply-rooted cause for the flourishing of culture. The vessel sometimes appears to be of coarse ware, but the essence is usually exquisite.

What is this essence? It would not be convenient here to study in passing the complex conditions of the scientific greatness of Germany; and besides, we could say nothing new. Let us confine ourselves merely to my impressions of those days.

Superior culture seems to me to be the fruit of individual and social education combined. In the university one is taught to work; but in the social medium, the product of the state, one is taught something better: respect and admiration for the man of science. To no purpose does the university student receive an efficient technical training and along with it the noble and patriotic desire to collaborate in the common labour of civilization, if, at the same time, he does not look about him with contempt for laziness, abhorrence for sham and intrigue, appreciation for superior merit, and reverence for genius.

Education and justice! That is the ultimate secret.

CHAPTER VII

My activity continues with increasing vigour. Some studies on the development of the nervous system (medulla and cerebellum). A curious arrangement in the muscle fibres of insects. My explorations in the olfactory bulb justify fully the doctrine of contact. Interesting discoveries in the cerebral cortex of mammals. Distinguished scientists who approve, confirm, or popularize my ideas. Some disappointments and unpleasantnesses.

The years 1890 and 1891 were periods of intense labour and of most gratifying rewards. Encouraged by the applause of Kölliker and convinced that I had finally found my proper path, I attacked my work with positive fury. The only explanation is that I was desirous of carrying conviction by the overwhelming volume of my communications. During 1890 alone, I published fourteen monographs, without counting the translations. To-day I am astonished by that devouring activity, which took aback even the German investigators, who are the most industrious and patient on the globe. My tasks began at nine o'clock in the morning and usually continued until about midnight. And the strangest thing is that the work gave me pleasure. It was a delicious rapture, an irresistible enchantment.

It is an actual fact that, leaving aside the flatteries of self-love, the garden of neurology holds out to the investigator captivating spectacles and incomparable artistic emotions. In it, my aesthetic instincts found full satisfaction at last. Like the entomologist in pursuit of brightly coloured butterflies, my attention hunted, in the flower garden of the gray matter, cells with delicate and elegant forms, the mysterious butterflies of the soul, the beating of whose wings may some day—who knows?—clarify the secret of mental life.

In some way or other, the simple admiration of the cellular form was one of my greatest delights. For even from the aesthetic point of view the nervous tissue contains the most charming attractions. Is there in our parks any tree more elegant and luxuriant than the Purkinje cell of the cerebellum or the *psychic cell,* that is the famous cerebral pyramid? The diagrams in Figs. 28 and 32, necessarily fragmentary, in which are illustrated respectively the ingenious architecture of the cerebellum and that of the retina, hardly permit one to guess the supreme beauty and the elegant variedness of the nervous pleasance.

Besides, the emotion of discovery is so sweet and so comforting! There is a quality so gently caressing to vanity and pride (human weaknesses with which one must always reckon) in the slightly self-worshipful sensation of discovering hidden islands or virginal forms which seem to have been awaiting since the beginning of the world a worthy contemplator of their beauty.

How many times during those years of investigative fever was I kept awake by the excitement of the newly discovered fact! How often, after an exhausting task and a profound sleep, such as wipes out physiological arrears and clears away the clouds from the slate of the brain, there welled up with the dawn, as if written by an invisible hand, the solution of a problem of morphology or of connection which had been anxiously sought! To-day I cannot well understand how that continual intellectual tension and that daily mental unrest did not upset my health. Undoubtedly, the sovereign satisfaction of doing something useful is a dynamic tonic of the first order.

I should not like to weary the reader by talking of my work in detail; for if telling a story is a pleasure, listening is patience and sometimes annoyance and boredom. Briefly, then, in almost telegraphic fashion, I shall state what was accomplished in 1890.

In my inmost heart, I regard as the best of my work at that time the observations devoted to *neurogeny,* that is to the embryonic development of the nervous system. I may be pardoned if, despite my promise of brevity, I point out a few of their antecedents.

"Since the silver chromate yields more instructive and more constant pictures in embryos than in the adult, why" I asked myself, "should I not explore how the nerve cell develops its form and complexity by degrees, from its germinal phase without processes, as His demonstrated, to its adult or definitive condition? In this developmental course, will there not, perhaps, be revealed something like an echo or recapitulation of the dramatic history lived through by the neuron in its millennial progress through the animal series?"

With this thought in mind, I took the work in hand, first in chick embryos and later in those of mammals. And I had the satisfaction of discovering the first changes in the neuron, from the timid efforts at the formation of processes, frequently altered and even resorbed, up to the definitive organization of the axon and dendrites. Also, in harmony with the fundamental biogenetic principle of Haeckel, I found that the nerve cell repeats in its individual development, with some simplifications and omissions, the permanent forms discovered by Retzius and Lenhossék, in the ganglia of the invertebrates.

It is unnecessary to say that if the problem of the morphology of the neurons appeared obscure before the publication of the memorable works of Golgi, that of their embryology was still darker. In the form of provisional solutions, there were current the most arbitrary speculations. The point which it was most urgent to clarify was how the nerves are formed and as a result of what mechanism the axonic processes connect, without errors or wanderings, with their terminal structures (motor end plates, cutaneous sense organs, etc.). Despite the abundance of conjectures, two theories divided between them the majority of votes.

According to Küpffer, His, and Kölliker, the neuroblast or primitive nerve cell, produces the nerve by giving off a bud or process, the axon, which they supposed to grow freely through the other tissues to attain the terminal apparatus, where it was supposed to end by independent ramifications.

On the other hand, Hensen and his followers denied categorically such a free growth, claiming (in order to explain the perfect adaptation and correspondence existing between the central end stations and the peripheral sense organs) that the neuroblast undergoes from the beginning a series of incomplete divisions. In the first place, after the nuclear division, the central cell body and the peripheral receptive organ are supposed to be produced; afterwards the nuclei are supposed to migrate while the protoplasm between them remains continuous, that is to say, one half of the cell with its nucleus would remain, *ab initio*, in the skin or the peripheral sense organ, while the other half would be situated in the embryonic nerve centres (Fig. 42, *A*). Thus the growth

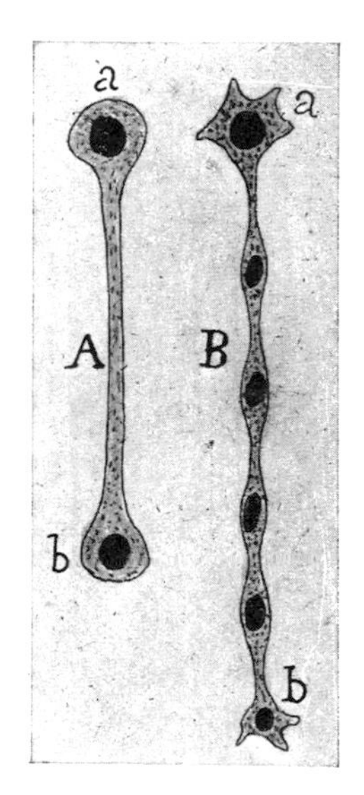

FIG. 42. HENSEN'S THEORY OF THE DEVELOPMENT OF THE NERVE FIBRES AND PERIPHERAL SENSORY MECHANISMS. *A*, neuroblast in process of elongation; *B*, chain of nuclei united by protoplasmic bridges; *a*, central cell; *b*, peripheral cell.

of the nerve would occur not through the continuous increment of a free extremity, but by means of a progressive stretching of the intermediate bridge of protoplasm. Fially new proliferations, originating exclusively in the nuclei, would develop from these organs the very long chain of the peripheral nerve.

As a variant of this hypothetical conception of Hensen may be regarded a certain theory which has been held since early times and was renewed a few years ago by Beard, Dohrn, Durante, Cornil, Bethe, and others in whose view the axons, and hence the nerves, are supposed to be produced by the differentiation and fusion of a long chain of neuroblasts which have migrated from the centres or from the ectodermal membrane (Fig. 43). In the opinion of

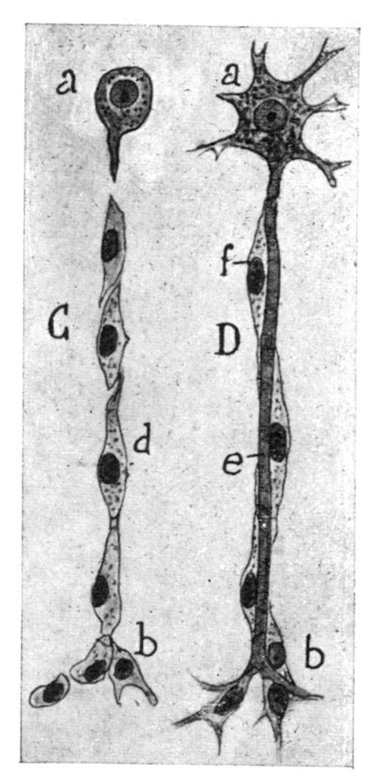

FIG. 43. CHAIN THEORY UPHELD BY BEARD, DOHRN, ETC. *C*, series of independent neuroblasts; *D*, the neuroblasts were supposed to form pieces of axon which finally fuse with each other and with the central cell (*a*); *b*, elements producing the peripheral ramification.

these scientists, the embryonic axis cylinder, far from being the offshoot in the course of growth of the protoplasm of one nerve cell, would represent the common histogenetic product of many ectodermal elements. In Figs. 42 and 43 there are presented diagrammatically the principle features of these two theories in the controversy.

My investigations, which were immediately confirmed by Lenhossék and Retzius, contributed to the clarifying of the debated question, definitely supporting the theoretical conception of Küpffer and His, and establishing finally upon a firm foundation the doctrine (which was already very probable in view of the recent morphological discoveries) of the genetic unity of the nerve fibres and of the dendrites. In effect, the preparations which I obtained in the earliest stages of the chick embryo (from the second to the fourth day of incubation), revealed clearly that, once the germinal or indifferent stage is past, the nerve cell first sends out the axon or primordial process, as His had divined, and only later produces the dendrites and the collaterals of the nerves. All these processes appear continuous with the cell body and increase successively, maintaining their individuality until they reach their adult length and finally connect with the other elements (muscular, epithelial, or nervous) with which they have to maintain a physiological relationship.

It is true that the illustrious His had already observed the axon of the neuroblast at an earlier date. The methods used by the Leipzig neurologist, however, did not permit him to discover the form of growth of that process nor to detect the moment of appearance of the dendrites. Besides, he did not and could not see, with the unreliable technique, of those days, the ultimate tip of the nervous expansion in the course of its growth, and so long as such an observation was not made, the severe objection of Hensen, "no one has seen in the embryo the free ending of a nerve in the course of its growth," preserved its full force.

I had the good fortune to behold for the first time that fantastic ending of the growing axon.[1] In my sections of

[1] Professor His was enchanted with my discovery of the *growth cone,* as he told me in one of his letters. His satisfaction was justified when it is remembered that, thanks to this discovery, the objections of Hensen were refuted and the monocellular conception of continuous growth of the axon and other processes of the neuron was solidly established.

the three-days chick embryo, this ending appeared as a concentration of protoplasm of conical form, endowed with amoeboid movements. It could be compared to a living battering-ram, soft and flexible, which advances, pushing aside mechanically the obstacles which it finds in its way, until it reaches the area of its peripheral distribution. This curious terminal club, I christened the *growth cone.* Confirmed by Lenhossék,[2] Retzius, Kölliker, and Athias, and later by Held, Harrison, and others, it is to-day one of the common facts of nervous development (Fig. 44, *a*).

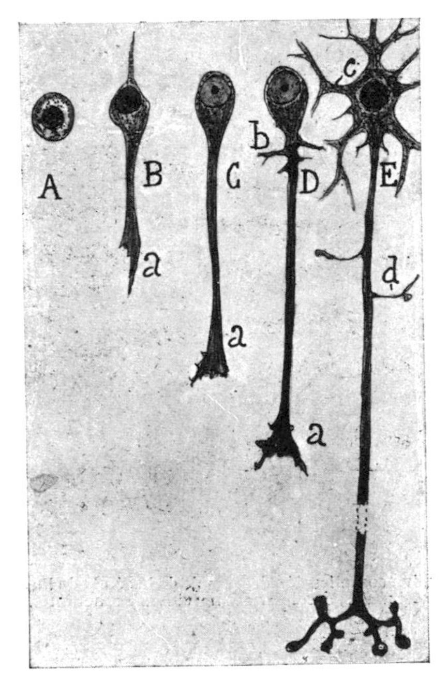

FIG. 44. ACTUAL DEVELOPMENT OF THE NERVE FIBRE ACCORDING TO THE OBSERVATIONS OF HIS AND OF MYSELF. *A,* primary embryonic nerve cell; *B,* bipolar phase, with the beginning of the growth cone; *C,* phase of the neuroblast proper; *D,* appearance of dendrites; *E,* modelling of the latter and formation of the collateral and terminal branches of the axon.

[2] It is only just to acknowledge that, with the exception of the growth cone, almost all those discoveries were also made independently by Lenhossék, although my communication saw the light before his. See Lenhossék: "Zur

With equal ardour and success I next attacked the ontogenetic development of the cells and fibres of the cerebellar cortex. In such a suggestive region several interesting problems were calling urgently for solution. How do the afferent fibres grow and how are the contactual connections organized between the climbing fibres, for example, and the stems of the Purkinje cells? During the development of the cerebellum, does not the metaphorical expression *climbing arborization* perhaps imply a real and actual action of climbing?

The facts which had been gathered in the cerebella of new-born animals answered in the affirmative. The axons of the conductors referred to, upon arriving from distant centres, smell out, so to speak, the bodies of the Purkinje elements, which they embrace by means of varicose nests which are the rudiments of the future arborizations. Once in contact with it, the branches of the nerve nests actually climb along the main stem and the dendrites, until they produce finally the complicated plexus characteristic of the adult conductors. It is unnecessary to say that this phenomenon, so significant for the neuron theory, was confirmed afterwards by other authors (Retzius, Kölliker, van Gehuchten, Athias, C. Calleja, Azoulay, etc.).

I was attracted also by the question how a pyriform neuroblast, devoid of processes, is converted into the prodigious tree, a sort of hedge, of the Purkinje cell. My curiosity was fully satisfied by the discovery of the primordial phases of this development, of which a representation is given in Fig. 45. Indeed, incidentally, I came upon an interesting biological fact. I noticed that every ramification, dendritic or axonic, in the course of formation, passes through a chaotic period, so to speak, a period of trials, during which there are sent out at random experimental conductors most of which are destined to disappear (Fig. 45, *a*). Like a miner who digs blindly in search of a lost

Kenntniss der ersten Entstehungen der Nervenzellen und Nervenfasern beim Vogelembryo,'' *Verhandl. der X inter. mediz. Kongresses,* Bd. II, p. 114, Berlin, 1890.

vein, the protoplasmic buds try various roads to reach their proper end. Later, when the afferent nerve fibres have arrived, or when the neurons mould themselves and attain in due time functional solidarity, the useful expansions remain and become fixed and the useless or exploratory ones are reabsorbed. In this case nature proceeds like the gardener who guides and cares for the well directed shoots and prunes off the defective or superfluous ones. For life abhors the redundant and shows itself peculiarly miserly in respect of protoplasm and of space.

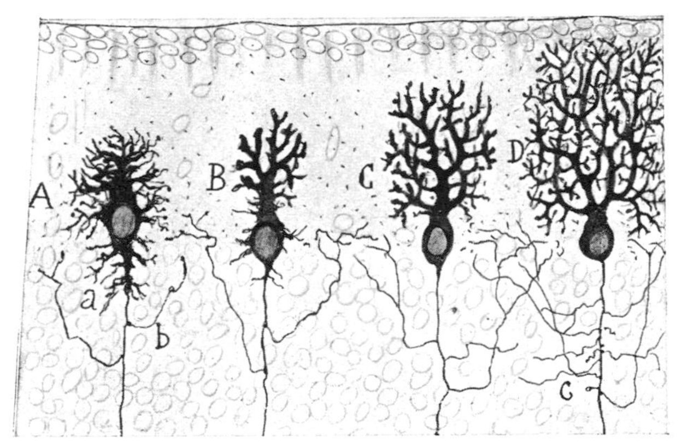

FIG. 45. SUCCESSIVE PHASES IN THE COMPLICATION OF THE BRANCHING OF THE CELL OF PURKINJE. *a*, temporary dendrites; *c*, luxuriant axonic collaterals.

Another curious phenomenon of migration and metamorphosis resulting from irresistible impulses and in spite of the greatest obstacles was revealed to me in the young or undifferentiated granules of the cerebellum of new-born mammals.

In Fig. 46 are reproduced schematically some of these curious cotillons of the granules. It had been known for a long time that the young or undifferentiated granule (germinal phase), along with other nerve cells in their early stages, occurs in the superficial zone of the cerebellum (Fig. 46, *A*) (*peripheral granules*), and has an irregular polyhedral form. Nothing, however, was known of its later development. My observations revealed that the granule emerges from this indifferent condition by turning first into a horizontal bipolar cell, that is by sending out two long processes in opposite directions (*4*) which are disposed parallel with the cerebellar laminae; later, from the deep side of the cell body there extends a descending process which draws into itself a good part of the protoplasm, including the nucleus, and thus changes the cell from a horizontal bioplar to a radial or vertical bipolar (Fig. 46, *5*

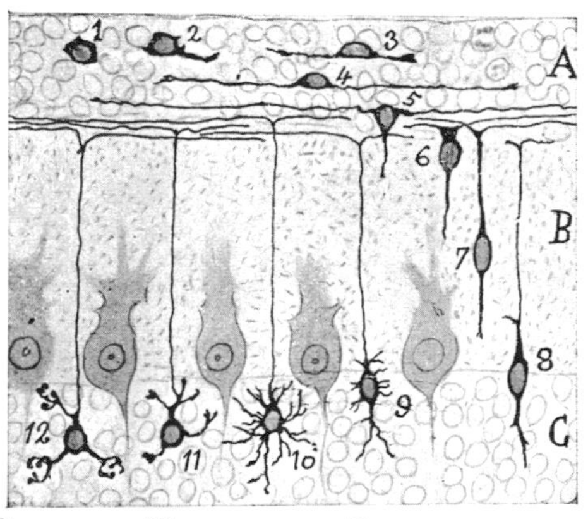

FIG. 46. SUCCESSIVE MIGRATION AND TRANSFORMATION OF THE GRANULE CELLS OF THE CEREBELLUM. 1, primary embryonic cell; 2, 3, appearance of polar outgrowths; 4, formation of a horizontal bipolar cell; 5, 6, appearance of a descending outgrowth; 7, 8, phase of vertical bipolarity; 9, 10, production of provisional or trial dendrites; 11, 12, formation of the definitive processes.

and *6*). Finally, the appearance of the slender dendrites and the definitive modelling of the cerebellar granule coincide with the laborious arrival of the cell body in the deeper regions (*9*, *10*).

All these surprising developments appear directed to fixing at once the position of the parallel fibres on the corresponding parts of the dendrites of Purkinje. It is observed, in effect, that the first expansions of the granule in the tangential bipolar phase are none other than the delicate terminal branches of the future axis cylinder (the parallel fibres). Whence it is seen that the nervous branches differentiate before the axon which sustains them, just as the latter precedes the dendrites.

The metamorphoses of the granule cited (confirmed afterwards by Lugaro, Retzius, Athias, and other scientists) reveal some of the essential steps of the developmental mechanism of the neurons, and also present difficult and transcendental problems. What mysterious forces precede the appearance of the processes, promote their growth and ramification, stimulate the corresponding migration of the cells and fibres in predetermined directions, as if in obedience to a skilfully arranged architectural plan, and finally establish those protoplasmic kisses, the intercellular articulations, which seem to constitute the final ecstasy of an epic love story?

Here is an unfathomable enigma, concerning which, however, I shall later on expound a certain hypothesis—the neurotropic theory—which was received sympathetically by many neurologists, although premature and inadequate, like all theories which aim to scrutinize the shadowy abyss of the deeper causes of development.

I do not wish further to abuse the patience of the reader by detailing the contents and range of other communications of 1890. These were concerned with the muscular tissues of insects, the nerve fibres of the heart, the structure of the cerebral convolutions, the origin and termination of the olfactory nerves, the structure of the nerve ganglia, the giant cells in leprosy, etc.[3]

I have already said that the years 1890 and 1891 were my Palm Sunday. The generous reception which my ideas received from distinguished scientists produced a full confidence in the revelations of the method of Golgi and in the accuracy of my descriptions. Consequently there developed a considerable literary movement. Everybody wished to contribute something to the enrichment of the new neurological doctrine which was sponsored in Germany by

[3] In the original about two pages are devoted to a summary of the results. (Translator's note.)

masters of such eminence as His, Waldeyer, Kölliker, and Edinger. The scientists of the Latin and Scandinavian countries followed later. In Italy, Lugaro and Tanzi adopted the new ideas in spite of the overwhelming authority of Golgi; in Belgium, van Gehuchten; in Switzerland, von Lenhossék[4]; in Sweden, Retzius; in France, Azoulay, Dejerine, and especially the famous professor of the University of Paris, the amiable Matías Duval.

It would be long and tedious to cite all the discoveries, articles of propaganda, or confirmatory studies with which outstanding neurological authorities supported the modesty of my scientific research. I shall mention only a few of them, almost all of which appeared in 1891.

One of the first scientists converted to my ideas was the professor at Louvain, A. van Gehuchten, a renowned cytologist of the school of Carnoy, later transformed, by a sort of induction, into an ardent cultivator of neurology. It may be permitted to copy here a few paragraphs of his famous jubilee discourse, in which the Belgian scientist recounts the first steps of his initiation:

"It was the time," says van Gehuchten, "when the method of Golgi at last received practical application. The new facts revealed by this procedure were to revolutionize the anatomy of the nervous system. The laboratories of anatomy were in a ferment. We all wished to carry our stones for the new edifice which, under the brilliant direction of Cajal, became so magnificent. Not only had the technique of the method been simplified, but the results procured were more constant and more decisive."

"The committee organizing this celebration has asked me how I conceived the idea, twenty-five years ago, of directing my scientific activity to studies of the nervous system. Wishing to answer you, I have tried to live again in imagination the first years of my university teaching. It was in 1888. I was corresponding with Cajal in connec-

[4] The celebrated Hungarian histologist, now professor in the University of Budapest and one of the few scientists surviving from that generation of investigators. He has been referred to in previous chapters.

tion with papers which each of us had published upon the finer structure of the muscle cell. One day he wrote to me announcing that he was abandoning his investigations upon muscles in order to devote himself to the nerve centres, basing his decision upon the fact that he had obtained remarkable results from the application to embryos of one of the formulae of the method of Golgi, which had been discovered in 1875. I tested his statements and came to the conclusion that he was right. . . . The first step had been taken, other workers followed naturally.''

As a matter of fact, the work done by van Gehuchten as an outcome of that suggestion was of the utmost importance, covering a great part of the nervous system, especially in lower vertebrates. Confining ourselves to the confirmatory studies published at that time by the Belgian savant, we may mention some eloquent semipopular lectures pronounced before the Belgian Microscopial Society and a certain extensive monograph devoted to the study of the spinal cord and cerebellum, in which the author, besides corroborating the facts discovered by me and by Kölliker adds new descriptive details and important interpretations.

It was to the distinguished Belgian scientist that I owed my becoming rapidly known in the French-speaking countries. In later pages I shall have to return to treat of the scientific discoveries of the ill-fated master,[5] since in succeeding years our activities often ran parallel, attacking the same subjects and contributing to the elaboration of the same concepts.

[5] Still young and in full mental vigour, Professor van Gehuchten died in Cambridge (September, 1914), in the famous university hall of which various fugitive Belgian scientists were cordially received. The lamented master was one of the many victims of the awful war which laid waste civilized Europe from 1914 to 1918. The burning of Louvain had ruined him materially and intellectually. The University destroyed, the library burned down, his magnificent collection of scientific preparations and apparatus in ashes, and himself a wanderer, far from his home land, van Gehuchten fell into a state of melancholy and profound depression. According to information given me by Professor Havet (another Belgian emigré), a slight operation (for appendicitis); which he would have been able to support perfectly in ordinary conditions brought on a cardiac seizure which was followed by death.

Two distinguished German investigators continued this work of diffusion and popularization: Waldeyer and His. The first published in a Berlin medical weekly a methodical and very clear exposition of the new ideas which he illustrated with a profusion of diagrammatic drawings. The word *neuron* (the nervous unit) is his, and in it he summed up the idea of the individuality, morphological, physiological, and genetic, of the ganglionic cell defended by His and by me.

Also His, the renowned embryologist of Leipzig, of whom I have already spoken with well-deserved praise in earlier pages, summarized the new concept of the minute structure of the centres in a suggestive pamphlet illustrated with numerous diagrams. Naturally, in explaining the morphological facts pointed out by me and by Kölliker, he recalled that in earlier embryos the neuroblasts behave as independent elements, develop by a process of growth, and are capable of migration.

Likewise interesting as a work of propaganda was the study of this subject by Küpffer,[6] one of the most celebrated anatomists and embryologists in Germany, and an active supporter, as has been said already, of the conception of the genetic unity of the nerves. Although it was published at a later date (1894), it is mentioned here as a representative work for spreading the new ideas in neurology.

The works of the scrupulous Retzius [7] were extraordinarily important. This savant grasped the idea of transmission by contact all the more eagerly since, in his earlier memoirs on the structure of the sense organs, he had shown himself hesitant in accepting the reticular theory. Be-

[6] *Medizinische Wochenschr.*, Bd. 41, März, 1894.

[7] *Biol. Unters. Neue Folge*, Bd. 1, Stockholm 1890; ibid., Bd. 2, 1891; ibid., Bd. 3, 1892. This great master and affectionate friend died in the full flower of his scientific activities in 1919. Like many who believed in human perfectability, Retzius was an indirect victim of the European war, that is of the heartrending spectacle of a civilization collapsing from lack of moral background and of high ideals. I still remember the piteous words with which he closed his last letter, written on his death bed: "I die despairing, for I have lost my faith in the destinies of humanity."

sides, he had already applied Ehrlich's method (methylene blue) to the nervous system of invertebrates and found, in perfect agreement with my views, that the terminal arborization of the nerve fibres in the ganglia never forms a net, but appears perfectly free and enters into close contact, in the molecular substance, with the dendrites of other neurons. Later, having used chromate of silver according to my directions, he confirmed and amplified in a series of magnificent monographs almost all the facts which I had described in the development and in the adult structure of the nervous centres. Particularly interesting is the building up of the neuron idea with relation to the structure of the sense organs, as expounded by this scientist in 1892.[8] In recalling his valuable support of those days, it would be ungrateful not to mention that it was at the instance of the Swedish master that my works received their first academic distinction, membership in the Royal Academy of Medicine of Stockholm, before which he delivered several lectures summarizing my investigations, as well as those of Golgi and Kölliker.[9]

Soon afterwards, Lenhossék, the professor at Basle, who had been so reserved at first, also intervened. Besides a very important work on the nervous system of the earthworm,[10] in which, like Retzius, he found in the invertebrates corroboration of the law of contact, this savant published a superb book on the spinal cord of mammals.[11] confirming

[8] *Biol Unters.*, N.F., Bd. 4, 1891; Bd. 5, 1892.

[9] This he told me in a charming letter of June 25, 1891. "I have often explained," he said, "your beautiful discoveries in our scientific and academic societies, and finally you have been made a member of our *Academy of Medicine*, etc."

[10] Arch. f. Mikr. Anat., Bd. 39, 1892.

[11] Lenhossék: Der feinere Bau des Nervensystems im Lichte neuster Forschungen," *Fortschr. d. Med.*, Bd. 10, 1892. Separately in 1893 and revised and enlarged in 1894.

It is very comforting to see how certain noble and honourable characters can change their opinions. The distinguished v. Lenhossék, so cautious and perplexed at first, wrote to me in 1890 words which, after discounting the usual exaggerations of courtesy, were very pleasant and encouraging, "Your repeated outstanding discoveries," he said in a letter which I have preserved, "inspire me with great admiration for your genius. I consider your findings as the most important advances which have been made in the past decade

my observations and greatly enriching our knowledge besides.

In France, I had the good fortune to gain as a supporter Dr. L. Azoulay, a young man of great talent, who confirmed not a few of my conclusions about the structure of the cerebellum, the cerebrum, and the spinal cord and later became the generous translator of my books into French and one of my best friends; and the brilliant Matías Duval, professor of histology in the Faculty of Medicine at Paris, who carried his belief in my ideas so far as to order the diagrams in my neurological publications to be reproduced in large wall charts for the purpose of teaching. Those who heard his highly eloquent lectures at that time (Duval was a scientific expositor of the highest order) relate that one of his favourite phrases in introducing his lectures on the nervous system was: "This time, light comes to us from the south, from noble Spain, the country of the sun. . . ." Similar words of friendship he repeated later in the foreword with which he sponsored before the French public the translation of my lectures in Barcelona.

Although published later (1893), there may be cited also, for completeness, an article of popularization issued in France by Dagonet[12]; the eloquent doctrinal exposition of Tanzi, professor in the Faculty of Medicine at Florence[13]; the summary of Bergonzini[14]; and, finally, the benevolent presentation of my ideas given by the famous Edinger in his classic book on the comparative anatomy of the nervous system.[15]

in the domain of microscopic anatomy. Professors His and Kölliker also, with whom I had a long talk recently in Basle, and various other colleagues concur in this opinion. *I regret sincerely that I did not formerly realize the full importance of your works, and that I showed towards them an unjustified scepticism, which I hope you will have overlooked.*" Unfortunately, as I have said before, men of this moral calibre are not common among scientists.

[12] *La Medicine Scientifique,* 1893.

[13] I fatti e le induzione nell odierna istologia del sistema nervoso. Reggio-Emilia, 1893.

[14] *La Rasegna di Science Mediche.* Anno 1893.

[15] Vorlesungen über den Bau der nervösen Centralorgane, 4 Aufl., 1893.

There were not only success and gratification, however, during 1890 and the following years; I had also unlooked for vexations and misfortunes.

One of these, in the scientific field, was my polemic with Professor Camilo Golgi, who, in an article published in the *Anatomischer Anzeiger*,[16] claimed priority in the discovery of the collaterals in the spinal cord. In this paper the master of Pavia, in a quite sharp and unfriendly tone, exhumed a certain brief communication published in 1880 in a local periodical at Reggio-Emilia (Italy) and absolutely unknown to scientists. In this article—which seems to have been forgotten by Golgi himself, since he does not refer to it in his great work on the nervous system (1885)—there appears a paragraph of three lines in which there are really mentioned the famous transverse branches sent forth by the fibres of the white columns. Up to the present time, in spite of diligent efforts, I have been unable to procure for myself the modest and unknown local medical Bulletin in which this discovery is announced.

I replied politely,[17] freely conceding to him the priority in the discovery, while lamenting that a fact of such great importance should have seen the light only in a regional medical review unknown to the scientific world. Also I took advantage of the occasion to publish a summary of the most important conclusions drawn from my studies and criticised severely the theoretical speculations of the Pavia savant (the merely nutritive rôle of the dendrites, the diffuse interstitial nerve net, the functional significance of the two types of neurons, the vegetative office of the neuroglia, etc.).

The just reclamation by Golgi naturally diminished my list of discoveries in the spinal cord. The balance in my favour, however, was sufficient to console my *amour propre*, which had received somewhat of a shock. Considering only the chapter on the collaterals, there still appeared as my personal possessions the description of the manner of ter-

[16] Anat. Anz., Bd. 5, 1890.
[17] *Ibid.*, Bd. 5, 1890.

mination of these fibres in the gray matter, their connections by means of pericellular nests with the motor and funicular neurons, their varying arrangement in the different columns, and, finally, their participation in the formation of the white and gray commissures.

From such mischances no investigator, not even the best acquainted with the bibliography, can ever be entirely free. How can it be avoided that through negligence, for convenience of publication, perhaps to assure an early date of appearance, a scientist may publish or *inter* (there are cases!) for a number of years in an obscure local bulletin, or in the transactions of a modest provincial academy, an interesting fact which he has recently discovered? Certainly, it is an obligation resting upon cultivators of science to publish our work in reviews or archives which are universally known, so as to facilitate bibliographic search and to avoid disagreeable surprises. But who has not committed at some time this sin of negligence?

My other troubles belong to the domestic order and would not interest the reader. My eldest son, who gave promise of being a lad of intelligence, took seriously ill with typhoid fever, from the after effects of which, besides a partial paralysis of his mental development, there sprang the germs of the cardiac affection which, fifteen years later, carried him to the grave. Then, one of my daughters, the first born in Barcelona, was a victim of the inexorable meningitis, contracted during convalescence from measles. In large and humid cities every illness is dangerous on account of the perpetual assaults of the tubercular bacillus which is carried in suspension with the dust and disseminated profusely through unscrupulousness in the handling of milk and meat.

Poor Enriqueta! Her image, pale and suffering, lives in my memory associated by a strange and bitter contrast with one of my finest discoveries: that of the axis cylinders of the granules of the cerebellum and their continuity with the parallel fibres of the molecular layer. Perchance in such distressing circumstances anguish was the sovereign sharpener of my wits. Continually awake, exhausted with fatigue and distress, I developed the habit of drowning sorrows during the small hours of the night in the light of the microscope, so as to lull my cruel tortures. And one bitterly fateful night, when the shadows were beginning to fall on an innocent being, there suddenly blazed forth in my mind the splendour of a new truth. But let us not renew the memories of sorrow. Besides, who cares about these things? We are human beings, and therefore suffering, physical and mental, waylays us continually; even apart from time, the terrible and inexorable enemy of life.

CHAPTER VIII

My work in 1891. With the collaboration of van Gehuchten, I formulate the principle of the dynamic polarization of the neurons. I complete my earlier observations on the brain and the retina and commence the analysis of the sympathetic ganglia. Unexpected success of my popular lectures on the fundamental structure of the nervous system. Examinations for the chair of histology in Madrid. My removal to the capital in 1892.

The fever of work and the mental tension were somewhat lessened during the year 1891; nevertheless, the harvest of observations still attained a certain importance. As we shall see shortly, the lessening of my activity was due to the loss of time in preparing for my examinations for the chair in Madrid.

There are two things to be recognised in my work in 1891; the elaboration of theory and the accumulation of observations of fact.

In the realm of theory, I regard as the most fortunate of my conceptions the principle of dynamic polarization, which was already contained in embryo in my speculative efforts of 1889.[1] It is a pleasure to acknowledge that in the elaboration and formulation of this concept Professor van Gehuchten had an important share.

The reader will permit me a little history.

There is no histologist or physiologist who, as he contemplated the complex form of the nerve cell with its two kinds of processes, the dendritic or short and the axonic or long, has not asked himself the following questions: What is the direction of the nervous impulse within the neuron? Does it spread in all directions, like sound or light, or does it pass constantly in one direction, like water in the watermill?

It is true that the physiologists had already brought

[1] R. Cajal: Conexión general de los elementos nerviosos, 1889.

forward, in connection with this problem, one important fact, namely: that, in the motor axons, the nervous discharge produced by the cells in the anterior horn of the spinal cord is transmitted exclusively in a cellulifugal direction, that is from the cell body to the motor end plate or peripheral termination of the nerve; and generalizing the assumption a little arbitrarily, certain neurologists—Gowers, Bechterew, Kölliker, Waldeyer, and others—attributed to all the axis-cylinders this same type of conduction.

As for the manner of conduction of the dendritic processes, there was no definitely formed opinion. Many authors doubted even their ability to transmit the current at all. (Golgi's conception of the purely nutritive role of the dendrites will be recalled). Only the physiologist Gad supposed, though without sufficient objective basis, that the dendrites might perhaps transmit the nervous impulse in a cellulipetal direction, that is, from the points of these processes to the cell body.

The appearance in 1889 and 1890 of my works on the retina, the olfactory bulb, the cerebellum, and the spinal cord changed the aspect of the problem, making it approachable by histological methods. Two advances, one objective the other theoretical, gave assistance in the task. The first was the absolute demonstration of the conductive power of the dendrites; the other was the homology which, on the ground of morphological comparisons, I (1889) imagined to exist between the thick peripheral processes of the sensory cells and the dendritic prolongations of the central neurons.

For example, glancing at Figs. 47 and 48, we observe that in the visual membrane (bipolar cells, rods and cones, and ganglionic cells) and in the olfactory apparatus (Fig. 48), the thick processes of the cells, comparable as a whole with the dendrites, are always directed towards the external world and evidently conduct towards the cell body, while the axon or cellulifugal prolongation is directed towards the central nervous organs. Proceeding by induction, it was natural to attribute similar dynamic properties to the dendrites of the multipolar neurons in the cerebral hemisphere, the cerebellum, and the spinal cord. This idea I expressed, though somewhat diffidently, in 1889, in my paper in *La medicina practica.*[2]

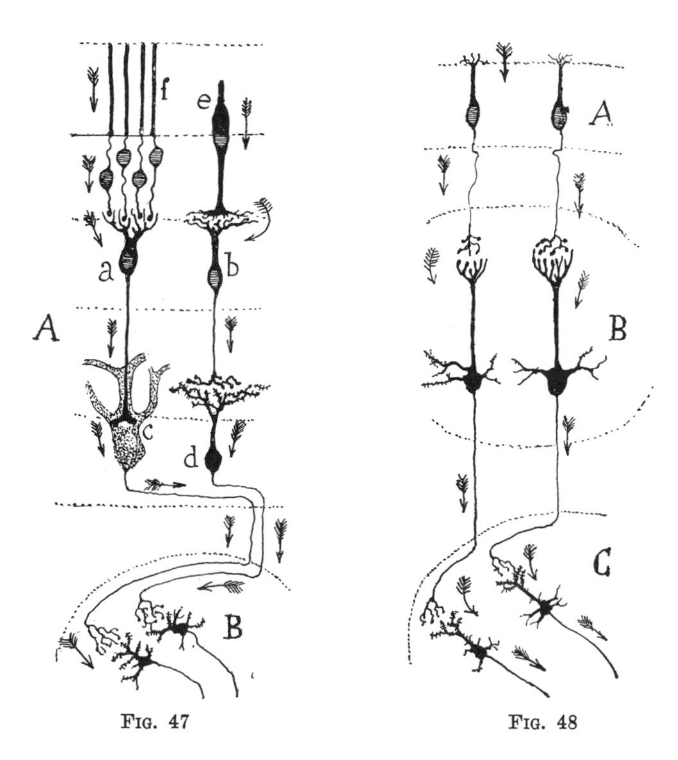

FIG. 47 FIG. 48

FIG. 47. Diagram to show the direction of the nervous impulse in the retina of the vertebrate. *A,* retina; *B,* external geniculate body; *a,* rod bipolar cell; *b,* cone bipolar cell; *c, d,* ganglionic cells; *e,* cone; *f,* rods.

FIG. 48. Diagram to show the direction of the nervous impulse in the olfactory mucous membrane and centers. *A,* olfactory mucous membrane; *B,* olfactory bulb; *C,* pyriform lobe of the brain, to which the tracts from the bulb run.

[2] "The role of the dendrites as receptors or collectors of impulses," I said, "is indubitable in two cases at least: in the olfactory glomeruli, where the nerve fibres arising from the nasal mucous membrane enter into relation with the dendritic tufts of mitral cells, and in the Purkinje cells of the cerebellum, of which the protoplasmic ramifications come into contact with parallel fibres from the granules."

I lacked at that time the confidence to elevate the formula to the level of a general law. It must be recognized that, notwithstanding the advances made in our knowledge of the structure of the sensory pathways, thanks to the investigations of Golgi, my own, and those of Kölliker, Tartuferi, Retzius and Lenhossék, and others, such a generalization would have been premature.

Besides, it appeared to me that certain facts were definitely contrary to the supposed exclusively cellulipetal conduction of the dendrites and cellulifugal of the axons. One of these was the existence in various nerve centres of vertebrates, and particularly in the optic lobe (birds and reptiles), of concentric zones in which only dendritic processes came together. In such cases it was necessary to admit contact between dendrites of diverse origins and hence conduction indifferently cellulipetal or cellulifugal.

The other serious difficulty depended upon the cells of the sensory or spinal ganglia, in which the peripheral conducting branch, which is indisputably cellulipetal, is exceptional in that it takes on in the adult all the structural and morphological characters of the axis cylinder.

Disheartened by such difficulties, I abandoned the question, which I considered prematurely proposed and perhaps insoluble by histological methods.

Two years later, that is in 1891, there appeared an interesting paper by van Gehuchten,[3] in which, incidentally and in a note, there was a criticism of my daring identification of the dendrites with the receptor processes of the sensory cells, as well as of the physiological consequences of such a theory.

"It appears difficult to us," says this scientist, "to admit the otherwise very ingenious hypothesis of Cajal, according to which the peripheral prolongations of the sensory ganglionic cells (he refers also to the bipolar olfactory cells, the retinal cells, etc.) would be a dendrite, while the central process would represent a true axon.

[3] "La moelle epinière et le cervelet," *La Cellule,* T. VII, 1891.

Ramón y Cajal has arrived at this hypothesis by comparing for example, the bipolar elements of the olfactory mucosa with the elements of the spinal ganglia.

"The idea of considering the peripheral process as dendritic is ingenious in that it establishes easily a functional difference between the dendritic and the axonic processes. The dendrites would conduct celluluipetally and serve to transmit to the cell body the nervous disturbances coming from neighbouring elements; while the axis cylinder would provide cellulifugal conduction, destined to put the nerve element from which it extends into relation with the others.

"To admit this hypothesis, however, it would be necessary to change completely our idea of the dendrites and to admit that one of these may become the axis cylinder of a nerve cell, which it seems to us difficult to accept."[4]

The reading of this incidental critique by the savant of Louvain attracted my attention and caused me to meditate anew upon the subject. Rightly do the psychologists affirm that, in connection with an idea which is repeatedly apperceived or considered, our successive states of consciousness are always different. Between the first and the later grasping of the concept, the mind has made various acquisitions; certain objections lose their force; difficulties which were apparently insuperable vanish away; and finally, new associations of ideas are forged. This is what happened to me on that occasion. The precision with which the savant referred to stated the problem altered the course of my thoughts, and the doubts and criticisms expressed by him, instead of deterring and dissuading me, produced the oppo-

[4] And yet when I, thanks to my studies and reflections, later on convinced all the scientific men of the reality of the polarization, rejected by van Gehuchten, the latter, who had neither brought forward facts in support of that conception nor devoted his efforts to overcoming the obstacles which stood in its way, afterwards claimed priority in the discovery as if I—as is confirmed by his own words—had not collaborated in the solution of the difficult problem. And many sheep of Panurge, who are never lacking in the laboratories, followed him unknowingly. Certainly pride or vanity sometimes clouds the clearest intelligence and eclipses the nobility of the noblest characters!

site effect. An obsession with the subject pursued me, and, full of hope and courage, I asked myself: "Why must not that formula be correct? Is it not plausible to think that with different morphological characters there correspond somewhat diverse functions? And could not this diversity, produced by physiological adaptation, be exclusively cellulifugal conduction for the dendrites and cellulipetal for the axons? Let us examine it again."

I submitted the facts in opposition to a much more careful and thoughtful study. The first obstacle—the existence of zones in which only dendrites came together—vanished entirely upon the examination of certain preparations of the optic lobe and the cerebrum of reptiles, birds, and amphibians made by my brother, who was ardently engaged at the time in analysing the nerve centres of the lower vertebrates.[5] There, where in former years I had found only dendrites, the sections referred to showed rich plexuses of axon terminations.

The second obstacle (the axonic character of the external or cellulipetal process of the spinal ganglion cell) was overcome by a rational interpretation based upon well established facts of embryology and phylogeny. It is true that in the higher vertebrates the outer process of the sensory cell has the character of an axis cylinder; but if we descend the animal scale (worms, moluscs, crustaceans, etc., Fig. 49, *A, B*, as proved by the investigations of Retzius and Lenhossék) or go back to the early stages of the embryonic condition, we shall readily recognize that the ganglionic or sensory cell assumes not the monopolar form characteristic of the higher vertebrates (mammals, reptiles, and amphibians), but the bipolar, like that of the elements in the olfactory mucous membrane or those in the retina. It thus presents a thick external process, a receptor of afferent impulses, devoid of a medullary sheath and hav-

[5] On a suitable occasion I shall speak of the important investigations of my brother upon the comparative histology of the nervous system. Those of his publications in which at that time I found valuable data for establishing the principle of dynamic polarization are entitled: *Investigaciones de histología comparada en los centros opticos de los vertebrados.* Thesis, Madrid, 1890, and *El encéfalo de los reptiles.* Zaragoza, 1891.

ing all the characters distinctive of dendrites, and a slender internal process directed towards the centres and possessing the attributes of an orthodox axis cylinder. From all this, it is inferred that, in the course of ontogenetic and phylogenetic development, a primitive process, strictly dendritic in both its dynamic and its morphological aspects, may acquire, by progressive adaptation, the structural but not the dynamic characters of an axis cylinder. Or, in other words, the anatomical features of the processes of the neurons are not primary facts imposed of necessity by the law of evolution but are secondary conditions of an adaptive character and are related mainly to the length of the conductor. For example, the possession of an insulating myelin sheath in the dendrites (in the sensory cells of the ganglia) is related not so much to the direction of the nerve current as to the considerable length of the conductor. Figure 49 shows the development of form and position which

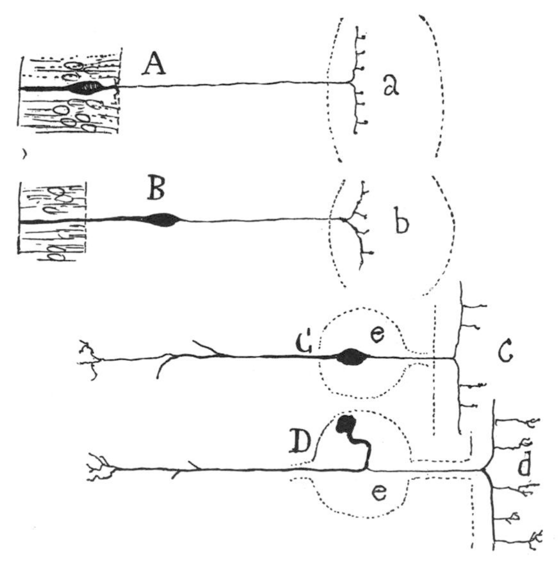

FIG. 49. Diagrams showing the changes of situation and morphology undergone by the sensory cells in the animal series. *A*, sensory cell of the earthworm (the cell body, as demonstrated by Lenhossék, lies in the epidermis); *B*, sensory cell of a mollusc (after Retzius); *C*, sensory cell of a lower fish; *D*, sensory cell of amphibian, reptile, bird, or mammal.

the sensory cell body has undergone during its phylogenetic history. It is seen that, as development progresses, this body first abandons the skin, confining itself to deeper organs, and when it is situated near the spinal cord (reptiles, amphibians, birds, and mammals) there begins another migration by virtue of which the nucleus lying between the two processes, central and peripheral, slips out towards the cortex of the ganglion while the processes thereafter rise from their pedicle of origin with the anatomical attributes of axons.[6]

This morphological evolution of the sensory neurons is reproduced during the embryonic development of the mammals and birds.

These difficulties being surmounted, and a histological analysis of the structural plan of the sensory pathways more exact than any made up to that time having previously been carried out, I was led to the following pronouncement,[7] which was received sympathetically by many neurologists and even by van Gehuchten himself.[8] *The transmission of the nervous impulse is always from the dendritic branches and the cell body to the axon or functional process. Every neuron, then, possesses a receptor apparatus, the body and the dendritic prolongations, an apparatus of emission, the axon, and an apparatus of distribution, the terminal arborization of the nerve fibre.* And as this course of the nerve impulse through the protoplasm implies a certain constant orientation, something like a polarization of the waves of excitation, I designated the foregoing principle: *the theory of dynamic polarization*

In such difficult fields, however, the full truth rarely

6 This curious displacement of the body, that is of the nucleus which seems to get away from the principal channel of the nervous impulse, as if facilitating the creation of direct routes, was later explained from the utilitarian point of view on the basis of the laws of economy of space and time of conduction.

7 *Congreso médico valenciano*, sesión del 24 de junio de 1891. Published also in the *Revista de Ciencias médicas de Barcelona*, núms. 22 and 23, 1891.

8 "Nouvelles recherches sur les ganglions cérébro-spinaux," la Cellule, T. VIII, 1892.

emerges at one stroke. It is pieced together, little by little, through many trials and corrections. In spite of its breadth, the principle stated was not applicable to all the known cases of neuronal morphology. It failed to cover the cases of many neurons of invertebrates and those of some elements of vertebrates, particularly certain nerve cells with arcuate axons arising far from the cell body discovered by me and by my brother in the optic lobes of lower vertebrates. Only later, in 1897, did I hit upon the realization that, contrary to the general opinion, the soma, or cell body does not always take part in the conduction of the nerve impulses which are received. The afferent wave is sometimes propagated directly from the dendrites to the axon. I had then to substitute for the preceding incorrect formula this other, which I designated *Theory of axipetal polarization: The soma and the dendrites conduct in an axipetal direction, that is, they transmit the waves of nervous excitation towards the axon. Inversely, the axon or axis cylinder conducts in a somatofugal or dendrifugal direction, carrying the impulses received by the soma or by the dendrites towards the terminal arborizations of the nerve fibre.* Consequently the currents flowing into the axon do not pass through the soma except when the latter is between the dendritic and the axonic apparatus.

This formula is applicable to all cases without exception, as well of vertebrates as of invertebrates, as well in the adult as in the embryo. Thanks to its complete generality, it constitutes a valuable key to the interpretation of the courses of the currents in neurons of the nerve centres. This fact was recognized by distinguished scientists, who did me the honour of accepting it without reservations.

I shall, however, discuss its advantage later on. For the present, I shall limit myself to copying here two diagrams (Figs. 50 and 51) in which the reader will be able to recognize easily how, in fact, this formula is applicable alike to the difficult cases neurons of which the dendrites spring from the base of the axon as occurs in invertebrates, cells with hooked axis cylinders, adult spinal ganglion cells, etc. and to the ordinary types of neurons in the brains of mammals (Fig. 48). The arrows mark the directions of the currents.

The reader will forgive me if I have lingered too long over the description of the stages of my reflections upon neuronal dynamics. I have wished to show by a typical

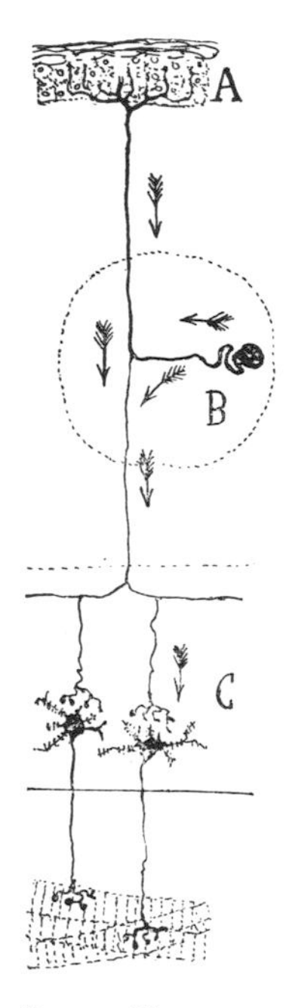

FIG. 50. SCHEME OF THE COURSE FOLLOWED BY THE CURRENTS IN SENSORY-MOTOR PATHWAYS. While the formula of axipetal polarization is conformed with, the supposition that the stalk of the sensory cell, contrary to the theory, conducts in both cellulipetal and cellulifugal direction is avoided. *A*, skin; *B*, spinal ganglion; *C*, spinal cord.

example the course followed in the elaboration of a theory; to narrate how the obstacles, apparently insuperable, which close the path to a rational conception, may be surmounted when one returns repeatedly to the subject, eliminating errors and analysing the contradictory facts to the bottom; and how, finally, the first theoretical outline is refined and purified by reflection, gaining progressively in general applicability until it embraces all cases.

In the field of concrete facts, I consider the best of my work in 1891 to be the observations in the retina, the cerebral hemisphere, and the sympathetic trunk.

The retina has always shown itself generous with me. A more or less important advance in the knowledge of this

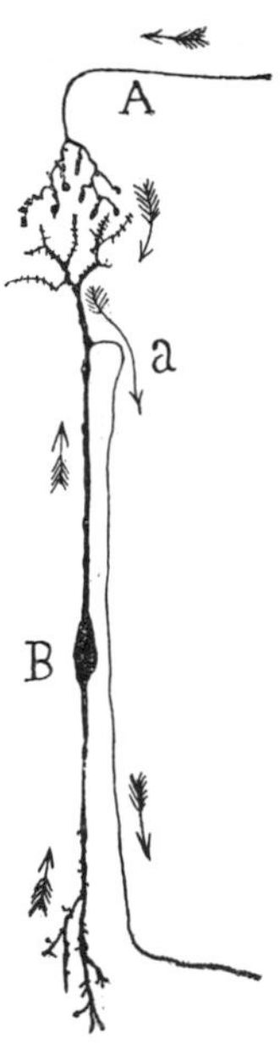

FIG. 51. THE COURSE OF THE CURRENTS IN THE CROSIER CELLS OF THE OPTIC LOBE OF FISHES, AMPHIBIANS, AND REPTILES, where the axon originates from a dendrite far from the cell body. This is well explained by the theory of axipetal polarization.

membrane marked each analytical effort in spite of the formidable competition offered me by Dogiel, the great Russian histologist, who at that time was successfully applying the methylene blue method of Ehrlich to the same subject. There is no occasion to specify here all the minute details of morphology and connection discovered during that campaign in the visual membrane of fishes, amphibians, reptiles, and mammals. In order not to weary the reader, I shall pick out only one of the points of most interest from a physiological viewpoint. I refer to the existence of two types of bipolar cells related to the two varieties of visual receptor elements known.

It is well known that, since the time of Johannes Müller and M. Schültze, physiologists and anatomists have recognized in the retina of vertebrates two orders of receptor cells: the *cone,* for diurnal or chromatic vision, and the *rod,* for crepuscular or colourless vision. The excitation of these latter cells produces an image with little detail, comparable roughly to an ordinary photograph out of focus (the rods do not occur in the central macula, the region of maximum visual acuity); while the stimulation of the cones, elements particularly concentrated in the *fovea centralis,* gives coloured pictures, detailed and brilliant, like a photograph in colours on an autochrome plate. In fishes, nocturnal birds, the mouse, etc., the rods predominate; in other animals there is a preponderance of cones (diurnal birds, reptiles, etc.). By a singular privilege, man unites the chromatic vision of the eagle and the crespuscular of the fish.

Now then, my observations, correcting the ideas expressed by Tartuferi and Dogiel, had shown that at their inferior ends, extending towards the plexiform zone (see Fig. 52, *c, d*), the rods and cones terminate not in nets, as these savants had declared, but freely and in different ways: the descending prolongations of the former end in a little free knob; while the thick expansions of the latter end in all vertebrates by a brush of branching horizontal rootlets (Fig. 52, *z*).

This important point established, I proposed a very simple question to myself. Since the impression received by the rod is different from that taken up by the cone, it is necessary from every point of view that each of these specific impressions should be conveyed through the retina by a separate channel.

If there were validity in the conclusions of Tartuferi

and Dogiel, according to whom the second link in the visual chain was supposed to be represented by a single type of bipolar in complete, substantial continuity outwards with the terminal segments of the rods and cones and inwards with branches of the ganglionic cells (internal plexiform layer), the ingenious expedient according to which nature has organized two classes of specific photoreceptor cells would be completely frustrated; since, from the second visual neuron onwards, both impressions, that of colour and that of black and white, would have to combine as they ran together through the same channels.

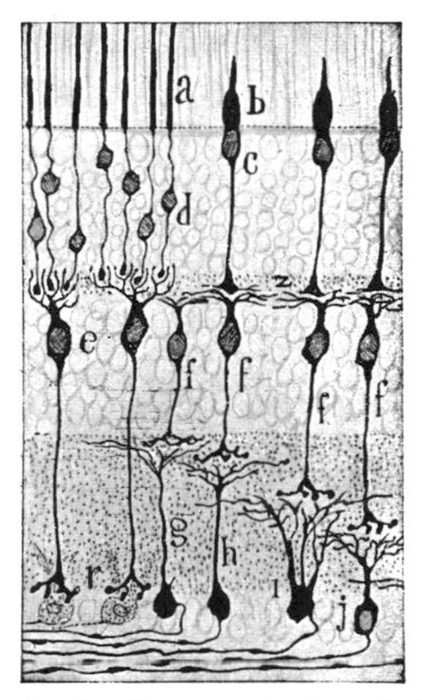

FIG. 52. Diagram showing the separate channels through the mammalian retina for the impulses received by the rods and those received by the cones. *a*, rods; *b*, cones; *e*, rod bipolar; *f*, cone bipolar; *r*, *g*, *h*, *i*, *j*, ganglionic cells.

When we reason with common sense and lift the war club determined upon vigorous action, nature ultimately hears us. Knowing what I was looking for, I began to explore eagerly and repeatedly the retina of fishes and of mammals (animals in which the differentiation between rods and cones reaches its maximum); and finally, as the reward of my faith, there deigned to appear most clearly and brilliantly those two types of bipolar cells demanded by theory and guessed by reason. In Fig. 52, *e, f,* I show schematically the respective channels from the rod and from the cone through the retina. Observe how one variety of bipolar makes a contact through its ascending dendritic tuft with a group of terminal bulbs of the rods; while the axonic or deep process of the same cell, forming a warty foot, connects below with the body of a certain giant ganglionic neuron. Remark also how the bipolar cell for the cone enters into an individual connection with the branching foot of a cone, by means of its external tuft; while its deep axon, spreading out in horizontal ramifications, comes into relation with the terminal branches of the medium and small ganglionic cells (Fig. 52, *g, h, j,* and Fig. 47, *b*).

It would be impossible to mention here all the other fortunate discoveries in the retina of fishes, amphibians, birds, and mammals.

Another of the studies into which I put most enthusiasm and analytical effort was that devoted to the cerebral cortex of reptiles, amphibians, and mammals. In truth, the subject attracted me with singular force. Devotion to the cerebral hemisphere, enigma of enigmas, was old in me, as I have already shown in earlier chapters. But I desired to penetrate further into that field and to determine so far as possible its fundamental plan or at least to complete an inquiry similar to that carried out some years previously in the cerebellum. But, alas! my optimism deceived me. For the supreme cunning of the structure of the gray matter is so intricate that it defies and will continue to defy for many centuries the obstinate curiosity of investigators. That apparent disorder of the cerebral jungle, so different from the regularity and symmetry of the spinal cord and of the cerebellum, conceals a profound organization of the utmost subtility which is at present inaccessible. Not merely the monumental cerebrum of *homo sapiens,* but even the more modest one of the reptile and of the amphibian—what am I saying!—even the so much disdained and so diminutive cerebral ganglion of the insect, apparently a mere reflex machine, opposes to analysis insuperable obstacles.

In the difficult warp of the brain, it is possible to advance only a step at a time and even so, in order to be fortunate, the advance trenches must be dug by men like Meynert, Golgi, Edinger, Flechsig, Kölliker, Forel, and others.

But my youth of those days, quite confident and perhaps somewhat presumptuous, knew nothing of the salutary fear of error; and I launched myself upon the undertaking with confidence that in that dark thicket, where so many explorers had lost themselves, I should be permitted to capture, if not lions and tigers, at least some modest game disdained by the great hunters. The fruit of this study was the revelation of a number of important details of cortical structure.[9]

Some of these observations rapidly became known thanks to my taking the precaution to publish them in French, taking advantage of a certain Belgian histological review, *La Cellule.*

Soon afterwards, Retzius, Kölliker, my brother, Edinger, Schäffer, etc., confirmed these results and extended them in certain points.

The last of my researches in 1891 was devoted to the structure of the sympathetic trunk. This inquiry, which is considerably weaker than the others, proves clearly the enormous influence of mental preoccupation upon the intellect. At the time, I was preoccupied with the examinations for the chair of histology in Madrid. The anxious preparation for the tests, the interruptions to which these were subjected, the fatigue of my repeated journeys to the capital, broke up the continuity of my analytical efforts and deprived me of that peace of mind without which every human work usually turns out poor, contradictory, and lacking in clarity and force.[10]

[9] The author summarizes eight points which he considers the most important of his discoveries at that time. (Translator's note.)

[10] One of the causes of these uncertainties in the study referred to was the use of doves and pigeon embryos, in which it is impossible to follow the entire course of the dendrites. How many failures or only partial successes are due to an unsuitable object of study!

The investigation mentioned, however, came at the right time. The true morphology of the sympathetic neurons was then unkonwn. Various histologists (Remak, Ranvier, Kölliker, and others) had recognized dichotomous branchings in them; but the greatest uncertainty prevailed as to the character and termination of these. Did the sympathetic cell, of which the motor nature seemed indubitable, possess true dendrites and axons in accordance with the ordinary morphological pattern or, as certain neurologists suspected, were all its processes rather of an axonic nature, arborizing in the smooth muscle fibre? Or did it consist rather, in keeping with the somewhat undecided view of Kölliker (1890), of a group of axons and a complex of dendrites?

Impatient to reach the goal before anyone else, I feverishly explored the sympathetic ganglion of bird embryos and very soon succeeded in establishing the existence in their neurons of genuine dendritic prolongations, which ended freely in the depths of the ganglionic fabric. Deceived by the appearances, however, I attributed to each cell two or more axons (in harmony with a recent opinion of Kölliker) when really it emits only one. Soon afterwards, in a special study carried out upon the mammals, I rectified my error of my own accord and drew up a description of the true arrangement of the sympathetic elements. But this delayed rectification tarnished my work greatly, and although my new morphological conception saw the light before the appearance of the observations of van Gehuchten, of Luigi Sala, a pupil of Golgi, and of Retzius, to whom I had suggested the appropriate methodological formula (the procedure of *double impregnation* with silver chromate), I could not avoid their repreaching me, rightly, for my vacillation and contradictions, and to van Gehuchten was adjudged the merit of having finally solved the problem. A certain amount remained, naturally, to my credit: the existence of the collaterals of the fibres derived from the spinal cord (*primary motor fibres* of many authors and longitudinal trunks uniting the ganglia); the pericellular nests of dendritic origin; the recognition of various types of neuron, etc. Figure 53, a reproduction of an engraving in my publication of 1891, will serve to supply descriptive details which it would be inopportune to enumerate here.

Other publications of 1891 are listed in the bibliography.

At the end of 1891 the volume of my practical work and the sum of the theoretical conclusions drawn had attained sufficient proportions to form the material for a book. Some pupils and physicians of Barcelona who were acquainted with my ideas invited me to expound them before the Academy of Medical Sciences of Cataluña. I complied with their requests with pleasure and prepared for my lectures large wall plates in colours, representing diagrammatically the structural plan of the nerve centres and sense organs. I was given a favorable reception and some enthusiastic students had the courtesy to take down my explanations and copy my drawings, publishing in the *Revista de Ciencias Médicas* of the same city a series of articles which I carefully revised and retouched.

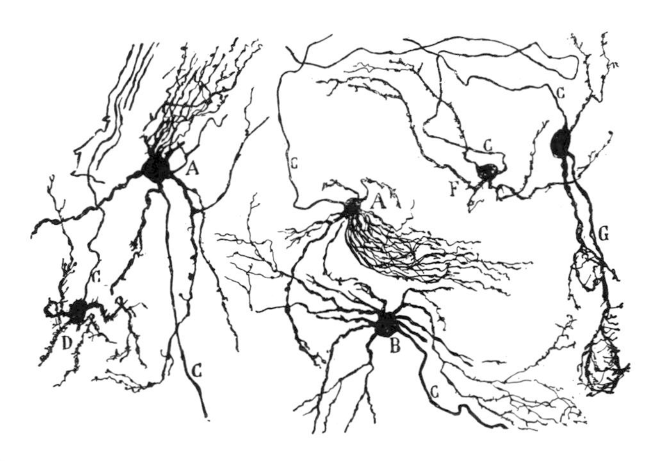

FIG. 53. VARIOUS CELLS FROM THE SYMPATHETIC GANGLIA OF THE DOG. The axons marked *C* are distinguished by the absence of branches. *A, B, D, F, G,* diverse morphological types of sympathetic neurons.

These articles, which saw the light in 1892,[11] had a succes which filled me with surprise, surpassing not only my hopes but even my dreams. I do not know how these lectures spread abroad, but in a short time there appeared translations or extensive paraphrases in various languages. Even the great W. His, professor of Leipzig, of whose good friendship I made acknowledgment in former chapters, suggested to me that they be translated into German. The German version, which appeared in 1893,[12] was made by no less a person than Dr. H. Held, then assistant to the master (whom he succeeded in the chair) and at present one of the major luminaries of German histology. As for the French edition, it was made by Dr. Azoulay, who translated conscientiously a text which I had specially revised and amplified. The little book, entitled *Les nouvelles idées sur la fine anatomie des centres nerveux* (Reinwald, Paris) and supported by a friendly prologue from the illustrious Professor Mathías Duval, of Paris, created a furor. In less than three months, two voluminous editions were exhausted. Such unexpected favour from the public suggested to me the plan, which I carried out in succeeding years, of writing an extensive book in which there would be taken up systematically and minutely the structure of the nervous system of all the vertebrates and there would be given an account, with the necessary background, of the whole of my scientific work. Of this formidable and patience-consuming work, upon which I was occupied earnestly for ten years, I shall treat farther on.

In April, 1892, my removal to Madrid took place. After examinations which lasted several months and were inter-

[11] Cajal: "Nuevo concepto de la histología de los centros nerviosos," *Revista de Ciencias Médicas de Barcelona,* numbers 16, 20, 22, and 23 of 1892, t. 18. The separate of these articles collected is dated the beginning of 1893.

[12] Cajal: Neue Darstellung vom histologischen Bau des Centralnervensystems. Translation by Dr. H. Held, *Arch. f. Anat. u. Physiol., Anat. Abt.,* 1893. As a foreword to this version Professor His announced that the German edition had been supervised by him and carried out by his assistant, who had an expert knowledge of the subject. Unfortunately Dr. Held was not sufficiently a master of Spanish and his version is full of errors and misunderstandings.

rupted by numerous incidents, I had the good fortune to be nominated unanimously for the chair of Normal Histology and Pathological Anatomy, made vacant by the decease of the unforgetable and meritorious Dr. Maestre de San Juan.[13] In the tribunal, under the chairmanship of Dr. Don Julián Calleja, there were judges of such prestige as Dr. Alejandro San Martín, Dr. Federico Olóriz, the Marquis of Busto, Don Antonio Mendoza and the professors of the subject, Doctors Cerrada and Gil Saltor.

My triumph was not easy, for I contended with rivals of great merit, especially one of them, for whose talents and culture I have always had the most candid admiration and cordial esteem.

As I have never allowed my self-love the slightest attempt at vanity or conceit, I must state here that my victory, which created such a stir at the time in medical circles in the capital, was due exclusively to two factors, to a certain extent impersonal and circumstantial: first, the thorough preparation obtained in teaching the subjects of the examination during four successive years; and, second, the credit and favour which my modest but numerous scientific publications (they already numbered over sixty) had attained among foreign scientists.

I deplored greatly having been obliged to return to the always cruel and irritating strife of competitive examinations in order to reach the Central University, the ideal of every provincial professor. However cultured and polite may be the weapons used in such contests, they always leave behind lamentable grudges and bitterness, cool friend-

[13] The most worthy Don Aureliano, whom we, his pupils, venerated so highly, succumbed to the results of an accident in the laboratory. A splash of caustic soda caused by the breaking of a flask occasioned the loss of his sight, which was succeeded by mental suffering so great that it carried off the master in a few months. Dr. Maestre was an excellent professor, who knew how to communicate his enthusiasm to those about him. I am indebted to him for unforgetable favours. After having sponsored me in the ceremony of investiture with the doctorate, he inspired me consistently in my efforts at research, strengthening my confidence in my own powers. The letters in which he acknowledged receipt of my publications were for me a moral tonic of the first order.

ships which have sometimes been cemented in community of tastes and interests, and prevent collaboration which might be very advantageous for national science.

In my case, to be professor in the Central University was at that time my only hope of satisfying with a certain amount of latitude my devotion to research and of augmenting my resources, which were seriously drained by the incessant expenses of the laboratory and of subscriptions to reviews, besides the support of a large family. My rivals were rich and eminent; they had fat and well-deserved practices and could afford to wait. But I, enveloped in my labours, had lost my clinical abilities almost entirely, and was consequently unfitted for professional practice, the sole occupation which can bring to the physician economic ease. Only in the decorous industry of writing textbooks, as lucrative for the professors in the capital as it is precarious for those in the provinces—an industry foolishly ridiculed by those who know only its abominable abuses—did I get a glimpse of the golden mean which would guarantee me, along with the precious mastery of my time, the supreme boon of independence of thought.

CHAPTER IX

My removal to the capital. My residence in the Calle de Atocha, near San Carlos. Sketches of some of my friends and colleagues on the faculty who are now gone.

When, coming back from the examinations, I rejoined my family, I found it augmented by another child. This was a cause of jubilation, although the appearance of a sixth offspring does not usually awaken as much enthusiasm as that of the first.

Among my fellow-professors at Barcelona the announcement of my triumph produced pleasant surprise, mingled, perhaps, with a little vexation. I seemed to perceive in some excellent colleagues a certain disappointment that they had not at the proper time done something calculated to retain me permanently in the Catalan capital.[1] These feelings of consideration and esteem, which honoured me so greatly, found a charming and enthusiastic expression in a banquet in my honour with which the Academy of Medical Sciences of Cataluña and my academic colleagues paid tribute to me who, for nearly five years, had had the honour of being their associate and collaborator. At the ceremony there were present also a number of professors of the Faculty of Sciences and the congenial fellow-members of the circle at the café.

It was with true regret that I had to leave such excellent friends and at the same time a city in which I found an atmosphere singularly favourable for the prosecution and publication of my scientific work. With no less sorrow did

[1] It was perhaps my esteemed friend Batlles y Beltrán de Lis who showed himself most vexed by my transfer to the capital, since he was anxious to create a position as microscopist for me in the Municipal Laboratory, which would carry fitting remuneration. The downfall of the liberal party, in the ranks of which he fought, and the consequent changes in the membership of the council, spoiled the kind plans of Batlles, for whose generous efforts I shall always be grateful.

I bid farewell to that famous group at the *Pajarera,* where in the company of García de la Cruz, Schwarz, Soriano, Villafañé, Castro Pulido, Castell, Odón de Buen, and others I had spent so many unforgetable hours.

The echo of my examination successes reverberated also in Zaragoza, arousing the enthusiasm, naturally, of my friends and compatriots. There, in the bosom of the family, where I broke the journey for a few days on my way to the capital, I enjoyed one of the purest and noblest satisfactions which it is possible to experience; the contemplation of the happiness and pride of my aged parents, those parents to whom the artistic and rebellious wanderings of their son had caused so many disappointments in other days. That joy was a beautiful compensation for their anxieties and a great consolation for me. How much I would have given that the lives of my progenitors might have been extended until 1908, the date of the most resounding of my triumphs! But the law of life is inexorable; to few parents is it given to witness the culmination of the careers of their children.

Also my excellent professors in Zaragoza celebrated my elevation to the University of Madrid. With a few exceptions, they showed themselves proud of their former pupil and the latter considered himself happy to have given cause for satisfaction to his masters. At their request, and in order to make some return for so many friendly courtesies, I gave two long lectures, illustrated with many pictures, explaining the more important results of my studies in the laboratory. Great was the surprise of my masters of former times to learn that indisputable scientific authorities of foreign countries had confirmed my modest discoveries and adopted my interpretations.

They naturally tendered me the tribute which was then the style, namely a banquet in my honour, with the inevitable toasts, infused not only with personal friendship but also with encouraging and patriotic hopes for the future of the newborn Spanish science. I remember that one of the most complimentary and effusive toasts was that of Doctor

Fornés, to whom I had gratuitously attributed some grudge against me.

I finally arrived in the capital of the monarchy in April, 1892, at the age of forty, eager for work and with my portfolio filled with scientific projects. According to my custom, I installed myself modestly,[2] as befits the scientific labourer who feels a *holy horror of a deficit,* as Echegaray says, and knows that ideas, like the white water-lily, flourish only in tranquil waters. I paid sixteen duros[3] a month as rent. Such restraint, which some censure as excessive and unfitting for a prince of the academic world, to borrow the phrase of a certain puffed-up and haughty professor, seemed to me necessary while I explored the territory and tried to accumulate the resources required for the education of my family and the complete development of my researches. For I have always considered dangerous and hindering the conduct of those professors who, recently arrived from some provincial corner, establish themselves in the capital like American dentists, squandering their modest savings in providing themselves with a carriage, an abode, and furnishings, in the hope of a wealthy clientele, which does not condescend to appear.

The habits of my new colleagues fitted in admirably with my mode of life. With inner rejoicing I saw that in the Faculty of Medicine as in the University at large nobody paid any attention to anybody else. "We live without knowing each other and die without mourning each other," as used to be said by Don Félix Guzmán, the professor of hygiene, who was much disgusted by this sullen spiritual aloofness between the collaborators in a common work. Similar expressions of sorrow I heard from Don Federico Olóriz who had recently been transferred to Madrid from his friendly and effusive home in Granada.

One must disillusion oneself. The capital cannot be for the hard-working and unpretentious man who enjoys the pleasures of social intercourse the celebrated "land of

[2] In no. 131 duplicado of the Calle de Atocha.

[3] Sixteen dollars.

friendship" of the poet. Hard and feverish is existence in the great cities: the greatness of the distances and the high cost of living necessitate hard work and the miserly taking advantage of every moment. To cultivate worldly relations involves a luxury which is permissible only to the rich and the idle. But, I repeat, this relative solitude of spirit, which so greatly vexed Olóriz, was always felicity to me. Coldness and indifference appear annoying when they really mean freedom and respect. "Certainly, no one thinks of me," I said to myself, as I saw at first that I was alone and lost in the immense crowd of the capital, "but, in return, what freedom of thought and work I enjoy! What an outstanding privilege it is to be able to prosecute our activities according to the dictates of our own inclinations without clashing with anybody!"

Notwithstanding my relative seclusion I had the good fortune to form and cultivate in the capital some, though very few, precious friendships. Passing over for the moment friends outside the teaching professions (of whom I shall treat elsewhere), I may mention Olóriz, Hernando, Letamendi, San Martín, Gómez Ocaña, García de la Cruz, and others.[4] It may be remarked that, with the exception of San Martín, all these friends belonged to the unassuming and despised group of professors who devoted their time to teaching and research, who had none of that intoxicating cupidity inseparable from the majority of the eminent clinicians. To the list mentioned I shall add also the names of Don Julián Calleja and of the Marquis del Busto. It was not my fortune to become intimate with these two eminent figures of San Carlos; but they are entitled to grateful mention here, as I owed to them unforgetable official support and favours.

The noble Marquis del Busto, professor of obstetrics, being desirous of assisting the laboratory of histology of San Carlos, turned over to it for many years, up to the time

[4] The sketches of these famous professors occupying about five pages of the original work have been omitted as being unlikely to interest the general reader outside Spain. (Translator's note.)

of his death, his emoluments as Clinical Director. Also the worthy Doctor Calvo y Martín, professor of surgery, in his enthusiasm for my modest successes in research and his desire to be useful to me, generously offered me accomodation for life in one of his houses, and honoured me besides with other attentions. However, I could not accept the offer of my kind fellow-countryman on account of my desire to live near the faculty of medicine (the house offered was in the Calle de Isabel la Católica).

Such were, in sum, those of my colleagues who have now disappeared for ever who had most influence upon me, either through their official support or through their guidance, and in all cases through their counsel and their regard.

CHAPTER X

Dangers of Madrid for the laboratory man. Temptations of scientific, literary and artistic dilettanteism. My spiritual recreations; walks in the environs of Madrid and the circle of the Café Suizo. New investigations on the structure of the brain. I begin the publication of my general work on the Structure of the Nervous System of Vertebrates.

Madrid is a city of the greatest danger for the provincial who is industrious and eager to extend the horizon of his intelligence. The ease and pleasantness of social relations, the abundance of talent, the attractions of societies, banquets, and café circles (tertulias), in which men of eminence in politics, literature, and science continually officiate as highpriests, the various theatrical presentations, and a thousand other distractions seduce and captivate the outsider, who finds himself suddenly demagnetized and bewildered. A complete metamorphosis has taken place in his life: the bee has been transformed into a butterfly, if not into a drone. Philosophy, art, literature, even politics and pastimes tug at his soul with a thousand taut and invisible threads. The busy worker has been succeeded by the charming intellectual Sybarite.

Moreover, the cerebral instrument, formed during many years of solitude and concentration, becomes dedifferentiated and blunted like a tool eaten into by rust: the special mentality brought from the remote provincial home is gradually reduced to the level of the mentality of the world at large. The callouses are lost and the hands become gloved, and the time slips away in admiring and imitating.

In vain we endeavour to make an end of the dangling, to abandon resolutely the road of Sybaris or Corinth, to return finally to the severe habits of former days: spurred by the sense of honour we get so far as to plan fine programmes of action. Unfortunately, they all die prematurely. "There is no time for anything!" we exclaim bitterly.

However, I made up my mind to close my ears at all costs to the song of the siren of the capital and to defend my time and work as much as in the provinces. And I finally succeeded, though not without offending nor without causing myself to be called unsociable, eccentric, and proud.

I am far from claiming, as I have already said repeatedly, that the man of science should be a Carthusian; rather I regard pastimes, excursions, the theatre, the Athenaeum, literature, clubs, etc., as necessary for him. But each must have its place, with restraint, and as tonics; when the mind needs them and not when others wish. Pure, but sanctified egoism, for without that no serious work is possible!

For these reasons, and as a compensation for the excessive concentration of laboratory life, I have always cultivated two distractions in Madrid: walks in the open air through the environs of the city, and the circles at the café.

The environs of Madrid! There is no need for me to make them known now, vindicating once more the much slandered Manzanares and the austere Castilian plateau. One must have the colour sense of a caterpillar always to miss the damp and uniform green of the northern districts and to fail to appreciate the penetrating poetry of the gray, the yellow, the brown, and the blue. Nor is it true that the succulent note of the green is entirely absent in the region of the capital. Far from being a desert and uncultivated, the surroundings of Madrid—the Retiro, the Moncloa, the Casa de Campo, Amaniel, the Dehesa de la Villa, El Pardo, etc.—are the most luxuriant and picturesque in the whole of Spain. We live in the lap of a mountain range of which the graceful outline embellishes our horizon and of which the breezes purify our atmosphere. In spring and autumn the Castilian plain presents itself covered with grass and dotted with flowers. Nowhere has the countryside more varied contrasts according to the seasons. Whatever be the preoccupation of the spirit, we can always find some quiet corner of which the peaceful beauty soothes the pangs of sorrow and opens up a new channel for our thoughts. How many little discoveries are associated in my memory with some solitary footpath of the Moncloa Park or with an ash tree on the banks of the Manzanares, or a little hill of Amaniel or of the Dehesa de la Villa, splendid lookouts to which the Guadarrama, standing out among its pine trees, displays all its august majesty!

The laboratory man, however, is suited not only by the physical terrain but also by the spiritual one, the congenial circle where, in the warmth of friendship and mutual confidence, there flourish the varied and spontaneous flowers of intellect.

It is true that my first sallies of exploration among the "tertulias" of Madrid were not very fortunate. I soon found in the *Café de Levante* a group of former acquaintances, mostly army physicians, whom I had known during the campaign in Cuba. Among these congenial companions there reigned a fraternal frankness and at times their conversation was lively, sparkling, and instructive. But an adverse fate pursued us: almost every day, fatally, irremediably, the comments turned to murmurs against the hierarchical superiors or to the promotions in the Army Medical Service; that accursed system of promotion by seniority, the destroyer of all noble stimulus and of all worthy ambition, an obstacle to justice, the refuge of idleness, and one of the worst calamities which we have suffered in Spain.

The evil had no remedy! Those worthy companions, who certainly were not entirely without ability, but who were petrified by the idle life of camps, barracks, and casinos, read nothing but the *Gaceta* and the *Boletín de Sanidad*.

Regretfully, I abandoned the society of comrades who recalled to my memory the excitements of war and youthful adventures across the Atlantic and sought another circle where I might recreate my mind and revivify the idle fallow land of my brain.

I think it was San Martín who introduced me to the circle at the *Café Suizo,* a gathering of ancient and glorious lineage, since there had belonged to it politicians, literati, and even distinguished financiers.

Although from the political and literary aspect the group referred to had deteriorated somewhat, it still enjoyed at that time well-deserved renown. From it, as is well known, emerged university senators, professors, rectors, counsellors, and even ministers. So famous and noted did the discussions of the group become that it often happened, with grave risk of indiscretion, that there were formed at neighbouring tables parasitic groups, or clubs of listeners, who, for the trifling price of coffee, acquired the right to become acquainted with our more or less extravagant chat and to gossip in perfect security.

Among those who met around the table there was naturally a predominance of the Galens, at the head of whom appeared Don Alejandro, but there were also lawyers, proprietors, university professors, and in fact men of every kind and condition. Anyone was admitted provided that he was presented by a formal member and on condition that he be governed by the three following rules: first, he must preserve in the discussion a due respect for persons; second, that he should discuss what he did not understand or understood but little (the effort was to avoid pedantic and academic bores); and third, that he should forget upon leaving all the nonsense and incoherencies brought forth by the stimulus of the coffee or by the disturbances of digestion. For it is important to observe that our gathering used to take place in the early hours of the afternoon, and seldom lasted more than an hour. By this arrangement, when we rose from the session, our minds were heated but still active for our daily work. It is a good thing to digress a little every day, but it would be dangerous to prolong the *diastole* of the mind at the expense of the *systole* of work.

With sorrow I recall today the changes which time and death have brought about in our beloved circle at the *Suizo.* These groups are living entities with youth, maturity, and decay; and like every organism, they feed, grow, assimilate, and excrete. New cells are incorporated, while other, alas! perish or wander away. And the dead are already legion!

I owe much to the delightful *tertulia at the Suizo.*[1] Besides unforgetable times of recreation and good humour, I learned many things there and overcame some of my defects. There we improved our minds a little, expounding and discussing hotly the doctrines of philosophers ancient and modern, from Plato and Epicurus to Schopenhauer and Herbert Spencer; and we rendered enthusiastic veneration to evolution and its high priests, Darwin and Haeckel, and abominated the satanic arrogance of Nietzsche. In the realm of literature, our table upheld naturalism against romanticism and the opposite, according to the speakers of the occasion and the humour of the moment. In turn, Pepe Botella and San Martín, the most musical of the gathering, used to wage colossal battles in favour of Wagner, when there were hardly any Wagnerites in Spain except the merry Peña y Goñi.

In an easy way, also, our group had a few dealings with politics. Without affiliating itself openly with any of the alternating parties, the table at the Suizo was always politically minded, in the best sense of the term. It commented, sometimes with passion and vehemance, but always inspired with intense patriotism, upon the great events of national life; it burst into shouts of indignation against the arbitrary and unjust actions of "bossism" and it wept tears of rage over the inconsequent and insensate actions which led up to the ignominies of 1895. There, naturally, were noisy echoes of the literature of the *regeneracion;*[2] signatures were collected for the famous manifesto of Costa, and the apostle of Spanish Europeanization, who died too soon, found support for his noble campaign. Convinced,

[1] This circle disappeared and scattered upon the demolition of the Café Suizo in 1920.

[2] Writers of this period who advocated abandonment of living in the past and emphasis on looking to the future, and material progress. (Translator's note.)

with the "hermit of Graus," that national prosperity must be founded upon "the school and the pantry," we expounded and contrasted repeatedly the methods of scientific pedagogy and the political proceedings calculated to overcome, or at least to decrease the lack of cultivation of our lands and of our brains. There, at a date not very distant, we were overcome with horror and execration, destroying the last relics of our youthful optimism, by the monstrous European war, which was not, as simple spirits touched with incurable charlatanism like to tell us, a conflict of commercial interests nor a struggle between two opposed conceptions of the State, but was very largely the bitter fruit of national pride, the inevitable clash between all-powerful military oligarchies, puffed up with arrogance and greedy for glory and dominion. There, in sum, even if at times we allowed ourselves to be captivated by the frivolous pleasure of inconsequence and gossip, we knew also how to rise frequently above the petty vexations of life, to feel ourselves more and more human and patriotic, and to advance a step or two along the paths of peace and love towards bright ideals.

It is time now to bring to an end this long digression (which may perhaps have relieved the reader after the tedious but unavoidable narrative of my undertakings in Barcelona) and to indicate briefly the laboratory work carried out in the capital in the years 1892 and 1893.

What scientific subjects drew my attention? There were, among other less profitable ones, the structure of the retina of fishes and birds, especially that of the fovea centralis; the organization of the hippocampus and of the occipital cortex of the cerebrum; and, finally, the arrangement of the sympathetic system. Yielding to a habit which was inveterate with me, I investigated these matters almost simultaneously. In general, such promiscuity is inadvisable. Nevertheless, in the natural sciences it is occasionally useful to concentrate the attention alternately on two or more fields of study; thus fuller advantage is taken of the material studied and the methods yield a richer harvest. Although it seems paradoxical, two or three subjects of study are less fatiguing than a single one. Persistently to pluck the same string finally becomes distressing. Besides, during the sacred fever, when one feels oneself in a productive vein, it is well to constrain fate and to corner, so far as possible, all the tickets in the lottery.

The reader need not fear a detailed exposition of investigations of 1892 and 1893 upon the subjects mentioned. I shall confine myself to mentioning only the most outstanding scientific advances.

1. I shall begin with the retina. As the reader will recall, my explorations in this region, which I found so fascinating, began in Barcelona. I desired, however, to complete and consolidate my earlier findings, embracing the whole vertebrate series in my observations; and I was especially eager to attack the problem of the structure of the fovea centralis, the retinal region of maximum sensitivity to colour and of the greatest visual acuity. By good fortune, there was no lack of material in Madrid. In fact, I made an arrangement with a professional animal-catcher, who provided me with living snakes, lizards, red owls, barn owls, crows, mergansers, salamanders, perch, trout, etc. Also a good friend in Cadiz was so kind as to send me several specimens of that most interesting creature, the chameleon, the jewel of reptiles, which is a regular inhabitant of the Cadiz dunes. With this abundant material my notebook became filled with interesting drawings and my notes overflowed with descriptive details. Such a rich harvest moved me to issue a communication on the retina of fishes, which was published, thanks to the kindness of the learned Don Ignacio Bolívar, in the *Anales de la Sociedad de Historia Natural,* and to publish later a voluminous monograph, which appeared in *La Cellule,* a Belgian biological review of high standing which has already been mentioned elsewhere. This last memoir, one of the most important which has sprung from my pen, was a voluminous

book which, a couple of years later, was considered worthy of the honour of translation into German.[3]

Remembering my promise to avoid prolixities I shall mention from among the new facts contained in the work cited only those which today, reading in cold blood and in the presence of the rich bibliography which has appeared since, appeal most agreeably to my vanity as a laboratory worker.

(*a*) In the whole vertebrate series, and especially in the fishes, of which the mode of vision much resembles that of mammals, there was confirmed the presence of the two types of bipolar cells, discovered a year before in the visual membrane of mammals, connected respectively with the rods and with the cones.

(*b*) The essential structure of the central fovea of the retina in reptiles and birds was laid bare, showing that each bipolar cell connects with only a single rod and a single ganglionic cell, not with several as in the rest of the retina, whence the indistinctness of vision in the latter.

(*c*) The development of the neuroblasts in the embryonic retina was shown to be the same as that described by His, myself, and v. Lenhossék in the spinal cord, and a hypothesis was proposed to explain the establishment of the specific connections between neurons in the adult. This latter conception will be discussed later.

2. Another of the themes to the elucidation of which I bent all my efforts was the structure of the hippocampus, or Ammon's horn, the oldest centre of association in the brain, the storehouse of olfactory memories and of the corresponding motor reactions.

B. Croce has said "that every scientific work is also a work of art," a statement akin to the oft repeated thought that "nature is the work of a divine artist." And this beauty is not only of the intellectual order, in the exquisite suitability of means for ends; in the natural sciences there often appear admirable plastic forms, as I have already remarked in earlier chapters. Hence it results that, how-

[3] Cajal: Die Retina der Wirbelthieren. German translation by Dr. R. Greef. Wiesbaden, 1894.

ever poor and incomplete may be the objective vision of the scientist, he will always preserve some reflection of natural beauty. He will even be able to affirm that the illogical and antiaesthetic elements in the scientific conception of a phenomenon necessarily imply error or misunderstanding in the ideas of the investigator.

But, leaving aside this line of thought, I may say that one of the stimuli which led me to scrutinize the hippocampus and the fascia dentata was the elegant architecture shown by the cells and the layers of these centres, as revealed by the illustrious Golgi in his great work. In fact, the hippocampus and the dentate fascia are adorned by many features of the pure beauty of the cerebellar cortex. Their pyramidal cells, like the plants in a garden—as it were, a series of hyacinths—are lined up in hedges which describe graceful curves. Examination of Fig. 54 will give some idea of this graceful stratification of the hippocampal

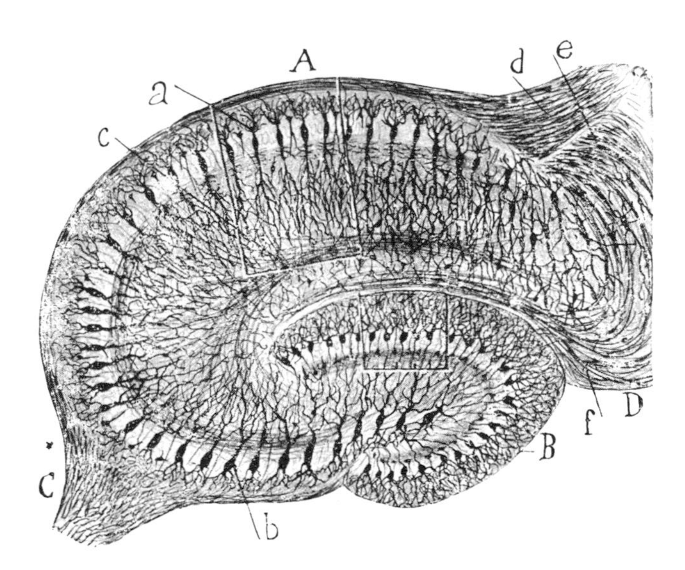

FIG. 54. Diagram of the architecture of the hippocampus and the fascia dentata as they appear in transverse sections. This figure shows the principal types of neurons described by Golgi and by Sala. *A*, hippocampus (Ammon's horn); *B*, dentate fascia; *C*, fimbria; *D*, subiculum; *a*, superior pyramid; *b*, pyramid of the inferior region.

neurons. It is unnecessary to remark that, taking advantage of the privilege of the first occupant, the celebrated investigator of Pavia was able to collect the most important anatomical data relative to the form and arrangement of the cells in the nervous organs under discussion; and the work of the master was completed at several points by his pupils Sala and Lugaro, as well as by Schäffer, the Hungarian histologist.

Nevertheless, there still remained much virgin ore for new workers. It was, especially, necessary to examine the cells with short axons, which had been inadequately studied by the savants mentioned, and it was important besides to attack the problem of the connections between the neurons, establishing so far as possible the pathways followed by the sensory or afferent impulses, an interesting task hardly touched by the scientists of the Italian school.

Such were the objectives pursued by me in the year 1892, with some good fortune, I believe. The results obtained caused me to prepare an extensive monograph, published first in the *Anales de la Sociedad Española de Historia Natural.* In the same year my work was considered worthy of the inestimable honour of being translated into German by the illustrious Kölliker, for his important review *Zeitschrift f. wissensch. Zoologie.* The interesting new points brought out included the description of several types of cells with short axons not previously noted, the demonstration of the courses and connections of the axons of the various types of cells and of the afferent fibres, and a description of the neuroglia.

3. My examination of the sympathetic system of the intestine was less important. Nevertheless, it includes a number of new facts, mainly the description of certain new types of cells and of the terminations of certain fibres.

In the year 1893 I published also less weighty works on the occipital cortex of small mammals and on malign tumors of the liver. Finally I sent to press some new observations on the structure of the spinal cord and of the sympathetic trunk.

CHAPTER XI

The Royal Society of London appoints me "Croonian Lecturer." My lecture before that society. Official banquets and other tributes. A visit to the scientific laboratories in London and a trip to the Universities of Cambridge and Oxford. I am created Doctor of Science "Honoris Causa." Personal impressions of English science and of the organization of English teaching centres.

In February, 1894, there reached me a communication from Dr. Foster, secretary of The Royal Society of London, inviting me, on behalf of that illustrious body, to deliver the discourse called The Croonian Lecture. This is an address upon a biological subject, for which the remuneration is fifty pounds sterling, and which was instituted by a certain English scientist with a view to bringing to London an investigator, either native or foreign, who was the author of some outstanding discovery. Always practical, the English scientific organizations are not satisfied to stimulate individual investigation from afar, adjudicating to the conqueror of a new truth the customary diploma of honour; they desire, in addition, to make the acquaintance of the author, to hear the exposition of his works from his own lips, and, above all, to examine and evaluate at first hand the methods of research by the aid of which the new fact was discovered. Directed towards an end so cleverly utilitarian, the English academies have created many prizes, all due to private initiative.

The resolution of The Royal Society took me by surprise. In truth, I was confounded and abashed by the flattering invitation, hesitating between frankly accepting it and courteously declining, as I feared that I should not measure up suitably to the honour which had been accorded me. In excuse for my hesitation, it must be remembered that The Royal Society of London is the most important scientific institution in Great Britain and perhaps in the whole world. The greatest scientists and thinkers of England have belonged to it. For a French or German professor to obtain the title of *Fellow* of an institution of such prestige, to be able to add to his cards the coveted initials F.R.S., is a supreme aspiration which is satisfied for very few. Besides, the Croonian Lecture had always been entrusted to investigators of the greatest ability, among whom I recall the illustrious Kölliker [1] and the admirable Retzius. Finally, by a culminating contrariety of fate, one of my daughters took seriously ill at the same time. My paternal instinct was disturbed and protested against leaving the patient, despite the encouraging prognoses made to tranquilize me by Dr. Hernando, the family physician and a generous friend of my family.

The comforting assurances of my colleague, the fortitude of my wife, who advised me to accept the invitation at any cost, an exceedingly kind letter from Dr. Foster, and another no less complimentary from Professor Charles Sherrington finally decided me. The last claimed generously, as a neurologist, the right to have me stay in his house. At the present time, my host, who was then young, can be regarded as the leading physiologist in England.

I commenced, then, in the midst of my anxieties, to write the lecture in French, since I had not a command of English sufficient for expressing myself fittingly in that language; then I collected my best preparations of the cerebellum, the spinal cord, the retina, the cerebral hemisphere, the olfactory bulb, etc., and having obtained the permission of my superiors in the hierarchy, I undertook the journey to England. In passing through Paris, I paid my cordial respects to my illustrious friend M. Matías Duval and had the pleasure of making the personal acquaintance of my translator, Dr. Leon Azoulay, who, with great kindness, revised

[1] A letter from the Professor of Würzburg, kindly informed me of the character of the ceremony and advised me to give my address, an essentially physiological slant. The illustrious Kölliker had pronounced the Croonian Lecture in May, 1862, discoursing "On the Termination of Nerves in Muscles."

and corrected the doubtful French of my pages. Finally, I arrived in London and put myself at the disposal of The Royal Society.

As the charming secretary of that body had already told me would be the case, the hospitality which I was accorded by Dr. Sherrington and his admirable spouse was of the pleasantest and overflowed with delicate attentions. No less generous and cordial was the reception accorded the modest Spanish investigator by Mr. Foster and other illustrious members of the Society, among whom I remember Schäffer, Klein, Bourdon-Sanderson, Horsley, Mott, and finally the very distinguished president, Sir William Thomson (Lord Kelvin), the inventor, as is well known, of the transatlantic telegraph, and one of the most frank, simple, and unassuming scientists whom I have ever known. Indeed, the simplicity and cordiality of the social relations of these scientists, the most eminent in England, their total lack of aloofness and of professional pride, the placidity and brightness of their private conversation, in contrast with the dignity and profundity of their scientific work, captivated me completely.

In his noble generosity, Mr. Sherrington, who was at that time professor of physiology in one of the faculties of Medicine in London (I think it was in Bartholomew's Hospital), undertook not only to entertain me and guide me in the formidable English Babel, but also to lend me useful and direct assistance in the preparation of my lecture. To this end, he had superb photomicrographs made from the most instructive sections, so that they could be projected, and provided me with everything required for making large scale diagrams in colour.

With such materials for demonstration, the reading turned out sufficiently clear and convincing, in spite of my nervousness. If my memory does not deceive me, it was pronounced on the eighth of March in the splendid mansion called Burlington House, the meeting-place of The Royal Society. My discourse took in the most fundamental of my discoveries concerning the morphology and connections of the nerve cells of the spinal cord, the ganglia, the cerebellum, the retina, the olfactory bulb, etc. And to put me in tune with the audience, in which physiologists and medical men predominated, and at the same time, to satisfy the English taste, which demands a practical or didactic value for everything, I concluded my oration by drawing from the facts explained various more or less probable physiological and even psychological interpretations.[2] These I shall treat elsewhere.

I should like to mention a detail which is not without value. That he might not lose the thread of the discourse, each auditor held in his hands, according to the English custom, a printed summary of its most important points. Nor must I forget another detail expressive of the exquisite courtesy of the Anglo-Saxons: upon the presidential dais, which was occupied by Lord Kelvin and various academic dignitaries, there shone the intertwined flags of England and of Spain.

At the end of the presentaton, I was warmly congratulated. Among those who grasped my hand effusively, I was pleased to recognize the Spanish Ambassador, Don Cipriano del Mazo, accompanied by his secretary, the charming son of Don Facundo Riaño, who was then an attaché of the Embassy, and by some other distinguished representatives of the Spanish colony. It was a day of pleasant and noble excitement, one of those which survive in the memory associated with sweet feelings of patriotism.

There then took place an uninterrupted series of entertainments, in which was brought out the friendly magnificence of Anglo-Saxon hospitality. It would be impossible to mention all the invitations received and the banquets attended.

Particular notice must be taken, however, of the banquet

[2] The English press published rather accurate extracts and the curious reader may consult among other reviews, *The Illustrated London News* of April 7, 1894.

of The Royal Society, at which there were present many guests from Cambridge and Oxford. At the time for champagne, there were enthusiastic toasts to English and Spanish science and declarations of cordial intellectual fraternity between the two nations. I still remember part of the eloquent discourse of Mr. Foster, a witty and original speaker, who flavoured his ideas with that fine salt of Anglo-Saxon humour, which is almost unknown with us. He said, among other things flattering to Spain and to me, that, thanks to my work, the impenetrable forest of the nervous system had been converted into a well laid out and delightful park, and that my researches had established connecting collaterals and motor end plates between the souls of Spain and of England, formerly kept apart by centuries of misunderstanding and indifference.

More intimate and less formal was the dinner held in the house of Dr. Paget, where I had the pleasure of meeting the most famous neurologists and medical men of the English capital.

I remember too the delightful trip to the cottage of my friend Dr. Schäffer, professor of physiology and histology in one of the London medical faculties. In this country house, surrounded with meadows and patches of woodland, enlivened by the play of children and the authoritative voices of the nurses, I had my first view of the ease, comfort, and elegance of the English home, as well as of the dignity with which scientists live and bring up their children in wealthy Albion.

It would be ungrateful to omit mention here of the intimate celebration and the splendid banquet held in the Spanish embassy and attended by the most distinguished members of the colony (among the guests was the learned and venerable Gayangos). When the time for toasts came, the host, Don Cipriano del Mazo, after praising my trifling merits to the point of paradox, intoned a most eloquent canticle to Spanish science and philosophy. His vibrant and emotional words moved us all, and especially me, so that I had hardly sufficient composure to thank him for his eulogies.[3]

Naturally, when the receptions and banquets were over, I devoted a few days to admiring the curiosities and beauties of the stupendous English capital: its rich and artistic monuments, the port and the wharves of the Thames, the British Museum, the Crystal Palace, the incomparable parks, etc. Not without deep emotion did I contemplate in Westminster the statue of Newton and the tomb of Darwin.

Needless to say, taking advantage of the good offices of my host, who was eager to please me, I paid instructive visits also to the chief educational institutions in the city, among others, King's College Hospital, Bartholemew's Hospital, the London Hospital, all centres of medical instruction, the Royal College of Surgeons, and finally the Royal Medical and Chirurgical Society. However, what most attracted my attention were the laboratories. There it was my good fortune to witness physiological experiments by Ferrier, Horsley, and Mott and to examine the histological preparations of Schäffer and of Sherrington. In this connection it will not be superfluous to give a few details.

In the English laboratories it was then very much the fashion to apply the method of secondary degenerations, associated with the so called stain of Marchi (colouring of the pieces of nervous tissue with osmic acid, etc.). This procedure, which they were employing with the aim of ascertaining the origins and courses of the principal tracts which connect the cerebrum and cerebellum with the medulla oblongata and spinal cord, is well known to require, as a primary condition, the performance of dangerous and difficult experimental operations on monkeys or dogs. One

[3] Among other expressions of exaggerated courtesy, I remember blushingly his saying: "In my extensive travels about the world, there have been three occasions when I have been most deeply impressed: one was upon viewing the cataracts of Niagara; another in Rome, gazing upon the Coliseum; and the third was in listening to the lecture of Cajal before The Royal Society."

of these carried out by Professor Ferrier on the macaque impressed me deeply both by the mastery of the manipulation and by the brilliance of the result; it was a case of total extirpation of both occipital lobes of the cerebral hemispheres. Thanks to the incomparable skill of the operator and to the perfect asepsis and hemostasis attained, the animal survived such an extensive removal and it was possible to explore, in due time, the secondary degenerations which took place. It is a fact that the English physiologists and especially Ferrier, the eminent scientist who shared with Hirtzig and Munk the discovery of cerebral localization, are prodigious experimenters.

When a foreign professor of some standing is travelling in England and puts himself in touch with her men of learning it is the thing to invite him to visit the important and historic universities of Cambridge and Oxford, where, as is well known, the intellectual youth and the most ancient aristocracy of the Anglo-Saxon race are given instruction. And if the distinguished foreigner has been selected to deliver the Croonian Lecture or has received some other academic distinction, then it is customary to confer upon him in either Oxford or Cambridge, according to the field of study of the candidate, the degree of Doctor, *honoris causa,* an academic ceremony performed with great solemnity with the students in attendance.

This was my experience. In the early days of my sojourn in London, I received polite missives from the Vice Chancellor of the University of Cambridge and from the indefatigable secretary, Mr. Foster (who belonged to the staff of that institution), asking me courteously to accept an honour so outstanding.

To this end, a number of professors, among them the afore-mentioned secretary of The Royal Society, accompanied me to the historic city on the Cam, and lodged me in a splendid building belonging to King's College. After a day's rest, visiting and admiring the beautiful Gothic chapel of the college, its excellent laboratories, its ample class rooms, its rich collections, its broad playing fields spread out upon both banks of the river, and other objects of interest, the hour of the solemn academic function arrived.

It took place, if I remember correctly, on the fifth of March, a few days before my lecture to The Royal Society, in the magnificent convocation hall of the Senate House. As everyone knows the devotion of the English to tradition, it is unnecessary to say that the ceremony was carried through with due regard to the most ancient canons. There were present the Vice Chancellor, the local and academic dignitaries, the faculty, and many members of the aristocratic colleges affiliated with the university. Masters and students wore the traditional robes of the doctor, consisting of a kind of toga or red gown and a special cap, the top of which is finished with a pyramidal attachment having a square base.

Likewise complying with custom, the candidate, who was a little nervous, also wore the quaint vestments. There were music by Beethoven and a Latin discourse from the orator in the mediaeval style. When the words of presentation were ended the Vice Chancellor, turning to the candidate, declared that, in consideration of his merits, the university conferred upon him the degree of Doctor of Science. During the ceremony, I had to inscribe my signature—with a feather pen, so as not to break the traditional usages even in the smallest detail—in the great roll of honour in which appeared the names of all the graduates *ad honorem*. And finally, when the academic solemnity was over, there was a great banquet in King's College, followed the next day by an intimate private dinner in the beautiful residence which Doctor Forster owned outside the town.

Of my visit to Oxford, the admirable Gothic city, the inestimable jewel of the Middle Ages, where every house is a historic shrine and each college rivals in richness and magnificence a royal palace, I will only say that I was overwhelmed by such marvels. What libraries! What museums! What Gothic chapels! What size, richness, and comfort in the students' quarters! In comparison with King's College, the delicate work of the renaissance, with Baliol College, with Corpus Christi College, and with Magdalen College, exquisite examples of the Gothic style, or with the grandiose John's College, half hidden by screens of ivy, etc., the finest of our official educational edifices seems a big, jumbled, mean erection. It is a pleasure to acknowledge that I was much fêted by the professors, especially by the learned Bourdon-Sanderson. Concerning this master, it delights me to say that I was as enchanted with the activity and the wise organization of his laboratory of physiology as with his ability and other personal endowments.

To avoid being wearisome, I shall omit the account of many other things in both Oxford and Cambridge which excited my admiration or awoke my interest. I shall mention only two instructive events of which I retain pleasant recollections.

As a tribute to the foreign professors of physiology assembled in Cambridge for the ceremony described above, the accomplished Langley, whose name has become famous through his important discoveries concerning the functions of the sympathetic system, invited us to witness one of his favourite experiments. In a cat under the influence of nicotine, the said professor with insuperable skill, had exposed nearly all the ganglia of the sympathetic trunk on one side. These ganglia, despite their small size, were very clearly visible, unobscured by blood, and free from the thoracic and abdominal viscera, which had been neatly displaced to one side, without damage, and fastened with aseptic clamps and threads. How, after such great injury, the heart still beat and all the vital functions of the animal remained almost undisturbed is an impenetrable mystery to me. He then applied a faradic stimulus to the ganglia (which is equivalent practically to stimulating the sympathetic fibres alone, since cocaine paralyzes the bodies of the nerve cells), and the contraction of the smooth muscles of the skin (*arrectores pili*) appearing in regular and successive cutaneous bands or rings showed beautifully not only that each ganglion innervates a special peripheral area, but also that this cutaneous zone is segmental, like the areas of distribution of the sensory ganglia.

My presence on the other occasion, which was equally instructive although of a mundane and social character, was due to a fortunate chance. There happened to take place in Cambridge at that time what is there called a *scientific conversazione,* a sort of inter-university social gathering for the popular exposition of the discoveries made by the English professors and for the promotion among them of that spirit of intellectual solidarity which is so lacking among the research workers of the Latin nations. To this end there assembled in a great hall of King's College professors from all the scientific centres of the United Kingdom, accompanied by their families and numerous invited guests. Before the session, each investigator arranged on a table the apparatus necessary for his demonstrations. The histologists and embryologists brought their microscopic sections; the physicists their recent scientific inventions; the chemists, samples of the substances they had discovered and diagrams of the mechanism of their formation; the bacteriologists, cultures of new species of microbes and preparations of pathogenic germs; the astronomers, drawings and photographs—especially spectroscopic ones—of the stars, etc. In this way, the scientific men, besides getting to know each other personally, shared in the spiritual experiences of their colleagues and helped mutually in the solution of the problems of the day. Besides, the lay public and the students receive the inestimable advantage of a science fresh, living, varied, and doubly suggestive from bearing with it the stimulus of novelty and from being explained by the authoritative, warm, and enthusiastic words of its author. I may add that, when the scientific demonstrations were over, there was a little music, bringing the session to a close with a concession to the young people, who entered into the pleasures of the dance.

Although the subject is quite well known and many good books have been written upon it, I should like to say a little about the English university institutions and their educational fruits. It is true that a month of hasty and superficial study, during which I was obliged by force of circumstances to devote more attention to the exposition of my own researches than to the appreciation of the work of others, was not sufficient for me to form a definite and well-founded judgment. I shall, therefore, limit myself to a mere personal impression based partly on what I saw and partly on what I was told by professors familiar with the problem of higher education.

My opinion could be summarized in the statement that in England the educational institutions are admirably organized for the production of *men,* but not for the formation of scholars. Nevertheless, scholars abound and often reach the highest pinnacles of originality and genius. In that nation, however, the most eminent scientists and thinkers owe little to the universities; they are privileged natures, which open up ways for themselves in spite of the defective and incomplete organization of the educational centres. For the investigator there is not, as in Germany, the direct product of the school, but is the indirect result of the cultivation of the individuality and of the building up of all the energies of the spirit. With some reservations, I might state that in the land of the Teutons the educational organization is more important than the man, while in England the man is more important than the organization. It would be desirable to know whether, in dealing with a race so admirably endowed as the English, the German method of instructing much and educating little would not yield even better fruit than the Anglo-Saxon method of educating much and instructing abstemiously. Perhaps the ideal, as many think, would be a perfect balance between the two pedagogical principles.

That the larger English universities and colleges, with their character of private institutions, their full liberty regarding their programmes, their power to choose masters even among those not equipped with professional degrees, and their strict subjection to the essentially utilitarian demands of their patrons, etc., leave something to be desired in respect of their function of moulding investigators is manifestly acknowledged by these same English masters, in that many of them had to put the final touches to their technical preparation and theoretical instruction in the most renowned German state schools. Some of them pointed out to me shocking deficiencies. In fact, as one turns over the programmes of studies of some of the medical faculties, one notes with surprise that in most of them the didactic effort is inspired by utilitarianism, or professionalism, even to a point where important theoretical disciplines included in the plans of study of the French, German, Italian, and even the Spanish universities, are completely absent or receive insignificant attention. To this influence is to be attributed the relative scarcity of histologists, pathological anatomists, embryologists, and bacteriologists in England as compared with Germany or France. Such a state of affairs, however, is tending to disappear. It is evident that during recent years many of the lacunae in the educational pictures have been filled in, especially in the organization of the universities of a modern character set up in London, Liverpool, Manchester and elsewhere, which are supported almost entirely by the state and are subject to its direct supervision. In these very new schools, without neglecting fitness for the best professional production, there has been conceded to pure or theoretical science—which fundamentally is the most perfectly practical of all, since it encloses the germs of every future application to the purposes of life—its due place, in imitation of the schedules of similar educational centres in Germany.

My mission to the British Isles having been fulfilled and my scientific and artistic curiosity satisfied, I started the homeward journey, but not before I had reiterated to my generous hosts, Dr. Sherrington and Dr. Foster, and to other professors who had heaped me with attentions, the expression of my hearty gratitude.

What a disenchantment it was to arrive in our Madrid, where, by an incomprehensible contrast, the utmost of Spanish culture is presented in the worst of educational edifices! My eye having become adapted to the image of such splendours and greatness, it saddened me to think of our mean and inartistic university, of the ancient and unhygienic College of San Carlos, of the dangerous shadows of the Clinical Hospital, of the liliputian Botanic Garden in the Paseo de Trajineros, and of the Museum of Natural History, always homeless and a fugitive from eviction by the Administration.

I was impressed with sorrow also at seeing our students scattered, with no corporate spirit, distributed in wretched, insanitary, and mean lodging houses, and turned over to a freedom very close to abandonment; and the professors themselves, entrenched in their chairs like owls in a belfry, unacquainted with each other and completely cut off from the noble aims of collaboration for a common institution, as if they did not form part of a single body and were not working for the same end!

As I stepped across the threshold of my house, my heart beat tumultuously. Through unforeseen circumstances, I had not been able to send word of my arrival. How should I find my daughter? Was the optimism of her mother's letters not perhaps a considerate artifice designed to inspire and comfort me in my daring mission? Fortunately, the predictions of Hernando had been confirmed. Though very weak and worn, the patient was already beginning to be really convalescent.

When, on the following day, amid the delight and tumult of the children, I unpacked the gifts which I had bought in London, I learned with surprise that I had been forestalled in this attention; the wife of Don Facundo Riaño, daughter of the learned Arabic scholar, P. Gayangos, with a delicate consideration which I shall never forget, had consoled the children in the absence of their father by presenting them with beautiful toys. Also, she lavished upon my wife, who was worn out and suffering from a month without sleep, the greatest attention and thoughtfulness. Blessed be that saintly woman, daughter and wife of learned men, whose virtues won her the esteem and veneration of all who had the happiness of knowing her!

CHAPTER XII

My studies during the years 1894, 1895, and 1896. New relations observed in the structure of the medulla oblongata, the pons, the thalamus, the corpus striatum, the pineal gland, the pituitary body, the retina, the ganglia, etc. Some observations on the structure of the protoplasm and the nucleus. To obviate possible objections, I succeed in confirming with the methylene blue method of Ehrlich the most important facts discovered with the aid of chromate of silver.

I fear to weary and even disgust the reader with the tale of my investigations during the triennium 1894, 1895, and 1896; and yet I must say something about them, even though very laconically, to avoid destroying the plan of exposition which I have been following.

Up to the present, it has been an easy task by means of simplified descriptions and schematic figures to give the reader an idea of my most outstanding anatomical findings. To this the organs studied lent themselves through their architectural regularity and relative simplicity. Now, however, we have to deal with inquiries carried out in nerve centres of peculiarly intricate structure, such as the medulla oblongata, the pons, the thalamus, the corpora quadrigemina, etc., organs with reason regarded by the student and even by the master, as the labyrinths of neurology. In studying such material it is essential, in order to avoid losing oneself in an entanglement of intercrossing pathways, to consult at the very beginning and with the greatest attention those topographic maps, based on the comparison of regular series of transverse sections, which have been constructed by the patience of Meynert, Schwalbe, Obersteiner, Flechsig, Cramer, Edinger, van Gehuchten, and many others. But, for reasons easily imaginable, it is impossible for me to reproduce these authoritative guides here without completely altering the character of this book. I shall not, then, abuse the patience of the reader who is little or not at all interested in neurological studies, and shall limit myself to giving a bibliographic list with a mere enumeration of the most interesting discoveries. A few figures will supplement so far as possible the arid laconicism of the text.

The principal exploration carried out during the period mentioned was aimed at gaining an acquaintance with the medulla oblongata, the wearisome labyrinth to which I alluded above. Nevertheless, there is no moorland, however bleak it be, which does not offer to the botanist some flower that is unassuming but of exquisite fragrance. In the hope of finding such, I adventured into this difficult domain, after first scrutinizing it macroscopically in regular series of microscopic sections taken from man, dog, cat, rabbit, and mouse. And, as usual, I also demanded from the method of Golgi applied to embryos and young animals, its most precious and decisive revelations. As a general result, the inquiries mentioned provided proof that in the medulla oblongata, pons, thalamus, etc., there hold sway both the anatomical law of *contact* between bodies and axonic arborizations and also the physiological law of *dynamic polarization.* As in the spinal cord, the sensory or afferent roots of the trigeminal, vestibular, acoustic, and other cranial nerves show the classic bifurcation into ascending and descending branches (except the sensory roots of the glossopharyngeal and the pneumogastric which have only descending branches); and at the same time, by means of terminal and collateral branches, enter into intimate connection with the bodies and dendrites of the motor neurons (nuclei of the facial, motor trigeminal, and oculomotor roots, etc.), forming the automatic apparatus of reflex movements.

Likewise, there are seen in the oblongata and the pons numerous association cells (medial longitudinal bundle, fibres of the reticular substance, etc.).

The well-known philosophical dictum, "Everything is one and the same," applies particularly to the structure of the nerve centres. Inspired by motives of extreme economy, nature delights in repeating itself. It is due to these providential uniformities of life that science is possible. The logical mind is comforted in its eagerness for simplicity and unity by the recognition that the organizing principle adopts the same means for like ends. "Unity of plan with infinite variety of forms" appears to be the motto of life. Like the architect, it conforms to the general lines of a certain style but reserves to itself the right to vary the ornamental motifs indefinitely. In consequence of this inexhaustible variety of expressions, there is no monotony or tediousness in the work of the investigator. For it is precisely these unexpected and ingenious adaptations, with which nature modifies her creations in each particular case, without violating the essential standards, that nourish the curiosity and keep alive the sacred fire in the laboratory man.

Unfortunately, I reached the mine a little late for great surprises and discoveries of the first rank. Edinger, van Gehuchten, and particularly Kölliker and Held had preceded me in the successful application of the method of Golgi to the structural analysis of the nuclei of the oblongata and the pons. Thus, I had to glean in a reaped field. Still, I was able to gather something. It was a patience-taking and unpretentious piece of work, of perfecting, of amplifying, of describing minute details, considerably more laborious than brilliant. I shall go over briefly a few of my principal contributions.

First, I may record the publication of an extensive monograph in the *Anales de la Sociedad Española de Historia Natural*. In it there were considered various neurological subjects: the structure of the pons Varolii, of the hypophysis, of the corpus striatum, of the acoustic centres, etc. It was shown that the cells of the pons send their axons into the middle cerebellar peduncles (Fig. 55, *b*, *c*) and receive collaterals from the pyramidal tract (Fig. 56, *a*, *e*), thus forming an important path (cortico-ponto-cerebellar path) connecting the cerebral cortex with the cerebellum. This was confirmed by Pusateri and other workers. In the corpus striatum, this study confirmed in mammals some ideas of Edinger as to the constitution of the *Stamganglion* of the lower vertebrates and the mode of origin of the descending cerebral pathways.

Another of my investigations of 1894 concerned a special region of the thalamus designated *the habenular ganglion,* a centre regarding which, in mammals, we had hardly more than gross data of microscopic anatomy. I studied it in the mouse, rabbit, cat, and other animals by the methods

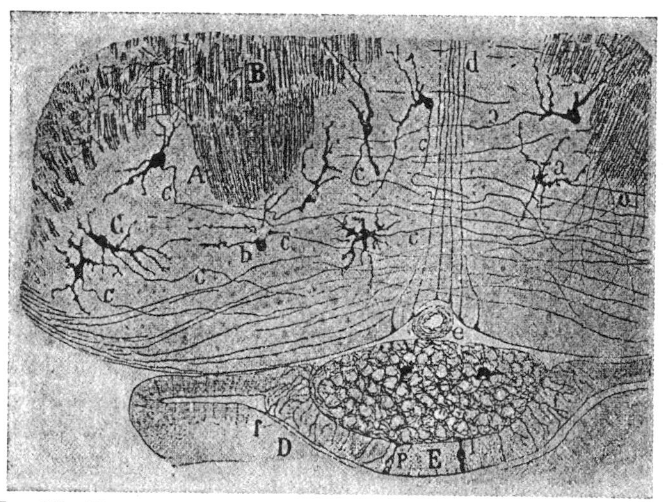

FIG. 55. PART OF A SECTION OF THE PONS OF A MOUSE, showing the origin of the middle cerebellar peduncles. *A*, pyramidal tract; *C*, cells of the pontine nucleus; *E*, epithelial portion of the hypophysis.

of Weigert, Nissl, and Golgi. Besides confirming in the mammals some important data obtained by van Gehucten in the habenula of the fishes, this work contains:

(*a*) histological proof of the existence in this centre of two clearly delimited nuclei, internal and external (Fig. 57, *A, B*).

(*b*) the discovery of the special morphology of the neurons composing the habenular nuclei (*A*) and of the entry of their very fine axons into the tract called *fasciculus of Meynert.*

(*c*) the finding in the internal nucleus of certain exceedingly dense pericellular nests or arborizations formed by the terminal ramifications of the axons of the *stria medullaris,* an important pathway belonging to the olfactory system (Fig. 58, *c*).

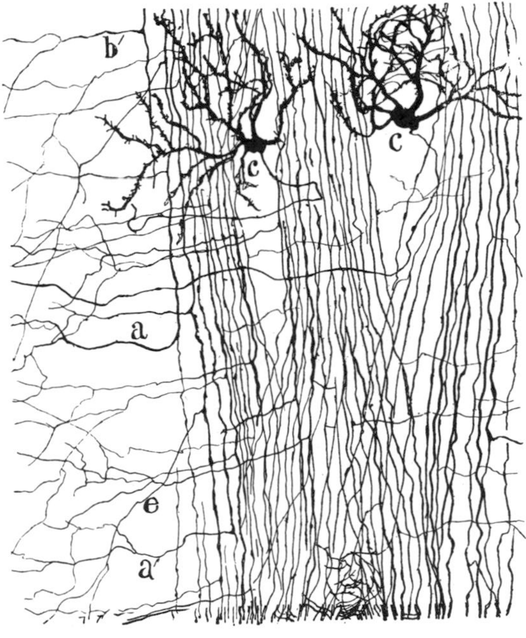

FIG. 56. LONGITUDINAL SECTION OF THE PYRAMIDAL TRACT OF A CAT WHERE IT TRAVERSES THE PONS, showing the collateral branches from this tract to the neurons of the pons, with which they enter into intimate contact.

Still richer in descriptive details and anatomical discoveries was the study devoted to the medulla oblongata, the cerebellum, and the origin of the cranial nerves, published in 1895, which almost forms a book in itself.[1]

[1] Among the points enumerated by the author as the most important in this work are the primary and secondary connections of the fifth nerve, connections of the superior cerebellar peduncle and of the optic nerve, ending of the bundle of Meynert, connections of the inferior olive, discovery of the commissural nucleus, afferent fibres to motor nuclei of nerves III, V, VII, XII, etc., ascending fibres in the medial longitudinal bundle, connections of the vestibular nerve, and bifurcation of axons from the mammillary body to form the tegmental tract and that of Vicq d'Azyr.

To complete the foregoing work on the oblongata, I gave to the press a couple of years later (1897) another communication also, in which are recorded various complementary observations, especially on connections from the spinal cord, etc.

Of other communications which appeared in 1895 I shall mention only the subjects: one concerned the structure of the deep nuclei of the cerebellum; the other, which was of

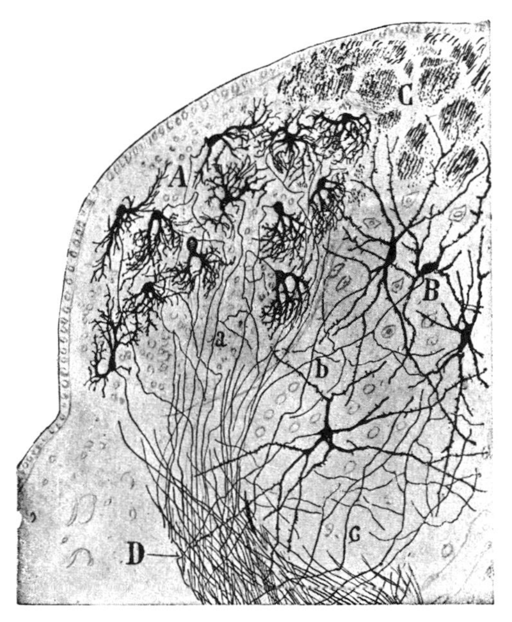

FIG. 57. CELLS OF THE INTERNAL (*A*) AND EXTERNAL (*B*) NUCLEI OF THE HABENULA. *D,* fasciculus of Meynert (fasc. retroflexus).

an iconographical character, but had a number of new descriptive details, was on the spinal cord. The most interesting feature of this last work was the preparation of large plates in colours copied from my best preparations.

During the year 1896 my activity rose to another peak like that of 1890, running feverishly through various divergent channels and expanding in some cases subjects already taken up. In one of these restudies, I attacked with new enthusiasm the retina, the oldest and most persistent of my laboratory loves. The new contribution was of a polemical character, constructed mainly to refute the theories of certain authors (Kallius, Renant, and Dogiel), who sought to revive in special forms the old and always reappearing theory of interneuronal networks. Faithful to my habit of not writing articles of pure controversy, I entered the lists armed with new observations of some value in the argument rather than with the trappings of dialectics.

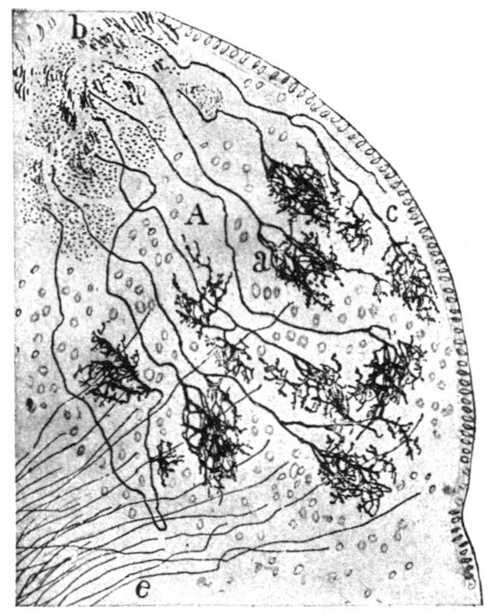

FIG. 58. FREE ARBORIZATIONS (*c*) distributed through the internal nucleus (*A*) of the habenula and derived from the olfactory pathway known as the stria medullaris (*b*).

Thus, after proving that the very rare cases of anastomotic fusion between dendrites, or between axons and dendrites, brought forward by these savants are mere optical illusions or artificial products of the reagents, I pointed out new and very clear arrangements of contact which are frequent in the retina of birds.

The structure of the nervous protoplasm and the organization of the nucleus of the neuron were also subjects of some study in 1896. These questions were then acute in all laboratories. The general morphology of the neuron having been precisely determined, it was urgent to examine its structure carefully, to ascertain the substratum in which the nerve impulse is produced and through which it circulates. Nissl, Dogiel, Levi, Lenhossék, Marinesco, Held, Lugaro, Holmgren, van Gehuchten, and many others had made interesting discoveries by the use of basic aniline dyes after fixation in alcohol (the method of Nissl), or the combination of acid aniline dyes with the basic ones, or, finally, variants of the old method of Altmannn, etc. There was little that I could gather in this field, which had been methodically explored and almost exhausted by my predecessors. Nevertheless, in the investigation referred to, some small contributions to knowledge of the structure of the neuron are set forth.

My duties as professor of pathological anatomy, entrusted with the official examination of material from clinics and autopsies, often obliged me to study and make specific determinations of tumors and neoplasias. The staining methods then in use, though valuable for many purposes, did not seem to me sufficiently efficacious and precise for purposes of instruction. Hence, I undertook repeated trials in histological dyeing, the outcome of which was a variety of formulae for trichromatic staining (yellow, blue, and red), capable of revealing in different colours the diverse histological components which make up tumors. One of the formulae which received most general acceptance among scientific workers was the so-called trichromatic method with basic fuchsin, picric acid, and indigo carmine. With it, the nuclei are coloured red; the collagen fibres pure blue or greenish blue; and the epithelial formations clear green, or yellowish or orange shades in different cases.

Having gained possession of singularly demonstrative tintorial procedures, I plunged into the study of certain tumors, particularly into the analysis of carcinoma, sarcoma, epithelioma, etc. Two papers on this subject appeared in 1896: one devoted particularly to the study of the structure of epithelial tumors, and the other aimed at demonstrating the local defenses developed by the organism against the invasion of the carcinoma or epithelioma.

In this same year, I published a little note in which, for the first time, the phagocytic capacity of the platelets of the lower vertebrates was demonstrated. Under certain conditions these blood corpuscles are capable of engulfing particles of carmine, microbes, etc.

Finally, to close this tedious list of papers, I shall mention yet one more communication, in which are considered the connections established between the nervous and the neuroglia elements (constellations or garlands of glia cells disposed around the soma of the neuron) and some original observations are brought forward.

My fury of inquiry during the aforementioned year 1896 was not yet fully satisfied with the study of the subjects mentioned. In the later months of that year I frequently turned with new ardour to matters which I had studied before; but this time I made use by preference of the valuable method of Ehrlich, to which Retzius, Dogiel, and their disciples owe so many and such splendid discoveries. As is well known, this procedure has the inestimable value of staining the nerve fibres and cells *in vivo*, or immediately after death, so that they stand out vigorously with a strong blue colour. Unfortunately the vital reaction of Ehrlich is so delicate and ephemeral that almost all fixing agents, and of course, alcohol, decolorize it.

It is true that the use of the new fixative, ammonium molybdate, introduced into the technique by A. Bethe, made possible the cutting of sections with the microtome, though with considerable inconvenience; but, with the exception of a few interesting experiments of Dogiel on the cerebellum of birds, no one had succeeded in obtaining, either by sectioning or by the examination of macerated pieces, instructive preparations of the central organs (cerebellum, cerebrum, spinal cord, etc.) of mammals.

I proposed at any cost to examine the structure of the spinal cord, the cerebellum, the cerebrum, the hippocampus, and other organs, by the methylene blue method, not only in the lower vertebrates but also in mammals. And, in fact, after several attempts, which led me to modify Bethe's method of fixation, I secured regularly sections which showed the organization of these regions pretty well.

It was not only the stimulus of scientific curiosity which led me to study Ehrlich's technique thoroughly, but there entered largely into my determination the desire, nay more, the urgent necessity to check through the revelations of a method which colours the cells and fibres while almost alive, the very clear and decisive, but somewhat capricious pictures produced by the method of Golgi. For, although most scientists accepted with complete confidence the very clear images of silver chromate, there were sceptics who suggested the possibility that some arrangements were artifacts, that is metallic deposits which did not correspond with preexistent structures.

It was therefore, absolutely necessary to show to everybody clear and decisive images, both of the spines on the dendrites and of other morphological features which I had discovered, by the use of technical methods entirely different from that of Golgi.

It was to this end that I directed persistent efforts at the close of 1896 and for almost the whole of 1897, during which time I made use almost exclusively of the methylene blue method of Ehrlich. My efforts, which were crowned with complete success, were varied, one turning upon the collateral spines, which had been denied, another concerning the neurons in the molecular layer of the cerebral cortex, and finally, the most extensive and important embracing the cerebellum, the cerebral cortex, the hippocampus, the spinal cord, etc.

The first communication demonstrated conclusively the existence of the dendritic spines in the pyramids of the cerebral cortex. In the most extensive and comprehensive paper, which was adorned with several phototypes, I succeeded in establishing, without the least possible doubt, the preexistence in the adult (rabbit, cat, dog, frog, and others) of the most important features revealed in embryos and young animals by the method of Golgi [collaterals of the white matter with their free arborizations (Fig. 59, *b*), axonic nests in the cerebellum and medulla oblongata, the morphology of the cerebellar granules, climbing and mossy fibres, etc.], thus refuting the sceptics with finality.

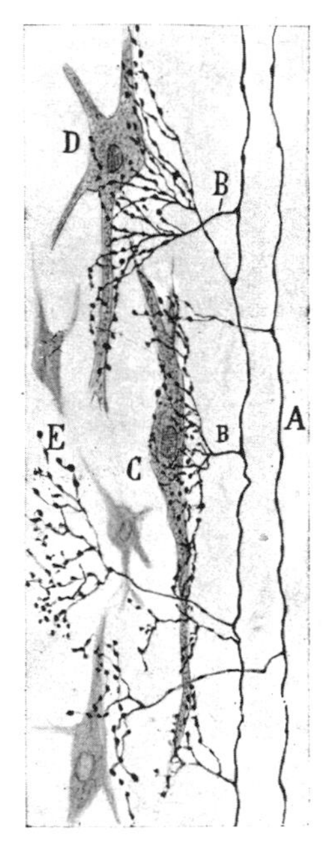

FIG. 59. NESTS FORMED ABOUT THE LARGE CELLS OF THE POSTERIOR HORN BY THE SENSORY COLLATERALS (Method of Ehrlich).

Besides these general results, of unquestionable critical value, the monograph cited contained several new observations. These were mostly concerned with the mode of origin of the bifurcations and of the collaterals (Fig. 60, *a*, *B*) which spring from constrictions in the nerve fibres, with the connections of the mossy fibres and other elements of the cerebellum, and with various types of terminations and cells in the other regions studied (Fig. 61, *A*).

The third monograph based upon the revelations of methylene blue was devoted to the cerebral cortex of the small mammals (cat, rabbit, and others) illustrating especially the structure of the first or plexiform layer, where, besides full confirmation of the results of the method of Golgi, there were described numerous new types of cells with short axons. Also, surrounding these, there is de-

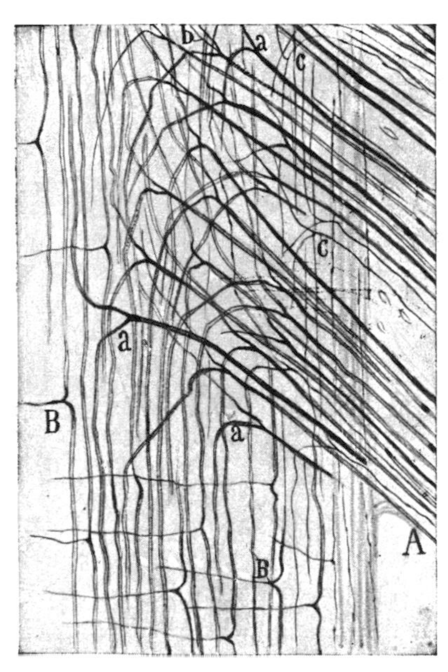

Fig. 60. The Bifurcation of the Sensory Root Fibres (*a*) and the collaterals of the white matter (*B*) in the spinal cord of the cat, as revealed by the method of Ehrlich. (Observe how the methylene blue confirms fully the revelations of silver chromate, the method of Golgi.)

scribed a special non-nervous net which was better studied later by Golgi, Donagio, Held, Bethe, and others and was the subject of much controversy. This is the *pericellular reticulum of Golgi,* so called from having been described exactly and minutely by this savant in 1898 (Fig. 62, *A, a*). Neither he nor his successors seem to have been aware of the true author of the discovery.

Finally, the last subject studied with the method of Ehrlich was the structure in the adult of the sensory spinal and cranial ganglia. In this investigation I had the collaboration, as preparator, of my assistant of the period, Don Federico Olóriz Ortega, the son of the eminent teacher of

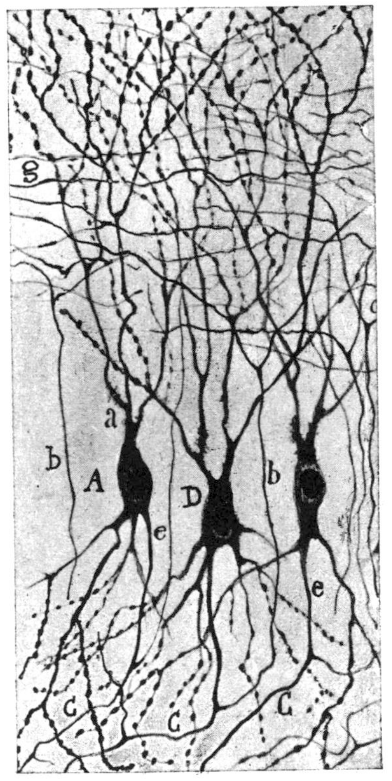

FIG. 61. LARGE PYRAMIDS OF THE HIPPOCAMPUS (Method of Ehrlich). *b*, recurrent axonic collaterals; *e*, axon. (The morphology corresponds exactly with that demonstrated by silver chromate.)

anatomy whom I have mentioned with deserved praise in former chapters. The monograph referred to, besides confirming in the cranial ganglia some discoveries of Dogiel as to the morphology of the unipolar cells in the spinal ganglia, contains an account of certain intracapsular, stellate cells of problematical nature, provisionally designated preganglionic satellite cells (Fig. 63, *A*, *B*) and a

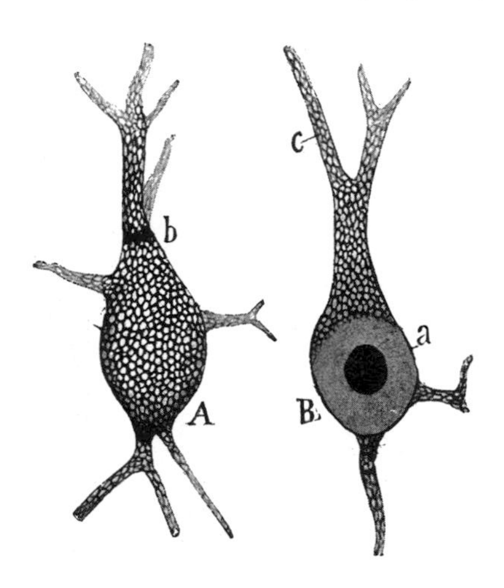

FIG. 62. CELLS WITH SHORT AXONS OF THE CEREBRAL CORTEX. *a*, superficial net on the cell membrane (Ehrlich's methylene blue).

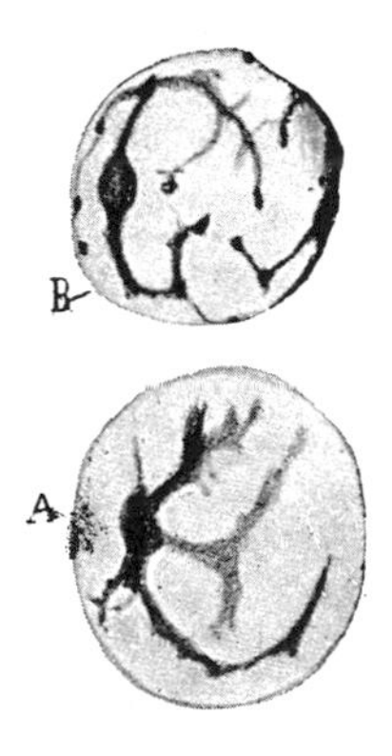

FIG. 63. SATELLITE CELLS ROUND THE SENSORY GANGLION CELLS OF THE CAT (Method of Ehrlich).

description of curiously complicated systems of nerve endings at the origin of the axons of the sensory cells.

CHAPTER XIII

Character sketches of some national figures: Castelar, Salmerón, Giner de los Ríos, Morayta, etc.

In order to interrupt the monotonous and insufferable narrative of my researches (I am not unaware that I am writing for two different publics), I am going to give my readers the rather brief and superficial impressions which I received of some notables of the capital during the years 1892 to 1896. The reader will understand that, as I was an enthusiast for the works and speeches of Castelar (we were almost all such during and after the *Gloriosa*), the most ardent of my desires was to know by sight the great tribune of the Revolution.

It was an unspeakable satisfaction for me to be presented in the *tertulia* of the great patriot by a fellow-student of mine, J. Gimeno Vizarra, then a professor in the University of Zaragoza, and editor of a *posibilista* daily (*Diario de Avisos*). At first, looking at the great man in his intimate circle, he did not give me the impression of a tribune of the people, but rather of a lofty and refined aristocrat. A glance about the room confirmed this first judgment. There hung from the walls numerous shields of honour, wreaths of gold, and pictures of great value, presented by reverent admirers or grateful Corporations. A multitude of *objets d'art* distributed here and there bore witness to the fine and lordly taste of their owner and to the veneration and generosity of his followers.

Like nearly all men of great ability, Castelar was short in stature. He displayed the obesity of the *gourmet,* his head was round and bald, his colour swarthy, his eyes large and dominating, his face clean-shaven, except for an imposing mustache in the style of Victor Emanuel, his voice strong and high-pitched; but when he spoke, he was transfigured, and acquired unsuspected elegance and distinction.

As those who heard him will remember, Castelar was not only the artistic, solemn, and somewhat theatrical orator of the great parliamentary debates; he was also a most facile, delightful, and picturesque conversationist. He might not convince, but he always fascinated or charmed. His coreligionists heard him with enchantment and, apparently, complete conviction. Eloquence is always right. Lulling them with his trills, the *Spanish canary* as Taine disdainfully called him, inhibited every effort at criticism and almost even the faculty of thought.

I also was in ecstasy before that torrent of sonorous words which sometimes, as they met and combined in synthesis, comparison, and contrast, produced unimagined splendours. Through that head, overflowing with imagery, there had passed the great figures of history and of literature; but there had passed also, leaving an ineffaceable trace, the romantic breath of Chateaubriand, Victor Hugo, Lamartine, and Michelet.

Gimeno presented me as a fervent follower of the study of the cells of the world, almost inscrutable, of the infinitely small, and as one more worshipper of his great talents as a writer and as a statesman.

"You do well," he said to me. "Life is a secret and the cell deserves our attention all the more in that we carry it within us and that it often influences our actions."

I boasted at that time, not without a certain amount of petulance, unshakably materialistic views; but, divining the sincere spiritualism of Castelar, I suppressed carefully an irreverent remark which came to my mind. "No," I should have replied to the incomparable orator if respect and veneration had not sealed my lips, "those tiny cells, which keep hidden in their minuteness the mystery of life, are *the whole man,* in his two aspects, rational and physiological. Unified by the division of labour, they react to the stimuli of the environment, give us the illusion of free-will, and, in fine, perform our actions in their completeness."

Afterwards, the conversation became general. Castelar, who delighted in talking, passed among the groups of his supporters, gave each some advice and encouragement, had, in a word, the desired promise and loyal consideration for everybody. But at times, descending from his august level of authority, he jested and satirized, not without wit, and even made sharp personal remarks. With what sorrow, I heard him criticise harshly Salmerón, whom I specially admired at that time! His words are still deeply engraved upon my memory, among them a comparison, perhaps not very respectful for the upright ex-president of the former Republic, but quite expressive and intentional.

"Suppose," he said, "that I put poison in this goblet. So long as it is there we are in no danger; but take care not to ingest the toxin, for then the catastrophe will happen. Well, then; Salmerón, the incorrigible doctrinarian, is the deadly poison of the republican banquet. So long as he remains outside our party, the danger is nothing; but so soon as we have the weakness to receive him, we bid farewell to the advent of the new Republic, of that orderly Republic which we all desire."

I confess that, in spite of my unmixed veneration for Castelar, the ill-feeling evidenced towards Salmerón disillusioned me considerably.

As I left the assembly, accompanied by my friend, I expressed the admiration which I felt for the magician with words and the indomitable patriot, whom I regarded also as an exalted character, unsullied, apart from some little personal prejudices, by pettiness or improprieties. But Gimeno, smiling slyly, cut me short with this disheartening remark:

"Friend Ramón: I share your burning enthusiasm for the politician and the patriot. We all revere him and trust that with his very ready ability to attract the sympathies of the army and of the conservative classes, we shall soon succeed in establishing a sound and stable republic. For the rest—do not deceive yourself. No one here has quite unsoiled hands, not even our leader, who, since he lives by his work, is supposed to be one of the least contaminated by the defects of spoils-distributing and favouritism. Castelar, I am sorry to say, is an irrestrainable spendthrift, and he is harassed by debts and besieged by unscrupulous persons. A little while ago, to pay off a pressing obligation, he used his powerful influence with the authorities to enable a certain creditor who owned a productive gambling house and was accused of homicide to flee abroad unpunished.[1] I shall not tell you anything else lest I discourage you completely.

I was stupefied at hearing of such contemptible actions. I was unable to understand how a man whose books paid splendidly, whose party associates filled his house with gifts of every kind, and who had no family (he was a bachelor and lived with a sister), would accept the more or less interested gifts or loans of an unscrupulous parasite.

The politician-philosopher Salmerón, to whom I had not the pleasure of being presented, I knew only in his lecture room. He was tall, slender, lean, and a little round shouldered, with noble features and eager searching eyes, which seemed to look right into one; his high and capacious skull was hairless, as if the fire of ideas had calcined the roots of the hairs; and his whole person shone with a certain attractive simplicity and a goodness and rectitude proof against temptations.

In his classroom, which I attended for about a month, he lectured "with supreme eloquence" (to quote the phrase of Castelar, who made a display in Congress of exquisite courtesy even to his worst enemies). He employed the Socratic method with his students. There was no maintaining a dogmatic attitude on the lecture platform; nor were there any oratorical mannerisms.

Every day he elucidated for his students, simply and paternally, some subject of logic, ethics, or metaphysics. He seemed to be preoccupied particularly with the theory of knowledge and the problem of criticism. Generally, the master confined himself to overcoming objections or dis-

[1] I do not guarantee the accuracy of this story, which, besides, was passed from mouth to mouth. It may have been a caluminous rumour which Gimeno had heard innocently, being deceived by ill-disposed persons.

sipating errors and obscurities. The aim of the professor, so far as I could understand, was to oblige his students to discuss things for themselves. Hence, rather than a course in metaphysics, the instruction acquired the character of a dialectic fencing bout and, especially, a strong inspiration to meditate earnestly upon the great problems of the spirit and of nature. When a boldly straightforward or somewhat presumptuous pupil defended warmly some questionable proposition, he kindly reminded him of the more or less probable solutions of the problem advanced by the various schools of philosophy. Everyone listened to him with profound respect; indeed more, with an unction almost religious. They took notes upon the ideas which escaped from the thinker in his eloquent improvisations, the more carefully since there was no text book or fixed programme.

What was the philosophy of Salmerón? I confess that, in listening to him for a month, I could not determine it; and, what is more, neither did many of his disciples know it definitely. On the whole, after talking it over in the halls with one of the most clear-sighted and judicious of them, I reached the conclusion that the former krausist, he of the difficult and labyrinthine definitions in the style of Sanz del Río, had become a positivist or perhaps an agnostic. The books of Compte, Littré, Huxley, Darwin, Haeckel, Herbert Spencer and above all, the inspiring lessons received directly from Claude Bernard during his stay in Paris had accomplished this almost incredible revolution. The glory of science had dissipated the mists of metaphysics, which, in the teaching of Salmerón, seemed to me to be reduced to a mere critical history of human thought.

In this case, the man was worth as much as the orator and the thinker. What a great pity it is that Salmerón did not write a book! We who loved and venerated him would have been able to establish from his works—I may presume—the wisdom and profundity of the master. To me, apart from his other merits, he had the privilege of all sincere men of talent: disinterestedly to change his mind.

To develop and to become purified: that is the touchstone of exalted characters and of great and noble understandings.

An excellent impression was produced upon me likewise by the learned lectures of Giner de los Ríos, the great teacher, whose ability was rivalled only by his modesty. He taught legal philosophy. He was so scrupulous intellectually and lived so far above the childish presumption of those instructors for whom only the subject they expound has importance, that a month after the beginning of the course he was still discussing with his students whether the conception of a philosophy of law was legitimate and acceptable.

In proof of his extensive culture, I have a reminiscence. Mingling with the group of many admirers which accompanied him, listening to his words, after he left the class, I dared to raise incidentally the unfathomable problem of inheritance and of the biological causes of death in the animal series. I had recently read Goette and Weismann, besides the highly suggestive books of Darwin and Herbert Spencer, whose biological principles fascinated me; and naturally I wished to shine before the group of spectators, defending the thesis that natural death, a phenomenon unknown in protozoa and microbes, constitutes an outstanding advance in the metazoa and vertebrates, brought about as a result of the federation of the living units, the division of labour, and the separation of the *soma,* or aggregate of the tissue cells, from the germ cell, which is virtually immortal and transmits the characteristics of the species.

This conception, now very commonplace but then quite new, expounded in a company of lawyers, offered all the piquant savour of scientific paradox. As was to be expected, my fellow-students for the moment heard me with astonishment. Their looks seemed to say: "Who may this bold fellow be, who presumes to unfold such absurd and daring ideas before the master?" But Giner, though unacquainted with the presumptuous intruder, defended me against my distrustful and scowling companions with admirable calmness and discretion, and explained in a neat and attractive manner the bold conceptions of Weismann, illustrating them with fresh and first-hand examples. In sum, he conveyed the impression that concerning all the great problems of inheritance, life, and death, the elderly professor had read much more than I.

In the classroom of the eminent teacher I witnessed one day the most notable act of modesty and intellectual honesty that I know of.

I do not remember what subject Giner was discussing. The variety of opinions brought out and the order and clearness of the exposition (it must not be forgotten that Giner was a great orator, but of the stuff, so rare among us, of the restrained, precise, and logical speakers) showed quite clearly that the master had prepared the lesson conscientiously. After a quarter of an hour, we noticed with surprise that his words, lucid and always at the service of his thought, became gradually halting and that the ideas lost vigour and clarity. There was a moment in which we admirers feared that, perhaps as a result of some pathological condition, the professor was going to become incoherent. Conscious of his condition, Giner, without changing countenance in the least, broke off his lecture with this remark, which filled me with astonishment, accustomed as I was to the flowery and endless perorations of some professors: "I cannot continue the lecture, gentlemen. There exists a certain incompatibility between the excessive abundance of data, which muddle the memory, and expedition and correctness of expression. We never talk better than when we have studied little, nor worse than when we have devoted many early morning hours to the scrupulous preparation of a lecture. So let us leave the subject for another day."

Those of us who have lived for many years bound like galley-slaves to the oar of the daily lesson know just how true is the foregoing observation. For myself, I can say that I am never more fluent and verbose than when, after a long and refreshing sleep, I improvise a lecture without having consulted a text-book or talked it over with anyone. Naturally, persistent wakefulnes and lengthy and concentrated reading produce the opposite effect. It is only that almost all we professors would consider ourselves disgraced if we were to present the spectacle of our inability to fill the regulation hour, with something left over, though to do so, we may be obliged to ramble on foolishly, ignoring the sad protests of a weary brain, which goes round in circles and repeats platitudes, or jumps disconnectedly between the most interesting subjects.

Of my visits to other classes, I have less definite recollections.

I shall speak only of Menéndez Pelayo, who stuttered like Cervantes, but was so learned and eloquent that his students forgot his hesitant speech in gathering the rich honey of his vast and exhaustive literary studies; and of Morayta, professor of history, who, though he did not attain the richness of diction and of imagination of Menéndez Pelayo, expounded the history of Greece clearly and methodically, hurling anathemas against the aristocratic, conceited, and disagreeable Lacedemonians and intoning fervent canticles in praise of democratic Athens, the focus in which ancient culture was concentrated and of which the rays still light European civilization.[2]

In all the foregoing excursions through the university, the Athenaeum, and some political and literary circles, I gained something precious and incalculable: the measure of ability and the standards of good expository method. The reader will readily understand that, having been educated in a remote provincial region and lacking special aptitude for the art of beautiful speech, this standard, while it could not transform me nor improve me in essentials, was highly profitable for my later professorial activities.

[2] In the foregoing descriptions I have tried to revive the impressions received during my first years in Madrid, without adding any present judgment. Obviously, today, after thirty-one years have passed (I write in 1923), I should have to modify some opinions and even to put a damper on some enthusiasms.

CHAPTER XIV

Theories and facts. Rigidness and constancy of histological facts. Instrumental character of hypothesis. Advisability of cultivating it from time to time, but without trusting it too much. Physiological conclusions drawn from the morphology of the neurons. Histological explanation of habit, of mental progress in the zoological scale, of talent, and of genius. Conjectures on the mechanism of sleep, attention, and association. Rigid economy which holds sway in the creations of life; laws of parsimony of space, of material, and of time of conduction.

Whoever cultivates histology or its related branches, bacteriology and embryology, with more or less success will sometimes have heard his expository enthusiasm checked by such disconcerting comments as the following:

"A magnificent lucubration! But can such a beautiful picture be a true one? The histology of today affirms those things, but will the histology of tomorrow also maintain them? As biology develops, who will accept, a century hence, the present histological doctrines?"

I will reply frankly. He who makes such remarks, besides displaying inexcusable ignorance of the essentially objective character of the microscopic sciences, confounds pitifully the fact of observation, a fixed and permanent idea, with the theoretic interpretation, which is essentially mutable and adaptable.

To distrust the reality of histological observations is equivalent to supposing that the new species discovered by the naturalist runs the risk of immediate disappearance; that the ganglion, the gland, or the vessel detected by the anatomist is in danger of evaporating; or, finally, that the star found by the astronomer is threatened with sudden extinction. Can the nature of the instrument of observation change the reality of the facts?

It may, perhaps, be argued that, in spite of all this, there is sometimes disagreement about the facts in the histological sciences. It is true that a revising and slightly sceptical attitude was fully justified fifty or sixty years ago, when minute anatomy, still in its infancy, lacked precise and definitive methods of staining. But today, fortunately, things have improved radically. Besides the fact that scientific criticism has become more exacting and scrupulous, not granting its stamp of approval except to structural features revealed conjointly and with agreement by very different techniques; present-day methods of colouration, the so-called selective methods, provide images so clear, neat, and full of contrast with the colourless background, that it would be absurd to harbour the slightest doubt as to their pre-existence.

Naturally, as time goes on, the viewpoint from which they are regarded may change, as may the physiological interpretations attached to them, but without their objective character being impaired. At the present moment there is a preference for discussion of general physiological hypotheses and biological theories (the mechanism of heredity, of adaptation and variation, of sexuality, of the physiological rôle of the organs and tissues, etc.)—and these will be discussed as long as the science of life does not attain ideal completeness of its data nor mount to the sphere of ultimate causes. But, I repeat, the first hand histological datum, well described and presented, constitutes something fixed and absolutely stable, against which neither time nor men have any power.

To leave this doctrine fully appreciated, I shall cite a concrete example taken from my own modest neurological investigations. I refer to the neuron concept now held by the great majority of histologists.

Let us imagine that there is discovered an exquisitely selective method of colouration, through which there is revealed an extremely delicate system of anastomotic fibres, absolutely invisible with existing procedures, extending between my nests, and climbing or mossy fibres, on the one hand, and the bodies and dendrites of the neurons on the other. In such a case, the leaves would not represent the ultimate processes of the tree; the arborizations of the axons and the spines of the dendrites which I have described would be preterminal, instead of terminal.

Would anything have been lost with this marvellous advance? Would the nests, the end plates and calyces, the ramifications of the axons, the spines of the dendrites and many other arrangements of contact be converted thereby into figments of the intellect? By no means. These forms would preserve intact their objective value and their character as general anatomical facts. Only one thing would require to be corrected; the physiological interpretation. From the utilitarian point of view, such arrangements could no longer be justified by the need for assuring the passage of the impulses by multiplying the surfaces of contact. Consequently the hypothesis of transmission by contact would have to be replaced by another; that of propagation through continuity. And it would be necessary to ascertain in some other way the dynamic significance of the above mentioned structures. Once more the provisional character of our theoretical interpretations and the unavoidable need of revising and perfecting them in accordance with new discoveries would be made apparent.

Precisely from fear of these possible errors (the history of biology is full of them), I am a fervent adept of the religion of facts. It has been said innumerable times, and I also have repeated it,[1] that "facts remain and theories pass away"; that every investigator who trusts unduly in the solidity and correctness of general conceptions and disdains the direct study of reality runs the risk of leaving no lasting trace of his activity; that facts are our only positive possession, our real estate, and our best charter of nobility; in fine, that in the eternal mutations of all things, they alone will be saved—and with them, perhaps, a part, the best, of our individual personalities—from the outrages of time and the indifference or the injustice of mankind.

All this is obvious; but it is certain also that, without

[1] Cajal: Reglas y consejos sobre la investigación biológica.

theories and hypotheses, our tale of positive facts would be pretty insignificant, and would grow very slowly. The hypothesis and the objective datum are linked together by a close etiological relationship. Apart from its conceptual or explanatory value, theory contains an instrumental value also. To observe without thinking is as dangerous as to think without observing. Theory is our best intellectual tool; a tool, like all others, liable to be notched and to rust, requiring continual repairs and replacements, but without which it would be almost impossible to make a deep hollow in the marble block of reality.

For the anatomist, the histologist, and the embryologist, bound to the hard bench of analysis, the building up of general principles is, besides, in obedience to logical tendencies and almost unrestrainable impulses. It is extremely difficult to check the impulses of the imagination when it is pushed aside and loudly claims its turn to do something. It is forced upon us, moreover, by the very mode of action of our thinking mechanism, which is essentially practical and purposive, and presents to us every day the problem of the mechanical causes and the utilitarian motives. A structural or morphological arrangement having been observed, there invariably rises in our minds the question: "What physiological or psychological service does it render the organism?" In vain does common sense, battling with such tendencies, check our curiosity, reminding us that the problem has been presented prematurely, long before all the indispensable data have been procured. Such a discreet reflection, while it may make us more circumspect, does not, however, paralyze the process of theorizing. The fantasy goes on dauntlessly, building upon sand, as if it did not know the irremediable frailty of its work. And it is useless to affirm, with Goethe and many modern thinkers, that the search for final causes has no sense; that our task is to determine the *how* and not the *why*. Our mind, which for thousands and perhaps millions of years has been questioning nature purely for utilitarian and selfish ends, cannot change its mode of looking at the world all at once.

Nor must we forget that in the biological sciences, to arrive at the *how,* that is, at the physico-chemical process which moulds the organic arrangements, it is necessary to pass through the preliminary *to what end* of inexpert and insatiate curiosity.

All this is glaringly contradictory, but it is fatally human. Reason and feeling never were good friends. Those who feel such a speculative urge know only too well how ephemeral the work of the great systematizing finalists usually is in biology. And yet—

All the foregoing preamble, for which I beg the reader's pardon, is intended to excuse, so far as possible, my speculative cavorts—fortunately few in number—and to explain how an unconquerable fanatic in the religion of facts fell, from time to time, into the weakness of sacrificing to the idol of dazzling and fascinating theory, in spite of being at heart convinced of its irreparable fugaciousness and notwithstanding having declared repeatedly that 'if as a result of unrestrainable impulses we form hypotheses, we should try, at least, not to believe in them too firmly.' We must not become intoxicated with either our own wine or that of others.

My conscience being relieved a little by this spontaneous confession, I shall proceed to a brief account of the lucubrations of my imagination during the three years under discussion. And first comes the declaration that among the conjectures and hypotheses of my own invention there are some which appear to me worthy and easily defensible even now, after twenty-five years of ceaseless progress; and there are some, on the other hand, frankly improbable, temerarious, and inacceptable. I shall dwell upon the former, naturally, more than upon the latter, which deserve only oblivion. Finally, a few belonging to the first category rank, according to my judgment, in the class of solidly founded empirical laws.

My first work of a theoretical nature was one which bore the title *General Considerations on the Morphology of the*

Nerve Cell and which was sent to the International Medical Congress held in Rome in 1894.

This communication was concerned mainly with an examination of the laws governing the evolution of the nervous system in the animal series and an indication, so far as possible, of which centres have preserved potentially their pristine plasticity during the innumerable incidents of development, being capable of adapting themselves structurally to the ever more varied and complex conditions of the Cosmos, and which are the centres, essentially animal, that are, as it were, ankylosed by an age-old automatism and that, objecting to any accommodation, have brought their history to an end almost absolutely.

With due regard for brevity, I shall enumerate rapidly the principal conclusions in this communication.

(*a*) The embryonic development of nervous tissue recapitulates briefly, with some simplifications and omissions, its racial history, both in respect of the neuroglia and in that of the nerve cell.

(*b*) From the point of view of racial development, there are simultaneously in all vertebrates two nervous systems: the sensory (peripheral ganglia, retina, olfactory bulb, spinal cord, cerebellum, thalamus, corpus striatum, etc.) which has finished developing by differentiation and progresses only by extension; and the cerebro-cortical (gray cerebral cortex with its convolutions), which continues to perfect itself in the animal series both by extension and by structural and morphological differentiation of its elements.

(*c*) The law of morphological progress with increasing functional adaptation is expressed in the neurons by the formation and lengthening of new processes and, consequently, by multiplication and diversification of intercellular connections.

(*d*) On the basis of numerous comparative observations, it was affirmed that the size of the nerve cell body and the diameter of the axon are not related to physiological specialization but are proportional to the richness and the extent of the terminal arborizations and, consequently, to the amplitude and diversity of the connections.

(*e*) By comparing the morphology and relative abundance of axonic and dendritic collaterals of the cerebral pyramids in the vertebrate scale, the conclusion was reached that intellectual power, and its most noble expressions, talent and genius, do not depend on the size or number of the cerebral neurons, but on the richness of their connective processes, or in other words on the complexity of the association pathways to short and long distances. That abundance of white matter indicates richness of connections and, therefore, superior intellectual rank was a thesis already defended at an earlier time by Meynert and Flechsig, although, in the absence of methods selective of the cell processes, they, naturally, could found it only on the gross structure of the gray and white matter, as demonstrated by inefficient methods (carmine, haematoxylin, Weigert's technique, etc.).

(*f*) Adaptation and professional dexterity, or rather the perfecting of function by exercise (physical education, speech, writing, piano-playing, mastery in fencing, and other activities) were explained by either a progressive thickening of the nervous pathways (suggestion made by Tanzi and Lugaro) excited by the passage of the impulse or the formation of new cell processes (non-congenital growth of new dendrites and extension and branching of axone collaterals) capable of improving the suitability and the extension of the contacts, and even of making entirely new connections between neurons primitively independent.

This last hypothesis, which has considerable probability, and which lends itself, as the reader will imagine, to interesting rhetorical and psychological developments, was also enunciated, and illustrated with some examples and comparisons, in my London lecture of the same year.

Naturally, in interpreting pyschologically the features of cellular morphology, I was far from excluding the part which, in course of time, for the purpose of explaining histologically habit, talent, and genius, would have to be attributed to the most subtle warp of the nervous protoplasm, of the complexity of which our ever increasing knowledge had not reached the supreme culmination of today. The neurofibrils and the endocellular apparatus of Golgi were then unknown, and the discovery of the Nissl granules was still quite recent.

Inspired by the same spirit, I made public in 1897 another synthetic work, designed to inquire into the principles of a utilitarian character which seem to govern the infinite variations in form, size, position, and direction of the neurons and of the conducting fibres. I may say, in passing, that I had the honour of delivering a lecture upon the same subject in the Athenaeum of Madrid.[2]

All these fluctuations in situation and morphology, and even the formula of axipetal polarization itself, seem to be determined, from the teleological point of view, by these three economic principles:

(*a*) Conservation of material (development of the shortest path between two related regions);

(*b*) Conservation of time of conduction (a dynamic consequence of the preceding);

(*c*) Conservation of space.

In the foregoing works the speculative development follows the observed facts very closely. The general conceptions referred to (the law of progress in the morphology of the neurons, the hypothesis regarding functional adaptation, standards of economy regulating the disposition of the cell body, etc.) are legitimate deductions or plausible hypotheses. All are susceptible to confirmation *a posteriori*, by comparison with the infinite variety of neuronal forms.

This severe and salutary correspondence with empirical data does not shine forth, unfortunately, in another com-

[2] As a matter of fact, as a reward for this discourse and for a complete course given in 1897 and 1898 upon my modest scientific investigations, the illustrious President of the Athenaeum, Don Segismundo Moret, who always honoured me with his kindness, and the executive committee, zealous in stimulating and honouring every enthusiastic cultivator of science or art, accorded me the title of *honorary member*.

munication, published in 1895, on the histological mechanism of association, ideation, and attention. Passing over certain conceptions which I believe to hit the mark, unfounded imagination has run riot in this whole venturesome lucubration.

The useful ideas are that of *unity of impression* and, more especially, the law of the neural avalanche, which is formulated thus: every peripheral impression received by the dendrites (sensory) of a single cell is propagated towards the centres in the fashion of an avalanche; or, in other words, the number of neurons concerned in the conduction increases progressively from the periphery to the cerebrum, in the convolutions of which (tertiary sensory areas) is the base of the cone of general influx and the origin of new connecting pathways. From this anatomo-physiological law, which is founded upon numerous investigations on the organization of the visual, acoustic, olfactory, and other paths, Tanzi and Lugaro profited greatly in their explanation of the probable mechanism of hallucination, association of ideas, and other important psychological processes.

Conceptions such as the others enunciated fall rapidly into deserved oblivion, for science is interested only in ideas open to experimental verification and stimulative to further work.

In closing this chapter, I shall mention two events which were rich in results for the stimulation and prosecution of my scientific work.

The first was the establishment, at the cost of no small pecuniary sacrifices, of my *Revista trimestral micrografica*,[3] with the object of publishing rapidly, and without having to wait for the editors of national or foreign periodicals, the works in microscopy of the Laboratory of the Faculty of Medicine and at the same time to stimulate the efforts of my pupils. In this publication appeared many of the communications enumerated in the present chapter and nearly

[3] The first number saw the light in March, 1897.

all of those which appeared thereafter, until 1901, in which year, the annual entitled *Trabajos del Laboratorio de investigaciones biologicas* was founded with official backing.

The first numbers of the said *Revista* were almost exclusively written by its editor. A little later, when the beginning of a school had been created, I was efficiently supported by, among other enthusiastic followers, my brother, Pedro Ramón Cajal, then professor of histology in Cadiz, who contributed no less than eight extensive monographs upon various comparative neurological subjects (fishes, reptiles, birds, and amphibians); R. Terrazas,[4] a student interne, with his interesting studies of cerebellar neurogenesis and those on cartilaginous tissue; the young Mallorcan, Blanes Viale, a most outstanding student (he also died in his flower, before he had finished his course), with a certain careful study of the olfactory bulb; Sala Pons, a former pupil in Barcelona, with his studies on the cerebral cortex of birds and the spinal cord of amphibians; Olóriz Aguilera, whose collaboration in my inquiries into the structure of the ganglia I have already mentioned; Carlos Calleja who was then an assistant in the faculty and was the author of a valuable communication on the olfactory cerebral cortex; and finally, Isidoro Lavilla, the present professor in Valladolid, who contributed two important studies, one on the intestinal sympathetic system and the other on the acoustic centres of mammals.

The second occurrence, very flattering to me, was my unsought election to membership in the Royal Academy of Sciences of Madrid. There is an anecdote in connection with this designation, which I shall mention because it reflects much honour on the patriotism and independence of that learned body.

One of the more conspicuous academicians, who had returned from Berlin, told his associates that the great Virchow, then at the height of his splendour and glory, had

[4] This brilliant pupil died when he had just graduated as doctor in consequence of typhoid fever contracted in the first district of which he was titular physician.

surprised him with a question which he could not answer: "What is Cajal busy with just now? Is he continuing his interesting studies?"

Our exalted academician was confused and somewhat ashamed that interest should be inspired in Berlin by the work of a Spaniard of whom he had never heard and took steps to satisfy his curiosity when he returned to the Peninsula. From his conversations with the learned astronomer, Don Miguel Merino, the memorable perpetual secretary, there arose an agreement to propose and support my candidacy for a certain vacancy which was then being contested. I have then the unusual privilege of being an academician upon the nomination of R. Virchow and of Don Miguel Merino.

The preparation of my inaugural discourse, which took place in 1897,[5] gave me an opportunity to expound, *ex abundantia cordis,* some rules and counsels designed to awaken the taste and passion for scientific investigation in our young teachers, whose interests lay largely elsewhere. I devoted special effort to making laboratory work desirable and attractive, and to that end I employed simple, sincere language, overflowing with infectious enthusiasm and with fervent patriotism. Its success surpassed my hopes. Such a flattering reception did my fiery address receive among the university public and in the press that the official edition was rapidly exhausted and my excellent friend, Dr. Lluria, making up for my lassitude, considered it necessary to republish it at his own expense, generously destining the new and very large edition to be distributed gratis among the students and in various educational centres.

While I am on the subject of distinctions and honours, I may mention also that in 1897, I was elected to membership in the Royal Academy of Medicine of Madrid; that this illustrious body awarded me a few months previously the Rubio prize (1000 pesetas) for the publication of a textbook, then recent, *Elementos de Histología;* that, in 1896,

[5] Reglas y consejos sobre la investigación biológica. See bibliography.

the *Société de Biologie* of Paris spontaneously awarded me the Fauvelle prize (1000 francs) in recognition of my work; that about the same time, the famous University of Würzburg,[6] on the occasion of the inauguration of the new university building, conferred upon me, along with several illustrious professors, the degree of doctor *honoris causa;* that a couple of years before (1895), the Physico-medical Society of the same Bavarian city, at the suggestion, no doubt, of my illustrious friend, Dr. A. Kölliker, appointed me a corresponding member; and, finally, that I was honoured with the same distinction at that period by the Academy of Medicine of Berlin, the Psychiatrical Society of Vienna, the Biological Society of Paris, the Italian Psychiatrical Society, and the Academy of Medical Sciences of Lisbon, and others.

[6] As was recorded by the Neue Würzburger Zeitung, a newspaper which gave a detailed account of the celebration, the ceremony of inauguration of the sumptuous edifice of the *Alma Julia* was very solemn. There were present various ministers of the Crown, the Rector, the Deans of the four Faculties, and representatives of all the German universities. Many discourses were delivered, among them a very eloquent one by the Rector, Professor von Leube. At the end of the proceedings the honorary doctorates were conferred, this honour being shared with me, as concerns the Faculty of Medicine, by the illustrious master of Stockholm, Dr. G. Retzius, and the great reformer of organic chemistry, Dr. Fischer, of Leipzig.

CHAPTER XV

My production in 1898 and 1899. Depressed by the colonial disaster, my productive force diminishes. Literature of the Regeneration: its infertility in the correction of national defects. Theory of the intercrossing of nerves and the structure of the "optic chiasma" in the animal series. Other less important papers.

My scientific work during the year 1898 was rather scanty and poor in new facts. This is easily understood: it was the year of the lamentable and insane war with the United States; a war brought on by the greed of our industrial exporters, the rapacity of our overseas employees, and the pride and untamed egoism of our politicians. Occasion for it was undoubtedly given by hereditary defects of the national character, among others a mistaken sense of honour and a certain gentlemanly punctilliousness, excusable in individuals but absurd and antinational in a people; but, more than anything, we were swept to the catastrophe by the disgraceful ignorance of our alternating political parties concerning the real magnitude and efficiency of our own and foreign military forces. For, although it seems absurd, at that time deputies, newspaper writers, soldiers, and others, honestly believed that our machinery of war in Cuba and the Philippines—vessels of wood and an army of invalids—could measure itself advantageously against the formidable equipment at the disposal of the enemy. The misfortune of a country is not in its weakness, but in the ignorance thereof of those whose inexcusable duty it is to know it.

It is but just, nevertheless, to recognize that such dangerous ignorance of international truths had its exceptions. Apart from the masses—who, having poured out their blood fruitlessly in two cruel campaigns, desired peace at any price—there were, even in the Ministry, men, like Sagasta and Moret, who saw the abyss into which the blind covetousness of the plutocrats and the unconscientiousness of the military authorities were leading us.

Bitter it is to recall how politicians so perspicacious and intelligent as Moret, Sagasta, and Canalejas, filled with the saving truth, yet lacked in the supreme hour the public-spirited courage required to proclaim it and to oppose energetically the opinions and feelings of the Crown, the army, and the press! So dangerous and difficult it is to make clear in the eyes of the public, as Pi y Margall did unflinchingly, that a nation of ninety million inhabitants, with immense wealth and inexhaustible industrial resources and military equipment, was bound to crush utterly a country of the utmost poverty, of seventeen million souls, and drained besides by four desolating civil wars!

However, let us not dwell upon sad memories, but return to our subject.

The recollection of the colonial disaster is perpetuated in my memory by chronological association with the writing of a paper with philosophical leanings on the fundamental organization of the optic pathways and the probable significance of the intercrossing of nerves,[1] one of the most peculiar and enigmatic anatomical arrangements in the vertebrates.

We were summering at the time along with the never-to-be-forgotten Olóriz in the picturesque town of Miraflores de la Sierra. The little villas in which we were lodging adjoined and thus our families were like one. Often, tired of chatting or reading we used to engage in a game of chess, of which Don Federico was very fond. In memory of the lamented master, I include here an intimate photograph, taken by one of my children during a very strenuous game (Fig. 64). As the day drew on, surfeited with reading or tense from the excitements of the game, we used to relax our brains by strolling along the road which winds at the foot of the Najarra and climbs to the Marcuera to end in the wonderful Monastery *del Paular*. During such healthful

[1] Cajal: Estructura del quiasma óptico y teoría general de los entrecruzamientos nerviosos. 1898.

PLATE 18

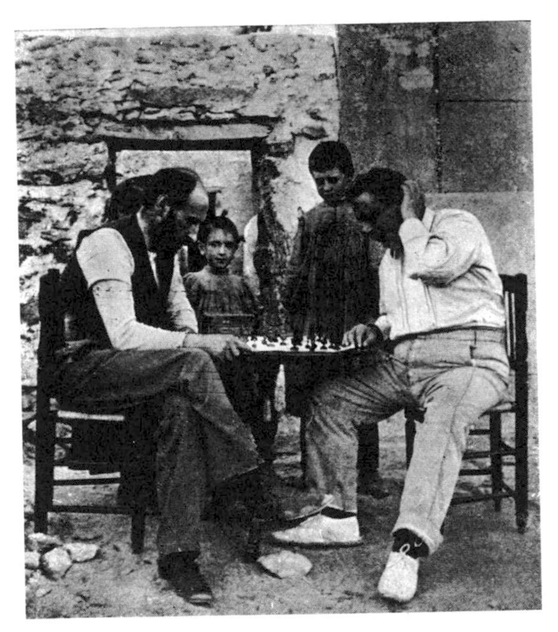

FIG. 64. DR. OLÓRIZ AND THE AUTHOR OCCUPYING THEIR VACATION LEISURE WITH A GAME OF CHESS (summer of 1898). I publish this picture in memory of the admirable professor, who departed this life far too early.

wanderings I used to enjoy imparting to my colleague the fruit of my meditations. Encouraged and confirmed by the approbation of my friend, I had almost completed the writing of my paper when in our peaceful retreat there fell like a bomb the dreadful and distressing news of the destruction of the squadron of Cervera and of the imminence of the surrender of Santiago de Cuba.

The tragic information interrupted my work brusquely, awakening me to bitter reality. I fell into profound depression. How could I philosophize when my country was in peril of death? And my brilliant theory of the optic decussation was laid aside *sine die.*

This weakening of the will—which was general among the cultured classes of the nation—drew me out of the laboratory, leading me, some months later, when the national consciousness emerged from its stupor, into the political arena. The press solicited urgently the opinions of all, great and small, as to the causes which had led to the dreadful catastrophe and the panacea for our ills. And I, like many others who were young then, listened to the voice of the newspaper siren and made a modest contribution to the excited and fiery literature of the regeneration, of which the eloquent apostles were, as is well known, the great Costa, Macías, Picavea, Paraíso, and Alba. Later the phalanx of the veterans was joined by some brilliant literary figures: Maeztu, Baroja, Bueno, Valle Inclán, *Azorín,* and others.

I believe sincerely that my declarations in *El Liberal, Vida Nueva,* and other daily papers [2] contained some just censures and pointed out some remedies which hit the mark. Nevertheless, today, at a distance of eighteen years, I can-

[2] As spiritual remedies I suggested the renunciation of international bullying, and of regarding as real progress what was really only a pale reflection of foreign civilization; the abandonment of the use of hyperbolical adjectives, of which we were always so prodigal in connection with our mediocre men; and, finally, the creation at any cost of an original culture. In the field of pedagogy I proposed the making of grants for study abroad to professors and doctors of ability; the addition to our university staffs of investigators of world renown; the abandonment of the weakening principle of seniority, with substitution of the German system of recruiting for the professoriate, etc., etc.

not reread those verbosities without some blushes. I am disgusted by some recriminations which were exaggerated or unjust, by the generally declamatory tone, and by a certain patriarchal and authoritative air unfitting in a humble scientific worker. What authority had a poor professor, far removed from social and political problems, to censure and correct?

Besides, rhetoric never checked the decadence of a country. We regenerators of '98 were read only by ourselves: like sermons, austere political preachings edify only those already convinced. The masses remain unmoved. It is sad to realize that truth does not reach the ignorant, because they neither read nor feel, and leaves cold, if not irritated, the adventurers and profiteers!

I see that I am again falling into tedious digressions. Taking up the thread of my narrative, I repeat that the dénouement of the colonial tragedy interrupted my meditations on the significance of the chiasma of vertebrates. At length, however, the waters receded to their channel and, recovering my equilibrium, I returned to my task with my old ardour. While my patriotism to Spain was humbled, my patriotism to the Spanish race remained alive and powerful and I may even say exalted. So I finally completed the paper referred to and went on planning new labours for the future.

The memoir cited, on the chiasma, comprises two parts: the first, exclusively anatomical, will always retain its value; the other, of a psychological nature, maintains views which were and still are subjects of lively controversy.

The anatomical inquiry was inspired by two radically revolutionary memoirs by Michel and by Kölliker which had recently appeared. There appears at times among scientists something like weariness of the consecrated truth. Iconoclastic and revolutionary fury extends even to the old. It is so tempting to the vanity to show that several generations of scientists have been wrong! Something of this sort must have been going on in the mind of Michel when he proclaimed, contrary to what had been generally believed since the time of Newton and is, besides, necessitated by undeniable physiological postulates, that the optic chiasma of man and the higher vertebrates (which have binocular vision of the fields common to the eyes) consists exclusively of crossed optic fibres; in consequence, the classic uncrossed optic tract, which joins each eye to the cerebral hemisphere of its own side, would be a mere anatomical illusion.[3]

In spite of the armament of histological proofs with which the savant cited supported his daring affirmations, the thesis of Michel caused general amazement. But the most serious thing was that some investigators of renown, and especially the venerable Kölliker, supported it with their prestige and even tried to bolster it up with new anatomical demonstrations. The drawings of the master of Würzburg, traced from irreproachable preparations by the method of Weigert, seemed conclusive. If this hypothesis prevailed, nevertheless, those of us who believed in the double optic path, an unavoidable physiological postulate, would have been unable otherwise to explain how we perceive only one visual image when the brain receives two almost identical (the requisite for vision in relief).

I was occupied at the time with the analysis of the visual centres of mammals and such a strange conclusion inspired me with invincible repugnance. It ought not to be, it could not be; unless nature, abandoning every law of higher harmony, delights in the superfluous and in the absurd. Appealing to observation, I proposed to study the matter thoroughly, attacking it with the most appropriate methods; the more so since, at the time, there were revolving in my imagination some conjectures aiming at a clarification of the enigma of the intercrossing of nerves. It is evident that before tacking my theory together I had to know definitely whether or not there existed homolateral fibres in the chiasma of man and of the primates.

I took the work in hand, then, making use of a wealth of material for study (fishes, amphibians, reptiles, birds, and

[3] Michel: Lehrbuch der Augenheilkunde, 2nd Aufl., 1890.

mammals). In place of the method of Weigert used by Kölliker (thin serial sections, in which the fibres appear cut off and are difficult to follow), I employed that of Ehrlich, with methylene blue, or that of Marchi (secondary degeneration after the ablation of an eye).

The result of such inquiries conformed absolutely with the traditional doctrine. Both techniques showed in mammals with binocular vision the existence of a very robust homolateral optic tract; in animals in which the presence of the said common visual field is hardly indicated (rabbit, guinea pig, mouse, etc.), the presence of a few homolateral fibres, the crossed ones predominating enormously; and, finally, in vertebrates with separate visual fields (fishes, amphibians, reptiles, and birds, in which vision is panoramic), the existence of a complete crossing over. The error of Michel and of Kölliker arose, as histological errors always do arise, from their having demanded of the method (that of Weigert) more than it could well give, filling in what was cut out in its revelations with over-venturesome interpretations. The drawings were correct, but the conclusions were erroneous.

Once the first important point had been determined, that is the unquestionable reality of the partial crossing of the primary optic paths, the time had come to see which of my conjectures as to the significance of crossings best squared with the variations in the organization of the chiasma and retina in the animal series and with the data and postulates of the physiology of vision.

We may state the problem just as my curiosity stated it then. It should be noted in passing that for the anatomical science of the period—with a closed horizon and confined to mere morphological description—there was no such problem. The pure anatomist, like the descriptive zoologist, is oblivious to all philosophical curiosity. When he has proclaimed that a crossing of the optic tracts is an anatomical rule in the vertebrates, he rests fully satisfied. This is incomprehensible mental inertia, for if anatomy and histology are to aspire to the rank of true sciences, it is essential that, like chemistry and astronomy, they concern themselves with the development of phenomena and become ever more dynamic and more causal.

Since I felt thus, I could abandon that passive and, as it were, beatific conformity which is the outcome of habit and extinguishes all etiological curiosity. I was profoundly surprised by one thing at which nobody else seemed to show surprise. The optic chiasma presented itself to me as something absurd or useless, which offends our sense of symmetry and of economy since, thanks to it, the optic conductors uselessly extend their course and create in the centres infinite compensatory complications.

"Would it not be simpler," I asked myself, "for each optic tract to debouch directly in the cerebral centres of its own side since the impression received by each retina arouses by preference motor reactions in the corresponding regions of the head, trunk, and upper extremity?"

But the apparent incongruities were repeated in the brain and in the bulb. The pyramidal tract of the cerebrum or of voluntary movements, the sensory columns coming from the cord and from the oblongata, the centrifugal bundles rising in the cerebellum also cross completely or nearly so.

And then, the absolute universality, the inevitable persistence of such decussations, which appear in the fishes and continue invariably right up to man! Actually, they are absent in no animal with lenticular vision, that is, provided with simple eyes in which the synthetic image is projected by a convergent lens. Recently I have recognized this crossing, although differently situated, in insects and cephalopods, of which the eye also conforms to the structural principles of the vertebrate.

"Perhaps," I thought, "the fundamental crossing of the optic tracts is necessarily bound up with the physical mechanism of vision. Let us seek then in this mechanism for the logical reason of such an organization. Once it is ascertained, nothing will be easier than to explain as compensatory and corrective arrangements, the primordial decussations of the motor and sensory pathways."

Rejecting other conjectures, I became possessed obsessively by the following thought: *Everything will have a simple explanation if it is admitted that the correct perception of an object implies the congruence of the cerebral surfaces of projection, that is those representing each point in space.* Hence, in order that the mental perception may be unified and may agree exactly with the external reality, or, in other words, in order that the image conveyed through the right eye may be continuous with that conveyed through the left eye, the intercrossing of the optic paths from side to side is quite necessary; a total crossing in animals with panoramic vision, a partial crossing in animals endowed with a common visual field.

The accompanying diagrams explain the foregoing theory clearly.

The first diagram (Fig. 65) shows the form and direction which the mental visual image would have had on the supposition that the optic nerves had not crossed. The incongruity of the two images is evident: that projected

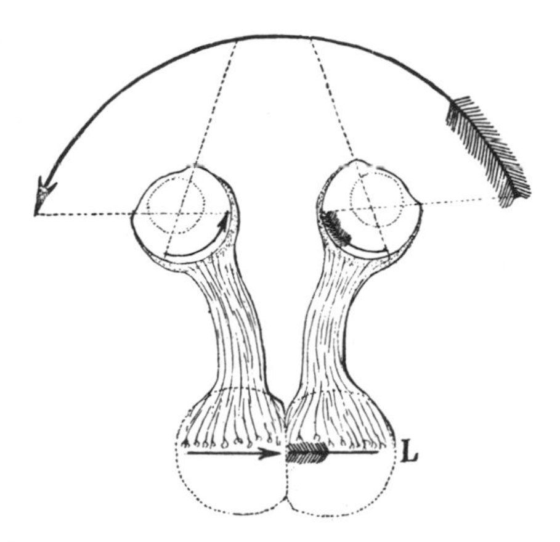

Fig. 65. Diagram to illustrate the incongruousness of the central projection of the images from the two eyes if there were no intercrossing of the optic nerves. *L*, optic lobes.

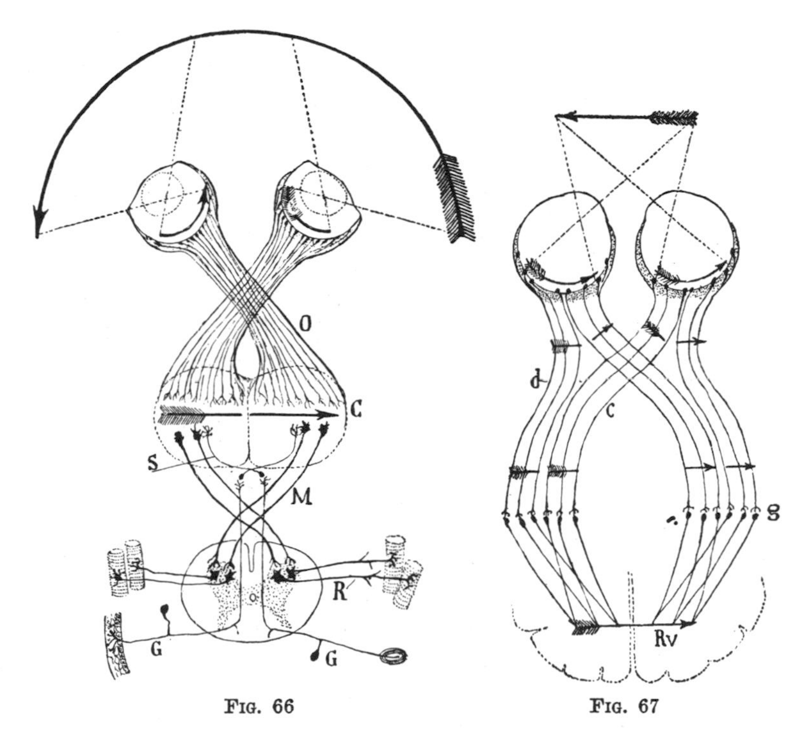

FIG. 66 FIG. 67

FIG. 66. Diagram to show the result of the complete intercrossing of the optic nerves in a lower vertebrate (fish, amphibian, reptile, bird, or mammal with panoramic vision). It will be seen that in consequence of this crossing the two central images form a continuous whole. *C*, primary and secondary visual centres; *G*, spinal ganglia and sensory roots; *M*, crossed motor pathway; *O*, crossed optic tracts; *S*, crossed central sensory pathway; *R*, motor roots of the spinal cord.

FIG. 67. Diagram to show how, in man and in mammals with stereoscopic vision, the central image is formed by combination of two representations of the object, transmitted by the two optic nerves. *c*, crossed optic fascicle; *d*, homolateral fascicle; *g*, external geniculate ganglion and pulvinar; *Rv*, visual region of the cerebral hemisphere, with the form of the mental projection.

through the right eye does not fit with that from the left eye, and it would be impossible for the animal to synthesize the two images into a continuous representation. The horizon would be presented as a panoramic view formed from two photographs, the right and left ones being laterally inverted.

Let us now examine the mental image resulting from the intercrossing of the optic nerves, an intercrossing adopted by nature in the case of lenticular eyes. Figure 66, *C*, shows with the greatest clearness that, thanks to the crossing, the two images, right and left, correspond and make a continuous panorama, the lateral inversion disappearing.

Things take place somewhat differently in the mammals, in which the double visual projection reproduces the same region of space. In these animals there exists the uncrossed tract (Fig. 67, *d*), through which the duplication of visual images is ingeniously avoided, while the advantages of the crossing are retained (Fig. 67).

Figure 66 shows also that the visual decussation has brought about the decussations of the principal voluntary motor and of the sensory paths.

This monograph contains also a description of an apparatus designed to make possible vision in relief of a double image projected by a lantern.

My ideas regarding the use of the decussations attained the flattering success of publicity. Besides being abstracted or reproduced in full by many foreign periodicals, they also had the honour of a good German translation, in book form, by Dr. Bressler; to this version a very kind prologue was written by the celebrated Professor Paul Flechsig, of Leipzig. Notwithstanding its defects, of which I am not unaware,[4] my theory suggested interesting studies. Among other researches it called forth that of Kölliker[5] already mentioned, rectifying former errors; that of Havet,[6] on the chiasma of crustaceans, which was fully confirmatory; and

[4] Honesty obliges me to confess that my paper contains doctrines of very unequal value. Today, after the passage of twenty-five years and the appearance of numerous investigations on the subject, I regard as a well-founded conception the explanation of the fundamental crossing of the optic nerves. I consider the corollary relative to the compensatory decussation of the motor and sensory paths as probable and plausible, no more; and some analysis and conclusions regarding the histological conditions of the perception of relief, as frankly hazardous.

[5] Kölliker: Neue Beobachtungen zur Anatomie des Chiasma opticum. Würzburg, 1899.

[6] Revista trimestral micrográfica, IV, 1899.

the very interesting one of Dr. Marquez,[7] in which the postulates of my conception were ingeniously and successfully applied to explaining the decussations of some motor nerves of the eyeball.

As was to be expected, the positive facts stated in my paper were received with applause and appreciated at their full value by the specialists in the field. But as to the theory proper, opinions differed. Lugaro and other savants advanced some ingenious objections and proposed other histological explanations. Without arrogance, I do not think that any of my opponents, former or recent, has succeeded in thinking of a more simple and natural purposive explanation of the fundamental crossing of the optic pathways in the lower vertebrates and of their incomplete crossing in man and mammals.

In connection with this theory it is important not to confound the conception of *usefulness,* which is undeniable in the immense majority of our organs and tissues, with that of *purposiveness,* a conception purely metaphysical, with the reality of which the biologist has nothing to do.

The remaining works of 1898 are listed in the bibliography.

[7] *Ibid.,* V, 1900.

CHAPTER XVI

My work during the years 1899 and 1900. New studies on the cerebral cortex, in which the human brain is attacked. Characteristic elements of the brain of man. Structure of the visual region. Studies on the auditory, tactile, and olfactory cortices. Establishment, by Dr. Cortezo, of the National Institute of Hygiene, of which I am appointed director.

I have already mentioned, in earlier chapters, some successful analyses of the cerebral cortex of lower mammals. Following up this road, it was natural that, sooner or later, I should attack the fine anatomy of the human cerebrum, rightly considered the masterpiece of life.

I felt at the time the most lively curiosity—of a somewhat romantic character—as to the enigmatic organization of the organ of the soul. "Man," I said to myself, "reigns over nature through the architectural perfection of his cerebrum. Such is his patent, his indisputable title of nobility and of dominion over the other animals. And if such a lowly mammal as the rodent—the mouse for example—displays a cerebral cortex of delicate and highly complicated construction, what an indescribable structure, what an amazing mechanism must not the convolutions of the human brain present, especially in the civilized races?"

In my inquiries, I was guided also by a certain directing hypothesis. The opinion generally accepted at the time, that the differences between the brain of lower mammals (cat, dog, monkey, etc.) and that of man are purely quantitative, seemed to me unlikely and even a little unworthy of the dignity of the human species.

On such a supposition, the superiority of the human brain would lie exclusively in the larger number of pyramidal cells and in the greater quantity of association fibres. But do not articulate language, the power of abstraction, the ability to form concepts, and, finally, the art of inventing ingenious instruments, a sort of extension of the hand and of the sensory apparatus, seem to indicate, even admitting fundamental structural correspondences with the animals, the existence of original resources, of something qualitatively new, in fine, and justifying the psychological nobility of *homo sapiens?*

Microscope in rest, then, I charged with my usual ardour to the conquest of the supposed anatomical characteristic of the king of creation, to the revelation of these enigmatic strictly human neurons, upon which is founded our zoological superiority.

To tell the truth, considering the inadequacy of the methods in vogue, the undertaking looked arduous and difficult, even devoting to it indefatigable patience and perseverance. Besides, it was necessary to overcome or to ignore moral and social prejudices which were very widespread and deeply rooted.

It is well known that the most exquisitely selective staining methods, like the procedures of Ehrlich and of Golgi yield good results only when they are applied to pieces of nervous tissue which are absolutely fresh, almost alive. And according to the requirements of the law, which consecrates outgrown and unfounded fears, the human cadaver does not come under the jurisdiction of the anatomist until twenty-four hours after death, when the extremely delicate and susceptible neurons and neuroglia cells have undergone serious alterations and have therefore lost their precious affinity for the reagents referred to (methylene blue and silver chromate).

In spite of everything, the reader will remember that the method of black colouration had already been applied successfully in man by Golgi and his followers. It has to be agreed, nevertheless, that such efforts, while they increased remarkably our neurological inheritance, were not able, perhaps as a result of the above mentioned limitations, to illuminate the more important wheels of the human cerebral machine, to wit; to determine the types of cells specific for each cerebral region, the general form of the interneuronal connections, and, finally, the manner of termination of the sensory conductors arriving from the periphery.

But in those days I was not greatly terrified by the obstacles. Determined to overcome them, I sought material for my studies in the Foundling Home and in the Maternity Hospital, domains in which, for obvious reasons, the tyranny of the law and the concern of the families are not very active. Thanks to the good offices of the staffs of these charitable institutions, and especially to the vigorous coöperation of Dr. Figueroa (an eminent physician, too soon lost to science) as well as the kindness with which I was favoured by the most worthy Sisters of Charity (who carried their amiability so far as to become autopsy assistants), my investigations went ahead as if on wheels. I am able to state that during a study of two years I had unrestricted disposal of hundreds of foetuses and children of various ages, which I dissected two or three hours after death and even while still warm.

My perseverance was finally rewarded and, in spite of many technical failures (definite infections hinder the reaction with the silver chromate), the harvest of new facts was bountiful. Before my persistent curiosity, the human cerebrum began to stammer some of its secrets. Unfortunately, these confidences were still quite fragmentary. But beginnings are made with small things.

Only in broad outlines shall I estimate my gains at that time. I shall mention, among other facts of a general character, the discovery of various new types of neurons with short axons, characteristic of the human brain; the definite observation, as I desired, of the terminal arborizations of the sensory fibres; the discovery of true pericellular baskets comparable to the elegant nests in the cerebellum and in the hippocampus; the discrimination of the various types of nerve cells of the molecular layer, etc. My principal aim, however, was to disentangle the structure of the sensory centres (*projection centres* of Flechsig). In each of them, my preparations showed with absolute clarity a specific and absolutely unmistakable texture, thus establishing upon immovable histological foundations the doctrine, then very much discussed, of cerebral localization.

Obviously the analysis of these centres proceeded by stages. It was a labour of many years, which was very incomplete, in spite of my perseverance. First, I explored the anatomy of the visual convolutions (calcarine fissure and neighbouring regions of the occipital lobe), the cerebral region upon which are projected the images collected by the retina. Later I examined the auditory, motor, and olfactory areas. For reasons which I shall explain in due course, I merely stepped over the threshold of the areas of memory (*association centres* of Flechsig) despite my burning curiosity, fed and further excited by my success.

Figure 68 shows the specific types of neuron which I

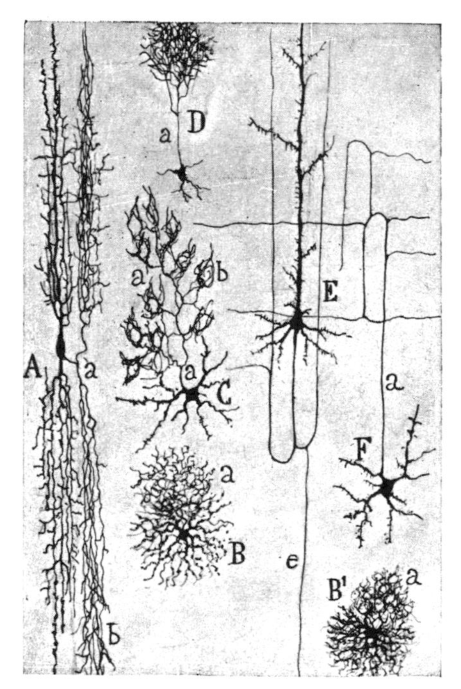

FIG. 68. Various types of neurons with short axons found in the cerebral cortex of the child of a few months. *A*, double tufted cell; *B*, dwarf element with short axon; *C*, basket cell; *D*, dwarf element with axon broken up into a tuft; *E*, pyramid with recurrent collaterals; *F*, cell with ascending axon dividing into very long horizontal branches.

found in almost all the cerebral areas of man. These elements, especially *A, B, E,* and *F,* are exceedingly numerous and can be considered peculiar to the human cerebrum. By this I do not exclude the possibility that some of them first appear, though with more primitive forms and sizes, in the cortex of the higher mammals, especially in that of the dog and that of the monkey. In any case, my investigations show that *the functional superiority of the human brain is intimately linked up with the prodigious abundance and unaccustomed wealth of forms of the so-called neurons with short axons.*

The various monographs [1] on the human cerebral cortex together made up a book which Dr. Bressler translated into German, and which brought me flattering eulogies from the great authorities in neurology.

Anyone interested in the descriptive details, overflowing with variations and niceties, which I collected patiently in the cerebral cortex during the years 1899, 1900, and 1901 should consult the German translation or, better still, my treatise in three large volumes: *Textura del sistema nervioso del hombre y de los vertebrados,* in the third volume of which I expound in more concise and orderly fashion, and with explanatory diagrams and figures not included in the corresponding memoirs, my ideas and discoveries on the structural plan of the brain of man and related mammals. Of this large book, however,—the principal work of my life—begun in 1899 and finished in 1904, I shall speak in due course.

In the year 1900, Don Carlos M. Cortezo, whose innovations in the Department of Public Health (*Direccion de Sanidad*) will never be sufficiently praised, founded the Alphonso XIII National Institute of Hygiene and had the kindness and generosity to appoint me director. He was not held back by the modesty of the sum appropriated in the state estimates for the great enterprise, nor by the absence of suitable quarters, nor yet by the lack of Spanish special-

[1] In the original text, the author devotes three pages to a summary of these. (Translator's note.)

ists in bacteriological and serotherapeutical studies. He probably believed that, when the need was created, adequate organs would arise to meet it, and he was not mistaken in his previsions.

My first inclination was to decline the honourable appointment, but at the time, the plague was ravaging Portugal and was liable to invade Spain. In such circumstances, I felt that it would be unpatriotic cowardice to refuse a charge which imposed upon me grave responsibilities and persistent zeal and activity. I had, besides, to organize the diverse sections of the Institute as quickly as possible, to draw up a plan of work, and, above all, to face boldly the delicate task of selecting the section heads notwithstanding the knowledge that, for the moment, despite the good will of the distinguished Dr. Cortezo, I could offer them no remuneration for their work. So I accepted the arduous commission.

When one proceeds in good faith and avoids personal friendships and favouritisms, he has gone a long way towards success. Acting then according to the well-known maxim that positions should be assigned to those who have demonstrated aptitudes and abilities in previous work, I placed at the head of the Section of Serotherapy Dr. Murillo, a person unknown to me, but of whose competence to deal with the problems of immunization I was convinced by his having worked in Germany with illustrious scientists. With a similar desire to make a success and to measure up worthily to the confidence reposed in me by my admired friend, Dr. Cortezo, I nominated respectively for the chieftaincies of the Sections of Bacteriology, of Expert Chemical Analysis, and of Veterinary Science, Dr. Mendoza, who was in charge of the laboratory of the Provincial Hospital, Dr. Gómez Pamo, Professor of Pharmacology, and Señor García Izcara, Professor of Veterinary Science; all men of known ability with whom I had not had any personal dealings and hence was not bound by feelings of friendship, which are often incompatible with justice. To these sections was added the former Institute of Vaccination, then directed by Dr. Serret.

As time went on, thanks to the definite support of the governments and to the zeal and persistent efforts of the Directors of Health (the enthusiastic hygienist, Dr. Pulido, the most worthy Dr. Cortejarena, and, more recently, the fervent, cultured and far-sighted Inspector General, Dr. Martín Salazar), the budding sanitary institution grew notably in scientific importance and in social efficiency. Many years later, when the inevitable phase of economic penury was over, three new sections were organized: that of Epidemiology, that of Parasitology, and that of the Health Park, in charge respectively of well-qualified specialists.

Today (1923) both on account of its efficient organization and on that of the multiplicity and effectiveness of its services to health, it can be affirmed that the National Institute of Hygiene is a credit to the nation and can take its place on a level with the best in other countries. In giving credit for collaboration, however, I must avoid omissions and injustices. The institution would not have been born without the bold and far-seeing initiative of Dr. Cortezo nor have attained its present splendour if a Minister of the Crown, Don Juan de la Cierva, with the energy and decision which he is in the habit of putting into every patriotic undertaking, had not included in the budget all at one time the appropriation necessary to erect the sumptuous edifice at Moncloa.

As for me, I put into it only the endless and tedious activities of administration, my good will, and the irrevocable purpose that the direction of the Institute should be carried on in an atmosphere of scientific probity and severe economy. And when, many years later (1920), I saw with satisfaction that the common work had a firm root in public opinion and had attained vigour and stability, I laid down the direction of the Institute, to which, being tired and ill, I could no longer attend as in happier days though I still rendered it the love and enthusiasm of former times. I entrusted it to a successor, young, competent, and able, and to strong and expert hands. It is a discreet maxim, in the words of Gracian, "To leave things well," that is to lay down our charges before our charges abandon us.

It was a pleasure and a comfort to me that this directorship should pass, as a result of competitive examination, to Don Francisco Tello, the best of my pupils and the most highly trained and intelligently eloquent of Spanish bacteriologists.

CHAPTER XVII

In connection with the commemoration of the decennial of its foundation Clark University (United States), a centre of higher learning, invites me conjointly with other European professors to give a series of lectures. Torrid heat of New York. My trip to Boston and Worcester (Mass.), where the university celebration takes place. Anglo-Saxon patriotism. Some spiritual causes of the war already mentioned between the United States and Spain. The educational institutions of Boston and of New York.

In June 1899, I was deeply engrossed in the aforementioned explorations in the human cerebrum when there reached my hands a courteous invitation from the American university of Worcester (Clark University) a centre of higher studies comparable with the Collège de France, to give several lectures regarding my investigations on the cerebral cortex. It was a case of celebrating a certain solemn academic festival, with many American and European savants present, to mark the tenth year since the foundation of this university, which was the outcome of private generosity, as the professional schools and establishments of higher culture usually are in the United States. To defray expenses of the trip, the official invitation enclosed a cheque for six hundred dollars.

I was deeply surprised and perplexed by the receipt of such a missive. I could not understand how a humble Spanish investigator should have been thought of in the United States, a professor belonging to a vanquished and humiliated race.

I was assailed by doubt. Could I reasonably accept such a compromised invitation a few months after the war, when Spain was still quivering with indignation and rancour after the iniquitous robbery of her colonies?

I consulted with the Minister of Education (ministro de

Fomento[1]), Marquis de Pidal, about the matter, and with several people whose opinions I valued highly; and contrary to what was to be expected, the Government, my friends, and even the political press (which commented upon the occurrence in words very flattering to me) advised me unanimously to accept the delicate and difficult commission.

Gladly would I have declined it. The more so as my health was far from flourishing at the time. As a result of a lingering attack of influenza or perhaps in consequence of the excessive excitement in the laboratory (each interesting discovery or what appeared so to me, cost me nights of sleeplessness), I suffered from palpitation and cardiac irregularities, with the consequent anxieties and fears. Obedient, nevertheless, to the urging of my friends and encouraged by the minister, who honoured me with an appropriate viaticum, I set out, accompanied by my wife so that she could attend to my attacks.

After passing through Paris, where I had the pleasure of calling upon professors M. Duval and M. Dejerine, and of embracing my good friends M. Azoulay and M. Nageotte, we embarked at Havre for New York in a ship of the French line. On board, I had the pleasant surprise of meeting the illustrious Dr. A. Mosso, Professor of Physiology at Turin, the great French mathematician M. E. Picard, professor in the Collège de France, and the famous Dr. A, Forel, who was then devoted to interesting studies on the psychology of ants. All these scientists had been invited, as I had, for the Clark celebration.

Needless to say, in such select company, the twelve days of the crossing passed very quickly. Professors Mosso and Forel, with whom I became very intimate during the journey, were revealed to me as most agreeable people as well as delightful conversationists. In our colloquies on board we discussed everything, divine and human; philosophy, science, art, politics, etc.

[1] The minister charged with encouragement of agriculture, industry, commerce, and public works, and until 1900 also with education. (Translator's note.)

In the middle of the month of June, we arrived in New York, the stupendous city of the skyscrapers, of the multi-millionaires, of the enslaving trusts, and of the suffocating heat. This last was for me a disagreeable surprise. I thought that grassy countries and maritime cities possessed the privilege of enjoying moderate temperatures during the dog days. And I, who in our Madrid, the typical city of sunshine and blue sky, felt myself enervated when the temperature reached 80° F. in the houses and 95° in the streets, was obliged, to my great discomfort, to endure 89° or 90° Fahrenheit in the hotel and 113° or 114° in the streets.

Nevertheless the Americans bear it as if it were nothing. Though they were pouring with perspiration, labourers and bricklayers were to be seen in the streets working strenuously. Oh, the steely fibre of the Anglo-Saxon race!

With that burning sun and the profusion of domestic installation of gas and electricity, it is easily understood that conflagrations are daily occurrences there. To my great distress, I had to witness one of these terrible disasters.

One day, at a most inopportune hour, fire broke out in the room of a guest on the first floor. Alarm suddenly spread among the men and nervousness and terror among the women. Some rushed frantically towards the main stairway, which was cut off by dense and suffocating smoke. With others, better advised, we took to the balconies, where American foresight, taught by tragic experience, had arranged long stairs for escape. But who could make a lady who is timid and nervous, like a good Spaniard, descend those aerial steps? Luckily the engines soon arrived and quickly extinguished the fire.

When the fright was over, I considered the curious incidents called forth by terror. From the point of view of individual psychology, there is nothing more instructive than a disaster. In flight, each one carries his idol in his arms: mothers their children, the newly wed their wives, actresses their jewels and valuables, merchants and bankers their portfolios and satchels. There is nothing like fear to reveal the true character and rapidly to value the goods of life.

I shall not fall into the temptation to describe the great American metropolis. I shall merely say that I admired Bartholdi's famous Statue of Liberty, the commercial suburb of Brooklyn, the bold bridge over the East River, the sumptuous palaces of Fifth Avenue, the famous cathedral of St. Patrick, of which I took some excellent photographs, the colossal buildings housing manufactures, industrial corporations, and great printing presses, the delightful beaches of Brighton and Manhattan, the incomparable Central Park, sprinkled with rock-crowned hills covered with magnificent trees, and, finally, the splendid stores in which everything is done by machinery and, by ingenious devices, the merchandise desired runs on aerial railways through endless corridors and floors, arriving in a few seconds, ready wrapped, in the hands of the customer.

It is a fact that in connection with these sightseeing visits to the great stores, I had regretfully to confirm a certain suspicion that I had regarding the feelings which had inspired the agression of the United States against Spain. In consequence of the cruel, unwise, and unsuccessful measure of concentrating the whole rural population of Cuba in encampments, the survivors who had not the courage to swell the armies of Maceo fled *en masse* to the United States (Key West, Tampa, New Orleans, New York, etc.), seeking work in the fields, factories, and business houses. Some of these unfortunates, mostly women, with whom I conversed in the work rooms and shops of New York, told us of heartrending abuses and cruelties. It is unnecessary to point out that the lamentations of so many thousands of fugitives, proclaiming and exaggerating beyond all probability the ancient Anglo-Saxon legend of Spanish cruelty, created in the United States an emotional condition which was easily exploited by the Cuban conspirators and by the imperialist or interventionist party.[2]

[2] In exculpation of this incompetent conduct of the Cuban authorities, it has been alleged that the same methods were employed by the highly cultured

The date of the academic celebrations at Worcester was approaching. Hence I put an end to my rambles and visits to scientific institutes and museums—which were then somewhat inferior to similar establishments in England and Germany—and set out for Boston, a city not far from the end of my journey. Throughout the trip in an express train I was accompanied by the same suffocating heat experienced in New York. It may be said in commendation of American civilization that the managements of the railways do everything possible to mitigate the discomforts of the traveller. To this end, besides other comforts, each car has a large supply of iced water, served free to the passengers by negro stewards, who are very courteous and solicitous.

On our arrival at Worcester, the heat wave, far from receding, had become intolerable. The burning breath of the atmosphere, hardly lessened during the night, as happens in very humid climates, made respiration impossible. I was a little feverish and somewhat congested. For this reason and because we had arrived at an inconvenient hour, I did not dare to notify the Rector; and so I spent the night—a sleepless one indeed—trying to relieve my raging headache with cold water compresses.

As a climax of ill fortune, the anniversary of Independence was being celebrated that day and a deafening clamour arose from the streets. Patriotic songs, stentorian cheers, and the reports of rockets were heard, and, above all, shots, now singly and now in volleys. At the windows and on the roofs, I saw many people like madmen discharg-

England in her treatment of the Boers. But, apart from the fact that one cruelty never justifies another previous and active cruelty, those who argue thus seem to forget that only powerful nations can commit certain excesses with impunity. Our Government, in authorizing the measures referred to in Cuba, acted as if Spain were the only country on the planet, or as if powerful and dominating nations which were neighbours of weaker states had not always invoked for their spoliations pretexts of humanity and civilization. The imperialism of the United States and its desire to annex adjoining lands were already notorious at that time. As for the catastrophe of the *Maine*, it was one pretext more, of which advantage was taken most skilfully and perfidiously.

ing rifles into the air. In the street, even the women were waving flags and shouting outrageously. Our traditional wrangles in the bull ring are child's play as compared with the frenzy and tumult of the American people on the famous Independence Day, on which, it may be said in passing, lamentable accidents always happen. It is a sad thing that men are able to express their jubilation only by making a noise! *A propos* of which I might ask: does the populace raise an uproar because it is happy or does it do so in order to make itself happy? The second seems to me truer than the first. For, say what one may, the manual labourer—and still more the brain worker—are at bottom sad and supremely weary animals. But let us drop impertinent reflections.

With dawn, that blast of folly and license ceased. When the forenoon was advancing and the effects of my insomnia had been somewhat relieved, I announced my arrival to the honourable president of Clark University, the distinguished psychologist and educationist G. Stanley Hall. In a short time there came to greet me and place himself at my service the genial secretary, who was also a professor of the university, a young man of culture as well as energy, as is shown by the following occurrence:

When I had ordered a carriage and told the coachman to take the baggage to the vehicle, according to the American custom, the elegant secretary addressed me courteously in these unexpected words:

"It is not worth while to trouble the coachman! Here am I to bring down the trunk."

And without listening to our protests, the stylish functionary tilted his immaculate silk hat smartly and, making a display of his unsuspected vigour and agility, carried down the large trunk and hand bag in a twinkling (together they weighed about ninety kilogrammes) and dexterously arranged them in the coach.

My wife was confounded by the sight of the patches of dust and the untidy creases which such a precipitate and rough task had produced in the irreproachable academic frock coat, and exclaimed:

"Why have you put yourself about? That was a matter for the porter."

"No," replied the smart *gentleman;* "that is the obligation of everybody. We live in America, the home of democracy, where nobody considers manual work a reproach or dishonour. Here we recognize only the nobility of talent and learning."

Here was an excellent lesson in legitimate and sane democracy. We may agree, however, that such persuasive propaganda is not within the power of everybody. It would not be enough to abandon aristocratic presumption and lordly fastidiousness; one would require also muscles of steel.

Directed by the secretary, the carriage conveyed us to the house of our host, a wealthy man of standing, an enthusiastic patron of the university and a prototype of that kind of patriotic philanthropist of which perfect examples are found only in England and in the United States; I mean to say men who are free of self-worship and of political sectarianism.

Our host, Mr. Stephen Salisbury, lived almost modestly, if one takes into account his great fortune, which he devoted to works of public benefit, culture, and benevolence. Inspired by feelings of tolerance and altruism which would surprise our pompous and fanatical men of great wealth, he founded two hospitals with a church for each, one for Protestants (he professed the reformed religion) and the other for Catholics. Besides, for the pleasure and instruction of his fellow citizens, he erected a sumptuous Museum of Art, the building of which, as well as most of the pictures, he presented to the municipality; he also gave to the public a certain park, valued in millions, and in addition was said, as I have already mentioned, to be one of the most devoted and generous patrons of Clark University, where he endowed chairs and instituted prizes. What men they are in these countries!

PLATE 19

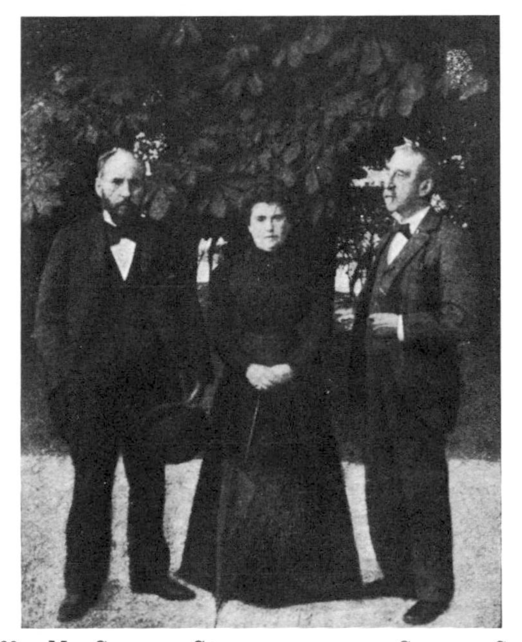

FIG. 69. MR. STEPHEN SALISBURY AND HIS SPANISH GUESTS.

The worthy Mr. Salisbury was descended from an English nobleman who had arrived in America with the first settlers and he dwelt in a commodious villa, where, it is superfluous to say, we were lodged and feasted like kings. Our host was approaching sixty-five and remained a bachelor, from horror, he told us, of the American woman, whose masculine tendencies and excessive freedom of movement (the feminist folly was then at its height) repelled him completely.

He had travelled in Spain and spoke a little broken Spanish. It is true that as he recalled the piquant adventures of his travels in Andulusia and extolled the charm and wit of the women of Cadiz, Seville, and Granada, he used to tell us that "in Spain only the women are talented." In his eyes, our men were deplorably inept and insignificant.

"I am delighted," he used to exclaim at times, "to entertain in my house a Spaniard who is endowed with common sense!"[3]

In the adjoining picture (Fig. 69) I reproduce a photograph of Mr. Salisbury and of his two Spanish guests taken by a valet who was an enthusiast in the art of Daguerre.

In his desire to be agreeable to us, and to enable my wife

[3] Unfortunately, this contemptuous opinion of the Spaniards cannot be regarded as pleasantry of an amiable and jocose table companion. It expresses a real feeling which is exceedingly widespread among the Anglo-Saxon people, upon which many of the dwellers in the Peninsula and Spanish-Americans should meditate. From my conversations with people of the United States, Englishmen, and Germans, I have become convinced—I am telling no secret—that, in the judgment of the laborious and energetic sons of the north, the Mediterranean nations, and especially the Portugese and Spanish, are composed of decadent races, degenerate morally and physically, who do not deserve any consideration. "Towards the South Americans we feel not the slightest sympathy," a certain United States professor told me confidentially, covering his thought with veils of euphemism.

I believe sincerely that we are calumniated; but I believe also that we Spaniards, Portugese, and Spanish-Americans do all that we can to justify the contempt and cupidity of the great nations with our grotesque tumults and insurrections, our disdain for science and great industrial undertakings—which prosper only when they are founded on original scientific discoveries—and our age-long lack of political solidarity (surrounded by very powerful and unified nations, we are divided up into twenty-one little states which regard each other with suspicion and hate each other cordially).

to penetrate into the pleasant intimacy of the American home, Mr. Salisbury had the kindness to introduce us to one of his friends, Mrs. Lawton, a widow gifted with real musical talents. (One of her sons had fought against Spain in Cavite.) She knew some Spanish and, in order to be able to get to know my wife, she reinforced her slender vocabulary by superintensive work during these days. Together, having become sincere friends, they visited orphanages, Catholic churches, and hospitals (to one of which Mrs. Lawton's mother, with that noble altruism so general in America, had left the funds necessary to endow a ward), the Ladies' Club, with magnificent social and reading rooms, the large department stores of the city, etc.

I also found a very pleasant and solicitous mentor for my rambles in pursuit of the artistic and picturesque in a certain somewhat eccentric Russian professor of mathematics, who displayed splendid long fair hair reaching his waist. Enamoured of Spain, he was very anxious to talk our language, which he praised warmly. His facility with tongues was amazing. In only two months stay in Granada he had learned Spanish without forgetting French, Russian, Polish, German, and Italian, which he spoke perfectly. His somewhat peculiar apparel was on a par with his flowing and romantic locks; but in that atmosphere of pleasant tolerance nothing shocked. His position was strengthened, besides, by his great ability with the theory of numbers.

The days from the fourth to the tenth of July were devoted to the events of the Decennial Celebration. These consisted of official receptions, banquets, trips to the educational institutions and to the picturesque environs of the city and, finally, the scientific lectures by American and foreign professors. A select audience gathered from all the States of the Union assembled in Clark University and faithfully attended the addresses.

Mine, three in number, concerned the structure of the cerebral cortex of man and the higher mammals, a subject which, as I have already indicated, I had been investigating during 1898 and 1899. My audiences were composed mainly of physicians, naturalists, and psychologists. Wishing to demonstrate graphically my recent discoveries in such a difficult field, I employed, as was my custom, large wall plates in colours. For those who were acquainted with neurological technique, I put on some demonstrations of microscopic preparations. I believe that I succeeded in satisfying the expectations of my hearers; in any case, I was loudly applauded.

The text of these lectures, along with all those delivered at the celebration, was printed at the expense of the university in a most luxurious volume, handsomely illustrated. At the beginning of each series of addresses appeared the portrait of the professor.

The closing Convocation, held on the tenth of July, was very solemn. There were read expressive letters of congratulation from the President of the Republic, Mr. McKinley, from several prominent members of the Senate and, finally, from many illustrious men of learning, native and foreign; the President, G. Stanley Hall, delivered an eloquent address in which he narrated the history of the university and then enumerated the scientific undertakings completed and outlined the programme for future investigations. There followed next a sort of sermon of an exalted tone delivered by the Reverend Dr. Vinton; and at the last, after the respective formal eulogies, we five foreign professors were ceremoniously invested with the degree of Doctor *honoris causa* (Doctor of Laws, according to the statement of the diploma), completing the proceedings with short speeches of thanks.

The rôle of guest, more or less illustrious, is a singularly compromising one in America. The people of the United States are not content with learning from the foreigner; they wish also to be judged by him. Whether we would or not, we had no remedy but to concoct answers to the following delicate questions:

"What defects do you see in our educational institutions? Will you be so kind as to point out the urgent reforms or the steps calculated to perfect the work of our university?"

Naturally, having due respect to courtesy and the impulse of gratitude, our judgments were unconditionally encomiastic; nevertheless, through the rhetorical foliage some useful reforms were indicated. I suggested for the teaching programme of the university two novelties: the creation of a laboratory for bacteriological investigation and that of another for experimental histology and pathology.

In this matter of interviews, however, I had worse luck than my companions. My position as a Spaniard made me the preferred mark of the political reporters. The newspaper women, especially, besieged me day and night. They wished me to tell them—a mere nothing!—the advantages or disadvantages which the United States might derive from the annexation of Cuba, Porto Rico, and the Philippines. It was like talking of the halter in the house of the hanged!

I got out as best I could from such inopportune meddling, but not without saying, perhaps because of my ill humor, several things that would have been better unsaid. I was amazed when I read my political statements in the local newspapers!

After all, I did not get off so badly in so far as I succeeded in warding off from my wife the assaults of those implacable female reporters (typical old maids and genuine representatives of what Ferrero called the third sex) determined at any cost to extract the opinion of Mrs. Cajal both on theoretical feminism and on the state in our country of the campaign for the emancipation of woman.

"In our country," I told them, "we are unfortunately so backward that women are still content to be *feminine* and not *feminists.* And apparently that is sufficient for their happiness and that of the home."

Not to abuse the patience of the reader, I shall pass over the entertainments, receptions, banquets, and attentions of every kind on the part of the illustrious president and the charming professors of Clark University of which both the foreign guests and the representatives of the American universities were the objects. As for what concerns me personally, however, it would be ingratitude not to mention the attentions and thoughtfulness which I received from Mr. A. Gordon Webster, the distinguished professor of physics, in whose house I had the honour of making the acquaintance of the genuine American woman, cultured, strong, a good housekeeper, and exempt from annoying feminist characteristics; and to speak of Dr. A. Meyer, a fervent admirer and a compatriot of A. Forel, in whose company I enjoyed the pleasure of visiting the principal institutions of public welfare, and particularly a magnificent hospital devoted to the treatment of nervous and mental diseases, a hospital where I could certainly appreciate the services rendered by the nurses, young, well-educated women, trained in the elements of medicine, who there, with advantage, take the place of our sisters of charity.

My departure from Worcester was preceded by an episode commonplace, no doubt, in every festival celebrated by young people in Anglo-Saxon countries, but productive of a profound impression upon me.

We had spent a day in the country, on the shore of a picturesque lake which serves as a reservoir for the drinking water of the city; and after a banquet at which professors and students were present, all the English and Americans present—there were over a hundred—rose to their feet and sang together with robust and vibrant tones first the American hymn and then the English "God Save the Queen." In the silence and darkness of the night, those stanzas raised lustily by the throats of all sounded to me like a sublime religious canticle. I was so deeply moved that my heart beat violently, a shiver passed over me, and tears were on the point of flowing.

The spectacle was both exciting and instructive. Those same men who, a few moments before, were chatting and laughing with that happy placidness which is an unmistakable sign of vigour and optimism, all agreed before separating that they were the sons of a common mother, noble

Albion, and that, therefore, they should feel themselves brothers in spirit and at heart. Who knows the patriotic hymn of the Spanish race?

Then I understood many things; and better than in the highly lauded book of Des Moulins I perceived wherein lies the much sung superiority of the Anglo-Saxon people. Builders of their greatness are, certainly, robust mentality and rectitude, and energy of character. Yet I regard as the principal factors two things totally unheeded in Spain and in the countries of our blood: education in patriotism and intensive inoculation with the spirit of unity.

Science, superior culture, administrative integrity, civic pride, military heroism, etc., are transformations of a single primordial force: the love of the race. In the happy English-speaking countries, patriotism appears as something spontaneous, profoundly mystical, like an irresistible fanaticism inoculated in childhood and fortified afterwards by political education.

Before returning to Spain, I visited several American cities and also, as a tourist and an enthusiast of the kodak, made the inevitable excursion to the wonderful cataracts of Niagara. Written about, eulogized, and photographed to satiety, it would be unpardonable now to pause to describe them.

Among the great cities visited during my sojourn in America, I retain a particularly vivid recollection of Boston, the capital of the state of Massachusetts, the most populous and highly cultivated region of the United States.

My visit to Harvard University aroused my sincere admiration and noble envy.

I was captivated by its masters, some as outstanding as Professor Charles S. Minot, of world-wide renown, by whom, be it said in passing, I had the honour of being led through the endless labyrinth of the university buildings. These splendid edifices occupy an enormous area in the populous suburb of Boston called, in memory of the celebrated English university, Cambridge.

It is impossible to describe here those admirable institutions, almost all founded and sustained by the gifts of outstanding citizens or of former students grateful for the instruction of their *alma mater.* I shall merely mention the magnificent Faculty of Medicine, with its rich anatomical and pathological collections (Warren Anatomical Museum) and its excellent research laboratories; the Faculty of Sciences, with the well-organized Jefferson Physical Laboratory; the University Museum, an enormous building which contains the collections donated by the celebrated naturalists, Agassiz, father and son; the Peabody Museum, an inestimable archeological collection; the Hemenway Gymnasium, a sumptuous edifice presented to the students by a wealthy citizen of Boston; the University Library, a pretentious palace where students and professors meet to consult not only scientific books but also the more important periodicals of the world; the numerous and sumptuous colleges (there are over seventy) where, after the English custom, the students live under the supervision of special professors and instructors; and the extensive fields for military training, tennis, football, etc., intended not so much for the physical development of the students as for the directing of their energies. Finally, to complete the list (a full one would occupy several pages), I shall mention the superb Memorial Hall, an artistic and monumental building filled with statues of famous men, adorned with portraits of benefactors of the university and with classical Greek, Latin, and English inscriptions, erected in memory of students killed in the terrible war of secession. In its spacious halls the student gatherings are held, and there they obtain moderately priced refreshments and receive at the same time—and this is the most delicately spiritual—an enduring lesson in exalted and comforting patriotism from contemplation of the legendary heroes of the race and meditation on their sayings and maxims.

My visit to the Library of the City of Boston, perhaps the richest and best organized in the world, was also particularly instructive. Despite the endless labyrinth of rooms, corridors, and aerial railways along which the books are carried; notwithstanding the legion of employees, linotypists, printers, illustrators, etc.; and in spite, finally, of the painful labour which may be imagined in the handling, classification, and cataloguing of several million books, pamphlets, and periodicals, the service is so quick and well organized that a few minutes after a request is made the volume reaches the hands of the reader. At the suggestion of my conductor, I tested it, asking for a certain copy of the first edition of *Don Quixote* preserved there as an inestimable jewel. Hardly three minutes passed before the precious copy was handed to me. I observed also, contrary to my expectations, that this library is very rich in Spanish books, ancient and modern, preserving even files of our principal newspapers.

In connection with the Spanish press, although the recollection is somewhat embittering, I should refer to a certain remark of the charming librarian, a man certainly of the highest culture, acquainted with the Spanish language and with the treasure of our classics (he had spent two years in Madrid on a fellowship, examining our archives and libraries), who had the kindness to show me all the departments of the famous institution.

When we reached the foreign periodical room, he stopped suddenly and, with a gesture of disgust, pointed out to me two Spanish dailies with large circulations and a certain satirical magazine, spread out upon a table.

"These papers," he exclaimed, "are responsible for half the blame for the recent war! They provoked us imprudently, calling us hucksters, sausage-mongers, and cowards! Telegraphed, translated, and commentated in our press, such coarse insults provoked deep indignation even in the friends and admirers of Spain, among whom I have the honour of counting myself!"

How distressing it was to hear such censures and to have to acknowledge their justice!

My sight-seeing concluded, I returned to New York to arrange the voyage back. Having to wait a few days for the arrival of the steamer, I was able to take advantage of them to study the educational institutions better and to inspect the novelties and industrial attractions of the tremendous city.

My first visit was to Columbia University, an enormous aggregation of large and magnificent buildings among which, besides the edifices destined for teaching, are a rich library, situated in the centre, the chapel, the gymnasium, the assembly theatre, lecture halls, dormitories, the Museum of Natural History, playing fields, etc. In other districts of the city are the Faculty of Medicine and Pharmacy, with admirable laboratories, libraries, dormitories, etc., and, finally, the University of New York, on University Heights, as it is called there, made famous by the celebrated Professor Morse, inventor of the telegraph bearing his name. A description of these admirable foundations, due, like most American educational institutions, to private munificence, would be interminable.

The picturesque outskirts of New York also attracted my attention, especially the famous military school of West Point, erected on an elevation with a splendid panorama over the Hudson. In this model academy, isolated and distant from the distractions and vices of the city, the cadets lead an austere, secluded life of intensive study and vigorous muscular development; an austerity lightened by the visits of their families and of many members of good New York society, who attend the private functions of the school on fixed days of the month, converse pleasantly with the young officers and give them the flattering impression that they are the chosen sons of their country and the hope for her future aggrandisement.

I wished to become acquainted also with the new industrial inventions of the nation endowed with the greatest genius for mechanical development and to examine briefly the new improvements of the phonograph and gramophone, with the advances introduced into the brilliant invention of Edison by the Italian Bettini. As will appear, my curiosity on this point involved a certain personal interest. Although it may appear strange, the present writer also, at that time, was incubating a certain improvement in the talking machine. According to the failing of all inventors, who are beings radically egoistical, I desired that the instrument should adhere invariably and immovably to the principles laid down by the celebrated wizard of Menlo Park.[4]

To justify myself, however, I must go back in my narrative and make a digression for which the reader will forgive me on account of the moral which it contains. In 1895 and 1896, the Edison phonograph and its variants (the graphophone of a certain Washington manufacturer and the famous amplifying diaphragms of Bettini) made a furore in Madrid. Thanks to the active propaganda of the Frenchman, M. Hugens, and especially to the sales facilities of the firm of Aramburo, which was like the casino of the enthusiasts for the cylinder, the cult of the phonograph spread like an epidemic, attacking even those who, like myself, were always refractory to the enchantments of music. The invention of Edison undoubtedly brought us delightful winter evenings, but it also led us to commit many abuses. Without the slightest scruple we assailed eminent artists, whose generosity we put to the test by obliging them to record romances, songs, and comic recitations. I remember that I and the charming Pepe Zahonero—a master of the art of persuading comedians, poets, and parliamentarians to record—carried our impertinence so far as to attack the famous Romero Robledo, who was so kind as to honour our horn by declaiming into it parts of his discourses, among others, one pronounced in defence of the Duchess of Castro-Enriquez, which he considered the best of his parliamentary successes.[5]

[4] *I.e.*, Thos. A. Edison. The original here has *Mungo Park*, which is evidently an error for Menlo Park. (Translator's note.)

[5] It is a fact that a certain forensic physician, having heard this eloquent declaration in my house, exclaimed: "Thus is history written!"

"What do you mean?

"Do you, by chance, suspect that the Duchess really maltreated the unhappy little girl?"

The talking machines of those days suffered from a serious defect, however. Enthusiasts of the phonograph will remember that when the impression in the wax of the cylinder was weak the voice was reproduced with timbre and modulation which were almost natural but with great weakness in volume, justifying the phrase of Letamendi, who called the phonograph *the talking rabbit*. If, on the other hand, in the desire to intensify the impression, one sang or talked close to the horn, the voice was screechy, strident, and unbearable for all sensitive listeners.

After a thorough analysis of the physical conditions of such an unpleasant defect,[6] there occurred to me the idea that if the engraving sapphire, instead of inscribing the sound wave as a varying depth of the groove, could produce it on a flat surface, tracing a continuous, wavy line on a plate of crystal or metal, it would be possible to intensify the sound greatly, to improve the purity of its quality and, finally to get rid of, or at least to lessen, the disturbing screech.

Enthusiastic over the idea, I entrusted to an unskilled machinist (in the absence of an expert mechanic) the construction of my disc phonograph, while I tried out practical methods of moulding gelatine, wax, or celluloid. Unfortunately, while the apparatus confirmed fully the new

"I am absolutely certain of it. I made the examination of the victim, and her skin was bespattered with bruises and contusions. In a paroxysm of anger the Duchess beat and kicked her horribly."

"How unscrupulous are politicians!"

"With reason did Romero say that this speech, through which the Duchess was absolved and cleared of all suspicion of excessive cruelty, was the greatest of his triumphs!"

[6] The cause of the stridency as is well known, is purely mechanical. As is shown by the most cursory microscopic examination of the grooves, it depends upon the fact that the engraving stylus, instead of making in the wax a continuous canal of varying depth, sculptures deep and isolated hollows, separated by spaces with no impression. Hence it is inferred that the diaphragm, in its energetic vbirations, engraves only half, and sometimes less, of the sound wave, without the secondary curves of the harmonic tones indispensable for a good reproduction of the quality. Such a defect is irremediable on account of the hardness of the material inscribed. The employment of a large cylinder diminishes somewhat, but does not overcome the defect.

principle of recording and its expected advantages, it worked deplorably. Called by more pressing occupations, I forgot the wretched machine, which I stowed away in the garret hoping for a mechanic capable of understanding me.[7]

Well, the apparatus which I had thought out and partly constructed in the years 1895 and 1896 I now found resplendent and recently launched before the public under the name of gramophone in a certain shop in New York. Spread afterwards over the whole world and exploited by the American Gramophone Company and its European subsidiaries, this machine was the foundation of a splendid business, running into very many millions.

It is not out of childish vanity that I refer to these matters, but in order that my biological, medical, or naturalist readers may learn at my expense not to squander time in pursuit of inventions outside the sphere of their own subjects. When we abandon the usual furrow, we always run upon the reef of being ignorant of, or knowing only

[7] Only in accessory motor arrangements and in the material used for moulding the discs (ebonite) did my apparatus differ from that launched by the Gramophone Company. I began by engraving on metal or crystal covered with a coat of wax and went on afterwards to obtain an electroplate, from which I took impressions in gelatine or celloidin. The movement of the reproducing diaphragm, which was set, naturally, at right angles to the disc with the impression, was brought about not by the disc itself, as in the needle gramophone, but by a clockwork mechanism, an arrangement less elegant and simple it is true, but having the advantage of preserving better the fine tracing of the inscription.

Later, I thought of another phonographic invention more complicated and difficult to carry out, *the amplifying photophonograph,* a description of which the curious reader may see in *La Naturaleza* for the year 1903. The recording of the sound wave is accomplished on a photographic plate by means of a double mirror attached to a vibrating membrane. From this negative is taken a positive on crystal coated with gelatine and sensitized, following the classic procedure of Poitevin for obtaining of carbon copies in relief. The sensitivity of the diaphragm was such (the ray of light taking the place of a lever) that speeches and musical performances could be recorded at a normal distance.

I was planning to produce this new apparatus when I learned that Edison himself had obtained a patent shortly before for an invention, if not quite the same, yet founded on the same principle. My evil star, or rather my gross ignorance of the phonographic patents registered in recent years, deprived me irremediably of the merit of priority.

superficially or incompletely the bibliographic and industrial background of the matter (registered patents of invention, etc.), as well as the intense and silent labour carried on by skilful engineers in the employ of the great industrial establishments of Europe and of America.

Under such conditions—further aggravated in our country by its being almost impossible to find workshops where delicate appliances and instruments of great precision are made—the cherished invention, in case it is fully realized, usually reaches the market with deplorable slowness and always with the wearing out of our energies and interest.

On the other hand, it is wise to distrust greatly the inventions of common sense. Logic is a gift so usual, so generously distributed! And although it may be humilating for the pride of the investigator, it has to be confessed that only chance discoveries are completely and absolutely our own. Exactly those in which we have had least share!

Oh, fortunate accident, the muse of the persevering and patient! How many who pass for geniuses owe to you their greatest conquests and the intoxicating flattery of fame!

CHAPTER XVIII

Afflicted by a severe cardiac affection, I resolve to live in the country, where I organize my laboratory. In my little house at Amaniel I am surprised by notification of the award of the international prize known as the Moscow Prize. Warm felicitations of my friends and colleagues, enthusiastic tributes from the students, and a commemorative ceremony in the University. My address to the young at the academic solemnity. At the instigation of the press, the Government agrees to establish a Laboratory of Biological Research. Some studies undertaken during 1900 and 1901.

In the year 1900 there took place an event which was of the utmost importance for my scientific future. The International Medical Congress, meeting in Paris, was so kind as to award me the important and coveted *international prize* (6000 francs). Instituted by the city of Moscow to commemorate the Medical Congress held there a few years previously, this guerdon was to be awarded to the most important medical or biological work published in the whole world during each triennium, or the interval between two medical assemblies. Upon the nomination of Dr. Albrecht of Vienna, and with the unanimous support of the members of the committee of award, it was decided to recompense with it my modest investigations. At the same session it was agreed also to hold the next Congress, in 1903, in Madrid.

As witnesses who were present would testify, the enthusiasm of the delegates and members of the congress from the Latin countries was great and sincere. The congratulations to our official representatives and the cheers for Spain resounded through the hall. In the name of our country and of Spanish science, Dr. Calleja, hesitating from emotion, delivered an eloquent and heart-felt address of thanks. It was almost—allow me the exaggeration of the remark—a racial celebration of the Spanish peoples, for congratulations upon the unexpected triumph were exchanged by the members of the congress from Spain and from the Spanish-American Republics.

When this took place in Paris, in the month of August of that year, I was spending the summer in my recently built cottage in the Quatro Caminos,[1] tranquilly pursuing my fascinating exploration of the structure of the cerebral cortex.

Although it is a matter of no importance, I may be permitted to explain why I chose to build my country house in a poor suburb, inhabited almost exclusively by labourers.

During the autumn and winter of 1899 my health left much to be desired. I was attacked by neurasthenia, with palpitations, cardiac irregularities, insomnia, etc., with the resulting mental depression. Such severe cardiac affections frequently attack people who are nervously fatigued, especially during that period of life when maturity is declining and the first weaknesses presaging old age begin to appear.

Naturally, my sufferings aggravated my temperamental gloom and hypochondria; and through a physiological and mental reaction I was seized by a violent passion for the country. All my desires were centered upon possessing a modest and retired cottage, surrounded by a garden and from the windows of which should be seen, by day the great peaks of the Guadarrama, and by night a broad stretch of sky not cut off by eaves nor choked by chimneys. Apart from the longed-for portion of the infinite, I desired to oppose to my *spleen,* in the form of a contrast in feeling, the surge of boisterous happiness which overflows on Sundays and sunny evenings from the garrets of Madrid to the democratic eating houses of Amaniel. There, far from the tumult of the capital, I should work to my taste during the summer months, surrounded by trees and flowers and in the midst of a colony of laboratory animals. There, finally, immersed in that soothing calm, my nerves would

[1] *The Four Roads.* A suburb of Madrid. (Translator's note.)

become settled and I should weave in peace the web of my ideas.

There is little to choose among the suburbs of Madrid for a nest for a romantic spirit, enamoured of picturesque vistas. Only the leafy ravines and the slopes in the neighbourhood of the Puente de Amaniel, with splendid views towards the Moncloa, the Guadarrama, and El Escorial promised an adequate setting for my little house.

Hence I bought a not very extensive garden in the said district of the Quatro Caminos and ordered the erection of a modest cottage, surrounded by a flower-garden, with a liliputian vine arbour and conservatory, terraced on a hill and exposed to the afternoon sun. And acting rashly, I put all my savings into the work.

My cure did little honour to the pharmacopeia. Once more there triumphed the best of physicians: instinct, that is, the profound *vis medicatrix.* For soon after I was installed with my family in the rural residence, my health improved markedly. At last there dawned in my spirit, with the new sap produced by sun, fresh air, and woodland odours, a cheerful optimism. And, in addition, there I was showered with unexpected satisfaction and good fortune.

It was, then, as I said before, in my modest orchard at Amaniel, situated in the Calle de Almansa opposite the little canal, that I was surprised by the exciting telegram of congratulation from Dr. Calleja and the kind and generous comments in the press reports.

Great was my delight at receiving the new distinction, and still greater when I learned that the honour was accompanied by several thousand francs, a benefaction by no means contemptible for an exhausted purse. The utmost of my desires would have been fulfilled if the elementary demands of courtesy had not obliged me to reply to thousands of telegrams of felicitation, post cards, and congratulatory letters. That downpour of congratulations—for which I was, naturally, sincerely grateful—lasted more than a month, compelling me to lay aside my favourite occupations indefinitely and to squeeze dry my poor imagination—almost empty of polite formulae—in adorning, varying, and blending to the limit of my ability the required expressions of gratitude and the inevitable protestations of modesty.

Among the felicitations, I must record, on account of the importance of their authors, the deeply appreciated telegram of Her Majesty, Queen Christina; the friendly letter of the President of the Ministry, Don Francisco Silvela; the no less kindly one of the Minister of Education,[2] the official communication from the City Council of Zaragoza, and many more. Nor would it be right to pass over the eulogistic articles in the political and professional press. There live, indelibly traced upon my memory, the eloquent biography written for the *Heraldo* by my eminent colleague, Dr. Amalio Gimeno; the graceful chronicle in *El Imparcial* offered by Mariano de Cávia, the master of fine words and patriotic thought; the laudatory articles in *El Liberal, La Epoca, La Correspondencia,* etc., and finally a certain panegyric, as enthusiastic as it was friendly, inserted by my friend Dr. Márquez in a medical periodical.

I shall omit, too, the visits of deputations, the official banquets, the private tributes[3] and the warm congratulations of friends.

Still, at the risk of prolixity, I may be permitted to mention a few other distinctions and official decorations.

At the suggestion of the Government, Her Majesty the Queen decorated me with the Grand Cross of Isabel the Catholic, the insignia of which were generously paid for by the students of the Faculty of Medicine, where, it may be said in passing, a solemn commemorative session was held.

[2] Ministro de Fomento.

[3] I should not like to pass over entirely the delicate and very thoughtful act of Señor and Señora Tolosa Latour, guardian angels of childhood, who inquired into the tastes of my children and presented them with fine toys and even objects of value (a kodak, the works of Campoamor, a music-box, etc.), in order that the recollection of the undreamed of triumph of their father should be associated in their memories with the sweetness of a satisfied desire.

A few months later I was granted the Grand Cross of Alphonso XII and was appointed a counsellor of Public Instruction.

The tribute, however, for which I am most profoundly grateful was the academic ceremony held a few months afterwards in the assembly hall of the University in the presence of the professors and students. Eloquent and enthusiastic addresses were given on that occasion by the Ministro de Fomento, who deigned to honour the function with his presence; the President, Sr. Fernández y González; and, finally, Don Julián Calleja and Don Alejandro San Martín.

My innate timidity suffered a most severe test at that time. That shower of exaggerated eulogies, based upon a noble feeling of patriotic satisfaction, moved me deeply. Foreseeing that in such a difficult moment my heart would be likely to paralyze my poor words, I made my acknowledgements in a written discourse, which was highly praised and recieved the honour of being reproduced, with flattering comments, by the political and professional press.

The following are the main paragraphs of this oration, which I reproduce because, besides containing some autobiographical data (motives inspiring my scientific work, etc.), they reflect with considerable fidelity the fervent eagerness for intellectual revival which the recent national misfortune had awakened in the university youth of Spain:

"*Gentlemen:* The tribute, as kind as it is sincere, which the Staff of the illustrious University of Madrid, presided over by the supreme director of education and the highly worthy representative of Her Majesty's Government, has been so good as to proffer me today places me in a most embarrassing position. The most elementary politeness obliges me to show myself grateful for the unaccustomed honour which you are conferring upon me; but it also demands of me, with the necessity of replying to you, a mental composure and an emotional calmness which are entirely incompatible with the solemnity of the ceremony and its extraordinary significance in my professional life. Permit me, then, upon this occasion, breaking custom in order to avoid the paralyzing affects of emotion upon speech, to have recourse to the written word. The brain disturbed by emotion is like the lake stirred up by the storm: the latter does not reflect clearly the stars in the sky and the trees upon its shores; the former cannot express the ideas and feelings which well up in the mind. There exist, no doubt, spirits of such temper that they can feel and think at the same time; but I, unfortunately, have a brain which is a slave to my heart, and I am permitted to think clearly only unbeknown to the latter.

"These sheets, then, serve me as a mask to hide my disturbed or discomposed expression. Taking refuge behind them, I will say without more preamble that your sincere and enthusiastic congratulations penetrate to the inmost recesses of my soul and that the unaccustomed testimonies of consideration and regard with which you have been pleased to exalt and overwhelm me will remain for ever engraved upon my memory, in the archives of sacred recollections, beside the joyful memories of childhood days and intertwined with the adored image of my mother.

"You undoubtedly exaggerate the importance of my writings and the success of my scientific work. They do not shine so brightly or go so far as your generosity imagines. Nevertheless, I understand well that the excess of your praises is designed for a higher end: in rewarding the modest investigator of today, you have wished, above all, to stimulate the scientific research of tomorrow. With patriotic foresight you have in mind, no doubt, what we might call the exemplary value of applause.

"You have referred kindly to the outstanding character of my faculties and to my unusual aptitude for the cultivation of science; and in all that you have shown more kindness than justice. I am really not a savant, but a patriot; I am a tireless worker rather than a calculating architect. The history of my merits is very simple; it is the quite ordinary history of an indomitable will determined to succeed at any cost. When, in my youth, I saw with sadness how greatly anatomy and biology had deteriorated in Spain and how few of my fellow countrymen had won a place in the history of scientific medicine, I made a firm resolution to abandon for ever my artistic ambitions, the golden dream of my youth, and to sally forth boldly into the international lists of biological research. My strength was patriotic feeling; my guiding star, the exaltation of the academic gown; my ideal, to augument the sum of Spanish ideas circulating in the world, garnering respect and sympathy for our science, and collaborating, finally, in the magnificent undertaking of discovering Nature, which is as much as to say discovering ourselves.

"The conquests made are quite modest; but if you esteem them somewhat, I dedicate them wholeheartedly to the Spanish university, as an offering from a reverent pupil to his *Alma Mater* and with the same noble pride with which the soldier dedicates to the Virgin who protects him in difficult situations the humble trophy won on distant strands.

"And, looking at things rightly, you receive what is justly yours. I am a son of the University; to her I owe what I am and all that I am worth; she taught me to love science and to revere its followers; she guided and supported me in my first experimental efforts, generously affording me, in proportion to her poor resources, the material means for my studies; she, finally, showed me, through a not very consoling present, a past splendid and glorious, and so inspired me with the unquenchable resolution to consecrate my life to the redeeming tasks of the laboratory so as to revive, so far as my powers would permit, the almost forgotten tradition of originality in medicine in our country.

"Fortunately, the Spanish university of today already feels eager for life and for renovation and wishes to travel resolutely along the road of progress. There is revealed in some of her masters, who were formerly devoted to their merely didactic function, a laudable desire to shake off foreign intellectual tutelage and to cooperate with their own personal efforts in the pacific conquest of nature and of art. Fortunately our classrooms, which have more than once been characterized as strongholds of the tyranny of texts and of routine of thought, have already opened to the vivifying breeze of the critical spirit and of universal thought, and in them shines with its own light a brilliant constellation of statesmen, scientists, humanists, and illustrious men of letters.

"Let us all prosecute the task of salvation with increasing ardour; let us work to make the University what it should be, both a factory of ideas and a focus of national education and culture.

"Today, this supreme summons to the heroism of deep thinking and of virile force is more urgent than ever. I address myself to you, the young, the men of tomorrow. In these recent mournful times our country has shrunk; but you should say: 'To the small country, a great soul.' The territory of Spain has diminished; let us all swear to expand its moral and intellectual geography. Let us fight the foreigner with ideas, with new facts, with original and useful inventions. When the people of the more civilized nations can neither discuss nor speak of philosophic, scientific, literary, or industrial matters without stumbling at every step upon Spanish expressions or concepts, the defence of our country will become a superfluous thing; its honour, its power, and its prestige will be completely guaranteed, for no one tramples upon what he loves, nor insults or depreciates what he admires and respects.

"I have spoken of our country and I wish that, upon such a solemn occasion, this should be the last word of my rambling discourse. Let us love our country even if it be only for her undeserved misfortunes. For 'sorrow unites more than does joy,' as Renan has said. Let us inculcate repeatedly into the young that higher culture, original scientific and artistic production, constitute a work of exalted patriotism. No more worthy of praise is he who fights with the rifle than he who wields the pen of the thinker, the retort, or the microscope. Let us do honour to the warrior who has preserved for us the home founded by our ancestors. But let us exalt also the philosopher, the man of letters, the jurist, the naturalist, and the physician, who defend and strengthen energetically in the noble lists of international culture the sacred heritage of our intellectual tradition, our language, our culture, in fine, our historical and spiritual personality, so much discussed and at times so greatly wronged by people of other lands."

Upon this occasion the press, which has always been very kind to me, did me an inestimable service. In its generous eulogies, it exaggerated, no doubt, the poverty of my instrumental equipment, and the disproportion between my economic resources and the results obtained. In any case, its agitation, the more welcome as it was spontaneous, created a certain state of opinion which was met diligently and generously by the Government of Don Francisco Silvela, who proposed to the cabinet, after consulting the opinion of him who was most interested, the foundation of an Institute of Scientific Research, where the humble laureate of Paris would be able to carry on his biological investigations on a broad scale and without economic impediments. The minister of public instruction, García Alix, and F. Villaverde, at the time entrusted with the portfolio of Finance, showed themselves remarkably enthusiastic over the idea and so expressed themselves to me.

The Government having decided to act upon the idea at once, the necessary recommendation to the Council of State was made immediately (the Cortes [4] were not in session) and there was appropriated for the purchase of equipment and the establishment of the laboratory 80,000 pesetas, leaving for the Cortes the legalization of the project and the ratification of the credits for equipment and personnel. With real munificence, Señor Silvela fixed the emolument of the Director at 10,000 pesetas, an excessive figure which, at my request, was reduced by the Count of Romanones, the successor of Sr. García Alix, when the Liberal party came into power, in 1901. The sanction of the co-legislative

[4] The Spanish parliament. (Translator's note.)

bodies having been obtained, the new centre of studies, under the designation *Laboratorio de Investigaciones biológicas,* was installed provisionally in a house in the Calle de Ventura de la Vega. Some months later, upon the initiative of the new Minister of Public Instruction, it was removed to permanent quarters in the Museum of Dr. Velasco.

Needless to say, the creation of this Laboratory fully satisfied my aspirations. Besides providing me with plentiful and completely up to date equipment, it did away with the deficit which, notwithstanding the support of the Faculty and the generosity of Dr. Busto, was caused by the purchase of books and scientific periodicals and, above all, by the publication of my *Revista trimestral,* which was continued as a new annual entitled *Trabajos del Laboratorio de Investigaciones biológicas.* Excellent paper, engravings and lithographs without restriction, and unlimited extension of the text in accordance with the manuscript available were the material gains secured, and as didactic advantages the daily more vigorous and reiterated collaboration of several assistants and students. Permit me to mention that in the *Trabajos* mentioned, which were established in 1902,[5] there have appeared up to today (1923) more than three hundred and fifty original monographs, which gives me the right and the satisfaction of thinking that the sacrifice made by the State has not been sterile for the progress of science and the credit of Spain abroad.

During the biennium 1900 and 1901, I sent to press several publications worthy of notice besides those on the acoustic and olfactory cortex already mentioned. These concerned the terminations of the auditory fibres, the thalamic connection of the central sensory tract (spinal lemniscus) and the other connections of the thalamus, the accessory olfactory bulb, the probable significance of the cells with short axons, the posterior quadrigeminal bodies,

[5] The first volume bears the dates 1901–1902, and the first papers appearing in the *Trabajos* are cited by the author in his bibliography under 1901. (Translator's note.)

etc. There were also a paper on some staining methods and one on a steroscopic invention.

The investigations of 1900–1901 were amplified and rounded out by those undertaken in 1902 and 1903. Being taken up with the organization of the cerebral centres and anxious to augment my assets with new facts in this *terra ignota,* I prosecuted the task of analysis with my habitual ardour, concentrating on the structure of the septum lucidum, the minute anatomy of the thalamus, with particular attention to the body of Luys, the mammillary body, and the tuber cinereum, and, finally, a certain enigmatic nucleus connected with the optic tract.

Afterwards, my activities were devoted to the cerebellar peduncles, elucidating various obscure points of their connections and secondary paths; I attacked, by the methods of Marchi and Golgi, the relations between the cerebrum, the anterior quadrigeminal bodies, and the thalamus; and, finally, I made some contributions on the staining of the myelin sheaths and the handling of sections.

I shall spare the reader the contents of these papers and, on account of their descriptive dryness, shall not even dare to mention them by title.

With the analysis of the centres of the cerebrum, I brought to a conclusion what we might call my programme of neuronal morphology and of breaking up new ground in the more or less cultivated territories of the brain and spinal cord. In the second half of 1903 a new cycle of investigations opened up for me. Thenceforward, my attention was drawn preferentially to the seductive problem of the intimate organization of the nerve cell and of the axis cylinder.

CHAPTER XIX

Participation of the Spanish histologists in the International Medical Congress held in Madrid in 1903. Communications of various foreign and native professors. Demonstration by Simarro of a new method for colouring the neurofibrils. Starting from this interesting procedure, I come by chance upon a very simple and constant formula for the impregnation of the neurofibrils, of axons, and of central and peripheral nerve endings. Story of the efforts directed towards the discovery of the new formula and the later perfecting thereof. Thanks to the new technical method, I am able to confirm and finally to consolidate earlier discoveries and to gather many new ones.

The year 1903 was one of the most active of the recently created Laboratory of Biological Research. A fever of work, comparable only with that experienced in the years 1889 and 1890, possessed me, absorbing all my faculties. No less than fourteen communications, some of them as voluminous as books, did I publish in that year, the second half of which I consider to have been the peak of my activity in scientific inquiry. Yet I was able during the hot weather to find enough time to undertake a trip through enchanting Italy, accompanied by my wife and sisters and bearing the indispensable camera, visiting Genoa, Milan, Turin, Pavia, Venice, Florence, Rome, Pisa, Naples, and other wonderful cities of the fatherland of art. Two fortunate events contributed very largely to this unusual display of energy: first the sessions of the International Congress of Medicine held in Madrid that spring, and later, about the month of October, the chance encounter of a certain formula for the impregnation of nerve cells and fibres which was singularly productive of new discoveries.

This International Congress compelled, naturally, the mobilization of all the forces of the Spanish enthusiasts for the work of the laboratory. It was important to play a part which should be as creditable as possible and we had to do our best.

For the meeting in Madrid there assembled numerous foreign scientists (Behring, Metchnikoff, Waldeyer, Frank, Veratti, Van Gehuchten, Henschen, Unna, Donaggio, and others) and not a few native and Spanish-American medical men.

Entrusted with the presidency of the section of Anatomy and Anthropology, I had plenty to do during those days of constant exertion in organizing and directing the sessions, completing my own and my pupils' communications, arranging soirées of microscopic demonstrations, attending banquets and other official enterainments. We all worked hard, in fact, to make pleasant to our illustrious guests their sojourn among us.

Among the eminent members of the Congress who took part in the proceedings of my section, several merit special mention, not only on account of their world-wide fame, but, also, because of the interest of their communications. Mr. Henschen, Professor at Stockholm, lectured in San Carlos on clinical cases of central blindness and the accompanying lesions of the occipital lobe of the brain, a subject intimately related to my histological studies upon the calcarine fissure. Professor Unna of Hamburg, the distinguished dermatologist, the originator of important methods of staining the epithelial and conjunctival tissues had the courtesy to attribute to me in a brilliant public address priority in the discovery of the plasma cells (my cyanophile cells found in syphilomas). The professor of Louvain, Mr. A. Van Gehuchten, an old friend of mine, presented to the Congress the first fruits of a procedure for demonstrating the course of the motor roots (the procedure of delayed retrograde degeneration). Dr. E. Veratti, a young man of great talent, pupil and assistant of Golgi, showed himself in various papers and discussions an enthusiastic defender of his teacher's ideas and methods; while the young professor of Modena, A. Donaggio made a favourable impression in the sessions for demonstrations, exhibiting most beautiful preparations of the internal framework of the neurons (the neuro-fibrils of Bethe) coloured by a technique of his own invention, which he did not care to divulge; and various other distinguished men also took part.

Among the Spanish members of the Congress—I refer naturally to the section of anatomy and anthropology—there deserve special mention Professor Anton, who gave an eloquent address upon some anthropological problems; and very specially Dr. L. Simarro, who in the presence of a large number of foreign savants demonstrated in the Laboratory for Biological Research excellent preparations of the neuro-fibrillar net impregnated by an original method which we shall consider later. Of less interest were the communications presented by other members including my own, one of which, of a polemical nature, concerned the venturesome reticular theories of A. Bethe whose method I had just finished trying out. In it I attempted particularly to promote and enliven the discussion on the important problem of the interneuronal connections and the minute structure of the nervous protoplasm, questions at that time of vital interest.

In the demonstration sessions, I exhibited many choice preparations showing the structure of the spinal cord, the cerebrum, and the cerebellum; preparations which were in agreement in spite of being stained by the methods of Golgi and of Ehrlich (pericellular baskets, collateral nerve bifurcations, etc.). With these I attempted to persuade the members of the absolutely objective nature of my interpretations concerning the method of termination of the nerve fibres in the gray matter.

Finally, for the sake of completeness as regards my personal part in the discussions, I have to mention also my address delivered in the great amphitheatre of San Carlos in the presence of numerous foreign scientists and honoured besides by the presence of the President of the Council of Ministers, Señor Fernández Villaverde. My lecture was upon the structural plan of the optic thalamus.

The second event referred to cannot be mentioned without looking backwards somewhat in the course of time and explaining some technical antecedents.

It is notorious that, in science as in art, each epoch has its dominant preoccupation which few succeed in escaping. Knowledge of the morphology of neurons and of the characteristic behavior of the axonal and dendritic processes being completed, or at least greatly advanced, the interest of the majority of neurologists turned toward the intimate structure of neuroprotoplasm. Along with other observers I also was swept away by the current.

Of course, the structural problem and the solution proposed during the years 1900–03 were old stories. Many years before, Max Schultze, Schwalbe, Ranvier, and more recently A. Dogiel (1898) had observed within the bodies of the nerve cells a certain enigmatic warp composed of fine granular fibrils which were prolonged into the protoplasmic processes.

The methods of the time, however, were inadequate to elucidate satisfactorily the relations of this intra-protoplasmic skeleton. Do such extremely delicate filaments constitute a net or run independently? Are they prolonged within the axons as far as the terminal arborizations? Finally, do there exist grounds for regarding them as intracellular pathways specially differentiated for the propagation of the nerve impulse?

The final answering of these questions necessarily involved the finding of some staining method which would be highly selective for the framework referred to. In the nerve cells of some invertebrates, leeches, for example, a Hungarian investigator, M. Apathy of Clausenburg, had the good fortune to stumble upon this much desired analytical procedure (a special formula for fixation using gold chloride) and to observe and demonstrate for the first time, intensely stained in violet, the neurofibrils or elementary conductive fibrils in question.

Unfortunately, the very complicated method invented by Apathy was not applicable to vertebrates. Its inconstancy, moreover, surpassed that of the most unreliable formulae of histological technique. All the neurologists who employed it had lamentable failures. When already, with the recession of the wave of enthusiasm, it was thought that those beautiful intra-cellular networks were perhaps something peculiar to the worms, there appeared within the fold another very original investigator. This was the physiologist A. Bethe, at that time professor in Strassburg, who restored the question to the order of the day, surprising us with an important memoir in which, by the aid of a special method (a combination of a mordant, ammonium molybdate, with a dye, toluidine blue), he demonstrated the neurofibrils of vertebrates, in particular those contained in the large cells of the spinal cord, ganglia, and cerebellum.

Fascinated by the importance and novelty of the revelations of Bethe, we all wished to take part in the enterprise, hoping for new and important conquests.

Adverse fate, however, continued in the ascendent. The complicated procedure of A. Bethe was not within reach of everybody. Like that of Apathy, it flourished only in the laboratory of its inventor or in the hands of a very few initiates. As for me, I obtained by dint of patience some mediocre and inadequate stains. Attributing the failure to my lack of skill as a preparator, I politely requested from the brilliant originator of the method, a typical preparation to compare with my own. Some weeks later I received, carefully packed, like precious objects, two preparations, one of the cerebellum, the other of the spinal cord of the rabbit.

"These preparations are exceptionally good," the Strassburg Professor wrote to me. "They have been made by the best of my students. Be careful in handling them and return them as soon as possible, as we have no others at present."

What a disappointment! The jewels of technique, those invaluable preparations, unpacked with emotion and examined with a palpitating heart, were no better than mine! Certainly within the nerve protoplasm the neurofibrils impregnated in violet could be observed, but they were so pale on the granular background of the matrix of the cytoplasm that it was impossible to recognize clearly their precise arrangement and their relations with other, extracellular structures. And upon such images had Bethe constructed a formidable theoretical edifice! In vain I toiled in search of the external course of the delicate filaments. Yet the Strassburg savant talked to us with surprising self possession of the direct continuity of these filaments with the pericellular net of Golgi (in reality discovered by me as already stated) a net itself interpreted arbitrarily (forgetting or ignoring all the terminations revealed by the methods of Golgi and Ehrlich) as the terminal portion of the nerve fibres.

I burned with desire to see the aforesaid neurofibrils in irreproachable preparations. Disillusioned regarding the fortuitous and inadequate techniques of Apathy and Bethe, unable nevertheless to attempt that of Donaggio, which was kept secret, and persuaded that for the vigorous colouration of such delicate threads it was necessary to resort to metallic reductions, I devoted myself persistently from 1901 to numerous attempts at impregnation. I made use sometimes of the reaction of ammoniacal oxide of silver discovered by Fajersztajn (1901), at other times of chloride of gold in the presence of tanin and pyrogallic acid, and at yet others of the haloid salts of silver and the photographic reducing agents introduced in microtechnique by Simarro (1900). The first fruits of this persistent labour were certain formulae of little importance for the colouration of the axons and of the myelin. The neurofibrillar skeleton, however, and the central nerve terminations, the main objective of my eager search, eluded me obstinately.

To such persistent efforts I was incited not so much by the hope of running across an easy procedure for the demonstration of the intraneural warp as by a desire to discover a formula for impregnation capable of producing intense and at the same time perfectly transparent colouration of the nerve cells and fibres. I longed to contrast once more the beautiful revelations of chromate of silver with those of other methods against which could not be urged the objection that they showed the cellular body and its processes as opaque silhouettes without suggestion of structure. Finally, I was inspired by the hope of procuring a powerful weapon with which to fence against many technical innovators who were irresistably inclined to the anarchistic vice of denying in the name of a new truth the truths already discovered by others.

After fruitless attempts with the foregoing methods, I devoted particular attention in 1903 to that of Dr. Simarro, the first author who succeeded in staining the neurofibrils by means of silver salts.

The sole result of all these efforts was the simplifying of the technique of the Spanish investigator, by eliminating the troublesome operation of poisoning the animals and getting rid of the disturbing action of light. In spite of everything, my hopes of bringing to the staining of neurofibrils constancy, vigour, and general applicability were disappointed. Essentially comparable with those of Simarro, my preparations showed nothing new.

At that time (August, 1903), with the excuse of resting my over-excited brain, I undertook the aforementioned pleasure trip to seductive Italy. The noble and sublime visions of art afforded thereby gave me the greatest delight, but from time to time there returned the anxieties of the laboratory, disturbing me in my contemplations. Before the pictures in a museum or at the foot of glorious ruins, I was seized persistently by hypotheses requiring experimental proof, technical projects apparently crammed full of promises.

One day, when the return journey was already commenced and my brain was vibrating with the vigorous shaking of the train there took possession of me with the obsessive strength of a fixed idea, a very simple hypothesis, which explained satisfactorily the failures of the method of Simarro and contained the germ (in case it should be confirmed) of an analytical resource as simple as efficacious.

Today I cannot understand why so obvious a thought had not occurred to me sooner. How true it is that the simplest solutions always emerge latest and that the constructive imagination before finding the good road, the eagerly sought for economic formula as Mach would say, begins by losing itself in the complicated.

This is the elementary and fruitful idea which flirted so much before revealing itself; the enigmatic substance which generates the neurofibrillar reaction must be purely and simply hot, free, nitrate of silver, capable of being precipitated by physical processes on the neurofibrillar skeleton modified by the action of the temperature. The chlorides and bromides of silver not only take no part in the reaction, but interfere with it. If the metallic deposit proceeds from the nitrate of silver in a colloidal medium, it results obviously that only a physical developer (pyrogallic acid or hydroquinone without alkali in place of the chemical developers rich in alkali used by Simarro) can precipitate the said nitrate upon the protoplasmic structures, leaving unchanged the disturbing bromides and chlorides, which are incapable of being reduced with the new developers. In order, however, to retain the free silver nitrate eliminated in the method of Simarro, it would be necessary to immerse not the sections but the blocks of nervous tissue in the silver bath and to increase the strength of the latter markedly. I have said that this project pursued me like an obsession. I was devoured by impatience and longed to find myself in the laboratory to put my schemes into practice. Genoa, Nice, Monaco, Marseilles—all the smiling and luminous cities of the famous *Côte d'Azur*—passed before my eyes leaving hardly a trace on my mind.

At my arrival in Madrid, I fell upon the experimental animals kept in my laboratory like a lion upon its prey. I tested the formula of which I had thought and its results were admirable. This first formula is summarized in the following simple steps: (*a*) direct immersion of the pieces of nervous tissue in silver nitrate; (*b*) heating for four days; (*c*) reduction of the silver salt in the block by means of a bath of pyrogallic acid kept in darkness with or without the addition of formalin; (*d*) washing; (*e*) alcohol; (*f*) imbedding in celliodin and finally sectioning. In sections placed in nitrate of silver I obtained no result. (It will be remembered that in the method of Simarro the staining was successful only in sections.)

Great were my delight and surprise. From the first attempts the neurofibrils of almost all the nerve cells of the spinal cord, medulla oblongata, ganglia, cerebrum, and cerebellum, besides numerous types of axonic terminal arborizations, appeared splendidly impregnated with a brown, black or brick red colour and perfectly transparent. Many dendrites ran in all directions across the tangled matrix of the gray matter, visible thanks to the intense dark brown colour of their little neurofibrillar bundles. As was to be foreseen, the undesirable reduction of silver chlorides and albuminates (striae of Fromman, constrictions, etc.) was conspicuous by its absence. Finally—and this was the greatest advantage—the colouration, besides being successful in all the nerve centres, gave constant results so long as my formula was followed strictly.

I remember still the admiring exclamation with which, a few weeks after the discovery, when a note explaining the formula had been published, van Gehuchten told me of the result of his first attempt on the brain of the rabbit. "Je n'ai pas dormi!" Nor did I sleep for several days, my brain throbbing with the outlines of new plans for work and anxious also over the ungrateful task of determining by experiment the optimum conditions for the reaction.

A preliminary note hastily published in the medical archives recently founded by Dr. Cortejo and Dr. Pittaluga, completed later by an extensive and careful monograph illustrated with engravings, made public rapidly the results obtained, which were confirmed and amplified greatly by many foreign investigators. Among the earliest to confirm them, to whom the method yielded a rich harvest of new facts, we remember Van der Stricht, Van Gehuchten, Michotto, Besta, Azoulay, Nageotte, Lugaro, Holmgren,

Retzius, Von Lenhossék, Schäffer, Umberto Rossi, Ottorino Rossi, Levi, Pighini, Legendre, Medea, Perroncito, London, G. Sala, and many others. With singular success the new formula was applied in Spain by my brother, R. Illera, Dalmacio García, and especially my assistant, Dr. Tello, who, in the exploration to which he subjected the nerve centres of lower vertebrates, besides reaping a rich harvest of new facts, discovered the curious phenomenon of a change in the neurofibrils during hibernation (fusiform transformation, etc.). Later it has been used with success by many others, among whom Achúcarro, Lafora, F. de Castro, D. Domingo Sánchez y Sánchez, Laura Forster, Lorente de Nó, Muñoz Urra, etc. are outstanding. From the formula under consideration have been derived a multitude of variants, some of which, like that of Levaditi, have been of service in the discovery of the microbe of syphilis.

In spite of its excellence and its ability to reveal the reticulum even in the smallest elements of the cerebrum and cerebellum, the method was still subject to certain defects. Nitrate of silver has mediocre qualities as a fixing agent and the modus operandi originally adopted very often colours the axons weakly and unevenly. If, however, the treatment of the pieces with silver nitrate is preceded by fixation for twenty-four hours in alcohol alone, in formol, or even better in alcohol with a few drops of ammonia added, this grave defect is corrected, vigorous and uniform colouration of both coarse and fine axis-cylinders being obtained, as well as of the majority of the central and peripheral arborizations in the nervous system. This new formula has, besides, the advantage of being applicable to all vertebrates and of producing excellent pictures in newborn or embryonic animals.

I trust that the reader will pardon the prolix details set forth concerning the investigations of technique in 1903, but the subject justifies the prolixity. Besides the fact that the new technique was the signal for a long series of laboratory studies published during twenty years, I cannot forget in writing these memoirs that I am read chiefly by those engaged in laboratory occupations. These will know how to excuse me and will perhaps thank me for a few descriptive details. I believe, moreover, that nothing inspires the new investigator so much as the honest narrative of the attempts carried out, of the vacillations, meanderings and strayings of the experimental work; in sum, of the artifices brought into play during the lengthy process of enquiry before reaching the desired solution. The novice will observe, finally, that success almost always represents a function and result of constant attention and persistent effort. When, burning with the sacred fire, he realizes how far chance enters into fortunate discoveries—chance deliberately sought and well taken advantage of, naturally—he will repeat doubtless, full of proud confidence, the well known exclamation of Corregio before a picture of Raphael "Anch'io son' pittore." Strange coincidence! Shortly after the publication of my formula, which was reached, as I have explained above, by starting with the analysis of the method of Simarro; the German Bielschowsky arrived at similar results making use also of nitrate of silver, but taking as a point of departure the method of Fajersztajn. Thenceforth, then, neurological technique possessed two analytical resources equally easy and fruitful; that of Bielschowsky, especially applicable to the human brain (frozen sections of blocks fixed in formalin), and particularly to its anatomo-pathological lesions, and mine, specially appropriate for the exploration of the structure of the nerve centres in mammals and lower vertebrates, sensory and sympathetic ganglia, nerve terminations, and embryonic development.

In after years various authors making use of my procedure altered it, as I have pointed out, to adapt it to new objects of study. Today at least twenty variants of my original formula are known.

CHAPTER XX

My discoveries with the new formula for silver impregnation during the years 1903, 1904, and 1905. Real arrangement of the neurofibrillar skeleton in the nervous protoplasm and in the pericellular arborizations; with the collaboration of Tello I demonstrate curious physiological variations of the neurofibrillar net under the action of temperature; and assisted by Don D. García, the neurofibrillar changes in rabies. Application of the method to embryos and fetuses, and study in birds and mammals of the structure of the nuclei in the medulla oblongata and the origin of the acoustic, motor, and sensory nerves. The neurofibrils of worms, particularly of the earthworm. Structural analysis of the motor end plates, of the neurons of the retina, and of other peripheral sense organs. Interesting morphological revelations secured in the sensory and sympathetic ganglia of man, etc.

It is a commonplace fact that scientific discoveries are a function of the methods used. A strictly differential technique having appeared, there follow immediately, in a logical series and in an almost automatic fashion, unlooked for clarifications of problems formerly insoluble or incompletely settled. And if this is true in respect of all the natural sciences, it is so most conspicuously in the realms of histology. For the histologist, every advance in staining technique is something like the acquisition of a new sense directed towards the unknown. As if nature had determined to hide from our eyes the marvellous structure of its organization, the cell, the mysterious protagonist of life, is hidden obstinately in the double invisibility of smallness and homogeneity. Structures of formidable complexity appear under the microscope with the colourlessness, the uniformity of refractive index, and the simplicity of architecture of a mass of jelly. The other natural sciences are more fortunate in that they work with objects of study which are directly accessible to the senses. Only histology and bacteriology are obliged to fulfil the preliminary and difficult task of making visible their special objects of study before they can commence the work of analysis. And in such a severe campaign they have to struggle, as I have already said, with two adversaries; smallness and transparency. The histologist can advance in the knowledge of the tissues only by impregnating or tinting them selectively with various hues which are capable of making the cells stand out energetically from an uncoloured background. In this way, the bee-hive of the cells is revealed to us unveiled; it might be said that the swarm of transparent and invisible infusorians is transformed into a flock of painted butterflies.

Hence, when chance permits an investigator to create a new selective staining method or to perfect in a fortunate way one already known, histology sensibly extends its horizon. The harvesting of new and significant facts, the cataloguing of forms and structures, is performed easily and refreshingly as if one reaped at will in a wheat-field sown by others.

Something of this sort was my experience in the systematic application of the formula of impregnation with reduced silver nitrate, of which the principal advantages are, as I have already said, its wide applicability, the transparency of colouration, the exquisite selectivity for the neurons, and the extraordinary simplicity of the procedure. This simplicity of the manipulations made it possible to concentrate a tremendous amount of work in a very short time, whence I was able to advance faster than Bielschowsky, Donaggio, and other illustrious introducers of methods which are very valuable but less rapid and convenient for the collection of new facts. The very clear and decisive preparations obtained at so little cost, besides revealing unknown morphological arrangements in various provinces of the nervous system and even in tissues of other kinds, enabled me to confirm anatomical data previously insecurely founded and to strengthen and establish somewhat controversial doctrines. It is unnecessary to say that during the last months of 1903 and through the following years I threw myself into the task, not merely actively, but with that impetuous enthusiasm, monopolizing and absorbing, which has earned me more than one dislike among my rivals.

Even in the first paper which appeared in my review the gleanings of new facts or of establishment of those little known were considerable. I shall mention here, in the briefest possible manner, only the most outstanding discoveries.

The first concerned the general problem of the architecture of the neurofibrils, which has already been referred to in the foregoing chapter in summarizing the ideas of Apathy and Bethe. My formula lent itself particularly well to this. As is shown in Fig. 70 the said framework is

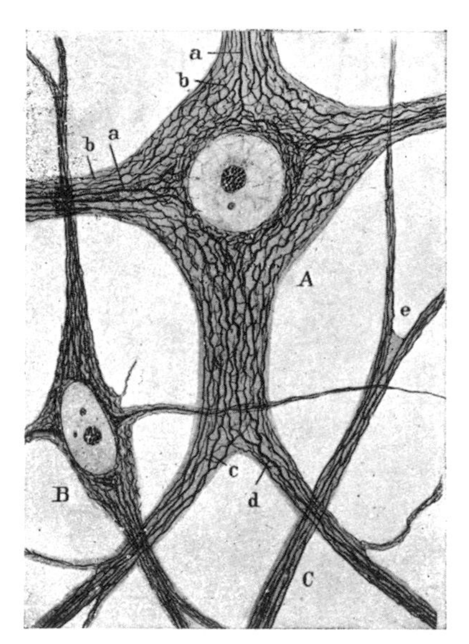

Fig. 70. Two Cells of the Spinal Cord of a Rabbit a Few Days Old. Observe at *a* and *b* indubitable branching of the intraprotoplasmic filaments and true net-formation. (Method of reduced silver nitrate.)

composed not of a system of independent threads passing from the cell body into the processes, as Apathy, Bethe, and Bielschowsky, and, to some extent, also Donaggio thought, but of a network. This arrangement was soon confirmed by a large number of authors.

My studies showed also that the neurofibrillar skeleton exhibits variations in arrangement according to the type of cell studied; and along with my assistant, Dr. Tello, I demonstrated that the neurofibrils change their appearance under physiological and pathological stimulation.

Almost at the same time I found that, under certain conditions, the new formula also produces excellent images of the so-called reticular apparatus of Golgi, and finally, of the neurofibrils in many terminal arborizations.

The last mentioned property was the more important since we lacked up to that time a reliable method capable of demonstrating and contrasting regularly the pericellular axonic arborizations revealed by silver chromate in the cerebellum and the spinal cord. When I saw the very beautiful preparations of the cerebellum, in which the basket endings, and the mossy and climbing fibres appeared bright and transparent, in energetic and varied hues, and stained completely, without any tintorial lacuna, my delight was immense. Shattered for ever were the objections of the sullen impugners of the method of Golgi, who were always suspicious that the silhouettes of the chromate of silver did not represent preexistent arrangements. Moreover, the colloidal silver does not only reproduce the classic forms of Golgi preparations but also brings out interesting and unexpected details of structure.

My eager curiosity led me next to try the new method of analysis repeatedly on embryos and recently born animals and I found that the colouration is obtained in nerve cells and fibres in the course of development even more constantly and intensely than in the adult. Many valuable observations were thus made in young birds and mammals.

The discovery of the curious modifications undergone by the neurofibrils when subjected to physiological stimulation led me to examine the reticulum in various pathological conditions. I hoped to discover some variation more or less typical of infective processes in the nervous system and capable of being utilized in diagnosis. These hopes were fully confirmed in the case of the nerve centres of animals suffering from rabies, in the study of which I was zealously assisted by D. Dalmacio García, chief of the Veterinary Section of the National Institute of Hygiene.

To round out the series of papers of 1904 I may cite one on the motor end plates of birds and mammals, one on the neurofibrils of the retina, and one on the ganglia of the earthworm.

The inventory of the work of 1904 would not be complete if I did not record that in that year I brought to a successful conclusion my great work in three volumes entitled *Histología del sistema nervioso del hombre y de los vertebrados*[1] (Madrid, 1899–1904). Of the amount of work put into it during the five years spent in printing it an idea maybe obtained from its 1800 pages of text in large quarto and its 887 original illustrations, almost all of large size. The reader will understand that in writing such a voluminous book, in which was summarized and rounded out the work of fifteen years, I sought honour more than profit. And without being guilty of immodesty or petulance, I may say that my calculations were not mistaken. There are works for which there is no greater reward than the consciousness of the personal esteem and the approval of the learned. On that occasion my exertions and efforts obtained the sole recompense to which I aspired; the respectful eulogies of the critics and the complimentary opinions of the most eminent scientists.

Being written in a language little known to scientists and containing an abundance of descriptive details, largely original, my book was honoured with various offers of translation. Among them, I recall particularly that of the firm of J. A. Barth, of Leipzig, and that of the house

[1] To attract purchasers, the publishers fixed the wholesale price of the three volumes at a little more than ten pesetas (fifteen for subscribers). Moreover, considering the essentially monographic character of the work, only 800 copies were printed. When I settled the account after the whole edition had been sold, I found that my losses exceeded three thousand pesetas.

of A. Maloine, in Paris. Finally, I consented to a French version in charge of my friend Dr. Leon Azoulay, a version which appeared in 1911 [2] and which may be regarded as a new work since I included in it all the fruit of my investigations up to that date.

I have said elsewhere, and I take pleasure in repeating, certain that the indulgence of the reader will excuse my weakness: the object of my work was, first of all, to create for myself an enduring stimulus to intensive work; foreseeing possible hours of discouragement and fatigue, I wished deliberately to give up my liberty by a formal engagement of honour made with the public. The book cited, moreover, was an expression of an egoism too human not to be forgivable. Fearful of oblivion and uncertain of followers capable of affirming and defending before strangers my modest scientific accomplishments, I was determined to combine into one organized whole the neurological monographs published during three lustra in periodicals at home and abroad, besides filling in with new inquiries the points not formerly considered. But before and beyond everything else, I desired my book to be—pardon the presumption—the trophy laid at the feet of the languishing science of Spain and the offering of fervent love rendered by a Spaniard to his despised country.

During the year 1905, my activities centered chiefly upon the architecture of the sensory and sympathetic ganglia of adult man and of some large mammals. Up to then the two methods for revealing the morphology of ganglionic neurons, namely that of Golgi and that of Ehrlich, had hardly been applied to the full-grown man. Hence the classic descriptions of Golgi, Ehrlich, Retzius, Dogiel, and others referred almost exclusively to embryos or young and small-sized mammals (mouse, rabbit, cat, etc., among mammals; chick, among birds). Considering the great changes undergone by all the nerve centres in their transition from the foetal stage to that of full maturity, one

[2] See bibliography, item 8.

wondered whether the human sensory and sympathetic ganglia might not have experienced important structural alterations during post-foetal development. But, for the elucidation of this point, histological technique prior to 1903 offered no reliable and effective method.

This methodological gap was happily filled by the new formula of impregnation, which has the inestimable advantage of staining intensely the sensory and sympathetic cells of adult man, even in material that is not very fresh.

Such an excellent property, besides the constancy and vigour of the colouration, permitted me, in my first exploratory efforts in the sensory ganglia, to discover a number of important facts of structure and to demonstrate certain changes in old age.

The strange types of neurons and the curious phenomena of sprouting described in the human ganglia attracted strongly the attention of histologists and pathologists, especially of J. Nageotte, who, thanks to penetrating explorations in the ganglia of tabetics by the method so often referred to, demonstrated new forms of pathological regeneration besides a notable increase of certain features pointed out by me in normal persons. The road having been opened up, a multitude of neurologists afterwards advanced along it with great success, among whom may be mentioned Levi, Marinesco, H. Rossi, L. Sala, Pacheco, Besta, Schäffer, Dustin, Ranson, Minea, Bielschowsky, Achúcarro, Castro, and others; some were animated by the desire to discover new normal forms, others were inspired by the hope of finding specific alterations associated with definite pathological processes. At the present time, the bibliography stirred up by my communication has extended to more than a hundred foreign publications.

No less unusual and disconcerting were the facts observed in examining the human sympathetic ganglia, as some of the adjoining illustrations testify (Figs. 71, 72). At the present time, a review of the investigations to which my inquiry upon the human sympathetic ganglia gave

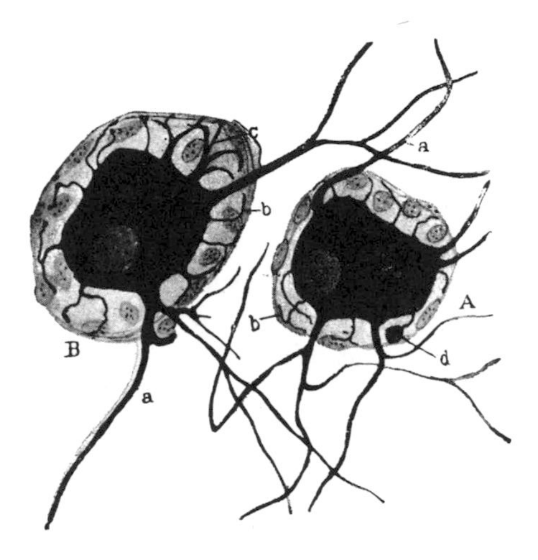

FIG. 71. CELLS OF THE SYMPATHETIC TRUNK OF MAN. Intermediate type with both short and long dendrites. *a*, axon; *b*, *c*, short dendrites.

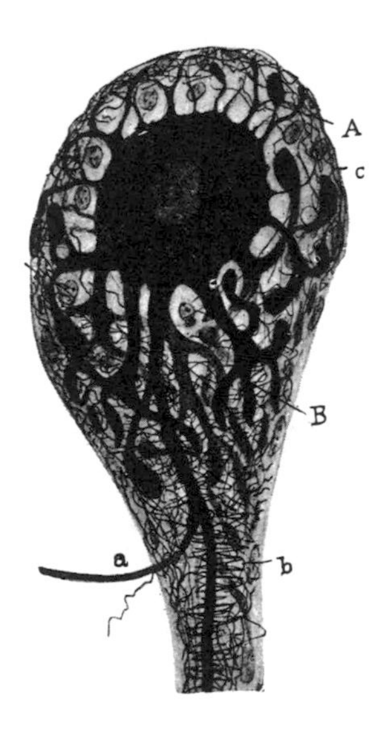

FIG. 72. HUMAN SYMPATHETIC CELL OF THE COMET TYPE.

rise would fill many pages. Without boasting, I can affirm that my investigations on the ganglia are among the most fortunate of my scientific work in the decade from 1903 to 1913.

Finally, I may close this decidedly tedious list of successful researches by mentioning a certain paper on the neurofibrils of the cerebellum and an essay on the effects of the new method on the structure of the striated muscle fibre. In the former, which is considerably more interesting than the latter, an account is given of observations with the new method on the stellate cells of the molecular layer of the cerebellum, of which the axon and the well known collaterals terminating in pericellular baskets are splendidly stained.

Among other points, certain developmental defects were signalized. These errors, which are not rare in the nerve centres, may have more significance than I attributed to them. It seems probable that the singular idiosyncracies of certain brains are due not merely to a chance augmentation or to a perfection by use of certain cells and pathways, but also to local failures of neuronal growth, as a result of which particular association systems may be extraordinarily weak or even absent.

CHAPTER XXI

Studies of 1905, 1906, and 1907. Investigations on the regeneration of the nerves and the central tracts. Controversy between the monogenists and the polygenists. The neuron theory emerges triumphant from the test to which it was submitted by the adherents of the chain theory. New studies on the genesis of the nerve tracts in the embryo, also strengthening the neuron conception. Facts demonstrating that the neurofibrils of the nerve cell consist of relatively autonomous living units.

The years 1905 and 1906 correspond with the zenith of my scientific career. During them fortune smiled upon me to the point of my attaining the highest rewards to which a man of science can aspire; and in the same period, besides contributions of less weight, I made observations which were decisive for the establishment of the neuron conception, at that time much discussed.

Let me begin by referring briefly to the most important of my laboratory work during these two years.

In response to stimuli of which I shall speak shortly, I devoted my attention in the first place to elucidating the always much discussed problem of the mechanism of regeneration of interrupted nerves and central nerve tracts; and afterwards (this was the task carried out in the second half of 1906) to studying with the new technique the genesis of the nerve fibres in the embryo, a subject intimately related to the preceding one.

Both studies were to meet a certain state of current opinion. After a long period of peaceful and almost undisputed supremacy of the neuron doctrine, the principal objective proofs of which, as the reader will remember, I had the good fortune to bring forth, there was reborn with incredible vigour in certain schools the old and almost forgotten error of reticularism and other similar speculative extravagances as, for example, the chain theory. It would appear that certain minds with a propensity to mysticism are troubled by simple and obvious truths. Temperaments of exaggerated arrogance seem determined to conquer fame not by the honourable and difficult road of discovering new facts, but by the much more convenient and expeditious one of denying or breaking down belief in the most absolutely demonstrated facts, in the name of utterly unfounded prejudices. Such an anarchical and calamitous passion, never completely eradicated from among biologists, reached its highest culmination, as I have just said, in the years 1900 to 1904. Then, however, the fanatics of reticularism adopted new tactics. Having little expectation, doubtless, of winning the victory in the open country of adult neuronal morphology, they chose for opposing neuronism the seemingly more propitious field of the regeneration of nerves and of embryonic neurogenesis.

Many were the bold adventurers who wished to fight in the shadow of the ancient banner unfurled by Gerlach and Meynert as far back as 1867. Discordant, and even antagonistic in many of their statements, they agreed only in an extraordinary and unanimous feeling of aversion for the doctrine of contact and of the independence of the nerve cells; a doctrine demonstrated to satiety, as we know, decades before by His, Forel, myself, Lenhossék, Retzius, Kölliker, van Gehuchten, Lugaro, Waldeyer, and Harrison, in the field of histology and normal histogenesis; and by Waller, Münzer, Ranvier, Vanlair, Ziegler, Stroebe, Forsmann, Marinesco, Langley, Mott, Halliburton, Segale, Purpura, and many others in the sphere of the degeneration and regeneration of nerves. Except the eminent Professor Nissl and an occasional other, the ranks of reticularism were made up of young enthusiasts as eager for reputation as they were uncritical in observation. I remember among them Büngner, Joris, Huber, Sedgwig, Ballance, Wietting, Marchand, Galeotti and Levi, Monckeberg, Durante, O. Schültze, and others, some of whom worked in times prior to 1900.

The leader and strategist of this brilliant host, by

the double right of talent and of critical fearlessness, came to be Alfred Bethe, a teacher in the University of Strassburg, who was justly famous on account of his impressive studies on the neurofibrils of vertebrates.

In 1903 the contagion of reticularism became so virulent and widespread, due mainly to the attractive statements of Bethe, that the illustrious Waldeyer was shaken in his faith as a neuronist, Professor Marinesco passed over temporarily to the opposing army and—who would have thought it!—even the brilliant van Gehuchten, one of the pillars of neuronism, weakened. The last, though not renouncing the orthodox doctrine entirely, made the following humiliating concession to the dissenters: "In the adult the nerve cell is perfectly individual, the product of a single neuroblast; but in pathological conditions, for example during the process of regeneration of a nerve, the new axis cylinders result from the fusion and differentiation of a chain of peripheral neuroblasts."

The quotation will show the reader to what a point the danger had grown. There were authors who regarded as definitely overthrown the brilliant conception of His and Forel. At length the reticularist chimaera showed itself so aggressive and employed, in its inconsistent objections, language so arrogant and so immoderate that the patience of the neuronists reached its limit. It was necessary to bring forward a corrective for the general aberration. A number of scientists, surprised at my silence and perhaps considering me to be the one most obligated to resume arms for the rights of truth, wrote to me in a tone of reproach: "What are you doing? How is it that you do not defend yourself?"

I have always felt an invincible repugnance for polemics. Precious time is wasted in them, which could be used better in gathering new facts. Besides, who does not know that truth, even though undefended, will prevail in the end? However, before the rolling tide of error and the reiterated urging of my friends I found myself obliged to make a halt in my progress and to descend to the palestra, bemoaning bitterly having to squander perhaps two or three years in pathological investigations the outcome of which could not be anything else than confirmation of truths demonstrated long ago by Waller, Ranvier, Vanlair, Stroebe, and many other scientists. At the end of the campaign, nevertheless, I had the consolation of seeing that the time had not been entirely lost. Besides strengthening various classical conclusions which were somewhat insecure on account of inadequacies of technique, I had succeeded in picking up a considerable number of original observations not lacking in value.

It would be unjust to forget that in this rude battle on behalf of truth I was not alone; I was accompanied by various eminent investigators who, like me, were roused by the boastings and temerities of the reticularists. I must mention particularly Perroncito, a favourite pupil of Golgi, who also applied the new method to the subject; Lugaro, a neurologist and psychologist of great ability; Medea, Marinesco and Minea, Tello, Nageotte, Krassin, and many more. Needless to say, the reduced silver method contributed decisively to the triumph of the good cause, this technique possessing the inestimable advantage in connection with the subject of the debate of staining completely and vigorously the buds or sprouts of the mutilated axons (central end), sprouts which it is possible to follow conveniently in thick sections through the scar and within the peripheral stump as far as the terminal structures themselves.

Let us recall now some antecedents of the problem of the regeneration of nerves.

The pathologists and physiologists of the first half of last century (Waller, Vulpian, Ranvier, Brown-Sequard, Münzer and others) made manifest the following fact: when a nerve trunk is cut in a young mammal, the portion thereof situated beyond the section (the peripheral stump) degenerates and dies rapidly, the remains of the axon and of the myelin being progressively resorbed; some months later, however, both the intermediary or internervous scar and the peripheral stump show numerous newly formed fibres which partially or completely reestablish the sensibility and motility of the paralyzed member.

By what histological mechanism is the destroyed peripheral stump restored and are the nerve endings in muscles and in sensory surfaces regenerated?

All the solutions suggested revolved about the two: the theory of continuity, or the monogenist theory, supported by Waller, Münzer, Ziegler, Ranvier, Vanlair, Stroebe, Kölliker, Mott, Halliburton, Harrison, and Lugaro; and the theory of discontinuity, or the polygenist theory, proclaimed by various physiologists (Vulpian, Brown-Sequard, and Bethe) and by a large group of pathologists and pathological-anatomists including Büngner, Wietting, Ballance, Stewart, Marchand, and Medea.

The supporters of the first solution maintained that the newly formed fibres in the peripheral stump represent simply prolongations, by means of sprouting and progressive growth, of the axis cylinders of the central stump, which were supposed to retain their full vitality thanks to their continuity with the cells of origin or trophic centres; while the adepts of the polygenic or second theory declared positively that the regenerated fibres result from the differentiation and successive transformation of the cells which ensheath the old nerve fibres (the nuclei and protoplasm in course of division of the cells of Schwann). These cells were supposed to be arranged at first in a solid chain or cord of protoplasm, within the links of which would arise progressively, by a process of differentiation respective pieces of axon which would later be fused into a continuous filament and finally connected with the free axonic extremities of the central stump.

In this state of the intellectual atmosphere, I undertook in 1905 my investigations upon the regeneration of nerves. They lasted about two years and were carried out on a large number of animals as, for example, the rabbit, the cat, and the dog. The results were published in several papers and afterwards in a German translation in book form.[1]

They provided detailed information as to the processes of degeneration and regeneration in cut nerves and showed that, within a few days after section, the ends of the fibres in the central stump give off branches in all directions (Fig. 73). Some of these, growing through the scar, reach the

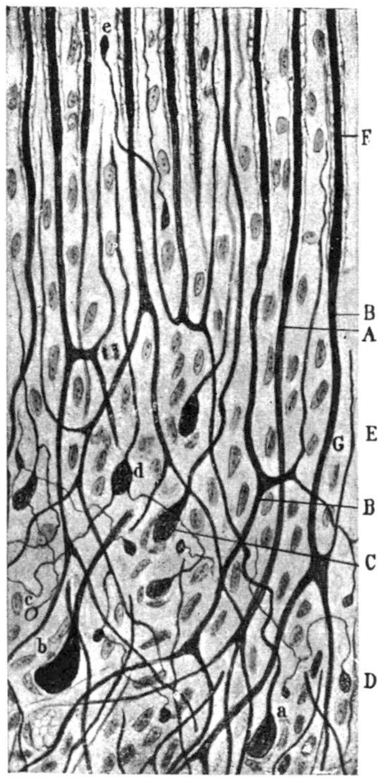

FIG. 73. CENTRAL STUMP AND BEGINNING OF THE INTERVENING SCAR OF A CUT SCIATIC NERVE SECTIONED THREE DAYS AFTER THE OPERATION. Cat a few days old. *F*, fibre of the central stump; *a*, terminal branch from a pre-existing axon.

cut end of the peripheral stump and extend through it to form the regenerated nerve, while the remainder degenerate.

[1] Bibliography, item 9. My inaugural discourse in the Academy of Medicine of Madrid, read on the 30th of June, 1907, also turned upon the subject of the regeneration of nerves.

I have already mentioned that a young Italian investigator, Aldo Perroncito, a pupil of the illustrious histologist of Pavia, also used the method of reduced silver nitrate (the value of which for pathologic-anatomical researches I had already announced in 1904) for the study of the regeneration of nerves. His conclusions coincided almost exactly with mine except that he had detected the existence of divisions and new branches in the central stump at an earlier date than I, namely on the second day after section, and had described perfectly the initial forms of the nerve strands and knots, noted by various authors and described in detail by me.

My work just cited on the regeneration of nerves had as its main object the procuring of objective proof that the new fibres appearing in the peripheral stump of a cut nerve represent incontestably buds from the axons of the central stump. On the other hand, the initial steps of the regeneration itself were somewhat neglected, i.e., the behaviour of the axons of the central stump during the first two days, a subject upon which much light was thrown, as I have just said, by Perroncito. A communication published in 1907 was designed to fill up this gap. In it, besides confirmation of some interesting facts pointed out by the young follower of Golgi, new facts were demonstrated, particularly concerning the behaviour of the degenerating fibres in the peripheral stump. Moreover, from some of the latter and some other facts was drawn a suggestion that the neurofibrils are composed of infinitesimal living units, the neurobions, which are able to grow and multiply relatively independently within the protoplasm.

As a result of these publications, a large number of authors returned to the neuron theory. Among the penitents we note Dohrn, Levi, Marinesco, and van Gehuchten. There soon followed confirmatory papers by Guido Sala, Nageotte, Minea, Lugaro, Dustin, Sala and Cortese, Modena, and above all by Tello, to whom we owe a brilliant study on the regeneration of the motor end plates and the sensory terminations. Nor must those be forgotten who upheld the monogenetic principle while making use of other methods: Krassin, Mott and Halliburton, Stewart, Poscharisky, Edmont, Stuart, and others. Opinion finally reacted vigorously in favour of the classic doctrine of continuous or monogenic development.

Even Alfred Bethe, the champion of the chain theory, showed himself somewhat conciliatory in his replies, which were not exempt from sharpness and acrimony, especially in a certain polemical work issued in 1907, no longer denying the regenerative capacity of the fibres of the central stump nor the arrival of its sprouts at the frontiers of the peripheral stump, but confining himself entirely to the defence of the necessity of the cooperation of the cells of Schwann of the latter segment to make effective the restoration of the nerve. Some time later, compelled perhaps by the irrefutable arguments adduced by Perroncito, Lugaro, Marinesco, and myself, the restless physiologist of Strassburg decided to abandon the field.[2] *Victis honos!*

I may add, further, that authorities of such prestige as Retzius, v. Lenhossék, Schiefferdecker, Edinger, Heidenhain, Verworn, Harrison, who looked on from afar, though with sympathetic interest, at the course of the debate, adopted in their writings, explicitly or implicitly, the monogenic doctrine, or that of continuity.

It is superfluous to say that the much abused neuron conception emerged from the test strengthened and dominant. Far from finding insuperable difficulties in the matter of nerve regeneration, as its adversaries expected, it met, on the contrary, new evidence in the light of which not a few puzzling phenomena of the structure and vegetative mechanism of nervous protoplasm received unexpected elucidation.

[2] This he told me a few years later, not without a trace of melancholy, in acknowledging courteously the receipt of my work in two volumes, *Estudios sobre la degeneración y regeneración del sistema nervioso.* Recently with a nobility of character which does him honour, he actually states that, at least in the majority of cases, the fibres of the peripheral stump proceed from the central one. (1923: Libro en honor de S. R. Cajal.)

The other paper referred to at the beginning of this chapter had to do with the origin of the nerves and of the processes of the neurons in the embryo. As was to be expected, I succeeded in corroborating with the new method all the interesting revelations made in 1890 with the aid of the chrome-silver reaction, and procured much new information regarding the manner of development and growth of nerve fibres, dendrites, etc., which was in complete accord with the neuron doctrine.

A resumé of these investigations (which were confirmed in principle by Held, as we shall see later) was communicated to the anatomical section of the International Medical Congress held in Lisbon in April, 1906.

I was burning with eagerness to try the new formula in the analysis of degeneration and regeneration of the central tracts, a subject upon which there had been published an infinity of monographs. Though with some differences in evaluating their observations, almost all the authors agreed that the regeneration of the white matter of the spinal cord, cerebrum, cerebellum, etc. is impossible, perhaps because of the absence of orientating elements or cells of Schwann. My observations, made in the optic nerve and in the spinal cord, confirmed the foregoing conclusion in principle, but demonstrated also that the incapability of regeneration is not a fatally irresistible law, but is a secondary outcome of a physical or chemical environment unfavourable for the growth of the sprouts. The central stumps of the cut axons also produce growth clubs and buds which penetrate the scar and from these cones there sometimes extend secondary projections which are richly subdivided. However, because of unknown causes, a few days after the lesion the recently formed axonic sprouts degenerate without crossing the scar and finally are reabsorbed.

During the year 1907 I sent to press also a number of other monographs, upon the contents of which I cannot linger here.

CHAPTER XXII

During the biennium 1905–1906 I am favoured with unexpected honours and rewards. The Helmholtz gold medal and the Nobel prize. Felicitations and tributes innumerable. Inconveniences of celebrity. My journey to Stockholm: ceremonies, festivities, and addresses. Meanness of our diplomatic representation. Moret, who always accorded me unmerited attentions, wishes to make me a minister. Astonishment of some politicasters upon learning that I declined such a coveted office.

In February, 1905, I received most gratifying news. In reward for my modest scientific works, one of the most eminent scientific bodies in the world, the Royal Academy of Sciences of Berlin, by a resolution passed at the end of 1904, had the kindness to award me the Helmholtz gold medal. Such flattering information reached me in a communication from the Minister of Foreign Affairs, accompanied by the official communication of the German Embassy in Madrid. A few days later this Embassy transmitted to me, along with the ordinance instituting the Helmholtz prize, two enormous medals; one of gold, weighing 620 grammes, the other of copper, a replica of the first. On the obverse side there appears the effigy of the great German physicist, and on the reverse the inscription: Ramón y Cajal, 1905.

At first I did not realize fully the importance and range of this honourable distinction. When I became acquainted with its antecedents by reading the ordinance cited, I was astounded to learn that this medal was awarded every two years to the author who had successfully accomplished the most important discoveries in any field whatever of human knowledge. With astonishment and blushes I read the list of the laureates.

The medal, instituted in 1892, during the life of the great German physicist, was adjudged to no less than E.

du Bois Raymond, Weierstrass, Robert Bunsen, and Lord Kelvin. And after the death of Helmholtz it continued to be awarded to such scientists as the following: in 1898, to R. Virchow; in 1900, to Sir G. G. Stokes; in 1906, to H. Becquerel; in 1908, to E. Fischer; in 1910, to J. H. vant Hoff; in 1912, to Schevendener, etc.; all luminaries of science, investigators and originators of genius. I blushed at figuring in the list of such glorious scientific innovators.

Without pressing my modesty to the point of claiming to be without merit—which would be an insult to the most learned Berlin Academy—I may be permitted to suspect that into the action of 1904 there entered largely the cordial regard and sincere esteem with which I was honoured by the illustrious Dr. Waldeyer, who signed, as Presidential Secretary, the aforementioned communication from the Academy.

The information having been made public by the press, which embellished it with generous and enthusiastic eulogies, I had to face the inevitable avalanche of felicitations and messages of congratulation, from that sent in the name of His Majesty the King by his secretary Señor Merry del Val to those received from the modest public bodies. All were received with fervent and cordial gratitude.[1]

A few months later, when my quiet and tranquil spirit was returning to the enjoyment of the delightful surprises of concentrated and unnoticed work, I was surprised one morning in October, 1906, when it was almost still night, by a laconic telegram sent from Stockholm and written in German. It said merely:

Carolinische Institut verliehen Sie Nobelpreiss.

It was signed by my congenial colleague Emil Holmgren, professor in the Faculty of Medicine. Shortly after, I received another telegram of congratulation from my intimate

[1] Special mention, among other tributes, is deserved by the artistic commemorative plaque presented by the students of the Faculty of Medicine of Madrid (January 26, 1905), a distinctive gift which was hung in my office with another precious jewel of Catalan silversmith's work which was presented to me in 1904 by the Academy of Medicine and Pharmacy of Barcelona.

friend Professor G. Retzius. Finally, after a few days had passed, there reached my hands the official communication of the Royal Carolinian Institute of Stockholm, the body in the hands of which rests the awarding of the Nobel Prize for the Section of Physiology and Medicine. Besides the inestimable honour which was accorded me, this prize had a by no means insignificant economic aspect. At the rate of exchange at the time, it was worth in real money approximately twenty-three thousand duros. The other half was very justly adjudicated to the illustrious professor of Pavia, Camilo Golgi, the originator of the method with which I accomplished my most striking discoveries.

If the Helmholtz medal, a purely honorary reward, caused me feelings of gratification, the Nobel Prize, as universally known as it is coveted by all, gave me a feeling of displeasure and almost of fear. I was tempted to refuse the prize as undeserved, irregular, and, above all, very dangerous for my physical and mental health. Interpreting literally the ordinance of the Nobel foundation, it appeared impossible to award it for the Section of Medicine and Physiology to histologists, embryologists, and naturalists. Hence, up to that time it had been adjudged only to bacteriologists, pathologists, and physiologists.

Facing the prospect of felicitations, messages, tributes, banquets, and other annoyances as honourable as troublesome, I made heroic efforts during the first few days to conceal the event. My precautions were in vain, however. In a short time the tattling press broadcast it to the four winds and there was no remedy but to get up on to a pedestal and make myself the focus of the gaze of everyone.

Methodically and inexorably the dreaded programme of attentions unrolled itself: telegrams of felicitation; letters and messages of congratulation; acts of homage of students and professors; commemorative diplomas; honorary elections to scientific and literary bodies; streets baptized with my name in cities and even in small villages; chocolates, cordials, and other potions of doubtful hygienic value, marked with my surname; offers of profitable participation in risky or chimerical enterprises; urgent requests for inscriptions for albums and autograph collections; petitions for appointments and sinecures . . . ; there was some of everything and to all I had to resign myself, at the same time grateful for it and deploring it, with a smile on my lips and sadness in my soul.[2] In a word, four long months were squandered in acknowledging felicitations, in pressing friendly or indifferent hands, concocting commonplace toasts, recovering from attacks of indigestion, and making grimaces of simulated satisfaction. And to think that, in order to guarantee my peace of mind and to avoid all possibility of popularity, I had deliberately chosen the most obscure, recondite, and unpopular of the sciences!

I must not, however, run into exaggerations which in the present case might sound like ingratitude, nor is it permissible to carry to the extreme the rights of egoism. It must be recognized that the honours rendered to men who in some way pursue the ennoblement of their country are ethically beautiful and efficiently exemplary; they arise from sentiments of unity and veneration too noble to be condemnable. Every well-bred person must be grateful for them and remember them. But we Latin people are extremists in everything. In contrast to the moderation

[2] Not all the tributes reduced themselves to courteous congratulations and transient effusions of commemorative banquets. Some had definite material value apart from their lofty spiritual significance. I may mention the great gold medal sculptured by the brilliant artist Mariano Benlliure, paid for by subscription among the students, the professors of San Carlos, and many Madrid physicians; the magnificent album, a true jewel of art, made precious by exquisite water colours, presented by all the organizations and active forces in highly cultured Valencia; the diploma of honour, admirably illuminated, sent by the Spanish physicians of Buenos Aires, who, desirous besides of collaborating in a material way in some of my scientific researches, opened a public subscription to finance the publication of one of my books (this work, published in 1910, I shall discuss later).

It is unnecessary to say with what lively gratitude I preserve all those and other generous gifts, which I keep proudly, as testimonies not only of my good fortune, but also of the fervent patriotism of many good Spaniards on both this and the other side of the ocean, who, inspired by the noblest spiritual unity, regard as their own every honour rendered abroad to one of their brothers.

and coolness of the northern peoples, we lack the sense of proportion and of balance, and what begins as a flattering attention ends by being wearisome importunity. In Spain —and Echegaray, Galdós, Benavente,[3] Cávia, and many others justly honoured can bear witness to the fact— in order to emerge safely from the attentions and tributes of friends and admirers, one has to have a heart of steel, the skin of an elephant, and the stomach of a vulture. The sweetness of the first moments is followed by a certain mild bitterness. Like vehement and rude friendship, among us fame bruises while it caresses; it kisses but it crushes. It deprives us of the ease of custom; it disturbs the peace of the spirit; it restricts the sacrosanct freedom of the will, turning us into the target of impertinent curiosity; it endangers humility, compelling us continually to think and speak of ourselves; and, finally, it alters the course of our lives, twisting it into capricious and useless meanderings.

In sincerity, I have to confess something which will perhaps make the reader smile ironically. As I suggested a little while ago, the Nobel Prize gave me more fear than pleasure. Medals, titles, decorations are distinctions relatively tolerated by rivals and adversaries. But a great pecuniary prize! The wealthy honour is something irritating and not easily endured.

There is, moreover, a large basis of truth for the very common saying that adversity follows good fortune as surely as the shadow follows the body. The two seem, in fact, to constitute alternating phases of the inevitable undulation of human destiny; and not through the influence of imaginary fates, but because excessive good fortune has

[3] When I write this I am cognizant that Benavente has been awarded the Nobel prize for literature. It is not a case of offering condolences to the great dramatist but rather of praying God to grant him the strength necessary to survive the endearments of his intimate confrères, as it was granted to Echegaray—another Nobel Prize winner—to bear during his melancholy later life the growing tide of a passionate criticism which was merciless towards the defects in the work of the master—imputable largely to the romantic tendencies of the period—and ignored perfidiously the incomparable beauties of thought and style which adorn it.

the unlucky quality of altering the feelings of men. As Seneca said—forgive the pedantry—in words which could not be improved: "In proportion as the number of those who admire one increases, those who envy one increase also. I devoted all my energy to raising myself above the common crowd, making myself notable for some particular quality, and I succeeded only in exposing myself to the missiles of envy and in uncovering to hatred the parts in which it could bite me."

How, I asked myself, would my foreign opponents take the gifts of my lucky star? What would all those scientists, whose errors I had had the misfortune to show up, say about me? How could I justify the preferences of the Carolinian Institute in the eyes of so many outstanding investigators who had been passed over and whose superior deserts I take pleasure in acknowledging? Finally, turning my eyes towards our beloved Spain, what should I do to placate certain professors—some of them from my own part of the country—for whom I was always a case of pretentious mediocrity if not a hard working fool? For, sad to confess, the greatest enemies of the Spaniards are the Spaniards themselves.

We shall soon see that my misgivings were justified and that the troubles began even during my sojourn in the Swedish capital. This was certainly not the fault of the Swedish scientists, who are models of courtesy and propriety, but of the strange character of the coparticipant in the prize, one of the vainest and most self-worshipful men of talent that I have ever known.

However, leaving aside premature comments, I must speak of my journey. The Statutes of the Nobel Foundation ordain that the laureates must attend personally the formal ceremony of bestowal of the prizes, which takes place every year on the tenth of December, the anniversary of the death of Alfred Nobel, and besides that they must explain and demonstrate in a public lecture the more essential of their scientific discoveries. Although dispensation from the journey was granted to our illustrious

Echegaray and to the great Italian poet Carducci in consideration of their advanced age, it was neither possible nor fitting for me to try to evade the custom which, besides, implies a due and polite testimony of gratitude to the Trustees of the Nobel Foundation and to the generosity of the Scandinavian people.

I set out, then, and arrived in Stockholm on the sixth of December, a few days before the commencement of the celebrations. After greeting effusively my good friends and colleagues of the Carolinian Institute, Doctor Retzius, E. Holmgren, and H. Henschen, I was introduced to the celebrated C. Golgi, who shared the prize with me, and to the other professors receiving awards, who had arrived from France and England. These were J. J. Thomson, to whom was awarded the prize for physics, on account of his penetrating investigations upon the nature of electricity, and H. Moissan, who received the prize for chemistry, in consideration of his invention of the electric furnace and his work on fluorine. I have already mentioned that the famous G. Carducci, the recipient of the prize for Poetry was excused from attending on account of ill health. Finally, the prize for Peace was awarded to the American Theodore Roosevelt. This decision produced great surprise, especially in Spain.

Is it not the acme of irony and humor to convert into a champion of pacifism the man of the most impetuously pugnacious temperament and the most determined imperialist that the United States have ever produced?

It must be pointed out, in exculpation of the circumspect people of Sweden, that such a strange decision was made by the Norwegian *Storthing,* to which the conferring of the prize for Peace is entrusted by a clause of the Nobel will.

The ceremony of awarding the prizes was a pompous event and one of the highest idealism. It took place, according to custom in the great hall of the Royal Academy of Music, which is adorned for that purpose with a bust of Nobel enwreathed with flowers. Upon the presidential platform were displayed the flags and emblems of Sweden and of the nations to which the laureates belonged. His Majesty the King presided, accompanied by the Princesses and the Princes, with their brilliant suite, and there were present the members of the Government, the diplomatic corps, the descendants of the Nobel family, high functionaries of the palace and of the army, representatives of the Swedish parliament and the civic government, professors and students of the University, and many very elegant ladies.

The ceremony was commenced by Professor Törnebladh, one of the Nobel Trustees, with a fine address, in which, after tracing the history of the foundation of the prize, he delivered a warm eulogy of science, closing by repeating the well-known maxim of Pasteur: "Ignorance separates men, while science brings them together." (What a pity that this fine maxim should have been contradicted by the monstrous war of 1914!)

The diplomas and medals were presented personally by His Majesty the King, who announced the candidates. In each case the president of the Academy responsible for the nomination eulogized in a brief and sentient oration the merits of the recipient. As was to be expected, the discourse in praise of the laureates in Physiology and Medicine was in the hands of the illustrious Count Mörner, president of the Carolinian Institute.

A few days later, the lectures by the recipients of the prizes took place. Upon the day set for mine, before a select and imposing audience I set forth the most fundamental results of my research work, adhering strictly to the facts and to the conclusions naturally suggested by them. According to my custom, in order to make myself clear even to the layman, I used a great many coloured plates of large size. My lecture was, I believe, to the taste of the public. In any case, it received very kind praises in the local newspapers.

In accord with precedent, the text of all the lectures was published some weeks later in a volume de luxe, adorned with most beautiful emblems in colours, with a reproduction of the medals, and with the portraits of the laureates, and enriched besides by the respective discourses of presentation by the sponsors and by the official representative of the Nobel Trustees.[4]

I must state that in the aforesaid lecture I made a cordial eulogy of my colleague, Professor C. Golgi, which was imperiously required by justice and by courtesy. I always rendered to him the tribute of my admiration and in all my books there may be read enthusiastic praises of the contributions of the savant of Pavia. I had the right, then, to expect from him equally friendly treatment on the occasion of his lecture on the neuron doctrine (*La doctrine de neurones*). Contrary to what we all expected, instead of pointing out the valuable facts which he had discovered, he attempted in it to refloat his almost forgotten theory of interstitial nerve nets.

He had the right to choose the subject of his address. The misfortune was that in defending his extravagant lucubration—which could be excused in 1886, when the basic facts of inter-neuronal connection had not been made known—he made a display of pride and self-worship so immoderate that they produced a deplorable effect upon the assembly. Not even incidentally did he allude to the almost innumerable neurological works which had appeared outside Italy, and even in Italy itself, since the remote date of his great work on the minute structure of the nervous system. For the anatomist of Pavía, neither Forel, nor His, nor I, nor Retzius, nor Waldeyer, nor Kölliker, nor van Gehuchten, nor von Lenhossék, nor Edinger, nor my brother, nor Tello, nor Athias, nor even his compatriot Lugaro had added anything of interest to his discoveries of former times. Likewise he considered it unnecessary to correct any of his old theoretical errors, or

[4] This elegant book is entitled: *Les Prix Nobel en 1906*. A separate impression of my lecture with magnificent reproductions of the wall plates was presented to me by the Nobel Foundation. Various scientific reviews reproduced my address, especially the *Archivio di Fisiologia* of Dr. G. Fano, vol. V, Firenze, 1907.

of his lapses in observation. Needless to say, in his drawings and descriptions of the cerebrum, the cerebellum, the spinal cord, the hippocampus, etc., there appeared none of the arrangements shown by me and confirmed by all authors; and when he showed a glimpse of one, it was artificially distorted and falsified in order to adept it, *nolens volens,* to his capricious ideas. The noble and most discrete Retzius was in consternation; Holmgren, Henschen, and all the Swedish neurologists and histologists looked at the speaker with stupefaction. I was trembling with impatience as I saw that the most elementary respect for the conventions prevented me from offering a suitable and clear correction of so many odious errors and so many deliberate omissions.

I have never understood those strange mental constitutions which are devoted throughout life to the worship of their own egos, hermetically sealed to all innovation and impermeable to the incessant changes taking place in the intellectual environment. What is more, neither can I conceive of any advantage in such egocentricity, for everyone is in the secret and knows what to believe. For such an attitude to be personally advantageous, within human limits, it would be necessary for progress to be paralyzed, for scientists to renounce the privilege of criticism, and for the mental level of investigators to fall so low that self-glorified talent would be able, by virtue of irresistible suggestion, to impose its individual visions dogmatically on everybody. But since to imagine all this is to take up an absurd position, I cannot conceive, I repeat, without appealing to psychiatry for adequate terms, of the psychology of such temperaments. What a cruel irony of fate to pair, like Siameses twins united by the shoulders, scientific adversaries of such contrasting character!

My colleague displayed the same olympic pride and pretentious mien in his toast at the official banquet. This solemn function was given by the members of the Nobel Foundation and was attended by the Princes and magnates, the diplomatic corps, and distinguished representatives of public and academic bodies. (His Majesty, who was very amiable to me, told me of his trips through Andalusia and praised handsomely the beauties of Spain and the character of its people.)

At the time for toasts, very discreet and eloquent speeches were made by various Ministers, the illustrious Presidents of the Academies and of the Nobel Foundation, and the representatives of the countries to which the recipients of the prizes belonged (except the representative of Spain, who apologized for his absence). Professor Sundberg gave in French a most gracious toast in my honour. Afterwards all the laureates responded courteously with speeches of thanks.

I do not think that I struck a discordant note in that concert of pleasant courtesy and graceful fraternity. In my brief remarks, delivered in French, I laid special emphasis on making sincere acknowledgements to outstanding investigators as worthy as, or more so than Golgi and I of the honourable guerdon.[5]

Besides the splendid official functions, I should mention also, for the sake of completeness, other attentions and considerations with which various distinguished scientists and the highly cultured and hospitable Swedish people in general sought to make our sojourn in Stockholm enjoyable. I may recall the banquet tendered to the laureates by Count Mörner, President of the Carolinian Institute, whose wife and daughters, prototypes of the splendid Scandinavian beauty, did the honours of the house marvellously; the intimate dinner given in my honour by Dr. Retzius, in whose house I had the opportunity to converse with his admirable wife and to become acquainted with the polished and elegant comfort of the Swedish home; the gala performance given for the foreign visitors in the Opera House; the excursion to the ancient University of Upsala—the Oxford of Sweden—; the visit to the skating rink, where the favourite sport of the far northern countries is cultivated;

[5] The complete text of the speech, in French, may be found in the original version of the present work. (Translator's note.)

the walk round the harbour and, in conclusion, the trip to the interesting Zoological Park, where, among other curiosities, there is exhibited a certain collection of rustic dwellings, with the ingenious household occupations in which the peasant family engages during the long northern winters.

To conclude the story of my journey to Sweden, of the inhabitants of which I preserve most pleasant recollections, I shall relate an anecdote and tell of an observation.

The separation of Norway still being recent, I ran the risk of remarking to a high dignitary, to whom I had the honour of being presented, with what surprise we in Spain had learned of the indifference of Sweden to the disruption of the common fatherland. My amiable companion, instead of bitterly bemoaning the fact, as I expected, merely replied, with a smile on his lips: "We should have been utter fools if we had upset our well-balanced budget and suspended the triumphant campaign on behalf of general culture and against alcoholism in order to maintain by force our union with the neighbouring country."

The observation concerns the sordid meanness with which Spain defrays the expenses of its representation abroad. While the Swedish minister in Madrid and the diplomatic representatives of France, of England, of Italy, and of other countries, in Stockholm are lodged in magnificent mansions, with the dignity suitable to their rank, the *chargé d'affaires* of Spain in that country subsists precariously on the second floor of a very unpretentious tenement. Such a shameful contrast caused a certain neglect which was noticed by many and was not at all flattering to our country. In keeping with courtesy and custom, each accredited foreign minister in the Swedish capital entertains his laureate compatriot with a private banquet at which are present the most select members of the colony of the corresponding nationality. All contributed this proof of consideration for their fellow countrymen honoured with the Nobel Prize —all except our Minister, who, lamenting doubtless, the lack of fitting surroundings and of adequate resources, evaded this act of courtesy. However, the omission was handsomely and gallantly compensated—despite the modesty of his resources—by the highly cultured Secretary of the Legation, Sr. R. Mitjana, who, I may say in passing, generously accompanied me in my strolls through the city and in my visit to Upsala (he spoke Swedish) and acted as the frankest and most fraternal of friends.

The case mentioned is not unique, unfortunately. In all the capitals which I have visited (except Paris) I have observed with sorrow that the Spanish Legation is the most lamentable and paltry. For the sake of national dignity, is there no way of rectifying somewhat such a degrading situation?

The third fortunate event—or that could have been so for me!—announced in the summary of the present chapter was the persistent determination of the illustrious Moret, at that time leader of the liberal party, to make me Minister of Public Instruction. Already in 1905, in some of our conversations at the Athenaeum, he told me of his wishes. I confined myself to thanking him, avoiding a reply with courteous evasions. The truth is that I neither felt myself to be a politician, nor was prepared for the arduous office of Minister, nor yet could I discover in myself, after careful self-examination, the gifts indispensable for worthy filling of a portfolio in our country.

The reader will remember that when, in 1905, Don Antonio Maura overthrew the conservative regime led by Villaverde, the liberal party came into power under the presidency of Don Eugenio Montero Ríos. Unfortunately the powerful political force formerly directed by Sagasta had lost its cohesion and had broken up into small groups, and at the head of each faction was a chief who aspired to the supreme leadership.

Meanwhile, there took place the shameful occurrences at Barcelona (the insolence of the Catalan autonomists of the "Cut-cut" and the patriotic, though inopportune indignation of the army). Montero Ríos had to resign and the chieftancy was transferred to Don Segismundo Moret, leader of the most important liberal faction. It must be recognized that, despite his great prestige, the illustrious democratic orator never commanded a sure majority. Resolved at any cost to restore the unity of the party, he conceived the plan, as soon as the festivities of the royal wedding should be over, of dissolving the co-legislative bodies and of having new elections. He wished to undertake with determination the reform of the constitution and to pass laws of a frankly democratic nature.

It was in March 1906 that, at a conference held in his house, the distinguished politician told me of his idea and expressed the desire that I should lend him my insignificant cooperation. I excused myself, as upon other occasions, by hiding behind my lack of parliamentary experience. But the eloquence of Don Segismundo was overwhelming. In words burning with sincere patriotism, he explained the great reforms of which the educational system stood in need, and extolled the honour which awaited the Minister who should convert them into laws; he added that men of science, too, owe themselves to the politics of their country, on the altars of which the peace of the hearth must be sacrificed, as well as the egoistic satisfactions of the laboratory; and he cited finally, to complete my seduction, the example of M. Berthelot and of other great scientists who did not disdain, in order to raise the cultural level of their nations, the portfolio of Public Instruction.

His warm exhortations made an impression upon my weak will. Excited in my turn by that captivating oratory, I had the weakness to point out to him some reforms calculated to waken the Spanish universities from their age-old lethargy: the engagement for a few years of eminent foreign investigators; the sending to the great scientific centres of Europe of the most brilliant of our young intellectuals, with the object of forming a nursery for the future teaching body; the establishment of great residential colleges attached to the Institutes and Universities, with suitable buildings, health-promoting games, zealous instructors, and other excellent features of similar establishments in

England; the formation, on a small scale and by way of experiment, of a sort of *Collège de France,* or centre of advanced research, where the most eminent members of our professoriate and the most profitable of those who had returned after being sent abroad would work comfortably; the establishment of pecuniary prizes for the benefit of professors who were successful teachers or were authors of important scientific discoveries, so as to counteract the dulling and discouraging effects of the principle of seniority, etc.

When I expected that Moret would show himself taken aback in the face of a plan of reform which involved asking the Cortes for large appropriations, he answered delightedly: "We are in complete agreement. Whenever the next election takes place, you shall be my Minister of Public Instruction." And, fascinated by the magic of his speech and the dominance of his talent, I did not contradict him.

A few weeks later (April, 1906) I attended the International Medical Congress at Lisbon. There, far from the bewitching presidential siren, I cogitated seriously over the weighty compromise in which I had become involved. And I ended by reaching the conclusion that, considering the disorganized condition of the Liberal Party, it was fantastic to expect the attainment of a decree of dissolution and hence was impossible to undertake the great work of our pedagogical and cultural elevation. In the eyes of my professional colleagues, and especially in those of the official politicians, I should appear not as a man of good will vanquished by circumstances but as one more case of vulgar ambition. This was repugnant to my feelings as a citizen and as a patriot.

In consequence of such reflections, I wrote to Moret withdrawing my promise and excusing my unreliability as best I could. The President was very angry with me. Nevertheless, he was sufficiently magnanimous to forgive my fickleness and a few months later he carried his benevolence so far as to elevate to the cabinet one of my friends, Don Alejandro San Martín. The highly cultured professor of San Carlos, with whom I had exchanged ideas as to the urgent university reforms, assumed the delicate task of sponsoring them, without abandoning, naturally, his own inspirations, some of them perhaps too radical (I refer, particularly, to the indirect suppression of the shameful independent teaching, a thing unknown abroad).

My easily made predictions were fulfilled completely. The discord which undermined the party sterilized the patriotic efforts of Moret so that he did not obtain the desired decree of dissolution. And, as was to be expected, the ministry of which I was to have been a member (after the crisis of June, 1906) existed anxiously and precariously in the midst of petty intrigues and internal dissentions. Finally, two months later, Don Segismundo fell, with the bitterness of not having brought about the fusion of his party nor accomplished any of the great democratic reforms which he was planning.

CHAPTER XXIII

My polemics with Held and Apathy. New Studies on neurogenesis in the medulla oblongata, the spinal cord, the retina, and other organs.

As the reader will recall, I remarked before that the Nobel Prize, granted to histologists for the first time in 1906, caused me more fear than gratification. I wondered what would be the reaction of those few scientists, not lacking in positive merits, whose errors of observation and of interpretation it had been my misfortune to demonstrate.

I was not long in finding out. In significant contrast to the great figures of neurology who, filled with noble generosity, hastened to congratulate me, a few histologists and naturalists who always distinguished me with their disdain or their unfriendliness rose violently against my modest person. It was high time, according to my pious confrères, to crush the neuron doctrine for good, burying at the same time its most fervent supporter. There was in their invectives so much injustice, they were accompanied by such virulent personalities, and they were, finally, so disproportionate to the insignificance of my polite observations of earlier times, that it would be ingenuous to believe that there was not a certain etiological connection between them and the award of the Nobel Prize.

In fact, it could not but be significant that my old friend H. Held, who was one of my detractors at that time, and whom I had certainly always treated with the consideration due to his tireless industry and his great merits (he had been an ardent supporter of neuronism and had even been the translator in 1894 of one of my books), should wax indignant just in 1907 [1] on the pretext that in a certain one of my communications, relating to the genesis of the neuro-

[1] H. Held, Kritische Bemerkungen zu der Verteidigung der Neuroblasten und der Neurontheorie durch R. Cajal, *Anat. Anz.*, Bd. 30, '07.

fibrils, I did not consider it pertinent to discuss or accept the ancient neurogenetic theory of Hensen, a conception definitely rejected a mere eighteen years before by eminent neurologists of the calibre of Kupffer, Ranvier, His, Golgi, Kölliker, Lenhossék, Retzius, Lugaro, Athias, and others. As for S. Apathy, the fiery naturalist of Klausenburg waited also until the said year 1907 [2] to feel himself aggrieved by the friendly objections which, in passing, his highly extravagant lucubration concerning the continuity of the neurofibrils in the worms had suggested to me in 1903.[3]

Understanding quite well the psychology of certain scientists, and the purpose of the new campaign, I made special efforts to conduct myself in my replies with perfect equanimity and justice, being persuaded that, in arguments of this kind, passion and reason are always present in inverse proportion. Hence, I ignored all the personal attacks and betook myself straight to the terrain of observation.

The central thesis of Held—a simple modification, on the other hand, of the old conception of Hensen—consisted in the claim that the growth cone of the embryonic axons does not grow freely towards its destination among the surrounding elements, which we thought had been demonstrated by Lenhossék, Harrison, and myself, among others, but that it traverses a channel through the interior of a preestablished system of communicating ducts. In the primordial spinal cord, such orientating conduits would be represented by the ependymal or epithelial cells; outside the cord, that is for the cones and axons extending out through the mesoderm, the ducts referred to would be constituted by radiating chains of primordial connective tissue cells. It may be remarked that in his new investigation Held made use of my procedure with reduced silver nitrate, except that in place of fixing the tissue in alcohol, with or without

[2] S. Apathy, Bemerkungen zu den Ergebnissen R. y Cajals hinsichtlich der feineren Beschaffenheit des Nervensystems, *Anat. Anz.*, 31, 1907.

[3] Cajal, Un sencillo método de coloración selectiva del retículo protoplásmico, etc., *Trab. del Lab. de Invest. biol.*, T. 2, 1903.

ammonia, as I did, he preferred to apply pyridin, the fixative in Donaggio's method.

It was easy for me, after studying the subject anew and with care, to demonstrate in irreproachable preparations the error of my colleague in Leipzig.[4]

The paper, or rather the diatribe of Apathy, virulent in nature and discourteous in form, and revealing, besides, an almost absolute ignorance of all my scientific work, was directed mainly, in favour of a certain peculiar conception regarding the origin and physiological significance of the neurofibrils of worms, to refuting my ideas concerning the arrangement and connections of these filaments—ideas shared fundamentally by almost all histologists who have investigated the matter.

The point upon which Apathy insisted particularly was his well known theory of neurofibrillar continuity. In the view of the Hungarian savant the neurofibrils and their elementary filaments represent the exclusive conducting agents of the nervous system. Sometimes scattered, sometimes grouped in compact bundles, the said threads are supposed to traverse chains of neurons without anastomosing, at least centrally. In the nerve endings they are supposed to turn back, forming loops or diffuse, continuous nets. The origins and terminations of the neurofibrils are thus alike pure illusion. Everything communicates with everything else.

To sustain such a very hazardous thesis, the Hungarian savant relied upon his excellent and very beautiful preparations of the ganglia of the leech and other worms. To refute him, I had recouse to an abundant supply of successful preparations of the same forms, which was an easy matter since certain formulae of the reduced silver method stain their neurofibrils splendidly.

Neither in the cells of the retina, nor in the sympathetic cells, nor yet in the sensory cells of the leech is it possi-

[4] Cajal, Nouvelles observations sur l'évolution des neuroblastes etc., *Anat. Anz.*, Bd. 32, 1908.

ble to perceive the slightest indication that the neurofibrils pass from one cell to another. Besides, my preparations show in the stomach and pharynx of the leech the unquestionable existence of sensory neurofibrils ending freely under the epithelial cuticle.

I believe sincerely, without fear of sounding a note of presumption, that the facts advanced by me as arguments against the quite discordant theories of Held and Apathy are incontestable in the present state of knowledge. At least, up to the present no one has been able to refute them. Moreover, in thoughtful Germany the neurogenetic theory of the Leipzig professor found very little echo. The great masters, such as Edinger, Waldeyer, Heidenhain, Schiefferdecker, and others emphatically disapproved of it or showed themselves cold towards it. In America, the celebrated Harrison and his school also rose against it vociferously, with an overwhelming mass of experimental evidence. In Italy, France, Holland, Austria, and Sweden, it did not gain, so far as I know, a single supporter.[5]

As for the violent Apathy, who threatened me at first with I know not how many crushing books and papers, he preserved thenceforward a silence which seems like an act of contrition.[6]

Here was another hard battle won for the neuron doctrine. Will it be the last?

I doubt it very much. The morbid desire to assert and to make prominent ones own personality, to be original above all things, wreaks ruin in our time. Following the course of least resistance, youth delights in reexamining values which it considers doubtful; and in the realm of science, instead of discovering new truths, it prefers to destroy its heritage of ideas from the past. It is so easy to

[5] Today Held is followed only by his immediate pupils. For in certain foreign schools the discipline is so strict that in theoretical interpretations the pupil can do only one of two things: agree with the master or leave the laboratory.

[6] I am informed by v. Lenhossék that the violent Apathy has passed away without any sign, so far as I know, of the least scientific activity during the last fifteen years.

build up with other people's material a theory of ones own, though it be a fantastic one!

How distressing it is to have continually to fight against other men to defend the truth, instead of fighting against nature to wrest new truths from it! But how can it be avoided? Who does not know that every scientific accomplishment dislodges some deeply rooted error and that behind it is usually concealed injured pride, if not enraged interest?

CHAPTER XXIV

Researches carried out in the decade 1907 to 1917. Comparative anatomical studies on the cerebellum, the medulla oblongata, and the origins of the motor and sensory nerves of fishes, birds, and mammals. Structure of the nucleus of the neuron. Survival of neurons removed from the organism. New investigations on degeneration and regeneration in the spinal cord, the cerebral hemisphere, and the cerebellum. Experiments in the transplantation of nerves. Observations in favour of the neurotropic theory. Production of artificial nerves in transplanted ganglia.

I propose in the present chapter to give a brief summary of the work accomplished during the years following 1907. This work was almost as intensive and varied as in the periods of greatest investigative vigour. To labour according to the inclinations of the spirit is an incomparable pleasure and solace. Moreover, I detest the unpatriotic egoism of those who, having attained the pinnacle, think only of lying down without further effort. Allow me the vainglory of saying that neither do triumphs enervate me nor do injustices hold me back; rather, after receiving a reward, I redouble my industry so as to deserve it and, when I fall into error, I work harder so that it may be forgiven me. And above all, the efforts, the discoveries, and the emotions of the laboratory captivate and delight me.

To summarize the contents of all the monographs and books published in the decade referred to would require not two chapters but another full sized volume. However, I take cognizance of the weariness of the reader, who must be sick of them if he has had the patience to watch the over-nice parade of so many descriptive details. Besides—why not acknowledge it?—the progressive assaults of age put a bridle upon my pen, which is daily more recalcitrant to my thoughts. Not in vain have seven and thirty years been passed flushed over the pages or growing pale over the ocular. The excitement of the unexpected fatigues the heart and eager and ceaseless attention carves deep ruts in the cerebral pathways; through them thought runs falteringly, and, when it runs against obstacles, produces less light than heat.

In almost telegraphic style then, I shall proceed to enumerate the experimental undertakings of more recent years. I propose, in order to avoid prolixity in my narrative, to omit the index which I have been drawing up of the matters treated in each monograph. Of some I shall say nothing. My plan will be to choose the facts of which I have the pleasantest impression or which promise the greatest theoretical return.

So as to proceed in an orderly fashion, I shall begin by grouping my writings into three classes: descriptive monographs, communications on technique, and books of assembly and coordination.

Histological Monographs. These develop a variety of subjects, the comparative and the pathological anatomy of the nervous system predominating, however.

The first series of communications, which appeared during 1908 and 1909, is focussed upon the comparative histology of the cerebellum, of the medulla oblongata, and of the acoustic ganglia, and the mode of origin and termination of the sensory and motor nerves of mammals, birds, fishes, etc. Such preferences are determined by mere convenience. I have already pointed out that, in young animals and advanced fetuses, the silver method introduced by me in neurological technique (fixation in pyridin, chloral hydrate, or ammoniated alcohol) gives outstandingly instructive results. With admirable clearness and variety of hues, it reveals both the voluminous neurons and their stout axis cylinders, which can be followed at will through the masses of gray matter which are less far advanced in development and hence are hardly stained. Advantage of this valuable quality has been taken in their comparative anatomical investigations by Tello, Beccari, Mesdag, Lenhossék, Winkler, Castro, Lorente and many others.

I shall select as I said, from the more important of the

structural data collected in two years of persistent labour and shall merely mention the following:

(*a*) Discovery of various terminal nuclei of the vestibular nerve in fishes, birds, and reptiles, with a new type of ending by contact (Fig. 74).

(*b, c*) Demonstration in embryos of the interstitial nucleus of the medial longitudinal bundle, and of the relations of the deep nuclei in the avian cerebellum.

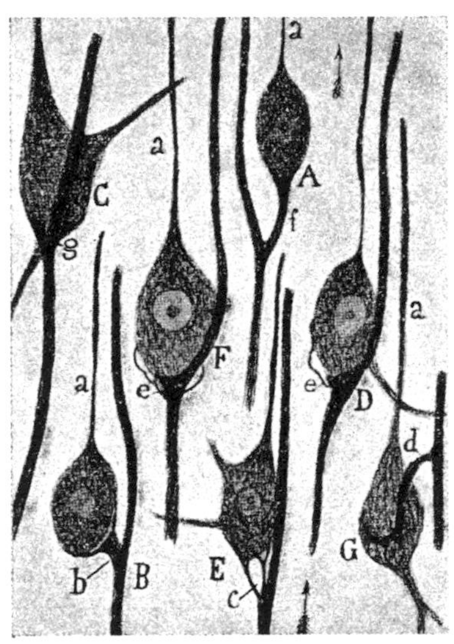

FIG. 74. Details of the manner of connection by contact of the vestibular nerve with the giant cells of the tangential nucleus of the bird. *A, D, F,* terminal plates and stalks in the vestibular nucleus mentioned; *a,* axons of the neurons.

(*d, e*) Discovery of new types of nerve endings in the cerebellum and in the internal ear.

(*f*) Analysis of the highly complex centres and tracts of the cochlear and vestibular systems in birds[1] (Fig. 75).

(*g, h*) Demonstration of connections of the reticular substance and of a crossed vagus root.

The investigations undertaken during 1910, 1911 and

[1] A German translation of the original (French) paper on this subject, with lithographs, was published in the *Jour. f. Psychol. u. Neurol.,* Bd. 13, 1908.

1912 were quite irregular, being spread over many and various subjects. I may cite: the structure of the nucleus, the autolysis and survival of neurons, the problem of neurotropism, the transplantation of nerves and ganglia, the technique of staining the platelets of the blood, methodological communications concerning the demonstration of the endocellular apparatus of Golgi and of the neuroglia of man, the structure of the cerebellum, etc. The principal theme, however, to which I devoted years of persistent labour and regarding which I collected most valuable data of great theoretical importance, was the degeneration and

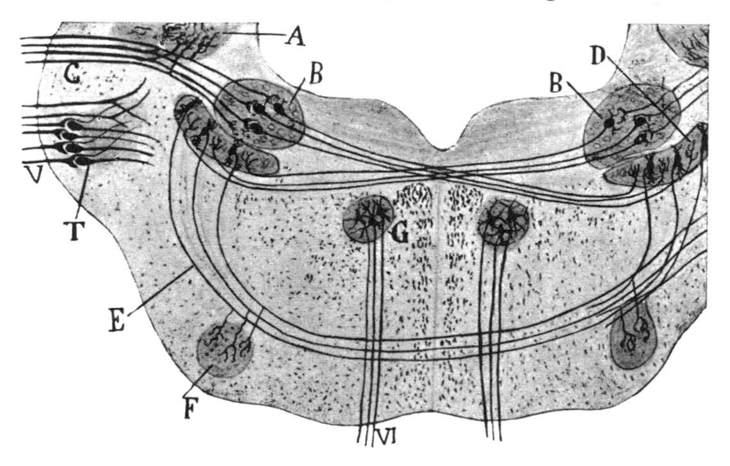

FIG. 75. Diagram of the acoustic centres and pathways in the medulla oblongata of the bird. *A*, angular nucleus; *B*, large-celled nucleus; *C*, cochlear or acoustic nerve; *D*, laminar nucleus; *E*, trapezoid body or secondary auditory path; *F*, superior olivary nucleus; *T*, tangential nucleus; *V*, vestibular nerve; *VI*, abducens nerve.

regeneration of the neurons and axons of the ganglia, the cerebellum, the cerebral hemispheres, and the spinal cord. As we shall soon see, these latter studies, which drew aside the veil a little from the intimate physiology of the neurofibrillar reticulum, corroborated the old neurotropic hypothesis formulated by me in 1892 and favourably received by many authors.

At the end of these pages will be found the list of the principle works referred to.

The harvest of new information regarding degeneration and regeneration of the spinal cord was very plentiful and extremely interesting. Some of the facts, of which I am about to give a brief account, as I have just remarked, form arguments of inestimable value in support of the doctrine of neurotropism. These prove that the production of outgrowths and their orientation through the various tissues are conditioned by the liberation round the cells and fibres of ferments which activate protoplasmic assimilation. These catalytic agents (neurotropic substances) are formed by the embryonic connective tissue, but more particularly by the cells of Schwann, which make up the sheaths of the ordinary nerve fibres, in the critical process of regeneration.

In normal conditions these lures are lacking in the central nervous organs and consequently the regeneration of the fibres of the interrupted white matter does not take place. But when favourable experimental conditions are set up, the tendency to regenerate which is latent in the fibres of the centres, awakes and develops extraordinary vigour.

In the spinal cord such favourable conditions are established often following the simultaneous section of the white matter and of sensory and motor roots. The liberation in the latter of neurotropic substances being initiated with the degeneration of the cells of Schwann, these substances diffuse into the columns of the cord, where the axons, formerly sluggish and apparently inert, grow actively. It is not rare to see them invade the thickness of the nerve roots and grow through them for long distances.

The same thing takes place in the cerebral hemispheres. As Tello has shown in his brilliant experiments, if a piece of degenerated nerve is introduced into a cerebral wound, the axons of the pyramidal cells, the most apathetic of nerve fibres and the most recalcitrant to any regenerative process, emerge from their inertia, swell up and send off very long shoots which penetrate the nervous implant with the same activity and power of growth which characterize the regeneration of the severed sciatic nerve.

Such facts, of great biological significance, definitely refute the generally accepted dogma of the essential irregenerability of the central tracts. Moreover, these and many other facts demonstrated at the same time teach us that the morphology of the nerve cells is not governed by immanent and fatal factors which are passed on by inheritance, as certain authors have maintained, but depends entirely on the actual physical and chemical conditions in the surrounding medium.

The majority of the investigations on regeneration and degeneration [2] were, as I have already indicated, collected in an extensive work in two volumes, one of the most important and detailed studies which it has been my privilege to accomplish. I should be guilty of ingratitude if I did not recall the fact that the cost of printing this work was defrayed by the generosity of the Spanish physicians of the Argentine Republic, who had the courtesy to write a foreword. As it is exaggeratedly eulogistic of my modest person, I shall not reproduce it here.

Oh, our noble, homesick, zealous compatriots who have emigrated, the flower of the race and the mirror of silent, persevering, and heroic industriousness!

In the midst of your tribulations, you dream of a great Spain, redeemed by culture and tolerance. I have an inclination to say that you are the only great and good Spaniards left to us. Distance, the mitigator of sentiment, has exalted in your spirits the sacred love of country. Distant in space but close to your hearts, Spain appears in your eyes as a star of the first magnitude; not as it is, but as you would that it should be. This is a noble passion in keeping with a magnificent programme; for just in so far as we all desire it with deep and sincere emotion, will Spain return to occupy in the world the place which she has lost.

[2] In the original of the present work, several pages are devoted to a summary of the most important points observed in these studies. (Translator's note.)

CHAPTER XXV

Continuation of the exposition of the work of 1912 to 1917. Some new research methods: that of urano-formol for colouring the endocellular apparatus of Golgi and that of gold-sublimate for the impregnation of the neuroglia of the protoplasmic type. Principal results obtained in the nerves and centres with these new formulae. Investigations on the eye and retina of insects. The retina of the cephalopods. Three books published during the years referred to. Some honorary distinctions received from foreign organizations.

INVESTIGATIONS ON TECHNIQUE. While I did not neglect my favourite studies on the important problem of regeneration in the nervous system, the years 1912 and 1913 were devoted mainly to methodological researches. These require attention, patience, and extraordinary laboriousness. When we apply a formula for selective staining originated by some scientist or other, we scarcely suspect the formidable amount of experimental work, the endless trials and tests which were required, in the first place, for the chance discovery of the new and useful reaction and, afterwards, for the task of determining exactly the optimum conditions for successful results. We should be inspired with heartfelt pity, rather than with base envy, by the rare triumphs in this class of inquiry. Oh, the feverish and impatient hours in which one anxiously awaits the fortunate reaction which flirts without surrendering! For the most serious thing about work of this kind is that whole years may be consumed in it without anything worth while being discovered. And I need not speak of the disappointment caused by the chance discovery of interesting reactions which afterwards, despite persistent trials, do not deign to reappear.[1]

[1] As an example of these fugitive reactions, which indicate the variability and delicacy of nerve chemistry, I may tell the reader of one of my most deplorable disappointments. In the years 1891 and 1892, I happened to im-

The comments serve as an explanation of the scarcity of papers in the years 1913 and 1914, a period of recrudescence of my researches in technique, a scarcity due also, as I shall relate shortly, to the fact that I was engaged at the time in writing two comprehensive books on very different subjects.

My first methodological preoccupation was an effort to discover some easy and constant procedure for impregnating with silver the reticular apparatus of Golgi, of which I had discovered in the muscle fibres of insects (1890) a probable representative.[2] The reader will remember that this intracellular reticulum was described by Golgi in nerve cells (1898) and afterwards observed in other tissues by his pupils Negri, Veratti, Pensa, Marcora, Vechi, and outside Italy by Holmgren, Retzius, Kopsch, Misch, Bergen, Weigl, and others.

However, the formula originated by Golgi and modified by his pupil Veratti was extremely uncertain and difficult. Nor did that of Kopsch (two per cent osmic acid) give full satisfaction. Somewhat more constant, though inapplicable to many tissues, was a certain variant of the reduced silver method, with which I succeeded, from 1903 onwards, in impregnating the reticulum referred to in invertebrates and in some epithelial cells of young mammals. Stimu-

merse pieces of the cerebrum of a young rabbit in a certain mixture of equal parts of 3 per cent potassium bichromate and 1 per cent gold chloride solutions. A few days later, sections of the pieces showed a splendid selective reduction of the gold salt in the Golgi apparatus (then unknown) of the cerebral pyramids. Enraptured with the wonderful results, I devoted myself ardently to reiterated trials to determine the conditions of success. Well, the confounded reaction *never appeared again!* I was guilty on that occasion of excessive scrupulousness and timidity, since I did not dare to publish my rare discovery; it seemed to me that it would be an abuse to announce a fact of which confirmation was, at the time, impossible. Had it not been for such considerations, the so-called reticular apparatus of Golgi, which the neurologist of Pavía discovered in 1898 (by means of a formula, indeed, which is notably uncertain), it would figure today among my assets and under my name.

[2] These nets, first seen by me in insects, and confirmed afterwards by Fusari in the vertebrates, have been regarded by Veratti, Golgi's assistant, as the internal reticular apparatus of the contractile cell. Other authors express the same opinion.

lated, no doubt, by these relative successes of mine, Golgi, who was working at the same problem, successfully modified my silver formula by the addition of arsenious acid as a fixative. The dark brown precipitate in the strands of the apparatus referred to was formed more rapidly and constantly than with previous formulae. By this means, the school of Pavía (Perroncito, Verson, Riquier, and others) and, abroad, Deineka, Legendre, and others extended our idea of the arrangement and significance of the aforesaid little intraprotoplasmic organ, and were able, besides, to attack the interesting subject of its changes during cellular multiplication (Perroncito and Deineka).

The new formula of the savant of Pavía still suffered from some drawbacks. One of them was the diffuse deposit of reduced silver which marked the useful reaction, compelling (Veratti) the employment of clearing agents which had an oxidizing action and were difficult to manage. Finally, the method still failed in some difficult organs.

By dint of trials and experiments, I stumbled by chance upon an excellent fixative—uranium nitrate. Through the use of this reagent, the colouration is obtained regularly in all tissues, especially when it is tried in young mammals. In nervous tissue, for example, splendid stains are procured, in which the net stands out clearly with a dark brown or coffee colour upon a clear and transparent yellow background.

Profiting by this unexpected discovery, I undertook a series of studies [3] on the apparatus of Golgi, as a result of which I was able to describe its form and relations in many types of cell where it had not yet been observed, its relations to the other constituents of the cell (Fig. 76), its embryonic development, and its behaviour in degenerating and regenerating neurons.

My repeated inquiries upon the technique of colouring the neuroglia selectively, stimulated considerably by the interesting work of Achúcarro (carried on in my labora-

[3] Among the series of papers, the very extensive monograph of 1914 (see bibliography) is undoubtedly the broadest investigative report yet published.

tory) upon the structure and connections of the human glia, led, in 1913, to my discovering the method of gold sublimate, a most simple procedure which allows one to impregnate specifically with a purple violet colour the two types of neuroglia of the cerebral cortex, and especially the "protoplasmic" form, or that with short processes, which is so notoriously refractory to the tedious methods of Weigert, Fano, Alzheimer, and others currently used by pathological anatomists.

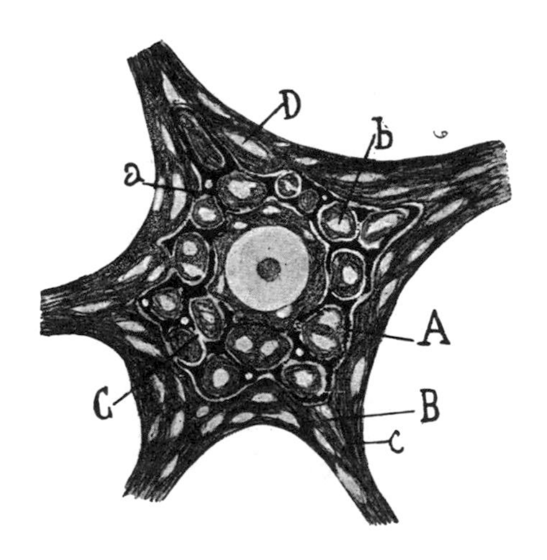

FIG. 76. Diagram of the Golgi apparatus in a motor cell of the spinal cord, with its connections with the other protoplasmic constituents. *A*, contents of the reticular apparatus; *B*, Holmgren's fibres; *C*, neurofibrils; *D*, Nissl granules.

Of its utility for the study of the pathological changes in the human glia, testimony is borne by the interesting works of Achúcarro and Gayarre on paralytic and senile dementia; of Lafora on the neuroglia of the dog in old age; of Achúcarro on the hippocampus and on the comparative histology of the neuroglia; and of Río Hortega on softening of the brain, etc. The method [4] is applicable not only to

[4] The formula for this and the preceding methods are given in the original work. They may be found also in the author's special papers and in his book on technique. (Translator's note.)

man but, in a measure, to all the vertebrates and even to invertebrates.

Thanks to the convenience of manipulation and the specificity of results of the new method of impregnation, I was successful in gathering a number of new facts and, especially, in establishing definitely certain doubtful and much discussed ideas upon the structure, development, and relations of the two types of neuroglia in man and mammals, as well as in demonstrating a third type of element, without processes, which will be mentioned again later.

BOOKS PUBLISHED. The most outstanding was my comprehensive work on the degeneration and regeneration of the nervous system.[5] This bulky work in two volumes, with three hundred and seventeen illustrations drawn from my preparations, constituted the principal undertaking accomplished during the years 1912, 1913, and 1914. It has already been mentioned. Such a considerable effort left me greatly fatigued; for it was not merely a matter of compiling synthetically all my investigations upon the subject but was largely a new work, as I explained in the foreword thereto.

The printing of this work having been financed by subscription of the physicians of the Argentine, the text is preceded by an enthusiastic and touching tribute (probably written by the learned physician and ardent patriot Dr. D. Avelino Gutiérrez, professor in the University of Buenos Aires) signed by forty-seven sympathetic colleagues, scattered through the whole territory of the Argentine Republic. Needless to say, each subscriber was as soon as possible sent a copy, printed on special paper and inscribed with a personal dedication.

What less could I do, to repay so noble and spiritual a tribute, than offer my compatriots of across the seas an original work, seriously considered and carefully written and illustrated?

[5] Cajal, Estudios sobre la degeneracion y regeneracion del sistema nervioso, T. 1, 1913, T. 2, 1914. English translation by May, 1928.

The second book (so I reckon it although it was published in the *Trabajos del Laboratorio*) centered upon the interesting subject of the retina and optic centres of insects. In this work my assistant, D. Domingo Sánchez, collaborated contributing mainly numerous and admirably made preparations.

As the reader will remember, my devotion to the retina is ancient history. The subject always fascinated me because, to my idea, life never succeeded in constructing a machine so subtilely devised and so perfectly adapted to an end as the visual apparatus. It is one of the rare cases, nevertheless, in which nature has deigned to employ physical means which are accessible to our present knowledge. I must not conceal the fact that in the study of this membrane I for the first time felt my faith in Darwinism (hypothesis of natural selection) weakened, being amazed and confounded by the supreme constructive ingenuity revealed not only in the retina and in the dioptric apparatus of the vertebrates but even in the meanest insect eye.[6] There, in fine, I felt more profoundly than in any other subject of study the shuddering sensation of the unfathomable mystery of life.

To contribute even with the slenderest ray of light to illuminating the dark abyss and with the object, besides, of completing my former book on the retina of the vertebrates with another comprehensive study on the retina and eye of the invertebrates, I undertook in 1915 this difficult research, which if my infirmities and physical decay will permit will continue for many years to come.

[6] By the well-known principles of gradual variation and selection of useful modifications it is not possible to explain satisfactorily many arrangements, for example: the transition in mammals from panoramic vision of a common field, with the sudden formation of a homolateral optic tract so as to avoid diplopia; the abandonment in the lower mammals of the excellences of the central fovea of the retina of reptiles and birds; the singular correspondences in the structure of the eye and of the retina in animals without phylogenetic relationship, for example, cephalopods and mammals; and in general, all the sudden and surprising correlations of the nerve centres which take place with each new adaptation of the sensory and motor organs to the environment.

The complexity of the insect retina is something stupendous, disconcerting, and without precedents in other animals. When one considers the inextricable thicket of compound or faceted eyes; when one penetrates the labyrinth of neurons and integrating fibres of the three great retinal segments viz. the layer of ommatidia, the intermediate or perioptic retina, and the internal or epioptic retina; when one discovers not one chiasma, as in the vertebrates, but three successive chiasmas of enigmatic significance, besides the inexhaustible supply of amacrine cells and centrifugal fibres; when one meditates, finally, on the infinite number and the exquisite adjustment of all these histological factors, so delicate that the highest powers of the microscope hardly bring them under observation, one is completely overwhelmed. And I, deceived by the unfortunate preconception of serial progress of zoological structures of similar function, hoped to find a very simple and easily studied architectural plan! It is indubitable that zoologists, anatomists, and psychologists have slighted the insects. Compared with the retina of these apparently humble representatives of life (hymenoptera, lepidoptera, and neuroptera), the retina of the bird or the higher mammal appears as something coarse, rude, and deplorably elementary. The comparison of a rude wall clock with an exquisite and diminutive hunting-case watch fails to give an adequate idea of the contrast, for the "hunting-case eye" of the higher insect does not merely consist of more delicate wheels, but contains besides various highly complicated organs which are not represented in the vertebrates. The adjoining figure (Fig. 77) is diagrammatic and shows only certain elements of each layer, that is of the three superposed segments or retinas, which I have designated: *retina externa, retina intermediaria,* and *retina interna.* The deepest ovoid organ may be regarded as the homologue of the optic lobe of vertebrates. This ovoid appears divided in the retina of the fly.

I shall not undertake to give here an idea of the objective contents of the book referred to. It must be read. I de-

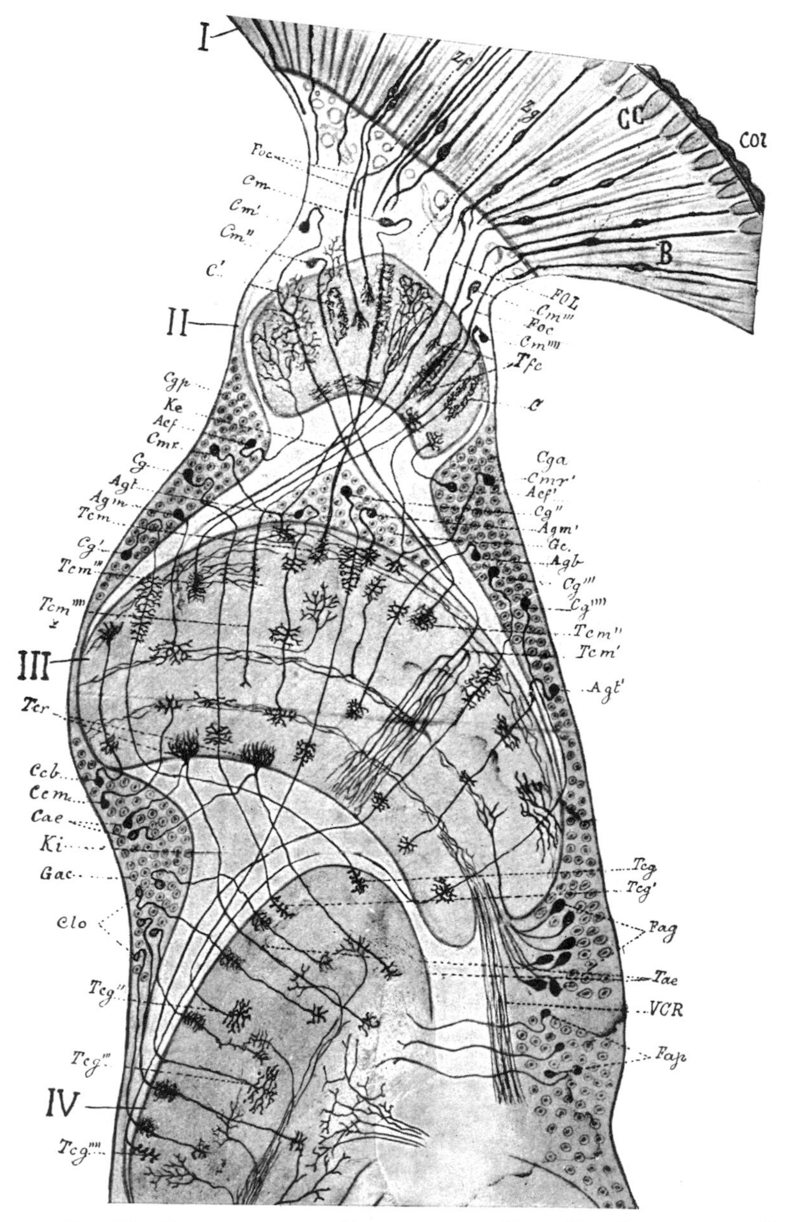

FIG. 77. DIAGRAM OF THE RETINA OF THE BEE. *I*, retina externa; *II*, retina intermediaria; *III*, retina profunda seu interna; *IV*, optic lobe; *Cor.*, corneolas; *CC*, crystalline cones; *B*, rods ending in the intermediate retina; *Cm*, neuron which receives the stimulus brought by the rods; *Tcm*, its termination in the deep retina; *Cg*, third neuron receiving the excitation, etc.

PLATE 20

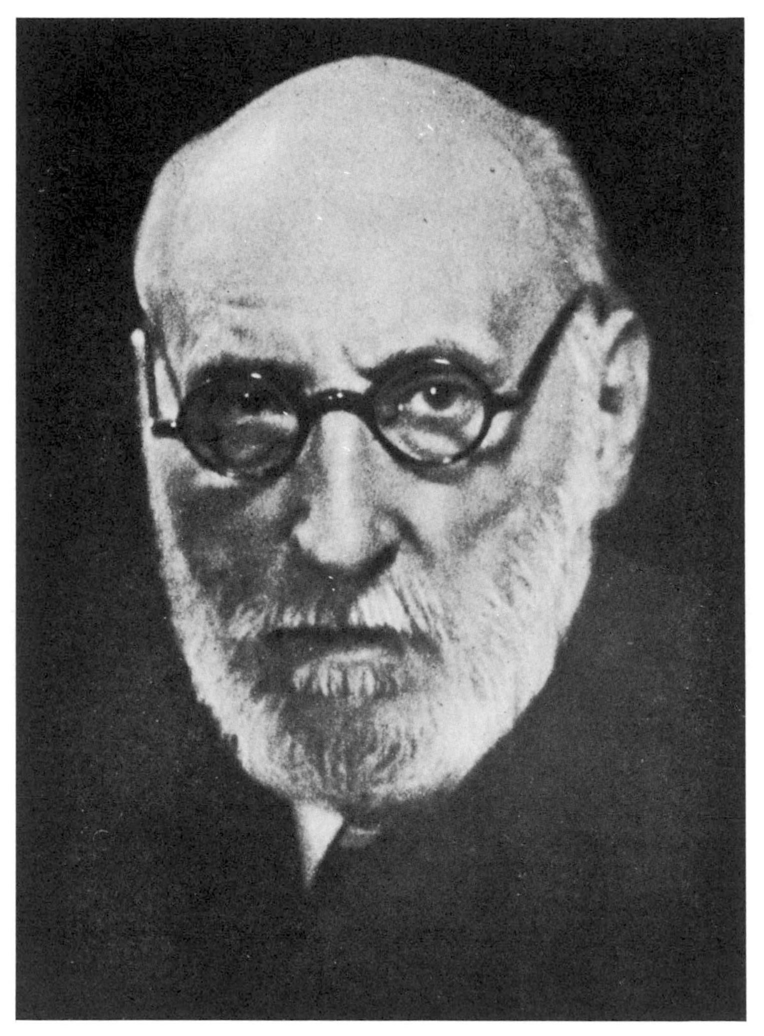

FIG. 78. THE AUTHOR AT THE AGE OF EIGHTY-ONE.

PLATE 21.

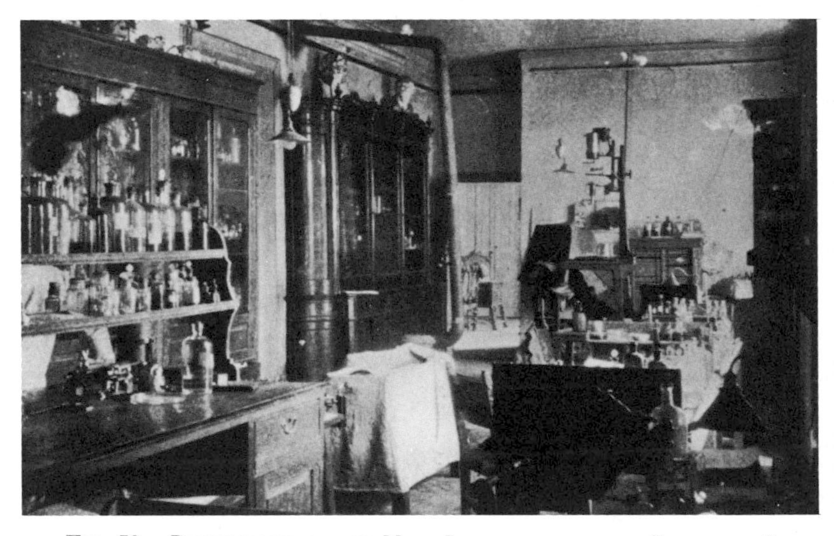

FIG. 79. PHOTOGRAPH OF THE MAIN LABORATORY OF THE INSTITUTO CAJAL TAKEN BY THE TRANSLATOR IN FEBRUARY, 1927. The open door in the background leads into the library, at the far end of which may be seen the closed door of the director's private laboratory. These are the quarters occupied by the Laboratorio de Investigaciones Biológicas from 1902, the new building of the Institute not yet being ready for occupation in 1927.

clare confidentially, for the benefit of those naturalists or histologists who do not disdain the study of the anatomy of the humblest creatures, that the original observations may be reckoned by dozens and that many problems of neuronal morphology and connection are satisfactorily and—I should like to believe—finally cleared up. And this is only a beginning. In my programme and that of my assistant, Sánchez, there is the intention of not stopping short of the discovery of the anatomical characteristic of instinct. Shall we triumph? . . . Since it is impossible to reproduce the hundreds of engravings which illustrate the monographs of Sánchez and myself I give here only the one simple diagram to let the reader judge of the subtilty and complexity of the animals the psychology of which, with a trifle of aristocratic disdain we characterize as instinctive. Fabre himself, whose opinion in the matter is not to be overlooked, attributed to insects not only instinct, which is like an innate understanding, but a certain amount of discernment, enabling them to triumph over unforseen accidents.

A vivid contrast to the foregoing books is another, published in 1912, on colour photography (*La fotografía de los colores*). The reader is quite familiar with my long-standing devotion to the art of Daguerre. Now I shall confess, in the bosom of intimacy, that by way of recreation or relief from more serious work, I engaged from time to time in some modest investigations on the theory and practice of the art of photography.[7]

The first motive was to contribute, with my modest undertaking, to making known among the devotees of colour photography the fundamental physical principles of this marvellous application of science. This I stated in the preface at the beginning of the work. "To deprive oneself of the theory," I said, "is to disdain half of the pleasure of colour photography, which consists in testing experimentally the precision of the scientific principles. The cultivator of photography of colours should not be a routine

[7] References to a considerable number of publications by the author in this field will be found in the bibliography.

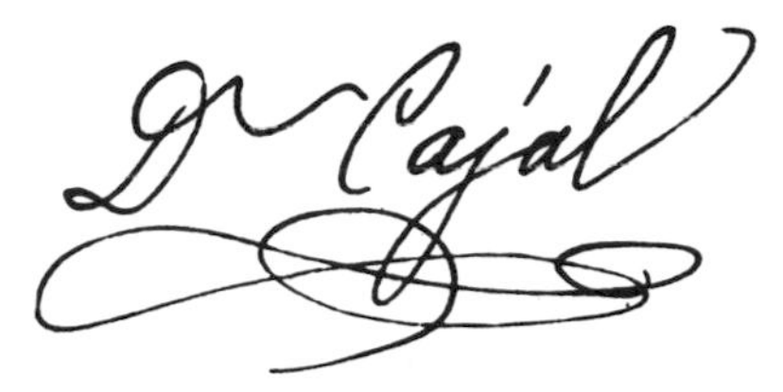

S. Ramón Cajal

Madrid 8 May 1931. S. R. Cajal

como tributo de consideracion
y afecto de su amigo
S. Ramón y Cajal

Madrid 23
Abril de 1934.

Fig. 80. Examples of the Autograph of the Author.

practitioner, merely adhering to receipts and formulae, like a carpenter who, moved by necessity, abandons the plane for the lens. Only he who knows is successful. The interpretation of the results obtained and the remedy for accidents and failures are to be found only in a clear understanding of the physico-chemical mechanism of each photographic operation.'' In truth my patriotic feelings were irritated excessively by hearing the nonsense talked by amateurs of undoubted culture (lawyers, physicians, engineers, etc.) when they discussed the probable causes of a false tone in the colour plates or the physical facts upon which the various three-colour methods are based. From this point of view of the making known in our country of the main principles of the commoner methods of colour photography, I sincerely believe that my book, written in clear and simple language, and illustrated with numerous original diagrams, filled a real need.[8]

The second motive belongs to the domain of the heart. To mention it renews in my mind most distressing recollections. The eldest of my sons, the one who most resembled me, alike intellectually and physically, had contracted very early in life a serious cardiac affection. Since he was given up by the doctors and unfitted for pursuing a profession, I established him as a bookseller, with the object of giving him occupation and dissipating so far as possible his deep depression. And in order to stimulate editorial efforts, a possible basis for future business undertakings, I wrote the first chapters of the book. Unfortunately the inexorable medical prognosis was fulfilled and the author was obliged *a fortiori* to become also editor. But let us not talk of sorrows. Why call up pains of which the only mitigant lies in forgetting!

For the sake of completeness I should also mention here a certain booklet of a literary character which appeared in

[8] One of the best chapters of the book is that on the principles and practical rules of the method of Lippmann, which contains a microscopic analysis of the structure of the plates of Zenker which produce the mixed colours and especially white.

1905 under the title Holiday Tales (*Cuentos de vacaciones*), and was signed with the nom de plume *Dr. Bacteria.* It contained five stories in the style of pseudo-philosophic *causerie,* in which with little novelty and in a clumsy style there are proposed and solved some problems of social ethics. Aware of the defects of the little work, I did not dare to offer it for sale, but restricted myself to presenting copies to those friends of whose kind indulgence I felt well assured. If at some time I have the necessary leisure, I shall perhaps reprint this book and offer it to the public after first expurgating from it cloying lyricisms and not a few defects of thought and style.

During these ten years I was favoured with numerous distinctions. To ignore them in an autobiography might be attributed to pride or ingratitude: to take a belated pleasure in enumerating them in detail would seem like childish vanity. I adopt a middle path and list them in an appendix. For all I wish to express my profound gratitude.

CHAPTER XXVI

Depressing effects of the world war. Disappearance during the war and the postwar period of almost all the few foreign scientists who read Spanish. Studies of recent years on the retina of cephalopods and the ocelli of insects. Contribution to knowledge of the initial developmental errors in the retina of the mammals. Observations of the epitheliofibrils of the ependyma, etc.

The mental disturbance produced by the horrible European war of 1914 was a very rude blow for my scientific activity. My health, which was already considerably weakened, became poorer and, for the first time, my enthusiasm for investigation cooled. During six years I remained cut off from communication with foreign laboratories and reduced to a monologue in which disgust and dejection were the fundamental key-note. Naturally, we continued working in my laboratory. My pupils, especially, made important discoveries. But in my will, shocked by the catastrophe, there rose for the first time that terrible "What is the use?" which enervates the best tempered volitions. I wondered whether in those monstrously tragic years there would be anyone who would read our works. In the face of the formidable struggle of Europe for world supremacy, what could the persistent labour of a group of modest Spanish biologists matter?

In these bloody crises of civilization, only those sciences are recognized which are placed with shameful submission at the service of the great destroyers of peoples. Yesterday it was the aeroplanes, colossal cannons, and asphyxiating and lacrimogenous gases; tomorrow it will be disease germs, epidemics spread from the clouds, poisoning of food and water.

Even from the economic point of view, the cultivation of pure science was very greatly hindered. All the instruments and reagents imported from abroad doubled or even tripled in price. The cost of printing as well as that of paper, photogravures, etc., was almost out of reach of the small appropriation of our laboratory. Only now, in 1923, has a minister, Sr. Salvatella, recognizing the penury of our resources, put an end to such a distressing situation, which would have got to the point of bankruptcy if the Board of Pensions and Scientific Investigations had not, from time to time, come to the rescue in respect of the most pressing material requirements. I should like to pay to the cultured minister the tribute of my most cordial acknowledgements.

As the acme of misfortune, when we entered upon the post-war period and international communications were reestablished we learned with sorrow that almost all the scientists who were acquainted with Spanish and had made known our works had passed away. I have already mentioned how van Gehuchten died in England during the horrible international strife. Almost at the same time there disappeared the venerable Waldeyer, Ehrlich, Nissl, W. Krause, Obersteiner, Dejerine, Brodmann, Alzheimer, Edinger, and Retzius. Then there followed Dogiel (perhaps dead of misery in the ignominious Russia of the Soviets), Obersteiner, Holmgren (the successor of Retzius), Humberto Rossi, and others. What need to continue?—the cortege of illustrious dead would be interminable.

I render to them all a heart-felt tribute of admiration and justice; but I wish to commemorate especially two scientific figures whose recollection still moistens my eyelids and reddens them with emotion: the most industrious, calm, and impartial L. Edinger, the famous neurologist of Frankfort, who so diligently and generously spread through Germany, in books and reviews, the works of my pupils and myself; and the eminent and indefatigable investigator G. Retzius, an old-time spirit in a modern brain, most brilliantly and unobstructedly open to all the truths discovered by his rivals and colleagues, without exception of nationality, race, or tongue. He was a descendant of Gustaf Wasa and, besides extraordinary intellectual gifts—to which I have paid tribute elsewhere—, he had inherited the nobility and the iron will of his lineage.

Fortunately there remain in Europe and America some, though few, men of great ability engaged in the pursuit of histology and, particularly, of neurology; I do not name them lest I should be unjust in omitting names entitled to glory. But for Spain the loss of some of the above-mentioned scientists was a true national bereavement; for they were just the ones who had taken the trouble to study Spanish and had taken a kind and, in some cases, enthusiastic interest in the discoveries made in our laboratory. The immense majority of the biologists of today are ignorant of the language of Cervantes. It is not surprising then that, in consulting the most recent neurological works, we find with sorrow that two-thirds of the modern contributions from Spain are absolutely unknown.[1] Hence one of the most urgent tasks of our young investigators will have to be the translation into English, French, or German of the more essential facts discovered in our country, many of which have been rediscovered by authors elsewhere, who were ignorant of our language, ten, fifteen, or even twenty years after they were announced in Spain.

The translations which I have recently inserted in German periodicals are a response to this pressing need, as is the intention, which will be accomplished this same year (1923), to publish the *Trabajos* of our laboratory in French or English, following the example of many Scandinavian, Dutch, Japanese, Hungarian, Polish, and other

[1] I do not print these bitter reflections in a spirit of criticism. I hasten to declare that the foreigners are right. There are only three peoples who enjoy the enviable privilege of using their native tongues in their scientific communications: the English, the French, and the Germans. Educated people of other countries have no choice, if they wish to make public their ideas, than to understand these three languages and to write in one of them. What right has Spain, a country of slender intellectual production, to try to impose the study of Spanish upon the Japanese, the Swedish, the Polish, the Russian, the Slovak, the Hungarian, the Dutch, the Rumanian, and the others who already spend most of their youth in mastering the three or four learned languages and write in them?

scientists. It is a very significant fact that the best known of my own work is that done just in those years when I used to publish my researches in French or German periodicals. A patriotism more ardent than well advised, and the illusory belief that the acquaintance with French and Italian—general among scientists—would provide facilities for reading scientific Spanish, were the cause of this fundamental error in tactics. To it was added another piece of stupidity—that of summarizing my earlier researches in an enormous French treatise (*Histologie du Système Nerveux de l'Homme et des Vertébrés*) which, on account of its high price (60 to 70 francs), could be acquired only by scattered foreign libraries and very few individuals.

As a typical example of the general ignorance of the rich Spanish bibliography, I shall confine myself to copying this paragraph from the Spanish translation of the work of Poirier, which is used as a text in our medical schools, where also—sad to confess—the work of Spanish histologists is very little known. "Basing his belief upon the results obtained with the methods of Golgi and Ehrlich, which stain the nerve elements in a mass of tissue even to their finest ramifications, Waldeyer, in 1891, wes led to consider the nervous system to be formed entirely of independent cellular units which he termed neurons." We may observe: (1) that His and Forel are not named, though they were the first authors who suggested, as a plausible hypothesis, the independence of the nervous ramifications, though without knowing how they terminated; (2) that neither am I mentioned, in spite of being the first who, independently of the theoretical lucubrations of the scientists referred to, piled up the unquestionable objective proofs of the way in which the nerve fibres terminate in the centres, that is: the formation of pericellular baskets, of excrescences for articulation, of contacts through climbing fibres, etc.; and this not merely in one communication but in more than two hundred monographs which embrace almost all the vertebrates and some invertebrates; (3) that there are forgotten likewise Kölliker, van Gehuchten, Lugaro, Retzius, Lenhossék, Havet, P. Ramón, Athias, Edinger, and innumerable other scientists who confirmed and extended my discoveries; (4) that Waldeyer, to whom histology is indebted for revelations of the utmost importance in other fields, *did not personally investigate the problem of interneuronal connections,* confining himself to making a popular review of my works in a German weekly and inventing the word neuron, etc.!

However, abandoning tedious digressions, I pass on to a brief review of my work in recent years.

One of the first works of the year 1915 referred to the fundamental plan of the retina of insects. It is a review of the extensive memoir already mentioned with some theoretical inductions.

There exists among the invertebrates an eye which bears a singular resemblance to that of mammals. It consists of a cornea, an ovular chamber, a lens, and a retina which, when examined by ordinary methods, exhibits a surprising likeness to that of vertebrates. Spurred by irresistible curiosity, I proposed to inquire how far this structural similarity really extended in animals so far apart in the zoological series, which, nevertheless, seem to have solved the problem of vision according to the same principles of physiological optics.

The investigations were carried out upon young and adult cuttle-fish and squid of three species during two periods in the marine biological stations at Palma (Balearic Islands) and Santander. From the facts observed, an apparently fairly well thought-out attempt was made to give a general physiological interpretation of the structure of the retina of the cephalopods, from which it was concluded that the retina of these animals has perhaps closer analogies to that of the insects than to that of the vertebrates.

In the following year (1918) appeared a discussion and critique of the diverse methods of obtaining stereoscopic photomicrographs and superposed coloured pictures corresponding to various focal planes. For the first time, the neurofibrils within the cells and various histological features refractory to photography were clearly photographed. I further added practical directions for the panchromatization and orthochromatization of plates, and for procuring coloured transparencies for projection.

The next publication was on the structure of the ocelli [2] and nerve pathways connected with them in some insects. From the many facts observed, an attempt was made to build up a hypothesis, still of a provisional nature, as to the physiological significance of the ocelli, which hypothesis may be summarized as follows:

The faceted eye is the organ for perception of colour and for precise (relatively, naturally) diurnal vision, both at short and at long distances, while the ocelli are a hyperphotosensitive apparatus for receiving indefinite uncoloured impressions of objects, useful only for orientating the animal at night or in the partial darkness of its nest or burrow.

It will be recalled that on various occasions I have defended the chemotactic hypothesis, or its analogues, to account, so far as possible in the present state of our knowledge, for the consistent orientation of the axons during the embryonic and foetal phases and for their invariable connection with particular cells. This is one of the deepest secrets of the process of ontogenetic or neurogenetic development.

In my former researches on the embryo, admirably confirmed and perfected by Tello, I concentrated almost entirely on the cells with long axons. Now, studying the cells with short axons in the retina of the mouse foetus, I showed that in their first periods of growth the cells are not subject to neurotropic influences, which only appear later. Moreover, I proved two facts of some importance which had already been indicated in earlier works: one is the migratory capacity of the body and processes, and the other the reabsorption of extensions which have reached

[2] The small simple eyes possessed by insects in addition to their large compound ones. (Translator's note.)

out excessively but been unable to acquire normal connections.

Another paper in the same year (1919) reported an extensive study of the development of sensory nerve endings in many different organs. The developmental mechanism was shown to be similar, with minor differences, for all the endings studied, and the diverse phases seem to be subordinate to the neurotropic influence of cells among which the nerve termination is established.

Two papers in 1920 were devoted to the technique of staining neuroglia and to a further description of that component of the nervous system, particularly of the mesoglia or microglia, which corresponds in part to the "third element" observed in 1913.

Other papers described the fibrils in ependymal cells, the structure of the cerebral cortex of the cat and of rodents, and new studies on technique, and advanced further proofs that regenerating nerve fibres grow freely, not through a syncytium.

Finally, there remains for mention a study of the senses of ants with particular emphasis on the question of how they find their way back to the nest. Among many other facts it is shown that there are great differences in visual power in ants, which include *visual, oligovisual,* and *olfactory* (blind) types. In reality the ant, like any higher animal, combines for its guidance all the sensory data at its disposal, without reckoning the internal impulses which arise spontaneously in association with earlier impressions preserved by memory.

CHAPTER XXVII

EPILOGUE

My teaching activity and spiritual multiplication. Outstanding pupils. The Spanish school of histology. Partial realization of my patriotic-scientific ideal. Aptitude of the Spaniards for scientific investigation. Feeling of duty done. Work of the author and of his pupils and immediate followers.

We are approaching the end of the present book. With as much clearness as is compatible with brevity I have explained the fundamentals of my modest labours and the conditions which inspired them.

As I have progressed in the narrative, my autobiography has become decreasingly personal. Regular work and the spirit of adventure are incompatible. Ever poor in events of interest, my life has been gradually absorbed by my work. The bee has been forgotten in the building up of the honeycomb.

Scientific activity would be incomplete if it confined itself exclusively to working upon material things; it operates also upon souls. That is a primary duty if the investigator belongs to the teaching body. Everyone has the right to expect that a considerable part of the labour of the master shall be employed in moulding pupils to succeed and surpass him. The fulfilment of such an important function is the highest patent of nobility of an investigator and his most outstanding right to the gratitude of his fellow men.

As I have explained in another book,[1] it is very important for the cultivator of science to work for his spiritual multiplication. In this way the life of the master is made full and fertile, since it carries potential new beings within it. "The task is doubtless wearisome," I said. "The activity of the professor bifurcates into the parallel currents

[1] Reglas y consejas sobre la investigación biológica.

of the laboratory and of teaching. Thus his troubles are increased, but his joys are also augmented. Besides nourishing lofty tendencies, he will enjoy the delights of mental paternity and will feel the noble pride of having fulfilled honourably his three-fold mission as investigator, teacher, and patriot. His life will not decline in melancholy solitude; rather, he will approach his end surrounded by a following of enthusiastic pupils capable of understanding his work and of making it, so far as possible, prolific and enduring."

It is unnecessary to say that I tried, though without any certainty of success, to mould my conduct according to this supreme ideal. Obviously, at the dawn of my career, I had to confine myself, by force of habit and of necessity, to the ranks of solitary workers; but I was always anxious, especially after the State placed in my hands a suitable and well-equipped laboratory, to found a genuinely Spanish school of histologists and biologists. And despite the lugubrious declarations of our decadence, both at home and abroad, and the kill-joys for whom science, like the aurora borealis, embellishes the sky of hyperboreal regions only, the dreamt of ideal has been in large part realized. The desired school of Spanish histology and neurology exists and is a permanent focus of activity. Its discoveries (excluding my own modest ones) have spread beyond the frontiers and its methods and inventions are applied in foreign laboratories. Moreover, they would be applied more widely if, recognizing the almost total ignorance of the Spanish language among scientists, we were to publish all our works in foreign periodicals. For it must be stated, although it proclaim our incurable indolence, that *hardly a third part of the Spanish histological publications is known abroad.*

The pretended incapacity of the Spaniards for everything that is not the product of fantasy or artistic creativeness, has been reduced to a vulgar calumny. When the dark sea appears tranquil in the night, a stirring of the waters is enough to make clouds of unilluminated noctilucas kindle their light and shine like stars. The like occurs in the social ocean. It is necessary to shake the thicket of sleeping cerebral neurons energetically; they must be made to vibrate with the excitement of novelty and infused with noble and lofty inquietudes. It has been sufficient that two or three of use (one the illustrious Dr. Simarro) should jolt the drowsiness of our young people for a constellation of worthy investigators to rise among us. I am ready to affirm, without fear of undue optimism, that, in certain fields of study which require ingenuity, patience, and perseverence, our compatriots rival if they do not surpass the most patient and persistent sons of the north. It is entirely a matter of awakening the scientific curiosity, which has slept through four centuries of mental slavery, and of inoculating by example the sacred fire of personal inquiry. We live in a country where scientific talent is not conscious of itself. It is the duty of the teacher to reveal and direct it.

The industrious young men to whom I refer are already legion, especially if we include those of the past with those of the present. Among the former ones (some dead in the flower of their youth and others unfortunately lost to national science in the *desert of the clinic*) I shall mention Cl. Sala, Terrazas, C. Calleja, Olóriz Aguilera, Blanes Viale, J. Bartual, I. Lavilla, E. del Río Lara, and Márquez.

Among the moderns it is a pleasure to me to name my brother, P. Ramón Cajal, F. Tello, N. Achúcarro, Domingo Sánchez, Rodríguez Lafora, Del Río-Hortega, Federico de Castro, and Lorente de Nó. This group of enthusiastic workers have already completed their training and are able to work alone and to triumph in the field of research. Many of the inquiries which I shall list shortly are the fruit of their own sole initiative. In process of formation, and giving promise of abundant fruit, are Arcuate, Fortún, Sacristán, Calandre, Sánchez y Sánchez, Ramón Fananás, Gil y Gil, Luna, Górriz, and others.[2]

[2] In recent years the abundance of devotees and the narrowness of the space available has necessitated the creation of new laboratories of histology. The most active of these offshoots of the *Laboratorio de Investigaciones biológicas* is that directed by Rió Hortega. In it several outstanding pupils have already distinguished themselves, such as Giménez Asúa, and Collado.

The list of papers by these investigators is a long one and within the common fervour for the religion of the microscope, each original mind has travelled along a different path.

Those named above have been my pupils in the broad sense of the word. All have had some part in my life and have shared in my emotions. All have heard me think with halting words during the absorption of my attention and in the brief parentheses of feverish work.

Nevertheless, it would be childish vanity and unjust pretentiousness to claim for myself the entire spiritual paternity of the present cultivators of histology in Spain. Several of them, especially Achúcarro,[3] Tello, Rodríguez Lafora, and Rió-Hortega, have markedly perfected their technical training and their intellectual formation abroad. From the German, French, and English Laboratories, they have brought to Spain, besides a mastery of the languages and bibliography, the latest methods of research and, what is worth more, the habit of self-criticism and the severe discipline of methodical work.

My chief role has been to foment their enthusiasm. It was always my principle to encourage and illuminate the will with full respect for individual tendencies. I always tried—and I am glad of it—to put as little pressure as possible on the minds of my pupils. Every opinion which was the outcome of an honest mental effort, especially if it has arisen from recently discovered facts, has inspired me with sympathy and respect, even though it might contradict fondly cherished personal conceptions. How was I to fall into the temptation to impose my own

[3] Spanish science has suffered an irreparable loss in the premature death of N. Achúcarro. An indefatigable worker, he combined talent and modesty and, what is rarer, a noble sense of justice towards merit in others. He knew that he was suffering from a mortal illness and yet he used to work with the enthusiasm of one who has before him an unlimited prospect of life. His last letter, infused with manly stoicism, gave me the utmost pain. Confined to an armchair by paralysis, he lamented only that he could not continue his researches in neurology. Unimaginable torture! To feel in ones soul the hum of a swarm of ideas and projects and to see before one only the eternal shadows of death! But the best of his work will persist; transformed and improved, it will continue to inspire the minds of his friends and pupils.

theories when I have given outstanding examples of abandoning them as a result of the smallest objective evidence against them? Far be from me that self-idolizing desire, the forerunner of irremediable senility.

Deeply impressed by these ideas; desirous of preventing my successors from becoming readers of a single book and hearers of a single master; and determined besides to obviate so far as possible any undesirable polarization of ideas and methods, I laid special emphasis upon my pupils enjoying the benefits of scholarships in the most outstanding foreign laboratories. It would be unjust to forget that, in this work of healthy patriotism and of refreshing doctrinal fresh air treatment, I have been solicitously helped by my worthy colleagues of the Pension Board, of which I am the unworthy president.

The results of such tactics have been excellent. On their return, the more outstanding scholarship-holders have made valuable conquests not only in the domains which I have preferably explored but also in other fields hardly touched in my laboratory; for example, that of pathological human neurology, in which Achúcarro, Lafora, and Río-Hortega have collected facts of great value. It is needless to point out that the scholarship holders mentioned have carried on their researches in my own laboratory and that my *Review* has been enriched and honoured by varied and interesting communications. Special mention is deserved by the too soon departed Achúcarro, who, thanks to the discovery of a new and fertile method of investigation (the tanin-ammoniacal silver method) and to his enviable didactic endowments, created in his turn an important school of pathological anatomy. His immediate pupils, Fortún, Gayarre, Sacristán, Del Río-Hortega, Calandre, and others, I look upon with the pride of a grandfather. The unexpected blossoming of this second and third intellectual generation demonstrates that the seed fell upon good ground. Everything gives assurance that the harvest of investigators will not be interrupted from now on. In their hands—and they know it—lies the future of histology in Spain.

I must draw to a conclusion. The impatience of the reader demands it; my weariness compels it.

I have aimed that my life should be, so far as possible, in accordance with the counsel of the philosopher, a living poem of intense action and of secret heroism on behalf of scientific culture. Poor is my work, but it has been as intense and original as my slender talents permitted. To judge it with some knowledge of the case, it will suffice to recall what Spanish histology was in 1880, when I made my timid beginnings, and what it is at the present time. Far am I—as I have already said—from overlooking precious collaboration of others, but it may be permissible for me to believe that my obstinate labour has counted for something in the present renaissance of biology in my country.

I consider it certain and even desirable that in the course of time my insignificant personality will be forgotten; and with it will, doubtless, perish many of my ideas. Nothing can escape from this inexorable law of life. In spite of all the allegations of self-love, the facts associated in the first place with the name of one man end by being anonymous, lost for ever in the ocean of Universal Science. In consequence the monograph, still impregnated with a human quality, will be incorporated, deprived of sentimentalisms, in the abstract doctrine of the general treatise. To the hot sun of actuality will succeed—if they do succeed—the cold beams of the history of learning.

But I have no right to afflict the reader with melancholy reflections. Let us repel sadness, which is mother of inaction. Let us devote ourselves to life which is energy, renovation, and progress, and let us keep on working. Only tenacious activity on behalf of truth justifies living and gives consolation for sorrow and injustice. Only this possesses the marvellous virtue of converting the obscure social parasite into a legendary hero.

I repeat, let us cultivate our garden—as Voltaire used to say—fulfilling so far as we can the double and austere duty of men and patriots. For the biologist, the supreme ideal consists in solving the enigma of his own ego, contributing at the same time to clarifying the formidable mystery which surrounds us. It matters not that our work be premature or incomplete; incidentally, until the long-sought ideal dawns, the world will gradually be made pleasanter for man. Nature is hostile to us because we do not know it; its cruelties represent revenge for our indifference. To listen to its inmost heartbeats with the fervour of passionate curiosity is the same as to decipher its secrets; it is to turn the ireful stepmother into the most tender mother.

In what nobler and more humanitarian enterprise could the intelligence be employed?

CHAPTER XXVIII

POSTSCRIPT

My retirement as a professor. In that connection there falls upon me a shower of distinctions and tributes. The Spaniards of America. Award of the Echegaray Medal. The book in my honour. The exaggerated generosity of Spain: Creation of the *Instituto Cajal* and reprinting of my works which were out of print.

I have hesitated considerably before writing this chapter. An enemy of exhibitions of vanity, and modest and retiring by nature, I am ashamed of any disproportionate or unmerited honour. I realize, however, that I write for the young and that I have no right to conceal tributes and distinctions, which by way of examples, may serve as incentives. Besides, he who writes a life must go to the end if he is not to defraud the reader.

Encouraged by these considerations, I go on to relate the most recent events.

When we have reached the age of seventy, the inexorable but foresighted law expels us from the class-room, cutting off forever the daily chat with our pupils. I do not regret that; I consider it wise and reasonable. Chill old age, with its disillusionments and its disabilities, is, with rare exceptions, incompatible with good oral instruction, which calls for quickness and sharpness of the senses, ready, enthusiastic, and vigorous diction, a vibrant and robust voice, agility of memory and of thought, and flexibility of attention capable of jumping instantly from the serene and lofty region of ideas to the vulgar and annoying requirements of maintaining order—an undertaking by no means easy in classes where there assemble four hundred youngsters the majority of whom regard study as wearisome vexation and desire impatiently to warm themselves in the light of the sun which glorifies the streets and gardens rather than in the light of knowledge.

All the same, I cannot complain of my students. Within and without the classroom, they always honoured me with unequivocal marks of respect and veneration, although stimulated by the spirit of mischief and by the desire for action of muscles taut and restless upon the hard scholastic benches.

Still less can I complain of the governors, of my friends, and of my professional colleagues. Towards my expected weaknesses of old age, they always showed an attitude of generous solicitude. Finally, upon the cessation of my labours as a teacher, these expressions of sympathy, always most pleasing, acquired the character of highly honourable and exaggerated tributes. To keep silent regarding the feelings of cordial esteem which inspired them on the excuse of discretion or modesty, would be a displeasing lack of appreciation and gross ingratitude. I shall speak of them shortly.

Before that comes a generous gesture on the part of the Government. Stimulated by some friends, the Minister of Public Instruction proposed, and the Cortes approved a large appropriation for the erection of a biological institute, which, through the benevolence of His Majesty the King, was christened *Instituto Cajal*. The work is already under way on the hill of San Blas, near the Astronomical Observatory. When the building is inaugrated, there will be installed in it, besides the Laboratory of Biological Research, which I have directed for the last twenty-two years, all the other biological laboratories supported by the Board of Pensions and Scientific Research. In place, then, of the mean and narrow quarters in which my students work, we shall have at our disposal in the future a magnificent palace not inferior to the proud foreign scientific institutes. There will live together, with mutual spiritual commerce, all those among us who are devoted to similar studies. I hope that community of quarters will be conducive of unity in aims and sentiments, and that, when they find themselves collaborators in the intellectual renaissance of our country, all will know how to give up our lamentable factionism and individualism, which lead to endless grudges and hard feelings. The persistent individualism represents—sad to confess—one of the gravest defects of the Spanish race.

I do not know whether the precarious state of my health will permit me to be present at the inauguration of the sumptuous institute. Perhaps the splendid building will be for me only a fine monument to my memory. It matters little. I contemplate with resignation the dark tunnel beyond which nobody knows whether there awaits us an everlasting and life-giving garden or a tragic and interminable desert.

I have referred above to an endless shower of tributes, all enthusiastic, kindly, and respectful, from Spain and from America. With more reason than Goethe, the sublime old man who preserved his enviable gifts to the end of his life, I could ask myself: "How can one find expressions of gratitude with which to reply in a varied and fitting manner to hundreds of letters, official communications, and messages?" So poor and monotonous is the language of sentiment in comparison with the language of intelligence!

Little, however, does awkwardness matter in formulating expressions of feeling which are individual and adapted to each case; what matters is to show heart-felt sincerity, vibrant with sympathy, even though this vibration be monorhythmic and express itself in commonplace phrases and formal acknowledgments.

Perhaps the most fervent and exaggerated compliments which arrived in connection with my academic retirement came from that Spanish America which never forgets the ancient soil of its ancestors and hastens to honour the distinguished men, however modest they may be, who have arisen among its people. I should be guilty of verbosity if I indicated here all the unmerited tributes from our America. I must confine myself to mentioning as a group the almost countless diplomas and messages which came from Mexico, of which the principal inspirer was undoubtedly my intimate friend Dr. Perrín, professor in the University of Mexico; the artistic busts erected in the Argentine Republic; the beautiful illuminated addresses received from all sides, and, above all, the public subscription, of the utmost educational value, taken up in Spain and in the Argentine in order to mark my jubilee by founding annual grants to outstanding students and professors for study abroad and in Spain. I may mention too the almost innumerable letters of congratulation, notices of meetings in my honour, erection of commemorative busts, etc. contributed not only by many American universities, but also by learned societies and cultural and commercial institutions entirely unconnected with teaching functions. This is a highly encouraging symptom. There exists in Iberian America such a precious treasure of veneration and love for the peninsular nations; it nourishes an eagerness so ardent and almost irritable to show to all the world the capacity for progress of the Spanish people; it feels, in fine, so lively an anxiety to promote, to make known, and to honour the true intellectual values of the latter, that there are moments when my relative pessimism regarding the destiny of Spain and its sister nations is dissipated. These splendid gestures open the heart to hope. They presage a possible spiritual coming together of Spain and America based, needless to say—and in this I agree completely with the illustrious American writer Blanco-Fombona—, on the absolute reciprocity of rights and interests, and excluding any distasteful and anachronistic pretension of overlordship. Such an approximation, which might assume the form of an alliance (including also Portugal and Brazil), is, at the present time, more than a common convenience; it is a vital necessity, a question of life or death for our stock.

If some day, laying aside jealousies and mutual disdain, which are evidences of reciprocal lack of understanding, the suggested alliance should be really established, we should have not only an invaluable instrument for peace and prosperity, but also a dike which might be insuperable against the insatiable greed and the overwhelming imperialism of certain northern peoples. But, alas, I fear that we come too late and that concord and spiritual intermingling between Spain and her daughters will rise in Spanish America only when it sees itself harassed, split up, invaded, and despoiled by its formidable and foresighted adversaries.

Asking the reader's pardon for these digressive unbosomings, I must continue my story by stating that I received similar sincere proofs of consideration and esteem in Spain itself from many Academies,[1] Universities, Institutes, normal and primary schools, provincial and civic governments, laboratories, clubs, etc. The list of such undeserved distinctions would fill several pages of this book. Some of them, especially those tendered by the school children, are deeply moving.

To dwell tediously and complacently on the enumeration of all the honourable tributes would be a childish display of presumptuous vanity. Even at the risk of appearing indifferent, unappreciative, or negligent, I must, then, pass over them with a gesture filled with heart-felt gratitude, without its detracting from my expressing to the tenderers my most sincere acknowledgements.

However, it is not permissible for me to omit, among so many extreme and exaggerated demonstrations, an extraordinary tribute offered by many Madrid colleagues. Forming a committee, they decided to open a nation-wide subscription to pay for the printing of an honorary volume written by my pupils and friends in Spain and abroad; to reprint, besides, my papers which were out of

[1] Although unrelated to my retirement, but coincident with it, I may record here the Echegaray Medal, awarded on May 7, 1922, by the Royal Academy of Science, in a session presided over by His Majesty the King, at which eloquent addresses were deliverd by Don Alphonso XIII, by the illustrious President of the body, Don Amós Salvador, and by my dear and venerated friend the learned naturalist Don Ignacio Bolívar.

print; and, finally, to accord me other attentions and tributes which, being so excessive as to make me blush, I do not know how to specify.[2] Of all these most charming manifestations of affection towards the retiring professor, none surpasses from both the spiritual and the utilitarian viewpoints, the aforementioned book,[3] in which there have had the kindness and generosity to collaborate with excellent and original communications foreign scientists of such prestige as M. v. Lenhossék, Cecile and Oskar Vogt, Jacques Loeb, Albrecht Bethe, C. Sherrington, A. P. Dustin, J. Boeke, Umberto Rossi, Ernesto Lugaro, M. G. Marinesco, V. Babes, Max Bielschowsky and Richard Henneberg, Karl Schäffer, Emil Holmgren, J. B. Johnston, I. Havet, M. Athias, C. v. Monakow, Celestino da Costa, Pierre Marie, E. Veratti, A. Prenant, Cl. Regaud and A. Lacassagne, B. A. Houssay, J. T. Lewis, R. Kraus, Chr. Jacob, C. Judson Herrick, and C. U. Ariëns Kappers.

Among the Spaniards are: P. Ramón, A. Pi y Suner, R. Turró, G. R. Lafora, P. del Río-Hortega, G. Pittaluga, J. Negrin, E. Hernández Pacheco, G. Marañón, F. Giménez de Asúa, Domingo Sánchez y Sánchez, M. Sánchez y Sánchez, J. Nonídez, A. de Gregorio Rocasolano, Fernando de Castro, Lorente de Nó, Manuel Bordás, O. Fernández and T. Garmendia, J. Mouriz, J. Ramón Fañanás, G. Loez Ortín, Sadi de Buen, and Miguel Fernández.

Needless to say, I am eternally indebted to the initiators of and subscribers to the fund for this honorary volume, among whom there stand out the Conde de Romanones, Dr. C. M. Cortezo, Dr. Amalio Gimeno, Don F. R. Carracido, Dr. Recassens, Dr. Francos Rodríguez, Don M. Sotomayor, Don G. Marañón, Don Blas Cabrera, Dr. G. Pittaluga, and, especially, Dr. Tello, upon whom rested the burdensome task of compiling the communications re-

[2] The translator will take it upon himself to mention that among these was the erection of a large and beautiful monument in the Parque del Retiro, the principal public park of Madrid.

[3] *Libro en honor de D. Santiago Ramón y Cajal.* Two volumes published by the *Junta para el homenaje a Cajal,* Madrid, 1922.

ceived, correcting the proofs, and preparing Spanish summaries of the English and German papers.

Some of the veteran foreign contributors have recently passed away before receiving the two volumes of the honorary book. Great was the loss to science. I refer to the illustrious professors E. Holmgren and Umberto Rossi. Many others who preceded them, like Waldeyer, Edinger, van Gehuchten, Retzius, and others, would undoubtedly have offered me a further testimony of their unquenchable friendship if inexorable fate had not closed the way to them during the war or the postwar period. Glory and honour to the fallen and joy to those who still live, gathering their strength, in their glorious old age, in the cause of scientific progress and the intellectual elevation of their respective countries!

These almost posthumous tributes to a modest worker in biology have for an old man a flavour of bitterness mingled with sweetness. They tell him nobly, gently, and discreetly that he has virtually finished his scientific career; that, having reached the mountain top, there is nothing for it but to roll down hill, swept along with dizzy swiftness by the hurricane of time in complicity with the restrictions and sufferings of decrepitude. Lacking or weak in the divine power of creation, there rises within him, filled with melancholy recollections, the consciousness of having lived too long. He has committed the sin of being too persistent, laughing at the ambuscades of sickness and the warnings of overwork. Weakness of memory, opening up an abyss between the present and the past, compels him to regard himself objectively, to look at his maturity as at that of another person almost incomprehensible and completely shut off from him. The sense of continuity is lost or attenuated so that when he reads his writings he wonders at his ingenuous old ideas, the pride and vainglory of youthful inexperience. He is different, and perhaps worse, for what he has gained in experience he has lost in enthusiasm and faith.

Like every old man, I also feel all those poisoned wounds of the heart and brain. They are the knocks of time at the door, time which is the implacable devourer of life. But I neither will nor should cease my efforts, and in order not to fall into mental inertia—a kind of anticipated death—I continue working, though I may have to confine myself unpretentiously to rounding out my earlier researches, which is for the old man the line of least resistance. I have besides the unavoidable duty of directing my pupils, inspiring them with unquenchable confidence in their own powers and robust faith in indefinite progress. Science, like life, grows ever, renewing itself continually without running against the wall of decrepitude in its creative impetus. It is a great stimulus to the young to know that the mine is inexhaustible and that all, if they firmly desire it, can transmit their names to posterity and add a blazon to the escutcheon of the race. For all those who are fascinated by the bewitchment of the infinitely small, there wait in the bosom of the living being millions of palpitating cells which, for the surrender of their secret, and with it the halo of fame, demand only a clear and persistent intelligence to contemplate, admire, and understand them.

CHAPTER XXIX

Conclusion by the Translator

The last years of the author were passed in rather close retirement and in continuation of the work to which he had so strenuously and fruitfully devoted his life. He retained the directorship of the institute which bears his name, and each day proceeded from his house in the Calle de Alfonso XII to the laboratory, where he continued to guide and inspire an enthusiastic group of younger investigators, both Spanish and foreign, giving unstintingly of himself at all times.

His devotion to reading remained unabated to the end. Writing also occupied him and a number of papers appeared, mostly confirming and consolidating the results of his earlier studies. A book on microtechnique was prepared in collaboration with Dr. Fernando de Castro, and two other books also were published shortly before the author's death—a new edition of "Café Chat" (*Charlas de Café*) and "The world as seen at eighty" (*El mundo visto a los ochenta años*).

Health, however, deteriorated and sleep, long elusive, as we have seen in foregoing pages, became increasingly difficult to obtain. The spirit of the master, nevertheless, remained undaunted in spite of suffering and, writing to the translator in October, 1932, he said, "I am confined to bed but am improving. I hope to recover my strength, if not fully, at least in part, so as to be able to continue my work." In later letters, the signature became less firm and the tone less hopeful.

Though physically weak, he preserved until a few hours before his death the full vigour and clearness of his intellect, receiving with pleasure the visits of pupils and intimates and discussing current events with them at considerable length.

Finally, at eleven o'clock on the evening of the seventeenth of October, 1934, the last curtain fell and the world of science lost one of her greatest and most striking personalities.

On account of the disturbed political conditions at the time, the funeral lacked official ceremonies, but it was attended by a great concourse representative of all classes of society, including the workers' organizations, in which the deceased was highly esteemed. The remains were laid in the Necropolis at Madrid, according to the expressed wish of the departed, by the side of those of his wife.

The country which Don Santiago Ramón y Cajal had loved so dearly and for which he had laboured so indefatigably did not, however, ignore, even officially, the passing of her famous son and among the posthumous honours paid him was the issue of a special mourning postage stamp bearing his portrait. Also a republication of all his works has been undertaken by the government.

The first anniversary of his death was marked by ceremonies in the various academic Faculties and in other scientific centres and was observed by the press of all persuasions, while a beautiful monument with a portrait bust was unveiled in the patio of the Faculty of Medicine (San Carlos).

WORKS BY THE AUTHOR

BOOKS

1. Manual de Histología normal y técnica micrográfica. Obra ilustrada con 203 grabados originales, 1.ª edición, Valencia; 1889, 2.ª edición, 1893.
2. Manual de Anatomía patológica general, seguido de un resumen de Microscopia aplicada a la Histología y Bacteriología patológicas (con numerosos grabados originales, en negro y color), 1.ª edición, Barcelona, 1890; 2.ª edición, Madrid, 1896; 3.ª edición, Madrid, 1900; 4.ª edición, 1905; 5.ª edición, Madrid, 1909; 6.ª edición, 1918; 7.ª edición, 1922.
3. Elementos de Histología normal y de técnica micrográfica. Madrid, 1897. 7.ª edición, 1921.
4. Les nouvelles idées sur la fine anatomie des centres nerveux. Con numerosos grabados y un prólogo del Dr. Mathias Duval. Paris, 1894.
5. Textura del sistema nervioso del hombre y de los vertebrados. (3 volúmenes.) Madrid, 1897, 1899 a 1904.
6. Cuentos de vacaciones (Narraciones pseudocientificas). Madrid, 1905.
7. Studien über die Hirnrinde des Menschen. Leipzig, J. Barth, 1906.
8. Die Retine der Wirbelthiere. Versión y prólogo del Dr. Greeff. Berlín, 1894.
9. Studien über Nervenregeneration. Leipzig, 1908.
10. Histologie du système nerveux de l'homme et des vertébrés. (Translation by Dr. L. Azoulay), 2 vol. en 4.° mayor. Paris, 1909–1911.
11. La fotografía de los colores: Fundamentos científicos y reglas prácticas. Madrid, 1912.
12. Reglas y consejos sobre la investigación biológica. Discurso leído con ocasión de la recepción del autor en la Real Academia de Ciencias Exactas, Físicas y Naturales, en la sesión del 5 de diciembre de 1897; (7 editions).
13. Estudios sobre la degeneración y regeneración del sistema nervioso. Madrid, 1913–1914, 2 vol.
14. Recuerdos de mi vida. T. I. Mi infancia y juventud. T. II. Historia de mi labor cientifica. Madrid, 1901–1917.
15. Charlas de café (pensamientos, anécdotas, confidencias). Madrid, 3rd Ed. 1923.
16. Manual técnico de Anatomía patológica. (In collaboration with Dr. Tello, to whom the most important part is due.) 1918.
17. Études sur la neurogenèse de quelques vertebrés.
18. Discurso leído con ocasión de la recepción de la Medalla Echegaray (May 1922).
19. Técnica del sistema nervioso. Madrid, 1932. In collaboration with Dr. Fernando de Castro.

20. Regeln und Ratschläge zur wissenschaftlichen Forschung. München, 1933. (Translation of No. 11 by Prof. Misckolezy.)
21. Histology. (English translation by Prof. Fernán-Núñez from the 10th Spanish edition of No. 3, with collaboration of Prof. Tello.)
22. El mundo visto a los ochenta anos. Madrid, 1934.

SCIENTIFIC MONOGRAPHS

1880

23. Investigaciones experimentales sobre la génesis inflamatoria. Zaragoza. Con dos láminas litografiadas, 1880.

1881

24. Observaciones microscópicas sobre las terminaciones nerviosas en los músculos voluntarios de la rana. Zaragoza, 1881. Con dos láminas litografiadas por el autor.

1885

25. Estudios sobre el microbio vírgula del cólera. Zaragoza. Septiembre de 1885. Con ocho grabados.
26. Contribución al estudio de las formas involutivas y monstruosas del comabacilo de Koch. *La Crónica Médica.* Valencia, 20 de diciembre de 1885. Con un grabado.

1886

27. Contribution à l'étude des cellules anastomosées des épithéliums pavimenteux stratifiés. *Internationale Monatsschrift f. Anat. u. Histol.*, Bd. III, Heft. 7
28. Estructura de las fibras del cristalino. Notas de laboratorio. *La Crónica Médica.* Revista quincenal de Medicina y Cirugía prácticas. Valencia, 20 de marzo de 1886.

1887

29. Tejido óseo y coloración de los cortes de hueso. *Boletin Médico Valenciano.* Enero de 1887.
30. *Notas de laboratorio:* I. Textura de la fibra muscular de los mamíferos. *Boletín Médico Valenciano.* Junio de 1887.
31. II. Fibra muscular del ala de los insectos. *Boletín Médico Valenciano.* Junio de 1887.
32. III. Músculos de las patas de los insectos. *Boletín Médico Valenciano.* Agosto de 1887.
33. Sobre los conductos plasmáticos del cartílago hialino. *Crónica Médica de Valencia,* 20 de abril de 1887.

1888

34. Observations sur la texture des fibres musculaires des pattes et des ailes des insectes. *Internationale Monatsschrift f. Anat. u. Physiol.,* Bd. V, Heft 6 u. 7.

35. Estructura de los centros nerviosos de las aves. Con dos láminas litográficas. *Revista trimestral de Histología normal y patológica.* Barcelona, 1.° de mayo de 1888.
36. Morfología y conexiones de los elementos de la retina de las aves. *Revista trimestral de Histología normal y patológica,* número 1.° mayo de 1888.
37. Terminaciones nerviosas en los husos musculares de la rana. *Revista trimestral de Histología normal y patológica.* Mayo de 1888.
38. Textura de la fibra muscular del corazón. *Revista trimestral de Histología normal y patológica.* 1.° de mayo de 1888.
39. Sobre las fibras nerviosas de la capa molecular del cerebelo. *Revista trimestral de Histología normal y patológica.* 1.° agosto de 1888, Barcelona.
40. Estructura de la retina de las aves (continuación del trabajo publicado en el núm. 1.° de la *Revista trimestral de Histología normal y patológica*), agosto 1888.
41. Nota sobre la estructura de los tubos nerviosos del órgano cerebral eléctrico del torpedo. *Revista trimestral de Histología normal y patológica.* Agosto 1888.
42. Estructura del cerebelo. *Gaceta Médica Catalana,* 15 de agosto de 1888.

1889

43. Coloración por el método de Golgi de los centros nerviosos de los embriones de pollo. *Gaceta Médica Catalana,* 1.° de enero de 1889.
44. Nota preventiva sobre la estructura de la médula embrionaria. *Gaceta Médica Catalana,* 15 de marzo de 1889.
45. Nota preventiva sobre la estructura de la médula embrionaria. *Gaceta Médica Catalana,* 31 de marzo de 1889.
46. Dolores del parto considerablemente atenuados por la sugestión hipnótica. *Gaceta Médica Catalana,* 31 agosto 1889.
47. Estructura del lóbulo óptico de las aves y origen de los nervios ópticos. *Revista trimestral de Histología normal y patológica,* 1.° marzo 1889 (números 3 y 4). Barcelona.
48. Contribución al estudio de la estructura de la médula espinal. *Revista trimestral de Histología normal y patológica,* marzo 1889.
49. Sobre las fibras nerviosas de la capa granulosa del cerebelo. *Revista trimestral de Histología normal y patológica,* marzo 1889.
50. Conservación de las preparaciones de microbios por desecación. Revista *trimestral de Histología normal y patológica,* marzo 1889.
51. Sur l'origine et la direction des prolongations nerveuses de la couche moléculaire du cervelet. *Intern. Monatsschrift. f. Anat. u. Phys.,* 1889, Bd. VI, Heft. 4 u. 5.
52. Sur la morphologie et les conexions des éléments de la rétine des oiseaux. *Anatomischer Anzeiger,* número 4, 1889.
53. Nuevas aplicaciones del método de coloración de Golgi. *Gaceta Médica Catalana,* 1889.
54. Conexión general de los elementos nerviosos. *La Medicina Práctica.* Madrid, 2 de octubre de 1889.

1890

55. Sur l'origine et les ramifications des fibres nerveuses de la moelle embryonaire. *Anatomischer Anzeiger,* número 3, 1890. Revised French translation of no. 48.
56. Sobre ciertos elementos bipolares del cerebelo y algunos detalles más sobre el crecimiento y evolución de las fibras cerebelosas. *Gaceta Sanitaria de Barcelona,* 10 de febrero de 1890.
57. Sur les fibres nerveuses de la couche granuleuse du cervelet et sur l'évolution des éléments cérébelleux. *Internationale Monatschrift für Anat. u Physiol.,* Bd. VII, H. I, 1890. Revised translation of no. 49.
58. Nuevas observaciones sobre la estructura de la médula espinal de los mamíferos. Barcelona, 1.° de abril de 1890.
59. Sobre la terminación de los nervios y tráqueas en los músculos de las alas de los insectos. Barcelona, 1.° de abril de 1890.
60. Sobre las células gigantes de la lepra y sus relaciones con las colonias del bacilo leproso. *Gaceta Sanitaria de Barcelona,* 10 de julio de 1890, número 11.
61. Sobre la aparición de las expansiones celulares en la médula embrionaria. *Gaceta Sanitaria de Barcelona,* 10 de agosto de 1890.
62. Sobre las terminaciones nerviosas del corazón en los batracios y reptiles. *Gaceta Sanitaria de Barcelona,* agosto 1890.
63. Sobre las finas redes terminales de las tráqueas en los músculos de las patas y alas de los insectos. *Gaceta Sanitaria de Barcelona,* 10 de octubre de 1890.
64. Sobre un proceder de coloración de las células y fibras nerviosas por el azul de Turnbull. *Gaceta Sanitaria de Barcelona,* del 10 de octubre de 1890.
65. Reponse a M. Golgi à propos des fibrilles collatérales de la moelle épinière et la structure générale de la substance grise. *Anatomischer Anzeiger,* número 20, 1890.
66. A quelle époque apparaissent les expansions des cellules nerveuses de la moelle épinière du poulet. *Anatomischer Anzeiger,* números 21 y 22, 1890.
67. Sobre la existencia de células nerviosas especiales en la primera capa de las circunvoluciones cerebrales. *Gaceta Médica Catalana,* 15 de diciembre de 1890.
68. A propos de certains éléments bipolaires du cervelet avec quelques details nouveaux sur l'évolution des fibres cérébelleuses. *Journal International d'Anatomie et de Physiologie,* Bd. VII, H. 11, 1890.
69. Origen y terminación de las fibras nerviosas olfatorias. Barcelona, 11 de octubre de 1890.
70. Textura de las circunvoluciones cerebrales de los mamíferos inferiores. Barcelona, octubre de 1890.
71. Sobre la existencia de terminaciones nerviosas pericelulares en los nervios raquidianos. *Pequeñas comunicaciones anatómicas.* Barcelona, 20 de diciembre de 1890.
72. Sobre la existencia de colaterales y bifurcaciones en las fibras de la substancia blanca de la corteza del cerebro. Barcelona, diciembre de 1890.

73. Coloration par la méthode de Golgi des terminaissons des trachées et des nerfs dans les muscles des ailes des insectes. *Zeitschrift f. wissenschaftliche Microscopie,* etc., Bd. VII, 1890. Revised translation of nos. 56 and 60.

1891

74. Sobre la existencia de bifurcaciones y colaterales en los nervios sensitivos craneales y substancia blanca del cerebro. *Gaceta Sanitaria de Barcelona,* 10 de abril de 1891.
75. Terminaciones nerviosas en el corazón de los mamíferos. *Gaceta Sanitaria de Barcelona,* 10 de abril de 1891.
76. Significación fisiológica de las expansiones protoplásmicas y nerviosas de las células de la substancia gris. Memoria leída en el Congreso Médico de Valencia. Sesión de 24 de junio de 1891.
77. Sur la fine structure du lobe optique des oiseaux et sur l'origine réelle des nerfs optiques. *Jour. internat. d'Anatomie et de Physiol.,* tomo VIII, fasc. 9, 1891.
78. Pequeñas contribuciones al conocimiento del sistema nervioso (Varias investigaciones sobre el gran simpático, retina médula espinal y corteza cerebral), 20 de agosto de 1891.
   I parte: Estructura y conexiones de los ganglios simpaticos.
   II parte: Estructura fundamental de la corteza cerebral de los batracios, reptiles y aves.
   III parte: Estructura de la retina de los reptiles y batracios.
   IV parte: Estructura de la médula espinal de los reptiles.
   V parte: La substancia gelatinosa de Rolando.
79. Nota sobre el origen y ramificaciones de las fibras nerviosas de la médula embrionaria. *La Veterinaria Española,* August, 1891.
80. Notas preventivas sobre la retina y gran simpático de los mamíferos. *Gaceta Sanitaria de Barcelona,* 10 de diciembre de 1891.
81. Terminación de los nervios y tubos glandulares del páncreas de los vertebrados (en union de Cl. Sala), 28 de diciembre de 1891. Barcelona.
82. Sur la structure de l'écorce cérébrale de quelques mammifères. *La Cellule,* Tomo VII, 1.e fascicule, 1891.

1892

83. Nota sobre el plexo de Auerbach de la rana. Barcelona, 13 de febrero de 1892.
84. Observaciones anatómicas sobre la corteza cerebral y asta de Ammon. *Actas de la Sociedad Española de Historia Natural,* Segunda serie, tomo I, Sesión de diciembre de 1892.
85. La retina de los teleósteos y algunas observaciones sobre la de los vertebrados superiores. Trabajo leido ante la Sociedad de Historia Natural en 1.° de junio de 1892.
86. La rétine des vertébrés. *La Cellule,* Tomo IX, 1.° fasc.

1893

87. Estructura del asta de Ammon y fascia dentada. *Anales de la Sociedad Española de Historia Natural,* Tomo XXII, 1893.

88. Estructura de la corteza occipital de los pequeños mamíferos. *Anales de la Sociedad de Historia Natural,* Tomo XXII, 1893.
89. Adenoma primitivo del hígado. *Revista de Ciencias Médicas de Barcelona,* 10 de mayo de 1893.
90. Beitrage zur feineren Anatomie des grossen Hirns. Translation of no. 83.
91. Los ganglios y plexos nerviosos del intestino de los mamíferos, y pequeñas adiciones a nuestros trabajos sobre la médula y gran simpático general, 23 de noviembre de 1893, Madrid.
92. Sur les ganglions nerveux de l'intestin. Review of the preceding by Dr. Azoulay. Société de Biologie de Paris (sessión del 30 de diciembre de 1893).
93. Pequeñas adiciones a nuestros trabajos sobre la médula y gran simpático general. Noviembre de 1893, Madrid.

1894

94. La fine structure des centres nerveux. The Croonian lecture. Proceedings of The Royal Society of London, Vol. 55.
95. Notas preventivas sobre la estructura del encéfalo de los teleósteos. *Anales de la Sociedad Española de Historia natural,* Tomo 23, 1894.
96. Algunas contribuciones al conocimiento de los ganglios del encéfalo. *Anales de la Sociedad Española de Historia natural,* Tomo 23, 1894.
97. Le Pont de Varole. *Bibliographie anatomique,* núm. 6, 1894. Resumé of article I of monograph 96.
98. Estructura del ganglio de la habénula de los mamíferos. *Anales de la Sociedad Española de Historia natural,* Tomo 23, 1894.
99. Consideraciones generales sobre la morfología de la célula nerviosa. *La Veterinaria Española,* números 5 y 20 de junio de 1894.

1895

100. Ganglions cérébelleux. *Bibliographie anatomique,* núm. 1. Enero de 1895. Résumé of article 2 of no. 96.
101. Corps strié *Bibliographie anatomique,* núm. 2. 1895.
102. Algunas conjeturas sobre el mecanismo anatómico de la asociación, ideación y atención. *Revista de Medicina y Cirugía prácticas.* Madrid, 1895.
103. L'anatomie fine de la moelle épinière. *Atlas der pathologischen Histologie des Nervensystems.* Berlin, 1895.
104. Apuntes para el estudio del bulbo raquídeo, cerebelo y origen de los nervios encefálicos. *Anales de la Sociedad Española de Historia natural.*
105. Evolution of the nerve cells. *Jour Nerv. & Ment. Dis.,* Dec. 1895.

1896

106. Beitrag zur Studium der Medula oblongata, des Kleinhirns und des Ursprung der Gehirnnerven. Translation with a foreward by Dr. Mendel, of no. 104, Leipzig. Ambrosius Barth. 1896.
107. Nouvelles contributions à l'étude histologique de la rétine et à la question des anastomoses des prolongements protoplasmiques. *Journal dè l'Anatomie et de la Physiologie,* 13 de noviembre de 1896.

108. Las defensas orgánicas en el epitelioma y carcinoma. *Boletín oficial del Colegio de Médicos de Madrid,* núm. 1896.
109. Las colaterales y bifurcaciones de las raíces posteriores de la médula espinal demostradas por el azul de metileno. *Revista de Clínica, de Terapéutica y Farmacia,* 10 octubre 1896. Tomo X.
110. Métodos de coloración de las neoplasias. *Revista de Ciencias Médicas de Barcelona,* 10 marzo 1896.
111. Estructura del protoplasma nervioso. *Revista trimestral micrográfica, número* 1, marzo 1896.
112. La fagocitosis de las plaquetas. *Revista trimestral micrográfica,* núm. 4, 1 marzo de 1896.
113. Sobre las relaciones de las células nerviosas con las neuróglicas. *Revista trimestral micrográfica,* núm. 1, marzo 1896.
114. Estudios histológicos sobre los tumores epiteliales. *Revista trimestral micrográfica,* núm, 2, junio de 1896.
115. Las espinas colaterales de las células del cerebro teñidas con el azul de metileno. *Revista trimestral micrográfica,* núm. 2, junio 1896.
116. El azul de metileno en los centros nerviosos. *Revista trimestral micrográfica,* números 3 y 4, 1896.
117. Allgemeine Betrachtungen über die Morphologie der Nervenzellen. *Arch f. Anat. u Physiol.,* Anat. Abt., 1896. (German translation of no. 99.)
118. Interpretaciones conjeturales sobre algunos puntos de Histofisiología neurológica. *Biblioteca de la Ciencia moderna,* Nov. 1896.

1897

119. Leyes de la morfología y dinamismo de las células nerviosas. *Revista trimestral micrográfica,* núm. 1, marzo de 1897.
120. Algo sobre la significación fisiológica de la neuroglia. *Revista trimestral micrográfica,* núm. 1, marzo de 1897.
121. Nueva contribución al estudio del bulbo raquideo. *Revista Trimestral micrográfica,* núm. 2, 1897.
122. Las células de cilindro-eje corto de la capa molecular del cerebro. *Revista trimestral micrográfica,* junio 1897.
123. Los ganglios sensitivos craneales de los mamíferos (en unión de D. Federico Olóriz Ortega). *Revista trimestral micrográfica.*
124. Terminaciones nerviosas en los husos musculares de la rana. *Revista trimestral micrográfica,* diciembre 1897.

1898

125. Estructura del quiasma óptico y teoría general de los entrecruzamientos nerviosos. *Revista trimestral micrográfica,* núm. 1, marzo 1898.
126. Algunos detalles más sobre la anatomía del puente de Varolio y consideraciones acerca de la doble vía motriz. *Revista trimestral micrográfica,* núm. 2 junio 1898.
127. Estructura fina del cono terminal de la médula espinal. *Revista trimestral micrográfica,* septiembre 1898.
128. La red superficial de las células nerviosas centrales. *Revista trimestral micrográfica.*

1899

129. Apuntes para el estudio experimental de la corteza visual del cerebro humano. *Revista ibero-americana de Ciencias médicas,* núm. 1, marzo 1899.

130. Estudios sobre la corteza cerebral humana.—I. Región visual. *Revista trimestral micrográfica,* núm. 1, 1899.

131. Estudios sobre la corteza cerebral humana.—II. Zona motriz del hombre y mamíferos superiores. *Revista trimestral micrográfica.*

132. Comparative study of sensory areas of the human cortex. Worcester, Mass., 1899.

1900

133. Estudios sobre la corteza cerebral humana.—III. Corteza motriz. *Revista trimestral micrográfica,* tomo V, núm. 1, marzo de 1900.

134. Estructura de la corteza acústica y circunvoluciones de la ínsula. *Revista trimestral micrográfica,* tomo V, números 2, 3 y 4. Diciembre de 1900.

135. Disposición terminal de las fibras del nervio coclear. *Revista trimestral micrográfica,* tomo V, números 2, 3 y 4.

136. La corteza olfativa del hombre y de los mamíferos. *Revista trimestral micrográfica,* núm. 4. Diciembre de 1900.

137. Contribución al estudio de la vía sensitiva central y de la estructura del tálamo óptico. (Con 4 grabados.) *Revista trimestral micrográfica,* tomo V.

138. Pequeñas comunicaciones técnicas. *Revista trimestral micrográfica,* tomo V, fascículo 3.°

1901

139. Estructura de la corteza olfativa del hombre y mamíferos. *Trab. del Lab. de Invest. biol.,* tomo I.

140. Textura del lóbulo olfativo accesorio. *Trab. del Lab. de Invest. biol.,* tomo I.

141. Significación probable de las células de axon corto. *Trab. del Lab. de Invest. biol.,* tomo I.

142. La vía de unión del cerebelo y médula espinal. *Madrid Medico,* Dec. 1901.

1902

143. Estructura del *Septum lucidum.* *Trab. del Lab. de Invest. biol.,* tomo I.

144. Sobre un ganglio especial de la corteza esfeno-occipital. *Trab. del Lab. de Invest. biol.,* tomo I.

145. Recreaciones estereoscópicas y binoculares. *La Fotografía:* Año 1901.

146. Estructura del tubérculo cuadrigémino posterior, cuerpo geniculado interno y vías acústicas centrales. *Trab. del Lab. de Invest. biol.,* tomo I.

147. Die Endigung des äusseren Lemniscus, &. *Ehrennummer des Deutsch. med. Woch. zum 70 geburtstage Leyden's,* April 1902.

148. Significación del tálamo óptico y constitución de las vías sensoriales centrales. *La Clínica moderna,* Zaragoza, 1902.

1903

149. Sobre un foco gris especial relacionado con la cinta óptica. *Trab. del Lab. de Invest. biol.*, tomo II.
150. Anatomía de las placas fotográficas. *La Fotografía*, núm. 17, febrero de 1903.
151. Las fibras nerviosas de origen cerebral del tubérculo cuadrigémino anterior y tálamo óptico. *Trab. del Lab. de Invest. biol.*, tomo II.
152. La doble vía descendente nacida del pedúnculo cerebeloso superior. *Trab. del Lab. de Invest. biol.*, tomo II.
153. Estudios talámicos. *Trab. del Lab. de Invest. biol.*, tomo II.
154. Plan de estructura del tálamo óptico. *Congreso médico internacional.* Madrid, 1903.
155. Método para colorear la mielina en las preparaciones del método de Marchi. *Trab. del Lab. de Invest. biol.*, tomo II.
156. Un consejo útil para evitar los inconvenientes de la friabilidad y arrollamiento de los cortes en los preparados de Golgi y Marchi. *Trab. del Lab. de Invest. biol.*, tomo II.
157. Consideraciones críticas sobre la teoría de Bethe, acerca de la estructura y conexiones de las células nerviosas. *Trab. del Lab. de Invest. biol.*, tomo II.
158. Sobre un sencillo método de impregnación de las fibrillas interiores del protoplasma nervioso. *Archivos latinos de Medicina y Biología*, 20 de octubre de 1903.
159. Sobre la existencia de un aparato tubuliforme en el protoplasma de las células nerviosas y epiteliales de la lombriz de tierra. *Boletín de la Sociedad Española de Historia Natural.* (Sesión de diciembre de 1903.)
160. Algunas adiciones a nuestro artículo anterior sobre la estructura del protoplasma nervioso. *Revista escolar de Medicina, etc.*, 15 diciembre 1903.
161. Un sencillo método de coloración selectiva del retículo protoplásmico y sus efectos en los diversos órganos nerviosos. *Trab. del Lab. de Invest. biol.*, tomo II.
162. Sobre la estructura del protoplasma nervioso. *Revista escolar de Medicina y Cirugía*, 1 noviembre 1903.
163. Sobre un nuevo foco subtalámico, al parecer de naturaleza centrífuga. (No bibliographic reference.) 1903. (Communication to the International Medical Congress, Madrid.)
164. Sobre las fibras cerebrales del tubérculo cuadrigémino anterior. 1903. (No reference, as for no. 163.)

1904

165. Algunos métodos de coloración de los cilindros-ejes, neurofibrillas y nidos nerviosos. *Trab. del Lab. de Invest. biol.*, tomo III.
166. Ueber einige Methoden der Silberimprägnirung zur Untersuchung der Neurofibrillen der Achsencylinder und der Endverzweigungen. *Zeits f. wiss. Mikroskopie u. mikr. Technik*, Bd. XX.
167. Variaciones morfológicas normales y patológicas del retículo neurofibrillar. *Trab. del Lab. de Invest. biol.*, tomo III.

168. El aparato tubuliforme (red de Golgi) del epitelio intestinal de los mamíferos. *Trab. del Lab. de Invest. biol.*, tomo III.
169. Un método de coloración de los cilindros-ejes y de las células nerviosas. *Revista de la Real Academia de Ciencias de Madrid,* tomo I, número 1, abril de 1904.
170. Asociación del método del nitrato de plata al embrionario para el estudio de los focos motores y sensitivos. *Trab. del Lab. de Invest. biol.*, tomo III, fascículos 2 y 3. Junio y septiembre.
171. La fotografía cromática de puntos coloreados. *La Fotografía,* número 37, octubre 1904.
172. Contribución al estudio de la estructura de las placas motrices. *Trab. del Lab. de Invest. biol.*, tomo III, cuadernos 2 y 3.
173. El retículo neurofibrillar en la retina. *Trab. del Lab. de Invest. biol.*, tomo III, fascículo 4.
174. Das Neurofibrillennetz der Retina. *Inter. Monatsch f. Anat. u. Physiol.* Bd. 21, H, 418. Festschrift für Dr. W. Krause.
175. Las lesiones del retículo de las células nerviosas en la rabia. (Trabajo hecho en colaboración con D. Dalmacio García.) *Trab. del Lab. de Invest. biol., cuaderno* 4.
176. Neuroglia neurofibrillas del Lumbricus. *Trab. del Lab. de Invest. biol.*, tomo III, cuaderno 4.
177. Variaciones morfológicas del retículo nervioso de invertebrados y vertebrados. *Trab. del Lab. de Invest. biol.*, tomo III, cuaderno 4.

1905

178. Tipos celulares de los ganglios sensitivos del hombre y mamíferos. *Trab. del Lab. de Invest. biol.*, tomo IV, fascículos 1 y 2.
179. Tipos celulares de los ganglios raquídeos del hombre y mamíferos. Nota leída en la sesión del 1.° de marzo de 1905. *Anales de la Sociedad Española de Historia natural,* 1905.
180. Las células estrelladas de la capa molecular del cerebelo y algunos hechos contrarios a la función exclusivamente conductriz de las neurofibrillas. *Trab. del Lab. de Invest. biol.*, tomo IV, fascículos 1 y 2.
181. Las células del gran simpático del hombre adulto. *Trab. del Lab. de Invest. biol.*, tomo VI, fascículos 1 y 2.
182. Coloración de la fibra muscular por el proceder del nitrato de plata reducido. *Trab. del Lab. de Invest. biol.*, cuadernos 1 y 2, tomo IV.
183. Diagnóstico histológico de la rabia. *Boletín del Instituto de Sueroterapia, Vacunación, etc., de Alfonso XIII,* núm. 1, marzo.
184. Sobre la degeneración y regeneración de los nervios. *Boletín del Instituto de Sueroterapia, etc.*, 1.ª parte, núm. 2, julio; 2.ª parte, núm. 3, septiembre.
185. Mécanisme de la régénération des nerfs. *Compt. rend. de la Société de Biol. de Paris,* Séance 11 noviembre 1905.

1906

186. Mecanismo de la regeneración de los nervios. *Trab. del Lab. de Invest. biol.*, tomo IV, cuaderno 3.°

187. Estructura de las imágenes fotocrómicas de G. Lippmann. *Revista de la Real Acad. de Cien. Exactas, Físicas y Naturates,* tomo IV, núm. 4, abril 1906.
188. Quelques antécédents historiques ignorés sur les Plasmazellen. *Anatomischer Anzeiger,* Bd. XXIX, 1906.
189. Sobre la policromía de los gránulos metálicos microscópicos. *Anales de la Sociedad Española de Física y Química,* tomo IV, 24 de noviembre de 1906.
190. Génesis de las fibras nerviosas del embrión y observaciones contrarias a la teoría catenaria. *Trab. del Lab. de Invest. biol.,* tomo IV, fascículo 4.° 1906.
191. Relación de méritos y trabajos científicos del autor. *Resumen de mis investigaciones hasta 1906.* Madrid, 1906.
192. Structure et connexions des neurones. *Conférence de* Nobel *faite a Stockholm le 12 décembre 1906. Archivos de Fisiologia,* volumen V, fascículo 1.°, noviembre 1907.)
193. Una modificación del proceder fotocrómico de Lumière a la fécula. *La Fotografía,* 1906.
194. Reglas prácticas sobre la fotografía interferencial de Lippmann. *Ciencia popular,* Barcelona, Noviembre de 1906.
195. Notas preventivas sobre la degeneración y regeneración de las vías nerviosas centrales. *Trab. del Lab. de Invest. biol.,* tomo IV, fascículo 4°., 1906.
196. Om neuronemas struktur och förbindelser. Dec. 1906. (Translation into Swedish of No. 192.)
197. Die Struktur der sensiblen Ganglien des Menschen und der Tiere. *Anat. Hefte,* 2te–Abt., 1906. (Translation and revision of No. 178.)

1907

198. Discurso leído ante la Real Academia de Medicina, en la recepción pública de S. R. Cajal, el día 30 de junio de 1907.
199. Notes microphotographiques. *Trav. Lab. Rech. biol.,* tomo V. fasc. 1.° y 2.°, abril 1907.
200. Les metamorphoses précoces des neurofibrilles dans la régénération et la dégénération des nerfs. *Trav. Lab. Rech. biol.,* t. V, fasc. 1.° y 2.°, abril 1907.
201. Note sur la dégénérescence traumatique des fibres nerveuses du cervelet et du cerveau. *Trav. Lab. Rech. biol.,* t. V, fasc. 3.°, juillet 1907.
202. Die Histogenetische Beweise der Neurontheorie von His und Forel. *Anatomischer Anzeiger,* Bd. 37, 1908.
203. Nouvelles observations sur l'évolution des neuroblastes avec quelques remarques sur l'hypothèse de Hensen-Held. *Trav. Lab. Rech. biol.,* t. V. 1907.
204. Quelques formules de fixation destinées à la méthode au nitrate d'-argent. *Trav. Lab. Inv. biol.,* t. V. 1907.
205. L'appareil réticulaire de Golgi-Holmgren coloré par le nitrate d'argent. *Trav. Lab. Rech. biol.,* t. V, fasc. 3.°, juillet 1907.

206. El renacimiento de la doctrina neuronal. *Gaceta Médica Catalana,* t. XXXI, núm. 724. Barcelona, 31 de agosto de 1907.

207. Una hipótesis sobre la constitución del retículo de la célula nerviosa. *Revista escolar "Cajal,"* año II, núm. 8. Abril de 1907.

208. Las placas autocromas Lumière y el problema de las copias múltiples. *La Fotografía,* Madrid, 1907.

1908

209. Las teorías sobre el ensueño. *Revista escolar "Cajal,"* año II, 1908.

210. L'hypothèse de la continuité d'Apathy: reponse aux objetions de cet auteur contre la doctrine neuronal. *Trav. Lab. Rech. biol.,* t. VI, fascículos 1.° y 2.°, juin 1908.

211. Sur un noyau special du nerf vestibulaire des poissons et des oiseaux. *Trav. Lab. Rech. biol.,* t. VI, fasc. 1.° y 2.°, junio 1908.

212. Les conduits de Golgi-Holmgren du protoplasma nerveux et le reseau péricellulaire de la membrane. *Trav. Laboratoire Rech. biol.,* t. VI, fasc. 3.°, août 1908.

213. Sur la signification des cellules vasoformatives de Ranvier. *Trav. du Laboratoire de Rech. biol,* t. VI, fasc. 3, 1908.

214. El ganglio intersticial del fascículo longitudinal posterior en el hombre y diversos vertebrados. *Trab. Lab. Inv. biol.,* t. VI, 1908.

215. Terminación periférica del nervio acústico de las aves. *Trab. Lab. Inv. biol.,* t. VI, 1908.

216. Los ganglios centrales del cerebelo de las aves. *Trabajos Lab. Inv. biol.,* t. VI, 1908.

217. Les ganglions terminaux du nerf acoustique des oiseaux. *Trab. Lab. Inv. biol.,* t. VI, 1908.

218. Influencia de la quimiotaxis en la génesis y evolución del sistema nervioso. Discurso inaugural de la Sección de Ciencias Naturales de la *Asociación Española para el progreso de las Ciencias.* Congreso de Zaragoza, 1908.

1909

219. Contribución al estudio de los ganglios de la substancia reticular del bulbo (con algunos detalles concernientes a los focos motores y vías reflejas bulbares y mesocefálicas). *Trab. del Lab. Inv. biol.,* t. VII, 1909.

220. Nota sobre la retina de la mosca. (M. VOMITORIA L.) *Trab. del Lab. de Inv. biológ.,* t. VII, fasc. 4.°, diciembre de 1909.

1910

221. Obtención de estereofotografías (proceder de Berthier-Ives) con un solo objetivo. *Revista de Física y Química,* 1910.

222. Nota sobre la retina de los muscidos. *Soc. Esp. de Hist. Nat.,* enero 1910.

223. Las fórmulas del proceder del nitrato de plata reducido y sus efectos sobre los factores integrantes de las neuronas. *Trab. Lab. Inv. biol.,* t. VIII, fasc. 1.° y 2.°, septiembre 1910.

224. El nucleo de las células piramidales del cerebro humano y de algunos mamíferos. *Trab. Lab. Inv. biol.*, t. VIII, fasc. 1.° y 2°, septiembre 1910.
225. Algunas observaciones favorables a la hipótesis neurotrópica. *Trabajos Lab. Inv. biol.*, t. VIII, fasc. 1.° y 2.°, septiembre 1910.
226. Algunos experimentos de conservación y autolisis del tejido nervioso. (Nota preventiva.) *Trab. del Lab. de Invest. biológicas*, tomo VIII, 1910.
227. Algunos hechos de regeneración parcial de la substancia gris de los centros nerviosos. *Trab. del Lab. de Invest. biológicas*, tomo VIII, fasc. 2.° y 3.°, diciembre 1910.
228. Observaciones sobre la regeneración de la porción intramedular de las raíces sensitivas. *Trab. del Lab. de Invest. biológicas*, tomo VIII, fasc. 2.° y 3.°, diciembre 1910.
229. Las plaquetas de la sangre impregnadas dentro de los vasos por el proceder del nitrato de plata reducido. *Trab. del Lab. de Invest. biol.*, tomo VIII, fasc. 2.°, 3.° y 4.°, diciembre 1910.

1911

230. Los fenómenos precoces de la degeneración traumática de las vías centrales. *Bol. de la Soc. Esp. de Biol.* Sesión del 24 de febrero de 1911.
231. Reacciones degenerativas de las células de Purkinje del cerebelo bajo la acción del traumatismo. *Bol. de la Soc. Esp. de Biol.* Sesión del 21 de abril de 1911.
232. Transformación, por efecto traumático, de las células del cerebro en corpúsculos nerviosos de axon corto. *Bol. de la Soc. Esp. de Biología.* Sesión del 16 de junio de 1911.
233. Los fenómenos precoces de la degeneración neuronal en el cerebelo. *Trab. del Lab. de Invest. biol.*, tomo IX, fascículos 1.°, 2.° y 3.°, julio 1911.
234. Los fenómenos precoces de la degeneración traumática de los cilindros-ejes del cerebro. *Trab. del Lab. de Invest. biológicas*, tomo IX, fasc. 1.°, 2.° y 3.°, julio 1911.
235. Fibras nerviosas conservadas y fibras nerviosas degeneradas. *Trab. del Lab. de Invest. biol.*, tomo IX, fasc. 4.°, diciembre de 1911.
236. Alteraciones de la substancia gris provocadas por conmoción y aplastamiento. *Trab. del Lab. de Invest. biol.*, tomo IX, fascículo 4.°, diciembre 1911.

1912

237. Proceder helicrómico por decoloración. Obtención de pruebas positivas estables con el azul de metileno. *Anales de la Soc. Esp. de Fisica y Quimica*, año X, febrero de 1912.
238. Fórmula de la fijación para la demostración fácil del aparato reticular de Golgi. *Bol. de la Soc. Esp. de Biol.* Sesión del 21 de junio de 1912.

239. Fórmula de fijación para la demostración fácil del aparato reticular de Golgi y apuntes sobre la disposición de dicho aparato en la retina, en los nervios y en algunos estados patológicos. *Trab. del Lab. de Inv. biol.*, t. X, junio de 1912.

240. El aparato endocelular de Golgi en la célula de Schwann y algunas observaciones sobre la estructura de los tubos nerviosos. *Trab. del Lab. de Inv. biol.*, t. X, fasc 4.°, agosto de 1912.

241. Sobre ciertos plexos pericelulares de la capa de los granos del cerebelo. *Trab. del Lab. de Inv. biol.*, t. X, fasc. 4.°, agosto de 1912.

242. Influencia de las condiciones mecánicas sobre la regeneración de los nervios (nota preliminar). *Trab. del Lab. de Inv. biol.*, t. X, fasc. 4.° agosto de 1912.

1913

243. Fenómenos de excitación neurocládica en los ganglios y raíces nerviosas consecutivamente al arrancamiento del ciático. *Trab. del Lab. de Inv. biol.*, t. XI, fasc. 2.°, julio de 1913.

244. El neurotropismo y la transplantación de los nervios. *Trab. del Lab. de Inv. biol.*, t. XI, fasc. 2.°, julio de 1913.

245. Sobre un nuevo proceder de impregnación de la neuroglia y sus resultados en los centros nerviosos del hombre y animales. *Trab. del Lab. de Inv. biol.*, t. XI, fasc. 3.°, diciembre de 1913.

246. Contribución al conocimiento de la neuroglia del cerebro humano. *Trab. del Lab. de Inv. biol.*, t. XI, fasc. 4.°.

247. Los problemas de la Biología celular. Asociación española para el Congreso de las ciencias. Congreso de Madrid. Discurso inaugural. (Demonstration that nervous protoplasm contains ultramicroscopic entities capable of growth and multiplication.)

1914

248. Algunas variaciones fisiológicas y patológicas del aparato reticular de Golgi. *Trab. del Lab. de Inv. biol.*, t. XII, 1914.

249. Eine neue Methode zur Färbung der Neuroglia. *Neurol. Centralbl.*, 1914.

1915

250. Variaciones fisiológicas del retículo de Golgi en algunos elementos epiteliales y mesodérmicos. *Bol. de la Soc. Esp. de Biol.*, Núm. 30, marzo de 1915.

251. Consideraciones generales sobre la polarización ontogénica y filogénica del aparato de Golgi. *Bol. de la Soc. Esp. de Biol.*, Núm. 30, marzo de 1915.

252. Contribución al conocimiento de los centros nerviosos de los insectos. Parte I, Retina y centros ópticos (con la colaboración de don D. Sánchez). *Trab. del Lab. de Inv. biol.*, t. XIII, 1915.

253. Plan fundamental de la retina de los insectos. (*Bol. de la Soc. Esp. de Biologia*, ses. del 19 de noviembre de 1915).

254. Significación probable de la morfología de las neuronas de los invertebrados. (*Bol. de la Soc. Esp. de Biol.*, ses. del 17 de diciembre de 1915.)

1916

255. El proceder del oro-sublimado para la coloración de la neuroglia. *Trab. del Lab. de Inv. biol.*, t. XIV, fascículos 3 y 4. Diciembre de 1916.

1917

256. Contribución al conocimiento de la retina y centros ópticos de los cefalópodos. *Trab. del Lab. de Inv. biol. de la Universidad de Madrid,* t. XV, 1917.

1918

257. La microfotografía estereoscópica y biplanar del tejido nervioso. *Trab. del Lab. de Inv. biol.*, t. XVI, 1918.
258. Observaciones sobre la structura de los ocelos y vías nerviosas ocelares de algunos insectos. *Trab. del Lab. de Inv. biol. de la Universidad de Madrid,* t. XVI, 1918.

1919

259. La desorientación inicial de las neuronas retinianas de axon corto. *Trab. del Lab. de Inv. biol.*, t. XVII, fasc. 1 y 2. Junio de 1919.
260. Nota sobre las epiteliofibrillas del epéndimo. *Trab. del Lab. de Inv. biol.*, t. XVII, fasc. 1 y 2. Junio de 1919.
261. Acción neurotrópica de los epitelios. *Trab. del Lab. de Inv. biol.*, t. XVII, 1919.

1920

262. Una modificación del método de Bielschowsky para la impregnación de la neuroglia común y mesoglia y algunos consejos acerca de la técnica del oro-sublimado. (*Trab. del Lab. de Inv. biol.*, t. XVIII, fascículos 2 y 3, diciembre 1920.)
263. Algunas consideraciones sobre la mesoglia de Robertson y Río-Hortega. *Trab. del Lab. de Inv. biol.*, t. XVIII, fasc. 2 y 3. Diciembre de 1920.

1921

264. Algunas observaciones contrarias a la hipótesis «syncytial» de la regeneración nerviosa y neurogénesis normal. *Trab. del Lab. de Inv. biol.*, t. XVIII, fasc. 4. Marzo 1921.
265. Una fórmula de impregnación argéntica especialmente aplicable a los cortes del cerebelo y algunas consideraciones sobre la teoría de Liesegang acerca del principio del método de nitrato de plata reducido. *Trab. del Lab. de Inv. biol.*, t. XIX, fascs. 1, 2 y 3. Octubre 1921.
266. Textura de la corteza visual del gato. *Trab. del Lab. de Inv. biol.*, t. XIX, fascs. 1, 2 y 3. Octubre 1921.
267. Las sensaciones de las hormigas. Real Sociedad Española de Historia Natural. Tomo extraordinario, publicado con motivo del 50 aniversario de su fundación, 1921, páginas 555–572. Also *Archivos de Neurobiología,* t. II, núm. 4. Diciembre 1921.
268. Estudios sobre la fina estructura de la corteza regional de los roedores. *Corteza suboccipital* (*retroesplenial* de Brodmann). *Trab. del Lab. de Inv. biol.*, t. XX, marzo de 1922, fasc. 1. Also *Journal f. Psychologie und Neurologie:* Berlin, 1923.

1922

269. Discurso leído con ocasión de la entrega de la medalla Echegaray, adjudicada por la Real Academia de Ciencias de Madrid. Abril de 1922.

1923

270. Quelques méthodes simples pour la coloration de la névroglie. Trabajo en honor del Dr. Monakow con ocasión de su Jubileo Universitario. Les Arch. Suisses de Neur. et de Psych., vol. XIII.
271. Discurso leído con ocasión de la recepción del Dr. Tello en la Academia de Medicina. (La quimiotaxis y las limitaciones y ventajas del criterio químico en las ciencias biológicas.) Enero de 1923.
272. Autobiografía. Tercera edición, con adición de varios capítulos y numerosos grabados. Mayo de 1923.

1925

273. Une formule pour colorer dans les coupes les fibres amedullées et les terminaisons centrales et périphériques. *Trav. Lab. Rech. biol.,* T. XXIII.
274. Note sur le reseau péricellulaire de l'épithélium pavimenteux stratifié de la langue. *Trav. Lab. Rech. biol.,* T. XXIII.
275. Quelques remarques sur les plaques motrices de la langue des mammifères. *Trav. Lab. Rech. biol.,* T. XXIII.

1926

276. Contribution a la connaissance de la névroglie cérébrale et cérébelleuse dans la paralysie générale progressive, etc. *Trav. Lab. Rech. biol.,* T. XXIV. (German translation in *Zeits. f. d. ges. Neur.,* Bd. C., 1926.)
277. Sur quelques lésions du cervelet dans un cas de démence précoce. *Trav. Lab. Rech. biol.,* T. XXIV.
278. Démonstrations photographiques de quelques phénomènes de la régéneration des nerfs. *Trav. Lab. Rech. biol.,* T. XXIV.
279. Sur les fibres mousseuses et quelques points douteux de la texture de l'écorce cérébelleuse. *Trav. Lab. Rech. biol.,* T. XXIV.
280. Notas tecnicas. Algunas precisiones sobre el proceder del formol bromuro y plata amoniacal para la coloración de la glia y microglia patológica. *Bol. de la Soc. Españ. de Biol.,* vol. XI.

1927

281. Sur la voie collatérale motrice du pédoncule cérébrale. *Trav. Lab. Rech. Biol.,* T. XXV.

1929

282. Un procédé simple pour impregner les gros et les fins axones dans les coupes de pièces indurées en formol, etc. *Trav. Lab. Rech. Biol.,* T. XXVI.
283. Considérations critiques sur le rôle trophique des dendrites et leurs prétendues relations vasculaires. *Trav. Lab. Rech. Biol.,* T. XXVI.

1932–3

284. Die Histologischen Beweise der Neuronenlehre. (German version by Dr. Miscolrky.) *Lehrbuch der Neurologie* von Lewandowsky, Vol. II, 1932–3.

1933

285. Neuronismo o reticularismo? *Archivos de Neurobiología*, Tome XIII, Madrid. (French translation entitled *Les preuves objectives de l'unité anatomique des cellules nerveuses, Trav. Lab. Rech. Biol.*, vol. XXIX.)
286. Les problèmes histophysiologiques de la rétine. *XIV Concilium Ophtalmologicum, 1933, Hispaniae.*
287. Die Neuronenlehre und die periterminalen Netze Boeke's. *Arch. f. Psych. u. Nervenk.*, Bd. 102, 1934.
288. Carrera literaria, méritos, titulos, condecoraciones, premios, distinciones y lista de trabajos de D. Santiago Ramón y Cajal, Catedratico jubilado de Histología normal y Anatomía patológica de la Universidad de Madrid. 2nda Ed.

In the last work cited the author lists eleven works published under the names of pupils for which he assumes practically full responsibility.

TITLES, DECORATIONS, PRIZES AND HONOURARY DEGREES OF THE AUTHOR

1. Distinctions Received in Spain

Member of the Royal Academy of Exact, Physical, and Natural Sciences of Madrid (Dec. 11, 1895).

Member elect of the Royal Academy of Medicine of Madrid (Nov. 13, 1897).

Member elect of the Royal Spanish Academy (June 22, 1905).

Member of the Spanish Natural History Society (President, 1896, and Honourary Member from 1898).

Honourary Member of the Athenaeum of Madrid.

Honourary Member of the Academy of Medicine and Surgery of Spain (April 18, 1897).

Honourary Member of the College of Physicians of Madrid (Jan. 1, 1897).

Counsellor on Public Instruction (Royal Order of May 18, 1900).

Grand Cross of Isabel the Catholic (Royal Order of Oct. 29, 1900).

Grand Cross of Alfonso XII (June 20, 1900).

Honourary Member of the Royal Aragonese Society of Friends of the Country (Nov. 9, 1906).

Honourary President of the Academy of Medical Sciences of Bilbao (Nov., 1906).

Illustrious and Predilect Son of the Province of Zaragoza (Aug. 20, 1900).

Corresponding Member of the Royal Academy of Sciences and Arts of Barcelona (Feb. 19, 1904).

Honourary Member of the Spanish Physical and Chemical Society.

Member of the Royal Academy of Medicine & Surgery of Madrid (June 30, 1907).

Senator elected by the Central University (University of Madrid). Later Senator for life appointed by Royal Decree of Feb. 14, 1910.

Counsellor on Health, etc.

Director of the National Institute of Hygiene of Alfonso XIII (1900).

Honourary Director of the Alfonso XIII Institute (National Inst. of Hygiene) (1920).

Honourary Professor of the University of Valladolid (Feb., 1922).

Honourary Member of the Royal Academy of Medicine and Surgery of Barcelona (May, 1922).

Honourary President of the Royal Academy of Medicine of Cadiz (May, 1922).

Honourary President of the Spanish Natural History Society (June 3, 1932).

Medal *Plus Ultra.*

Ribbon of the Order of the Republic (April, 1933).

2. PRIZES AND HONOURARY AWARDS AT HOME AND ABROAD

Prize awarded by the Provincial Council of Zaragoza for the studies on the etiology of cholera (Sept. 17, 1885).

Gold medal for exhibit of microscopic preparations at the World's Exposition at Barcelona.

Plaque presented by the Academy of Medicine and Pharmacy of Rome (1894).

Medal presented by the International Congress of Hygiene (1897).

Rubio Prize (1000 pesetas) for the publication of the book *Elements of Histology* (1897).

Fauvelle Prize (1500 francs) awarded by the Société de Biologie of Paris (1896).

Croonian Lecturer, Royal Society of London (March, 1894).

Special Lecturer (with four illustrious foreign professors) at the Decennial Celebration of Clark University, Worcester, Mass.

Moscow Prize (5000 francs) awarded by the executive committee of the International Medical Congress of Paris for the most important medical work published in the preceding three years (August, 1900).

Martínez y Molina Prize (4000 pesetas) for a work, *On the cerebral sensory centres of man and animals,* written in collaboration with Dr. Pedro Ramón (Jan. 25, 1902).

Helmholtz Gold Medal awarded by the Imperial Academy of Science of Berlin (1905).

Plaque presented by the medical students of Madrid to commemorate the award of the Helmholtz Medal.

Nobel Prize in Medicine for the year 1906.

Gold medal presented by the medical students of Zaragoza in memory of the Nobel Prize.

Gold medal presented by the Spanish Lovers of Progress in commemoration of the Nobel Prize, etc.

Commander of the Legion of Honour, Paris (1914).

Cross of the Order "Pour le mérite" Berlin (1915).

Echegaray Medal awarded by the Royal Academy of Sciences (April, 1922).

Book in honour of Don Santiago Ramón y Cajal on the occasion of his retirement (2 vols., 1922).

Member of the Order of the Crown of Roumania (1933).

3. Partial List of Foreign Honorary Degrees and Titles

Doctor of Medicine, *honoris causa,* University of Cambridge (March 14, 1894).

Doctor of Medicine, *honoris causa,* University of Würzburg (Oct. 28, 1896).

Doctor of Laws, *honoris causa,* Clark University (July 15, 1899).

Doctor of Medicine, *honoris causa,* University of Louvain (May 10, 1909).

Doctor of Medicine, *honoris causa,* University of Christiania (1911).

Doctor, *honoris causa,* University of Mexico (Sept., 1922).

Doctor, *honoris causa,* University of Bordeaux (Nov., 1922).
Honourary title of Doctor of the University of Paris (Nov. 29, 1924).
Honourary Doctor of the University of Strasbourg (May, 1925).
Honourary Doctor of Medicine of the University of Guatemala (May, 1925).
Corresponding Member of the Medico-physical Society of Würzburg (Jan. 26, 1895).
Corresponding Member of the Society of Medicine of Berlin (Sept. 25, 1895).
Corresponding Member of the Society for Medical Sciences of Lisbon (July 11, 1896).
Corresponding Member of the Society for Neurology and Psychiatry of Vienna (June 3, 1896).
Honourary Member of the Italian Psychiatric Society (Oct. 9, 1896).
Corresponding Member of the Société de Biologie, Paris (Feb. 13, 1897).
Honourary Member of the Royal Academy of Sciences of Lisbon (March 4, 1897).
Honourary Academician of the Academia Scientiarum Ulisiponensis (March, 1897).
Corresponding Member of the National Academy of Medicine, Rome (May, 1897).
Corresponding Member of the Conimbricensis Instituti Societas, Coimbra (June, 1898).
Honourary Member of the Society of Medicine of Ghent (Belgium) (April 3, 1900).
Honourary Member of the Academy of Medicine of Budapest (Dec. 14, 1901).
Honourary Member of the Society of Alienists and Neurologists of Kazan, Russia (April 9, 1902).
Honourary Member of the Academy of Medicine of Yourief, University of Dorpat (Dec., 1902).
Foreign Corresponding Member of the Academy of Medicine of Turin (May, 1903).

Honourary Member of the Academy of Medicine of New York (Feb. 4, 1904).

Honourary Member of the Imperial and Royal Academy of Medicine of Vienna (March 18, 1904).

Foreign Associate of the Academy of Medicine of Paris (May 23, 1905).

Honourary Member of the Royal Academy of Medicine of Rome (April, 1905).

Honourary Member of the Medico-chirurgical Society of London (1905).

Associate Member of the Société de Biologie of Paris (Dec. 16, 1905).

Foreign Corresponding Member of the National Academy of Medicine of Venezuela (Jan. 4, 1906).

Foreign Corresponding Member of the Société de Neurologie of Paris (Dec. 6, 1906).

Corresponding Member of the Academy of Rome, Regia Lynceorum Academia (1906).

Honourary Member of the Royal Irish Academy of Dublin (March 16, 1907).

Foreign Correspondent of the Royal Academy of Medicine of Belgium (July 20, 1907).

Honourary Academician of the Science Museum (Section of Biological Sciences) of the University of La Plata (Dec. 14, 1907).

Fellow of the Royal Society of London (1909).

Corresponding Member of the Royal Academy of Sciences of Turin (1910).

Honourary Member of the Berliner Medizinische Gesellschaft (Oct. 26, 1910).

Foreign Honorary Member of the Royal Academy of Medicine of Belgium (Jan. 20, 1911).

Corresponding Member of the Italian Society of Neurology (1911).

Foreign Member of the Royal Academy of Turin (1912).

Honourary Member of the Royal Society of Medical and Natural Sciences of Brussels (1912).

Foreign Associate of the Academy of Medicine of Paris (1913).
Honourary Member of the Conimbricensis Instituti Societas, Coimbra (1913).
Corresponding Fellow of the Royal Society of Edinburgh (1913).
Honourary Member of the Imperial University of St. Petersburg (July, 1914).
Foreign Member of the Swedish Royal Academy of Sciences (April, 1916).
Corresponding Member of the Institute of France (1916).
Honourary Academician of the Academy of Medicine of the National University of Buenos Aires (Aug. 14, 1919).
Foreign Member of the National Academy of Sciences of the United States of America (April, 1920).
Member Extraordinary of the Royal Academy of Sciences of the Netherlands (May 19, 1920).
Foreign Corresponding Associate of the Royal Lombard Institute of Science and Letters, Section of Medical Sciences (1921).
Honourary Member of the Academy of Sciences of Santiago, Chile (1922).
Corresponding Member of the Academy of Sciences of Bavaria (July, 1922).
Honourary Member of the National Academy of Medicine of Mexico (April, 1922).
Honourary Member of the Mexican Society of Ophthalmology (May, 1922).
Honourary Member of the Berlin Society of Psychiatry and Nervous Diseases (June, 1923).
Honourary Member of the Academy of Medicine of Bucharest (1923).
Corresponding Member of the Florentine Medico-Physical Academy (May, 1924).
Honourary Member of the American Neurological Association (June, 1924).
Honourary Member of the Neurological Society of Philadelphia (Nov., 1924).

External or Corresponding Member of the Hungarian Academy of Sciences (May, 1925).
Corresponding Member of the Academy of Sciences of Vienna (Math.-Naturw. Klasse) (May, 1926).
Honourary Member of the Hispano-American Ophthalmological Society (Nov., 1931).
Corresponding Member of the American Philosophical Society, Philadelphia (May, 1932).
Foreign Corresponding Member of the British Medical Association (April, 1934).

INDEX